A SHORT HISTORY OF
MEDICINE

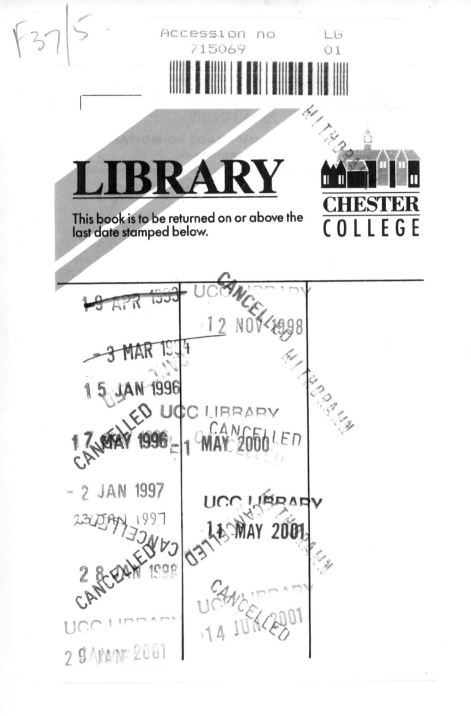

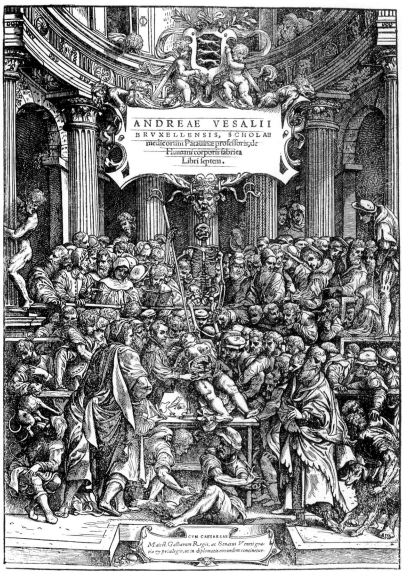

I. ANATOMY ANCIENT AND MODERN

Vesalius and the idealized anatomical theatre

(Title-page of Andreas Vesalius, *De humani corporis fabrica*, Basle, 1543. Copy in the
Wellcome Historical Medical Library)

(*See p.* 91)

A SHORT HISTORY OF
MEDICINE

BY

CHARLES SINGER

AND

E. ASHWORTH UNDERWOOD

SECOND EDITION

OXFORD

AT THE CLARENDON PRESS

1962

Oxford University Press, Amen House, London, E.C.4

GLASGOW   NEW YORK   TORONTO   MELBOURNE WELLINGTON
BOMBAY   CALCUTTA   MADRAS   KARACHI   LAHORE   DACCA
CAPE TOWN   SALISBURY   NAIROBI   IBADAN   ACCRA
KUALA LUMPUR   HONG KONG

PRINTED IN GREAT BRITAIN

PREFACE

SINCE the first publication of this book in 1928 Charles Singer made minor alterations in the text during successive reprintings, but, although he considered that a more extensive revision was desirable he was never able to devote the necessary time to this work. Some years ago he asked me to undertake the preparation of a new edition. He entrusted the writing of the work to me, and I am entirely responsible for the present book. It was gratifying to me that he was able to go through all the proofs of the text before his death, and I profited much from his helpful comments.

My intention was to preserve the original form of the book as far as possible, and for the period up to about the eighteenth century this has I hope been done. In this period various alterations and additions have been made, including a section on medicine before the Age of the Greeks. After the close of the eighteenth century my aim could no longer be achieved if even scant justice was to be done to the greatly increased output of important scientific researches in various countries during the modern period, and to the historical studies published during the last three decades. That part of the text dealing with the nineteenth and twentieth centuries is therefore entirely rewritten and greatly expanded, and at least the last two-thirds of the present book is completely new.

The great progress made in medicine and the medical sciences during the earlier part of the twentieth century is treated in some detail because I feel that for the student of medicine and the medical sciences these researches form a bridge between his current studies and advances made in the more distant past. Thirty years ago these researches were discussed in the larger textbooks of medicine and the medical sciences, but in the current textbooks they have had to make room for more recent work. It seems desirable that the student of medicine should appreciate the continuous evolution of the subjects which he is compelled to study.

In the space of this book it was impracticable to deal with all the many facets of the art and science of medicine. I have on the whole tended to treat the scientific aspects more fully because they are generally more difficult to understand, and because brief discussions of their history are rather unrewarding. In the clinical field a few of the specialities are chosen for discussion while others are completely excluded.

I am much indebted to Sir Francis Walshe for having read through my section on Neurology and for his helpful comments. Dr. R. A. Hunter gave me similar help in relation to the section on Mental Diseases. I am obliged also to Professor Bradford Hill for having discussed with me the draft of my concluding section on Vital Statistics and Epidemiology. To Dr. Margaret Rowbottom I am grateful for varied assistance, and particularly for help in the time-consuming task of ascertaining the dates of death of many who have but recently left the field of their labours. I am indebted to my wife for much help, especially in relation to proof reading and the checking of the Indexes. Finally, to the staff of the Clarendon Press I desire to express my thanks for their patience and great assistance.

1961   E. A. U.

ACKNOWLEDGEMENTS

Acknowledgement is made of the authors' indebtedness to Her Majesty The Queen for gracious permission to reproduce the Leonardo drawings which appear here as Plates VIII and IX.
The source of each illustration is given in its accompanying legend. Acknowledgements are gratefully made to the following persons or bodies for permission to publish the illustrations mentioned: Messrs. Alinari (Fig. 24); Messrs. Baillière, Tindall & Cox (Fig. 116); Messrs. John Bale, Sons & Danielsson (Figs. 50a, 106, 107); Bibliothèque de l'Arsenal, Paris (Fig. 68); Bibliothèque Nationale, Paris (Fig. 29); Bodleian Library, Oxford (Fig. 30); Boston Museum of Fine Arts (Fig. 10); British Museum (Plates IV, V; Figs. 6, 16, 38, 40, 62, 76); Messrs. Down Bros. and Mayer and Phelps (Fig. 101); Soprintendenza alle Gallerie di Firenze (Fig. 14); Messrs. Griffin & Co., Ltd. (Fig. 87); Herdersche Verlagshandlung, Freiburg im Breisgau (Fig. 27); The Controller, H.M.S.O. (Figs. 143, 144); International Publishers Co., Inc., New York (Fig. 85); Casa Editrice S. Lapi, Città di Castello (Fig. 28); Messrs. H. K. Lewis & Co., Ltd. (Fig. 139); The Louvre, Paris (Fig. 17); Sir Robert Macintosh, Oxford (Fig. 96); Mansell Collection, London (Fig. 5); Messrs. Albin Michel, Paris (Figs. 13, 33, 119); National Dental Association of America (Fig. 131); Oxford University Press (Figs. 92a, 108a, 109a, 111a, 112a, 126); Messrs. Pritchard Photographic Co., London (Fig. 101); Messrs. G. P. Putnam's, New York (Fig. 7); The Conservator of the Museum of The Royal College of Surgeons of Edinburgh (Fig. 136); The Royal College of Surgeons of England (Fig. 124); The Royal Society of London (Fig. 65); The Hon. Editors, Proceedings of the Royal Society of Medicine (Fig. 147); Society for Experimental Biology and Medicine, New York (Fig. 114); Messrs. G. Steinheil, Editeur, Paris (Fig. 1); University Press of Liverpool (Fig. 118); Messrs. A. Villani, Bologna (Plate VII); Yale University Press (Fig. 84).

CONTENTS

ADDENDA AND CORRIGENDA   xvi

I. THE DAWN OF MEDICINE

Medicine in prehistoric times   1

Medicine in Ancient Egypt   3

The medicine of Mesopotamia   9

II. ANCIENT GREECE

Origins of Greek medicine   16

The Hippocratic physician   27

Hippocratic practice   32

Aristotle   41

III. THE HEIRS OF GREECE

The Alexandrian School   48

Medical teaching in the Roman Empire   51

Medical services in the Roman Empire   55

Roman hospitals   56

Galen   59

The final medical synthesis of antiquity   60

IV. THE MIDDLE AGES

Byzantine medicine   67

The period of depression in Europe   68

Arabic medicine   73

The medieval awakening   76

The universities   78

Medieval anatomy, surgery, and internal medicine   80

Medieval hospitals and hygiene   84

V. THE REBIRTH OF SCIENCE

The anatomical awakening   88

The anatomical reaction on surgery   95

Concepts of disease   98

The rise of internal medicine   101

The first physical synthesis   111

The revival of physiology   115

Microscopical examination of the animal body   124
From alchemy to chemistry   135
The medical theorists   137
   (*a*) Iatrophysics   138
   (*b*) Iatrochemistry   142
   (*c*) Vitalism   143

VI. THE PERIOD OF CONSOLIDATION
The Reign of Law   145
The rise of clinical teaching   147
Anatomy and the Edinburgh School   150
Physiology passes to the modern stage   151
Some physiological advances   154
Discovery of the nature of the air   161
Morbid anatomy becomes a science   168
Clinical methods and instruments   171
Surgery and obstetrics   174
The beginnings of the science of vital statistics   179
Military, naval, and prison medicine   181
The Industrial Revolution   191
Communal disease and hygiene   196
Control and recognition of epidemic diseases   198

VII. PERIOD OF SCIENTIFIC SUBDIVISON
Origins and implications of scientific specialization 205
The revolution in preventive medicine   208
The transition to a physiological synthesis   236
The nervous system and neurology   239
Schools of clinical medicine   280
The experimental foundations of modern medicine   287
   (*a*) The work of Johannes Müller   287
      The electric phenomena of nerve   288
      The mechanism of muscular contraction   292
   (*b*) The work of Claude Bernard   294
   (*c*) The work of Karl Ludwig   299
   (*d*) Later physiological investigators   302
      Respiration   303
      Circulation   311

The blood 316
Biochemistry 319
The Cell Theory 320
Establishment of the doctrine of the germ origin of disease 326
· Anaesthesia 341
The revolution in surgery 351
Some modern surgical advances 362
Radiology and radium therapy 374
Bacteriology becomes a science 379
Some important bacteriological results 381
Discovery of the main pathogenic bacteria 390
Developments in bacteriology 395
The study of immunity 409
Some practical applications of immunity 433
Virus diseases 445
Rickettsial diseases 450
The conquest of the tropics 452
(a) Malaria 454
(b) Yellow fever 466
(c) Trypanosomiasis 481
(d) Leishmaniasis 487
(e) Plague 488
(f) Some other tropical diseases 492
The changed view of insanity 494
The new movement in psychology 512
Some modern physiological concepts of clinical import 515
(a) Ductless glands and internal secretions 515
(i) The thyroid 519
(ii) The parathyroids 534
(iii) The adrenals 538
(iv) The pituitary 541
(v) The gonads 549
(vi) The pancreas 551
(b) Histamine 555
(c) The chemical transmission of the nerve impulse 564
(d) Nutrition and metabolism 578
(e) Vitamins and deficiency diseases 610
(f) The function and diseases of the heart 622

The development of modern pathology 627

Knowledge of the eye and its disorders 640

The rise of paediatrics 650

The teeth and their diseases 659

The study and use of the natural drugs 671

    (*a*) The history of the pharmacopoeias 671

    (*b*) Contents of a modern pharmacopoeia 676

    (*c*) Active principles: alkaloids and glycosides 679

    (*d*) Pharmacology, the scientific investigation of drug action 684

Chemotherapy and allied methods of treatment 687

    (*a*) Protozoal and spirochaetal diseases 689

    (*b*) Bacterial infections 693

    (*c*) The antibiotics 693

Blood transfusion 698

The revolution in nursing 701

Collective medical data 710

    (*a*) Demography and vital statistics 710

    (*b*) Biometry and medical statistics 721

    (*c*) Epidemiology 727

EPILOGUE 742

APPENDIX: NOBEL PRIZEWINNERS 757

SELECT LIST OF REFERENCE MATERIAL 761

INDEX OF PERSONS 797

INDEX OF SUBJECTS AND PLACES 819

LIST OF PLATES

I. Anatomy Ancient and Modern · (*Frontispiece*)

II. The Asklepieion at Epidaurus · *facing page* 24

III. Aesculapius treating a girl · 25

IV. The Aqua Claudia, Rome · 56

V. The Isola Tiberina with church of San Bartolomeo, Rome · 57

VI. The miracle of Saints Cosmas and Damian, after Gallegos · 72

VII. Bologna in 1505, after Francia · 73

VIII. Drawings of the heart by Leonardo da Vinci · 88

IX. Drawings of the foetus in utero by Leonardo da Vinci ⎱ *between* 88

X. Skeleton, after Vesalius ⎰ *and* 89

XI. Muscle-man, after Vesalius · 89

XII. Muscle-man, after Albinus: superficial muscles · 152

XIII. Muscle-man, after Albinus: deep muscles ⎱ *between* 152 *and* 153

XIV. Vertebral column, after Cheselden ⎰

XV. Anatomical theatre at Bologna · *facing page* 168

XVI. Gravid uterus, after William Hunter · 169

XVII. Lord Lister on ligaturing the femoral artery · 360

XVIII. The Laboratory of the Liverpool School of Tropical Medicine, June 1899 · 456

XIX. Plague-fighters of the seventeenth and twentieth centuries · 488

XX. Claude Bernard carrying out an experiment · 552

XXI. The evolution of the clinical thermometer · 624

LIST OF TEXT-FIGURES

1. Neolithic trephined skull   2
2. The Ebers Papyrus   5
3. Imhotep. Silver statuette   6
4. Egyptian surgical instruments   9
5. The Code of Hammurabi   11
6. Clay model of sheep's liver. Babylonian   13
7. Bronze model of a liver. Etruscan   13
8. Babylonian surgical instruments   14
9. Map of Greece, showing main invasions   18
10. Votaress. Gold and ivory statuette. Late Minoan II   19
11. Aesculapius. Marble statue   21
12. Sources of Hippocratic medicine   23
13. Ruins of the Asklepieion at Cos   24
14. Hippocrates. Bust in the Uffizi, Florence   30
15. Instruments used by Greek surgeons   33
16. Greek vase showing double-spica bandage   35
17. Greek clinic shown on an Attic vase   36
18. Aristotle's Ladder of Nature   42
19. The parts of the uterus according to Aristotle   43
20. Embryo dogfish, after Johannes Müller   43
21. Aristotle's Qualities, Elements, and Humours   46
22. Physician of the Hellenistic Age   52
23. Roman surgical instruments   54
24. Roman advanced dressing-station   57
25. Dissections of the hands of Man and of Barbary ape   63
26. Diagram of Galen's physiological system   64
27. St. Luke represented as a physician   70
28. Surgical treatment at the Siege of Naples, 1194   72
29. Faraj ben Salīm translating Rhazes   75
30. Trephining the skull in the Middle Ages   80
31. Thong drill   81
32. Anatomical teaching in the fifteenth century   82
33. Bernard de Gourdon teaching at Montpellier   83
34. The Hôtel-Dieu at Paris in the sixteenth century   85
35. Paré's method of reducing a dislocated shoulder   95
36. Artificial arms and hands, devised by Paré   96

37. Tagliacozzi's method for repair of injury to lower lip 99
38. The four temperaments, represented c. 1500 102
39. Hyoscyamus, after Brunfels 104
40. Hyoscyamus, after Fuchs 105
41. An allegory of epidemic syphilis, 1496 107
42. Guaiac in the treatment of syphilis, c. 1580 109
43. Thermometer and pulsimeter, after Galileo and Sanctorius 116
44. Sanctorius in his balance 117
45. Valves in a vein, after Fabricius 118
46. Action of the valves in veins, after Harvey 121
47. Diagram of the circulation of the blood 122
48. Capillaries in frog's lung, after Malpighi 125
49. Chick embryo, after Malpighi 126
50. Leeuwenhoek's microscopes 127
51. Red blood corpuscles, after Leeuwenhoek 129
52. Capillaries in frog's foot, after Leeuwenhoek 130
53. Structure of voluntary muscle, after Leeuwenhoek 131
54. The first illustration of bacteria, after Leeuwenhoek 131
55. The first illustration of plant cells, after Hooke 132
56. Swammerdam's experiments on muscular contraction 134
57. Boyle's second air-pump 137
58. Sensory impression and motor impulse, after Descartes 139
59. Descartes's theory of nervous action 140
60. Analysis of arm movements, after Borelli 141
61. Arm movements in terms of the lever 141
62. Windmill ventilator designed by Stephen Hales 156
63. Beaumont's illustration of his patient's gastric fistula 157
64. Galvani's experiments on 'animal electricity' 158
65. The origin of the voltaic pile 160
66. Mayow's experiments on combustion and respiration 162
67. Priestley's apparatus for 'pneumatic chemistry' 164
68. An experiment on respiration by Lavoisier 167
69. Emphysema, and 'ossification of the lungs', after Baillie 170
70. Laennec's stethoscope 173
71. Sixteenth-century lying-in scene 175
72. Obstetric instruments 176
73. John Hunter's country house at Earl's Court 178

74. Graph of the population of England and Wales, 1670–1830   192
75. St. Bartholomew's Hospital, London, *c.* 1752   195
76. The pest-house, Tothill Fields, London, 1796   196
77. The quarantine station at Naples, after Howard   199
78. The hand of Sarah Nelmes   201
79. Industrial cottages, 1844   216
80. London death-rates, 1841–1924   221
81. Greenwich and the *Dreadnought* hospital ship, after Parrott   222
82. Origin and distribution of a spinal nerve   253
83. Diagram of a simple reflex   253
84. Cerebral localization after Grünbaum and Sherrington   259
85. Pavlov's apparatus for experiments on conditioned reflexes   268
86. Thomas Young's kymograph   300
87. Diagram of 'Pavlov's pouch'   303
88. Riva-Rocci's sphygmomanometer   312
89. The nature and origin of animal cells, after Schwann   323
90. Organisms found in souring of beer, after Pasteur   332
91. Sterilization in a flask with an open bent neck, after Pasteur   334
92. Anthrax bacilli   337
93. Screw-clamp for production of anaesthesia by nerve compression   342
94. Morton's ether inhaler   345
95. Snow's chloroform inhaler   346
96. Clover's chloroform inhaler   347
97. Shipway's apparatus for warm chloroform and ether   348
98. Lister's hand-operated carbolic spray   356
99. Operating table used by Lister   357
100. Trephining the skull in the sixteenth century   358
101. A modern abdominal operation   359
102. Spencer Wells forceps   363
103. Spencer Wells operating, *c.* 1875   364
104. Results of Macewen's osteotomy   369
105. Forlanini's original apparatus for artificial pneumothorax   372
106. Röntgen's X-ray picture of weights in a closed box   375
107. Röntgen's X-ray picture of his wife's hand   376
108. Diphtheria bacilli   382
109. Plague bacilli   383
110. Monthly incidence of Malta fever, 1905, 1907   386

111. Tetanus bacilli   388
112. Typhoid bacilli   389
113. Case mortality of laryngeal diphtheria, 1894–1910   435
114. Electron micrograph of poliomyelitis virus   450
115. Distribution of malaria in England and Wales, 1860   455
116. Life-cycle of the malaria parasite   458
117. Seasonal incidence of malaria in Italy, 1921–6   465
118. First illustration of *Trypanosoma gambiense*, after Dutton and Todd   484
119. St. Antony of Padua casting out a devil, after Mezzastri   495
120. 'The Retreat', York   498
121. Physical restraint used for lunatics in early nineteenth century   500
122. The 'baquet' of Mesmer   508
123. Charcot demonstrating a hysterical patient   510
124. Cretinous infant before and after thyroid treatment   526
125. Liebig's laboratory at Giessen, after Trautschold   580
126. Mackenzie's ink-polygraph   624
127. Position of the lens of the eye after Vesalius and after Fabricius   640
128. Couching a cataract, c. 1583   644
129. The Hospital for Sick Children, Great Ormond Street, 1882   656
130. Sixteenth-century dental instruments   660
131. Early artificial teeth   661
132. Artificial teeth after Paré and after Fauchard   662
133. Early dentures of the nineteenth century   664
134. Trade-card of a maker of artificial teeth, c. 1750   666
135. Ceremonial preparation of theriac in the sixteenth century   675
136. Alexander Wood's hypodermic syringe   686
137. Hypodermic syringe of c. 1860   686
138. The first illustration of the *Spirochaeta pallida*   690
139. Culture plate which led to the discovery of penicillin   694
140. Treating the wounded at Sebastopol, before the arrival of Florence Nightingale   705
141. Hospital ward at Scutari   707
142. Population of England and Wales, 1801–1951   714
143. Population of Great Britain by age-groups, 1891, 1947   718
144. Population of Great Britain by age and sex, 1891, 1947   719
145. Vital statistics of England and Wales, 1876–1955   720
146. The normal curve   724
147. Weekly incidence of cholera in Sheffield, July to October 1832   734

ADDENDA AND CORRIGENDA

(For minor variations of birth and death dates, compare the dates in text with those in name index; the latter are generally to be preferred. For death dates of those recently deceased, see name index.)

p. 165, l. 15   *For* sulphur dioxide *read* silicon tetrafluoride

p. 166, l. 36   *For* colorimeter *read* calorimeter

p. 183   *For dates of* Fabricius Hildanus *read* (1560–1634)

p. 234, l. 26   *For dates of* Joseph Kinyoun *read* (1860–1919)

p. 244, l. 4   *For dates of* Varolio *read* (1543–75)

p. 246, l. 7   *For* Magnus Gustav Retzius *read* Gustaf Magnus Retzius

p. 248, l. 7   *For* 1926 *read* 1906

p. 279, ll. 8, 9   *For* Déjérine *and* Déjérine-Klumpke *read* Dejerine *and* Dejerine-Klumpke

p. 284, l. 34   *For dates of* Addison *read* (1793–1860)

p. 315, l. 20   *For* Sidney *read* Sydney; *for dates read* (1835–1910)

p. 368, l. 13   *For dates of* Godlee *read* (1849–1925)

p. 371, ll. 32, 33   *For* Johann Metzger (1839–1900) *read* Johann Georg Metzger (1838–1909)

p. 377, l. 33   *For dates of* Finsen *read* (1860–1904)

p. 378, l. 29   *For* Franz Nagelschmidt *read* Karl Franz Nagelschmidt

p. 392, l. 10   *For* typhoid fever *read* glanders

p. 404, ll. 30, 31   *These lines to read* somatic antigens) unaffected. These facts were totally neglected till 1917, when Edmund Weil (1880–1922) and A. Felix (p. 405), who had been

p. 442, l. 12   *For* tetanus toxin *read* tetanus antitoxin

p. 448, l. 14   *For* Woodruff (p. 697) *read* Alice Miles Woodruff

p. 524, l. 17   *For dates of* John Byrom Bramwell *read* (1822–82)

p. 526, l. 12   *For* Hector Mackenzie *read* Sir Hector William Gavin Mackenzie

p. 553, l. 9   *For* glycosuria *read* hyperglycaemia

p. 557, ll. 9, 10   *For* Karl Vogt (1880–) *read* W. Vogt (fl. 1907)

p. 609, l. 1   *For dates of* Boyd Orr *read* (1880–)

p. 619, l. 8   *For* Walter Norman Haworth *read* Sir (Walter) Norman Haworth

p. 623, l. 34   *For dates of* Sir Arthur Keith *read* (1866–1955)

p. 638, l. 3   *For dates of* Kennaway *read* (1881–1958)

p. 639, l. 17   *For dates of* M. J. Stewart *read* (1885–1956)

p. 702, ll. 14, 15   *For* Mlle Le Gras *read* Louise de Marillac (1591–1662), Madame Le Gras

p. 715, l. 9   *For* Bertillon *read* Jacques Bertillon (1821–83)

p. 733, l. 21   *For dates of* Brownlee *read* (1868–1927)

I

THE DAWN OF MEDICINE

MEDICINE IN PREHISTORIC TIMES

SCIENTIFIC medicine began with the Greeks. But, just as there were brave men before Agamemnon, so there were men who practised the art of healing long before the time of the Greek physicians. The skeletons of prehistoric men and animals show that their bodies reacted to disease and to injury much as do our own. The art of writing, which gave us our first contemporary ideas about these matters, was invented about 5,500 years ago. Man had existed on this earth for about half a million years before that, and our knowledge of his culture, his way of life, and the diseases from which he suffered in these remote times is being gradually reconstructed from the relics which he left behind him.

The men of the Old Stone Age have left carvings in bone and cave paintings as evidence of their artistry. We may infer that there were also physicians or wound-healers in these early times, but the evidence for this has perished. Though the bones of men who lived in the enormously long Old Stone Age sometimes show signs of disease, so far none have shown any trace of surgery.

About 9,000 B.C. the New Stone Age began in the Near East. In north-west Europe it endured until about 2,000 B.C., when it was succeeded by the Bronze Age. The New Stone Age has provided archaeologists with much evidence that one surgical operation, at least, was very frequently performed. The operation was that of trephination, which consists in cutting an opening through the cranium or brain-case. The opening was often circular, but sometimes square. It varied in size from a tiny hole up to an opening about two inches in diameter. Trephination was performed on men, women, and children. Skulls are not infrequent which show that it was carried out on several occasions on the same individual, and we know something of the method employed. In classical Greece—as we shall see—a metal drill called a trephine was used to cut the hole, but the men of the New Stone Age had no such tools. The operator usually made a circular mark on the outer surface of the skull with a flint knife or scraper. With the same rude tool he then cut this mark deeper to form a groove, and at length a circular piece of bone was removed (Fig. 1).

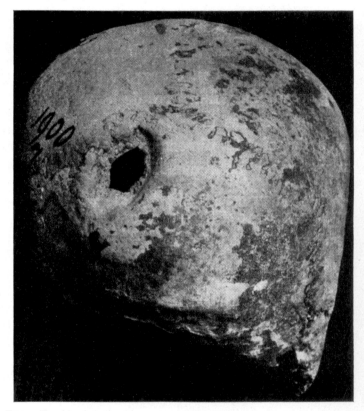

FIG. 1. Trephined skull, with recovery and partial regrowth of bone. Neolithic. Mus. National d'Hist. Naturelle, Paris. Collection Prunières. After Lucas-Championnière, *Trépanation néolithique*, Paris, 1912)

Why was this operation performed? The modern surgeon still performs it, most frequently on patients who have suffered fractures of the skull or on those who have increased pressure on the brain. Few prehistoric trephined skulls show any signs of fracture, so the operation must have been performed for some other reason. The life of prehistoric man was dominated by magical influences. In the New Stone Age certain nervous and mental conditions must have been attributed to a demon which had possessed the patient. This belief is still common in primitive races. Naturally the surgeon would seek to let the demon escape. It is conceivable that in some cases of what we now know as Jacksonian epilepsy—which is due to a spicule of skull bone pressing on the brain—the surgeon may have been lucky enough to trephine over the point of pressure. The symptoms would be relieved, and the successful result may well have helped to popularize the operation in other conditions in which its beneficial effect would to us appear doubtful.

There is another aspect to this primitive operation. At certain periods of the New Stone Age at least, the round plate of bone which was cut from the skull was not thrown away, but seems on the contrary to have been highly prized. It was hung round the neck as an amulet. Thus our earliest surgical operation is associated not only with the treatment of disease but also with its prevention.

MEDICINE IN ANCIENT EGYPT

The history of medicine begins in that strange land whose very existence depended on the rise and fall of the Nile. About the beginning of the third millennium before the Christian era its first dynasty was founded. Within the next four hundred years the pictorial signs which had been used to transmit ideas developed into something that may be called writing. It was soon discovered that writing material could be made from the papyrus reed. Our word paper is derived from the Greek word *papyros*. A mixture of soot, gum, and water was used as an ink for writing. Thus began the period of documentary history.

Our extraordinarily rich knowledge of the life and work of the Egyptians arises largely from their profound belief in immortality. Not only was the soul immortal; but it was believed that at some later time it would return to the body to continue the earthly life. It was therefore desirable to preserve the body and the dead person's treasured possessions. In the period before the first dynasty it was customary to bury the bodies in the desert sands, and in that rainless land they often remained well preserved for thousands of years.

About the beginning of the period of documentary history (*c.* 3,500 B.C.) Egyptians began to embalm their dead. It is from the mummies and the papyri and other articles entombed with them that we have gained our knowledge of Egyptian medicine.

The methods of embalming certainly changed during the centuries. The Greek historian Herodotus gives an account of the method as practised in the fifth century B.C. The brain was drawn out with a hook in fragments through the nose. Then an incision was made in the left flank, and certain organs were removed. The heart was left untouched. The body cavity was now filled with spices and the whole body was next placed in a solution of salts for about two months. Then it was dried, covered with a special paste, and wrapped in linen bandages. The organs removed were preserved in special jars.

It might be thought that this process would give the physicians some knowledge of anatomy. This was not so. The process was carried out not by physicians but by technicians. The crude knowledge of the organs which they obtained was almost confined to their external appearance. Nevertheless, the representations of organs often found in amulets and other figures indicate that the Egyptians may have known rather more about the structure of the body than their writings suggest.

The basis of our knowledge of the medicine of ancient Egypt is derived from the Medical Papyri. Only a handful of these have been recovered. The best known is the Ebers Papyrus, written about 1570 B.C. (Fig. 2). Copied from much older books, it is a series of recipes for named diseases, such as those of the stomach and heart. The Edwin Smith Papyrus, on the other hand, is essentially surgical. The conditions described are arranged beginning with those affecting the head, then those of the rest of the body in descending order. The writer does not describe how the operations should be carried out. Surgery in ancient Egypt was a craft which was handed down from father to son. Indeed, no Egyptian writings describe surgical procedures.

One of the most obvious features of Egyptian medicine was its association with religion. Several deities were specially connected with healing, and many methods of treatment had to be accompanied by an invocation to one of these gods. The patron deity of physicians was Thoth. The Ebers Papyrus says 'he gives to the physicians skill to cure'. The Greeks later identified Thoth with Hermes. Isis was often invoked as a provider of magical cures. Under the Roman Empire the practice of invoking her extended over nearly the whole

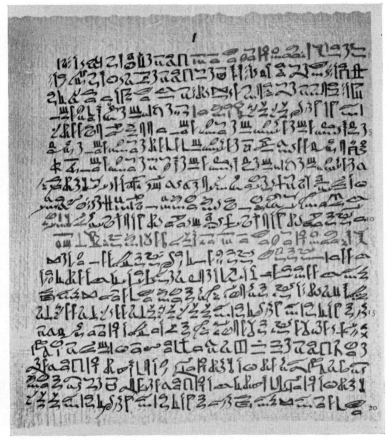

FIG. 2. The Ebers Papyrus: first twenty lines
(Facsimile by G. Ebers, Leipzig, 1875)

western world. Isis instructed her son Horus, who was regarded as the protecting deity against noxious animals. Another Egyptian god of healing represents a deified historic figure, the first physician whose name has come down to us. This was Imhotep, almost certainly a historical person, who lived about 2,700 B.C. (Fig. 3). He was vizier and principal architect to the court of King Zoser, and he was celebrated as a physician. Imhotep was later identified with the god Asklepios of the Greeks. Nevertheless, recent research casts doubts on the traditional belief that Imhotep was a physician.

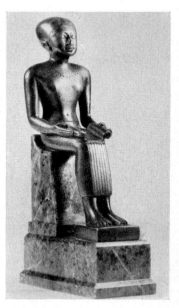

FIG. 3. Imhotep. Silver statuette (Wellcome Historical Medical Museum)

Although the Egyptians were a religious people, magic was inseparable from religion in their treatment of diseases. It is probable that the earliest physicians were really magicians, and that their cures lacked any trace of the rational element. The world was full of evil spirits which preyed upon mortals. Many diseases were supposed to be due to a demon having entered the patient's body, or having shot poisoned darts into the patient. Was not the easiest way to cure the disease to force the demon to depart? Hence the magician would cast a spell upon the demon. In the magical papyri the instructions given for doing this are very detailed, since for its success magic demands implicit adherence to set formulae. The spell must be repeated word by word, as the magician has been instructed. An invocation such as 'Get thee hence, thou breaker of bones' was common. It was better if the magician could address the invading demon by his name; or the disease might be addressed and ordered to desist. These charms were given in full. The magician might be instructed to put his hands on the patient, to hold his seal over the patient's head or to draw a magic circle round the patient's house. The spell might be said over a knotted cord, or an image of wood or clay, which was then given to the patient to wear. Such magico-medicine was practised in civilized communities very much later than the Egyptians, and indeed it is still being practised.

Drugs were often given along with or as part of the spell. There was some reason behind this. The demon might be considered as disliking hateful remedies, and hence the practice of giving foul substances as drugs. Indeed it is probable that the practice of giving drugs first arose thus, as many of the substances used could have had no effect whatever on the condition treated. Then it was found that, when a particular substance happened to be given in a certain disease, the patient got well. The association between cause and effect was noticed, and empirical medicine—which until recent times depended on trial and error in the use of drugs—had begun.

In the *Odyssey* of Homer, written possibly *c.* 800 B.C., we read that 'the fertile soil of Egypt is most rich in drugs, many of which are wholesome in solution, though many are poisonous'. This is certainly borne out by the large number of drugs mentioned in the papyri. Magic did not believe in running unnecessary risks; prescriptions contain many drugs, and several prescriptions are often given for the same disease. The Egyptian physician also had several methods of administering drugs. A common method was to give a mixture of drugs as a potion. The substances to be used were either boiled and strained, or pounded in a mortar. They were then often made up as a draught in milk, wine, or beer. Beer was itself frequently given as a remedy. Sometimes the drugs were made into pills with dough, or mixed with honey and given as a sweatmeat. Diseases of the lower bowel were treated with suppositories. Purgatives, enemata, and emetics were also used. Diseases of the chest were sometimes treated by inhalations, skin conditions with ointments. The physician compounded the remedies himself. There were many specialists, and those who concentrated on the treatment of eye diseases were very numerous.

The Egyptian physician used an astonishing variety of drugs not only from the mineral and vegetable, but also from the animal kingdom. Thus of the ox he used most parts. We would expect that the flesh, fat, liver, and brain might be employed, but gall, blood, and excrement were also given. Such remedies from various animals continued in use in Europe until the late eighteenth century, when even powdered mummy was still employed. As Sir Thomas Browne said: 'Mummy has become merchandize. Mizraim [Egypt] cures wounds, and Pharaoh is sold for balsams.' Salts of copper and antimony were frequently used, but herbs provided most of the ingredients of a mixture, notably the common household vegetables as beans, peas, onions, and leeks. Fruits such as figs, dates, and grapes were also common. The Egyptians discovered the value of certain drugs still in our pharmacopoeia.

Certain operations such as circumcision were carried out as a ritual and were rather in the domain of the priest than the physician or surgeon. The antiquity of such ritual operations is suggested by the fact that they were performed with flint instruments, though for other purposes bronze instruments were used. The surgeon was directly concerned with wounds which were always expected to heal with suppuration—and therefore with scarring. Practitioners did try to reduce the amount of scarring. Where the surgeon nowadays would suture the edges of the wound they tried to produce a similar result with adhesive plaster. Severe bleeding from a wound was stopped by the cautery. Abscesses were opened and drained. They did not trephine the skull or amputate limbs.

Authentic surgical instruments dating from ancient Egypt are rare. A relief of a collection of instruments which were possibly used for surgical purposes is illustrated in Fig. 4. The temple in which this relief is found was begun by Ptolemy VI Philometor (181–146 B.C.), and building continued for about four centuries. The relief itself probably dates from about 100 B.C. Reading the rows from above downwards and the instruments roughly from left to right, some of the instruments are as follows: First row: A probe-director (or a bifid probe), forceps, two saws, a double retractor, a cautery, and designs to represent bandages. Second row: Two cauteries, three probes, three forceps. Third row: Two forceps, two flasks, a strigil, two 'magic eyes', a balance for weighing, two growing plants. Fourth row: Two cupping glasses, an instrument case (cf. Fig. 23), a pair of shears, a sponge, two probes, and two scalpels (cf. Fig. 15). Though these instruments certainly date from the Alexandrian period, there is no evidence that in design they had changed radically from those employed in the period with which this chapter deals.

An important feature of Greek medicine was emphasis on a proper diet. The Egyptians, on the other hand, did not prescribe a diet, but their use of drugs had an important influence on the early Greeks. Physicians from Egypt were summoned to attend most of the monarchs of the ancient world, and many others travelled widely in the course of their profession. Greek scientific medicine owed much to

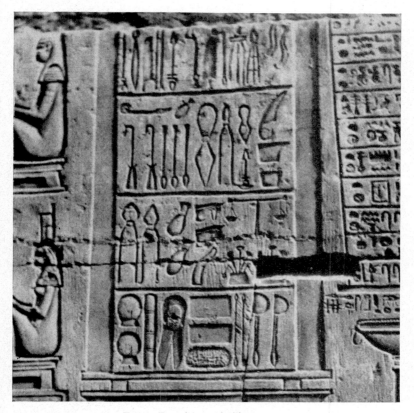

FIG. 4. Egyptian surgical instruments
(Relief, temple of Kom Ombo)

the empirical method which, though so closely associated with magic, was first recorded by the Egyptian physician.

THE MEDICINE OF MESOPOTAMIA

The civilizations of the valley of the rivers Tigris and Euphrates first arose about the same period which saw the dawn of civilization in Egypt. The primitive inhabitants of the south of Mesopotamia, the Sumerians, built the city of Ur and laid the first foundations of their science. About 2300 B.C. Sargon of Akkad conquered the Sumerians, and the great Babylonian age began. Like the great periods of some other city-states, it did not last long. The empire of Assyria was rising in the north, and this culminated in the greatness of Nineveh and absorption of the other Mesopotamian states.

Writing had been invented in Mesopotamia in Sumerian times. The wedge-shaped or 'cuneiform' signs were inscribed on soft clay tablets with a stylus. The tablet was sun-dried or baked in an oven. These tablets were bulky, and a book which, if written on a papyrus roll would occupy relatively little space, was much less portable and less easily stored if written on clay tablets. Nevertheless, a royal library often contained a very large number of these cuneiform texts. Most of the surviving medical texts were found in the library of King Ashurbanipal, who lived in the seventh century B.C. Many of these works were copies of much earlier texts. We have no reason to doubt the fact that medicine in Mesopotamia started as far back as in Egypt.

Like the medicine of Egypt, that of Mesopotamia was primarily magico-religious. Those who dealt with diseases were at first priests, and had been trained as such. They were divided into three classes: first were the diviners, who interpreted omens and foretold the course of the disease; next, the exorcists, who drove out the evil spirits which caused diseases; lastly, the physicians proper, who performed operations and administered drugs. After 2000 B.C. the physicians were ruled by a strict code of laws, that of Hammurabi, laid down about that time. Many of its clauses relate to treatment, and it thus forms the earliest known system of medical ethics. The code itself is cut on a block of black diorite, now in the Louvre, at the head of which is a carved representation of King Hammurabi receiving the code from the Sun-god (Fig. 5). When we regard these laws from the point of view of the physician, we may wonder how the Babylonians ever succeeded in keeping their medical men. While the rewards for successful treatment were clearly stated, the penalties for failure were severe. Here are some of the rewards and punishments:

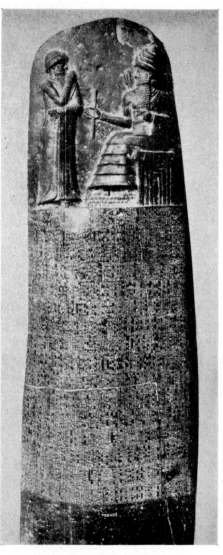

FIG. 5. The Code of Hammurabi
(Louvre. After R. W. Rogers, *History of Babylonia
and Assyria*, New York, 1915)

If a physician has treated a nobleman for a severe wound and has cured him, or opened an eye-abscess of a nobleman and has cured it, he shall take ten shekels of silver.

If he has treated a nobleman for a severe wound and has caused him to die, or opened an eye-abscess of a nobleman and has caused the loss of the eye, the physician's hands shall be cut off.

If a physician has treated the severe wound of a slave of a poor man and has caused his death, he shall render slave for slave.

If a physician has cured a shattered limb, or has cured a diseased bowel, the patient shall give the doctor five shekels of silver.

A magical procedure of the Babylonian priests, which had an influence on the future development of scientific medicine, was divination from the examination of the entrails of animals. These Mesopotamian peoples were accustomed to consult omens when about to embark on any important venture. The practice of examining the liver was probably reserved for matters of great political importance to the state, or to ascertain the probable result when an individual had a serious illness. In this process a sheep was brought to the temple and sacrificed. The priest examined the entrails, paying particular attention to the surface of the liver. Minor variations in its different parts were noted, and from the combined results the priest gave his forecast. Long training must have been needed to give the necessary experience. Although this method of consulting the oracles may not have given much knowledge of anatomical structure, it certainly fostered a tradition of close anatomical observation in a limited field, and so led on to true anatomy.

The various omens which could be given by examination of the liver are written in many Babylonian tablets. In addition, we have a number of models of the sheep's liver, the best preserved of which is illustrated in Fig. 6. This model dates from about the time of Hammurabi, c. 2000 B.C., and it was probably used for instruction in a temple school. The surface is divided into a number of squares, each of which has a prognostication written in it. The omen in any particular square was given by the priest if the liver of the sacrificed sheep showed an abnormality in that particular region. It is known that the Babylonian priests had special terms for all the main parts of the liver, including those named in the drawing. The art of divin-

ing from the state of the liver was highly technical. It spread over
much of the ancient world and gradually altered in character. By the
time that it reached Etruria it had lost any scientific background that

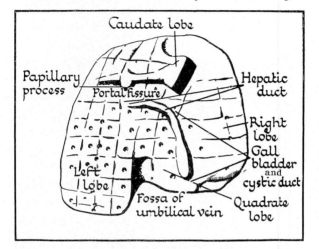

FIG. 6. Clay model of a sheep's liver. Babylonian, *c.* 2000 B.C. Sketch showing the
modern anatomical names of certain features in the model
(British Museum, No. 92668)

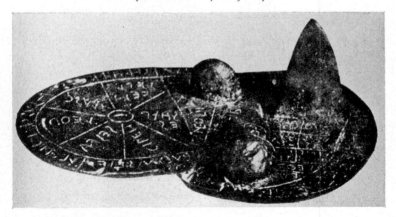

FIG. 7. Bronze model of a liver. Etruscan, *c.* third century B.C., found near Piacenza
(After Jastrow, *Aspects of Religious Belief and Practice in Babylonia and Assyria*, 1911)

it had ever had, and the bronze Etruscan model of a liver shown in
Fig. 7 bears, not written prognostications, but the signs of the
zodiac and other astrological symbols.

During the whole course of Mesopotamian medicine magic was of great importance. Many illnesses were supposed to be due to evil spirits from which the individual had to be protected. If the patient was suffering, the demon had to be exorcized by a suitable incantation. These evil spirits might be of several kinds, ghosts of dead persons, or spirits born from the union of a human being and a demon, or, again, mere spirits of evil. In his incantation the priest sometimes proceeded to name the different types of spirits in due order, so that his chance of addressing the spirit responsible for that particular illness was increased. Toothache was supposed to be due to the gnawing of a worm, to which the exorcizer addressed himself.

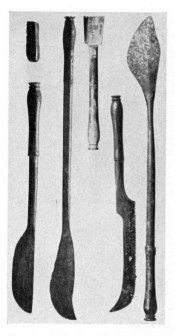

All these mysterious incantations and manual rites were often accompanied by the administration of drugs, a practice essentially rational. The materia medica of Assyria and Babylonia—like that of Egypt—was drawn from the vegetable, animal, and mineral kingdoms. Quite frequently the medical texts gave instructions for the preparation of the remedies. Fumigations and inhalations were used, and tubes were employed to blow the remedies into orifices such as the nose, ear, or bowel. Ointments and poultices were used for superficial conditions.

FIG. 8. Babylonian surgical instruments
(Collection of Prof. Meyer-Steinig of Jena)

These Babylonian physicians used about 250 plants and 120 mineral substances. In addition they employed many substances derived from animals. The vegetable remedies consisted of fruits, cereals, spices, resins, and gums, together with drugs prepared from other parts of the plant. The Assyrians also employed sulphur, in the treatment of skin diseases, and they had many remedies for diseases of the eyes. The animal remedies used were often of a disgusting nature; and many were certainly employed to sicken the demon and to induce it to depart from the person possessed.

We know little about the operations which were carried out or the men who performed them. No surgical texts have yet been discovered in the ruins of Assyria and Babylonia. It is probable that patients were bled and abscesses opened. Eye diseases were very common; and some of the diseases of the eyelids were treated by minor operations. Babylonian surgical instruments are rare. Three knives, a saw, and a trephine found at Babylonian sites are shown in Fig. 8. Beyond that we can say little of their surgery.

II

ANCIENT GREECE

(To about 300 B.C.)

THE Greeks not only started scientific medicine upon its course, but also provided the substantial basic elements of our anatomy, physiology, and pathology, and above all perhaps our conception of the bodily 'constitution', 'habit', or 'temperament'. It is from the Greeks that we derive almost all our medical nomenclature. When to this we add that our medical traditions are inherited through a direct and continuous chain from the Greek practitioners, it becomes evident that the debt that medicine owes to this marvellous people is great indeed.

This debt has become associated with two or three great figures. The names Hippocrates, Aristotle, Galen, are familiar to all. Yet it is not always recognized that these men were but the representatives of a widely extended and long-lasting system. Greek medicine was, in fact, like modern medicine, the result of centuries of carefully recorded, collated, and progressive research. Greek medicine first assumed a scientific aspect with the Ionian and Italo-Greek philosophers at the beginning of the sixth century B.C. It continued to make important advances until the death of Galen at the end of the second century of the Christian era. Thus the life-span of progressive and scientific medicine among the Greeks was not less than eight hundred years. With the most tolerant use of the words 'scientific' and 'progressive', we can hardly place the beginnings of modern medicine in Europe before the end of the fifteenth century. Thus our own system has only been developing its characteristic features for some four and a half centuries, which is but little more than half the course of Greek science.

It is evident, therefore, that we may have much to learn from the Greeks, not indeed in matters of actual fact or observation—for nearly all that is directly useful in their writings has been absorbed long ago into our medical literature—but in spirit and method. From a study of the character and course of Greek medical science we can gain hints of the snares and pitfalls and catastrophes into which the art of medicine may at times be led. Further, by study of the practice of medicine under conditions so different from ours, we learn something of what is truly permanent in the art of healing. Lastly, by tracing the growth of the science of medicine, as it arose among the Greeks and as it died in the hands of their less worthy descendants, we may take alike example and warning. We may learn to distinguish the healthy and vigorous growth of a science from the stunted and deformed products that are often acclaimed, even in our own times, as Wisdom's final word to Man.

It has been said that, 'save the blind forces of Nature, nothing lives or moves which is not Greek in origin'. The saying needs modification, for there is a thing which still lives and moves that is not Greek in origin, a blind force which is not a blind force of Nature. It is the force of superstition, of that age-old belief that Nature will give us something for nothing, which is expressed by the word magic. As we have seen, magic was important in the medical practice of the Egyptians and Babylonians. The Greeks as a nation were no more free from that contemptible fallacy than are the men of our own days. But the greatest of the Greeks stood wholly above such folly, and we can watch the Greek mind gradually lifting itself from that primeval mental attitude which is older than any known culture, older perhaps than any known race, the attitude of Nature-worship, or animism. To give an idea of how the 'sweet reasonableness' of the Greek mind gradually dissipated the animistic fog, a few words must be said about the history of the Greeks. Without that amount of history it would seem a miracle that Man ever became reasonable at all.

The medicine we call Greek might be described as the system which prevailed in ancient times in that half of the Mediterranean area which lies east and south of the Italian Peninsula.

Up to about 1400 B.C. most of the coast-lands of this Mediterranean area were inhabited by that very remarkable people, the Mycenaeans. These have left some extraordinary remains, the full significance of which has not yet been revealed. The general development of the Mycenaean civilization has, however, been outlined by modern

archaeological investigation. Its findings have resulted in a revision
of the story which Homer tells in the *Iliad*.

It would seem that the Hellenic peoples of the Eastern Mediterranean had become divided in culture, some adhering to the Mycenaean, others to the more modern 'Greek' type. Between these two

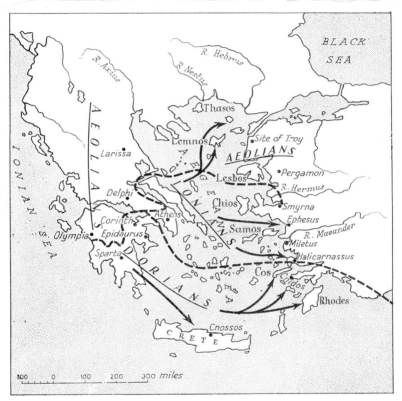

FIG. 9. Map of Greece, showing the direction and extent of the main invasions

there were doubtless gradations and conflicts, but the greatest of
these is reflected by Homer as the war of the Achaeans with Troy,
an event that must have taken place later than 1400 B.C. As a result
of this conflict the 'Greek' mode of life emerged within a relatively
short time. We are at the dawn of Greek documentary history. The
siege of Troy represents an attack by the invading Greeks on one of
the last Mycenaean strongholds. About 1000 B.C. the whole eastern

Mediterranean basin was being overrun by the Greek tribes coming in from the north of Greece. These Greeks were not a pure race, but a mixed multitude of invaders who came along several lines of advance. As always happens in such invasions, the conquered were not exterminated, but mingled with the invaders. Thus the Greeks, as they advanced, absorbed much of the culture and outlook of the civilization that they submerged.

In considering the history of rational medicine we are concerned chiefly with two main invading streams of Greek tribes: that of the Dorians, who passed towards Crete and towards the Island of Cos and the opposite peninsula of Cnidos, and that of the Ionians, who colonized most of the remaining part of western Asia Minor (Fig. 9). These two peoples were, between them, responsible for the main intellectual output of the Greeks of those early days. The medical system which they initiated first took shape in western Asia Minor, and thence became diffused over the whole of the Greek world. The Greek system of medicine which thus arose in Asia Minor had various roots, as indeed the medicine of a mixed people,

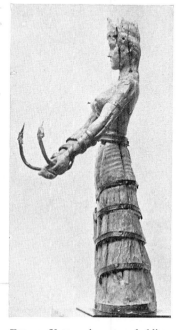

FIG. 10. Votaress in ecstasy, holding serpents. Gold and ivory statuette. Late Minoan II, *c.* 1400 B.C. (Museum of Fine Arts, Boston, U.S.A.)

living under very complex social conditions, was bound to have.

Firstly, there was the submerged civilization of the conquered Minoan folk. It is probable that the cult of the serpent—so constantly associated with Aesculapius and still used as a medical emblem—was of Minoan origin, for the serpent was a symbol much used in the Minoan religion (Fig. 10). It is probable too that some of the hygienic ideas of the Greeks were derived from the same source, for the Minoans had an excellent system of drainage. We can, however, say little on this head because the complete interpretation of the Minoan and Mycenaean records is still hidden from us.

Secondly, we have to remember that the shores of Asia Minor lie on the outskirts of the great civilization which had grown up in the valley of the Tigris and the Euphrates. The Greeks drew from that source much of their more superstitious beliefs, as well as some, at least, of their scientific method. On the one hand, the demoniac theories that bulk so largely in later Greek medicine doubtless came from Assyria and Babylonia. The medicine of the New Testament, for instance, with its casting out of devils, is of Mesopotamian origin. But, on the other hand, the Mesopotamian peoples had for long ages laid up a great treasury of observation, notably of astronomical data which were often applied to astrological ends. There was also some knowledge of the surface anatomy of certain organs derived from the practice of divination (p. 12). Working on the basis of these records, the Greeks were able to create a scientific method which appears as a prominent feature of their intellectual life in later centuries. Moreover, there was in Mesopotamia a standardization of both medical and surgical procedure which the nimble-witted Greeks were naturally quick to adopt. On its lower and less intellectual side, however, the Mesopotamian material was made to minister to Greek superstition and especially to astrological belief.

Thirdly, to the Egyptian civilization the Greek debt was also considerable. Many drugs were derived from Egypt and others were also suggested by Egyptian practice. The basis of Greek medical ethics too can be traced to Egypt. Some of the practical devices of Greek medicine, such as the forms of the surgical instruments, were of Egyptian origin. Nor can we neglect the statement made by the Greeks themselves, that mathematical knowledge—the test and index of all scientific growth—came to them first from Egypt. Lastly, we will recall that the Egyptians deified a physician, Imhotep (Fig. 3), in exactly the way that the Greeks deified their physician Asklepios (Fig. 11). Both Imhotep and Asklepios were, in fact, historic personages, and their evolution into gods presents many interesting parallels.

The Greeks of western Asia Minor, thus drawing material from many sources, came to develop, towards the end of the seventh

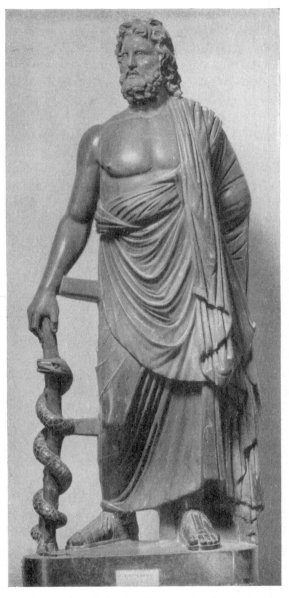

FIG. 11. Aesculapius. Marble statue found at Anzio
(Capitoline Museum, Rome)

century B.C., a philosophical system from which the whole of their science may be said to be a natural growth. Factors in this development were the medical schools of Cos, where Hippocrates was born, and of the opposite peninsula, Cnidos. These schools were in active operation by the sixth century B.C. By the middle of the fifth century they were important elements in the growing complexity of Greek life. Much of the Hippocratic Collection (p. 27), which contains the earliest Greek medical writings that have survived, must have been put together somewhere in the fourth century B.C., though its final recension is certainly later (Fig. 12). In that final recension Persian and Indian elements were also included, though to what degree is still very uncertain.

But the picture of the development of Greek medicine is not yet complete. Although we inherit the scientific spirit from the Greeks, and although they set a standard for all time of the purest and most disinterested type of medical practice, they are also in part responsible for some of the basest forms of medical jugglery that have afflicted and still afflict mankind. The medicine of the physicians was only one of their medical systems. There was a far lower form which gradually passed into the hands of the priests. The temple jugglery of Greece is ancestor, both by imitation and by direct tradition, of much medieval and modern medical miracle-mongering.

Furthermore, in ancient as in modern times, all medical men were not equally pure in aim or scientific in method. The practice of some Greek physicians was more than flavoured with magic. In justice, also, it must be said that not all priests were mere charlatans, and that there are traces of scientific method in the treatment of patients in the temples. There was, indeed, a relation between the practice of some of the physicians among the Greeks and that of some of their priestly magicians. We shall not attempt to determine the actual extent and nature of this relationship. For our purpose it is enough that the two systems were quite distinct in their most typical developments.

The temple system of Greek medicine was associated from an early date with a deity, Asklepios, whose cult became widespread in the Graeco-Roman world. Numerous representations of him have come down to us, and in them we see him gradually moulded to a

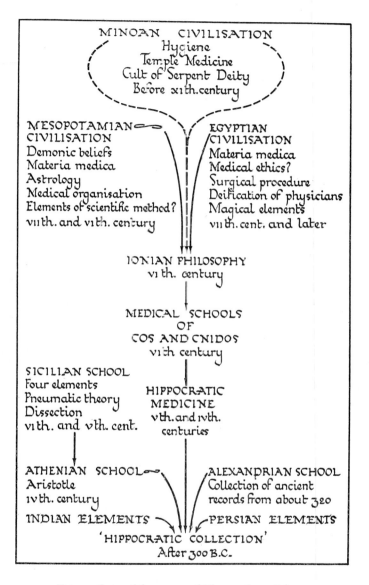

MINOAN   CIVILISATION
Hygiene
Temple Medicine
Cult of Serpent Deity
Before xith.century

MESOPOTAMIAN
CIVILISATION
Demonic beliefs
Materia medica
Astrology
Medical organisation
Elements of scientific method?
viith. and vith. century

EGYPTIAN
CIVILISATION
Materia medica
Medical ethics?
Surgical procedure
Deification of physicians
Magical elements
viith.cent. and later

IONIAN PHILOSOPHY
vi th. century

MEDICAL SCHOOLS
OF
COS AND CNIDOS
vith century

SICILIAN SCHOOL
Four elements
Pneumatic theory
Dissection
vith. and vth. cent.

HIPPOCRATIC
MEDICINE
vth.and ivth.
centuries

ATHENIAN SCHOOL
Aristotle
ivth. century

ALEXANDRIAN SCHOOL
Collection of ancient
records from about 320

INDIAN ELEMENTS   PERSIAN ELEMENTS
'HIPPOCRATIC COLLECTION'
After 300 B.C.

Fig. 12. Some of the sources of Hippocratic medicine

particular type. He becomes at last an aged man of noble, benevolent, and dreamy aspect, holding in his hand a staff around which a serpent twines itself (Fig. 11). The cult of the god Asklepios was carried on at numerous sites. The best known, both from literature and excavation, is Epidaurus. The conditions there are typical of those

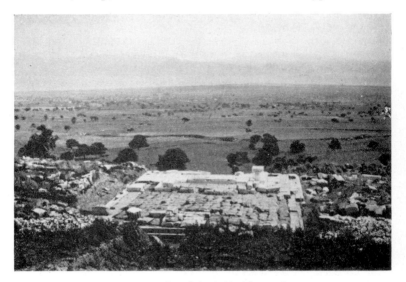

FIG. 13. Ruins of the Asklepieion at Cos
(After Laignel-Lavastine, *Histoire Générale de la Médecine*, vol. i, 1936)

in other Asklepian centres (Asklepieia), such as at Cos (Fig. 13). The principle was that the patient who visited the centre slept in a building with sacred associations. In the morning he related to the priest any dream which he had had during this incubation sleep; the priest interpreted the dream and advised the patient regarding the treatment, which was supposed to be prescribed by the god.

An illustration of a large model of the Asklepieion at Epidaurus, based on the extensive investigations and reconstructions of archaeologists, is given in Plate II. It shows in the left background a circular building, the *tholos*, which covered the sacred spring. This structure was built about 350 B.C. by the architect Polykleitos, and in classical times was considered to be the most perfect building in Greece. On the right of the *tholos* and separated from it by a few trees is a build-

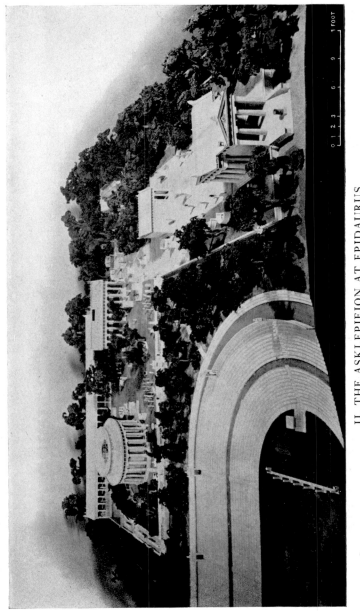

II. THE ASKLEPIEION AT EPIDAURUS

(Reconstruction after Defrasse and Lechat. Model in the Wellcome Historical Medical Museum)

(See p. 24)

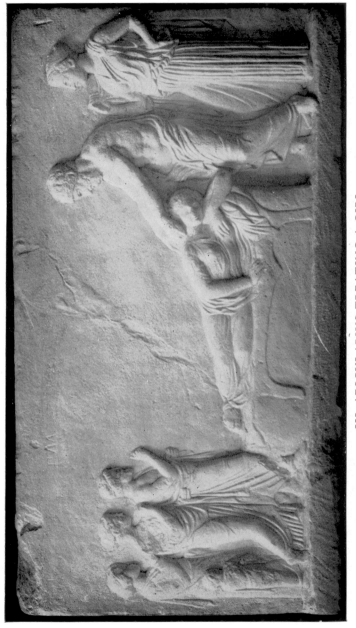

III. AESCULAPIUS TREATING A GIRL

(Athens Museum. Reproduced from a cast in the Wellcome Historical Medical Museum)

(See p. 26)

ing showing eleven columns along its side. This was the temple of
Asklepios built about a century earlier. It contained the famous
statue of the god. Behind these two buildings is seen a long building
with many columns, a roof and open sides. This was the *abaton*
which contained individual shrines and couches, on which the
patients had their incubation sleep. On the right of the model are
shown certain buildings used for special physical methods of treatment and for other purposes. In the left foreground of the photograph is shown part of the open-air theatre which still stands. It was
considered the finest in Greece.

It was the custom for a patient who was cured to leave at the
Asklepieion a votive offering, consisting of a representation in stone
of the affected part. Numerous offerings of this type have been recovered. He often left, too, a written testimonial to the value of his
cure. The temple priests had sacred snakes which accompanied them
when they visited the patients during the night. The snakes licked
the wounds and other lesions of the patients. It is possible that the
patients were given drugs, and that during their fitful sleep they
mistook the priest for the god himself. Ancient statues frequently
represent the god as bearing a staff round which is entwined a sacred
snake. But the association of the serpent with healing is a very old
belief; and it is worth while to note that to this day the symbol of
the profession of healing is a snake entwined around a staff, although
it is connected with supernatural healing and not with rational
medicine.

The cult of Asklepios seems to have arisen before the beginning of the fourth century B.C., and to have been widespread
and influential by the middle of that century. In 293 B.C. the plague
was raging in Rome, and messengers were sent to bring a sacred
serpent from Epidaurus. When the ship arrived in the Tiber, the
serpent—incarnating the god—swam ashore to the Island of St.
Bartholomew (the Insula Tiberina). This was regarded as an omen,
and an Asklepieion was built on the island (Plate V and p. 57). The
cult of the god now developed rather differently from the cult as
practised in Greece; in this book, when the Roman god is referred to,
he will be given his latinized name, Aesculapius.

While in its early stages the healing methods practised at Epidaurus and other Asklepieia were probably purely supernatural, physicians gradually came to be associated with the priests, and rational forms of therapy came to be practised. These included diet, drugs, baths, massage, and exercises and games in the stadia. The relief showing Asklepios treating a girl (Plate III) probably refers to the practise of massage.

Epidaurus is about thirty miles from Athens. It lies between two considerable ranges of hills, and the country bears still, in its customs and place-names, some remnants of the ancient cult. One tradition tells that a certain maiden, Koronis, being with child by Apollo, brought forth the infant Asklepios on the mountain above Epidaurus. There is still a village named Koroni hard by. She fled to conceal her shame and left the child on the mountain, where it was tended by a goat and watched over by a dog. The infant performed various miracles which we need not pursue, though a temple arose on the site where he is said to have wrought them. One of his miracles, however, has a wider interest and is worth recounting. A certain Hippolytus, falsely accused of impure relations with his stepmother, was slain by the gods in answer to the curses of his father, Theseus. Raised from the dead by the wonder-working Asklepios, he reappears in legend at the Arician grove in Italy. 'There', says a Greek chronicler of the second century A.D., 'he became a king and devoted a precinct to Artemis, where, down to my time, the prize for the victor in single combat was the priesthood of the goddess. The contest was open to no freeman, but only to runaway slaves.'

The son slain by his father and then rising from the dead; the runaway slave seeking sanctuary with Artemis in her grove, allowed his liberty and elevated to the priesthood there; the priesthood held only so long as the priest can guard it in mortal combat against the next runaway slave; this succession of slave kings and priestly murders has touched the imagination of the poets and artists in ancient and in modern times. The sacred grove of Artemis stood by the side of the lake of Nemi:

> the still glassy lake that sleeps
> Beneath Aricia's trees—
> Those trees in whose dim shadow

The ghastly priest doth reign,
The priest who slew the slayer,
And shall himself be slain.

It is a picture utterly out of accord with the general trend of classical mythology. Long ago scholars saw therein a remnant of a submerged faith, that ancient 'Nature worship' which survived among the Greeks, and survives with us. From this incident is named that great classical work of anthropology by Sir James George Frazer, *The Golden Bough*. By this story and by all that it implies, by all that learning has drawn out of it and associated with it, the history of medicine comes into contact with the brooding spirit of savage man. Into that dark realm we shall not enter in this volume.

History is the tale of the spirit of Man unfolding itself. This process is always slow, often imperceptible, sometimes retrograde, yet over long periods of time it is sure. Where no evolution of the spirit can be traced true history cannot be written; wherefore no man can write a history of human folly. Irrational man, driven by disease and fear of death, exhibits the same follies in all ages. The medical follies and superstitions of our own days are as in those when Aesculapius claimed men's allegiance. His garments and his names are changed, his temples are transformed, his priests assume other titles, but his face is the same, and he works the same wonders with about the same success. It is of rational medicine that we have henceforth to speak.

THE HIPPOCRATIC PHYSICIAN

We turn to the other side of the picture. Nothing could be in greater contrast to the orgies of the savage, the dark ways of the magician, or the charlatanry of the priests, than the serene spirit of wisdom which pervades the best Greek medicine. The finest presentation of that system is to be found in a group of about seventy works that have been associated together since antiquity under the name of Hippocrates. It is known as the Hippocratic Collection (or Corpus). These works consist of textbooks on special subjects (both for physicians and laymen), lectures for the use of students, and notebooks in which the material is not presented in a literary form. It will naturally be asked, 'Which of these works is by the man

whose name they bear?' To that question, alas, no definite answer
can be given. There is no single work which we can state with
confidence to be the composition of the Father of Medicine, and
possibly none is. These books are the work of a number of authors,
belonging to different schools, holding various and often contradictory views, living in widely separated parts of the Greek world
and writing at dates divided from each other, in the most extreme
cases, by perhaps five or six centuries. The opinion has been expressed that the Collection is really the library of the Hippocratic
School at Cos. Of the finest books of this collection we can but say
that they contain nothing inconsistent with a Hippocratic origin,
that their ethical standpoint is in accord with the Hippocratic ideal,
and that they are the work of physicians of great intellectual power
and experience.

If we ask what is known about Hippocrates himself, and if we seek
information rather than entertainment, our answer will be almost
as meagre. Hippocrates is no mythical figure, for he is mentioned
with great respect by his younger contemporary, Plato. He was the
son of a physician, and was born at Cos about 460 B.C. The most
active period of his life thus began about 420 B.C. His death is
placed between 377 and 359—the latter would make him 101, an
appropriate age for a great physician. He led a wandering life, and is
heard of at Cos, Thasos, Athens, in Thrace and elsewhere, and
lastly at Larissa in Thessaly, where his grave was long shown.
Among his pupils were his two sons, and his son-in-law. Of the
work of the latter we have a fragment preserved both by Aristotle
and in the Hippocratic Collection itself. That is all that is really
known about the Father of Medicine.

If critical examination has dealt thus hardly with the Hippocratic
writings and with Hippocrates himself, what is left which may surely
be derived from the Greek medical system? The answer is that
medicine has from the Greeks two great things: the picture of a
man and the institution of a method.

The man is Hippocrates himself. His figure, gaining in dignity
what it loses in clearness, stands for all time as that of the ideal
physician, for the ideal is there and is clearly set forth in these great
writings, whether or not we discern the details of his earthly features.

Calm and effective, humane and observant, prompt and cautious, at once learned and willing to learn, eager alike to get and give knowledge, unmoved save by the fear lest his knowledge may fail to benefit others—both the sick and their servants the physicians—incorruptible and pure in mind and body, the figure of the greatest of physicians has gained, not lost, by time. In all ages he has been held by medical men in a reverence comparable only to that which has been felt towards the founders of the great religions by their followers. This conception of the Hippocratic physician has been of incalculable spiritual value to the medical profession in the twenty-four centuries that have passed since his death.

Generations of students have remembered the calm, righteous, and dignified features of the British Museum bust to which the name Hippocrates had been attached for centuries. But authoritative criticism had long been levelled against this attribution, and it must be recognized that this bust is not a portrait of Hippocrates. In recent years a named, but badly damaged, bust was discovered at Ostia, and it is identical in type with a perfect, but unnamed, bust which had long been in the Uffizi Gallery at Florence. Both of these busts are Roman copies of a Greek original, now lost. The Uffizi bust (Fig. 14) must therefore be regarded as the best extant portrait of the Father of Medicine. Here too the features are calm and dignified, and they suggest the determination and singleness of purpose which, we feel, must have been elements in the character of this great physician.

So much for the man. We turn now to the method.

The method of Hippocratic medicine is that known today as the experimental or, better, experiential. It was employed among the Greeks for centuries after the death of Hippocrates. Then came a time when a social and philosophical upheaval prevented its further prosecution. For the thousand years that followed the break-up of the Roman Empire the medical practice of Europe was at best a corrupted imitation and misunderstanding of the Hippocratic teaching; at worst it descended to a low level of animism and magic. Then there was a rally. Slowly—very slowly at first—the foundations of modern science were laboriously laid. Among the first elements in this scientific renaissance was the recovery of the Hippocratic works.

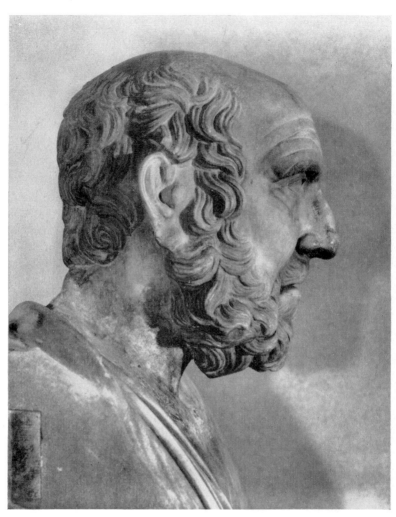

FIG. 14. Hippocrates

(Bust in the Galleria degli Uffizi, Florence. Reproduced by kind permission of the Soprintendenza alle Gallerie di Firenze)

In the centuries that followed this renaissance the very words of the Hippocratic Collection were taught in the medical schools in a spirit that was anything but that of Hippocrates. Gradually, however, a better understanding crept into men's minds. The spirit of those writings and their methods and observations now came rightly to be exalted above the works themselves. The works themselves were later dropped from the medical curriculum. They are no longer used in any medical school. But if we turn again to contemplate the Hippocratic treatises, we may recognize in them the modern process of careful record of data and cautious inference from them—that collation of experience from various sources obtained by various methods with which we are now so familiar. We may even see in full force the actual process of case-taking, bedside instruction, and the clinical lecture. These methods are practised much in the way in which we know them, and are set forth with a conciseness and beauty of language and a loftiness of ethical tone which have not since been surpassed. To such a collection medical men must always return. No part of it is more impressive than the Oath with which the name of Hippocrates has long been associated.

The Hippocratic Oath, in its present form, is perhaps of later date than Hippocrates. Yet parts of it may be even earlier than he, and some suggestion of it is perhaps to be traced in the teaching of Pythagoras (c. 530 B.C.). The later date of the Oath in its modern form by no means removes the interest of this grand ethical monument. No passage better reflects the spirit of the Hippocratic physicians. The Oath is clearly designed for a youth entering on his apprenticeship to such a physician.

I swear by Apollo the healer, invoking all the gods and goddesses to be my witnesses, that I will fulfil this Oath and this written Covenant to the best of my ability and judgement.

I will look upon him who shall have taught me this Art even as one of my own parents. I will share my substance with him, and I will supply his necessities, if he be in need. I will regard his offspring even as my own brethren, and I will teach them this Art, if they would learn it, without fee or covenant. I will impart this Art by precept, by lecture and by every mode of teaching, not only to my own sons but to the sons of him who has taught me, and to disciples bound by covenant and oath, according to the Law of Medicine.

The regimen I adopt shall be for the benefit of the patients according to my ability and judgement, and not for their hurt or for any wrong. I will give no deadly drug to any, though it be asked of me, nor will I counsel such, and especially I will not aid a woman to procure abortion. Whatsoever house I enter, there will I go for the benefit of the sick, refraining from all wrongdoing or corruption, and especially from any act of seduction, of male or female, of bond or free. In my attendance on the sick, or even apart therefrom, whatsoever things I see or hear, concerning the life of men, which ought not to be noised abroad, I will keep silence thereon, counting such things to be as sacred secrets. Pure and holy will I keep my Life and my Art.

If I fulfil this Oath and confound it not, be it mine to enjoy Life and Art alike, with good repute among all men at all times. If I transgress and violate my oath, may the reverse be my lot. [Slightly abridged.]

HIPPOCRATIC PRACTICE

Among the most remarkable features of the Hippocratic Collection is the feeling of contact with the patient which most of its works convey. This is naturally a special characteristic of the surgical works. One treatise, which bears the title *On wounds of the head*, has always drawn attention as showing special ingenuity and experience. The description of trephining is of peculiar interest, because the practice was known in prehistoric times (p. 1) and is still employed by savage and semi-civilized peoples. The process recommended for cases of fracture of the skull and injury to the underlying structures resembles, in many details, the modern surgical procedure.

When it is necessary to trephine a patient, make up your mind and judge as follows. If you have had charge of the case from the first, do not trephine the bone down to the membrane at once, for it is not desirable that the membrane be long exposed, lest it end by becoming rotten and fungous. There is also another danger, to wit that you wound the membrane with the saw during the operation, if you try to remove the bone by trephining immediately down to the membrane. Therefore, when the bone is almost sawn through and is already loose, cease trephining and allow the bone to come away of itself. While trephining, often remove the instrument and dip it in cold water. If you do not do this, the trephine, becoming heated by the circular motion and heating and drying the bone, may burn it and cause an unduly large piece of the bone round the sawing to come away.

So much for a normal case which comes to the physician's hands

directly after the accident. But in less fortunate cases he is not called
in so early, and the wound suppurates before he can bring his art to
bear upon it. In such a case he is advised to act as follows:

Saw the bone immediately to the membrane with a serrated trephine
[Fig. 15, *a*], frequently removing the trephine and testing with the

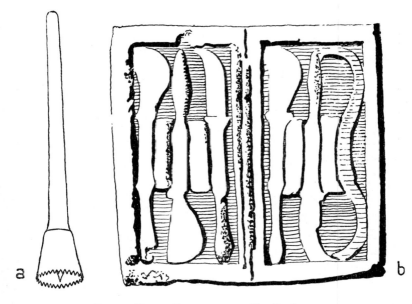

FIG. 15. Types of instruments used by Greek surgeons

(*a*) Simple trephine with centre pin.   (*b*) Case of scalpels.
(*a*) Sixteenth-century instrument of ancient type.   (*b*) Relief in the Asclepieion,
Athens.

probe all round along the track, for the bone is sawn through much more
quickly if it is already suppurating and penetrated by the pus. The bone,
however, often happens to be thin in places. Therefore be on your guard
not to apply the trephine at random, but fix it in the bone where it appears
thickest, frequently making an examination and trying to raise the bone
by moving it. And after removing it, continue such treatment as may
appear advantageous to the wound, according to circumstances.

Two types of trephine were used. One had a centre pin, and was
used until the serrated edge began to bite; the other had no centre

pin and was used to complete the cutting of the bone. A trephine was either held between the palms of the hands and rotated by the action of rubbing them together (cf. Fig. 100), or was rotated by a cross-piece and thong (cf. Figs. 30 and 31). No ancient Greek trephines have survived. For a Babylonian trephine, see Fig. 8.

Among the works of the Hippocratic Collection is a lecture notebook known by the title *Concerning the things in the Surgery*. It is written in very abbreviated style and consists of mere headings. Nevertheless, our attention is arrested by its startling modernness, when we read such a passage as this:

Operative requisites in the surgery: the patient; the operator; assistants; instruments; the light, where and how placed; the patient's person and apparatus. The operator, whether seated or standing, should be placed conveniently to the part being operated upon and to the light. Each of the two kinds of light, ordinary or artificial, may be used in two ways, direct or oblique.

Many illustrations on ancient Greek vases show that the art of bandaging must have reached a fairly high level (cf. Fig. 16). Consider also the following details:

The nails [of the operator] neither to exceed nor come short of the finger-tips. Practise using the finger-ends. Practise all operations with each hand and with both together, your object being to attain ability, speed, painlessness, elegance and readiness. Let those who look after the patient present the part for operation as you want it, and hold fast the rest of the body so as to be all steady, keeping silence and obeying their superior.

This passage reminds us of the operator and operating-theatre during the first half of the nineteenth century. At that time surgery had reached the frontiers beyond which it could not pass until the advent of the general anaesthetic. The great surgeons of that period were indeed outstanding for their technical ability and for the consummate speed and elegance with which they carried out amputations.

In the Hippocratic Collection the physician attended cases of every type, and did not refuse to do his best for a case because the use of an instrument was demanded. He was thus no specialist. But the mass of his practice lay with cases to which instrumental treatment was

inapplicable. In cases in which surgical intervention was not justified
the Hippocratic physician adopted for the most part what is called
an 'expectant' line of treatment. Realizing that, in general, the
tendency of the body is to recover, he contented himself with 'waiting on Nature'. This does not
by any means imply that he was
helpless, for much could be
done by nursing, regimen and
diet to aid the patient in that
conflict which he alone had to
fight. For the conduct of that
great battle wise and useful
directions are recorded. But believing in 'the healing power of
Nature'—the famous phrase is
used in the Hippocratic writings
—the physician was none too
eager to administer drugs. In
the state of knowledge of the
day this reluctance was well
judged. The Hippocratic drugs
were neither numerous nor complex. Some of them, however,
were very efficient, and their
judicious if reluctant use at the
right juncture saved many a life.
     A rough idea of the types of
patients seen by the Greek
physician is provided by the
illustrations on certain Attic

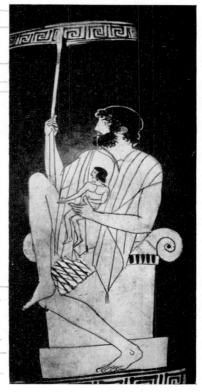

FIG. 16. Telephos wounded in the thigh,
showing a double-spica bandage
(British Museum, Vase E 282)

vases, such as is shown in Fig. 17. Here a young physician is seated
in the centre of the illustration. He is about to bleed a patient from a
vein at the bend of the elbow. The blood will be received in the large
bronze basin on the floor. Above the physician's head are three cupping vessels shaped like inverted flasks. In front of the physician
sits another patient with his left arm bandaged; he awaits treatment, or bleeding, or both. Behind this patient stands a female

who is possibly smelling herbs as a preventive against infection. Behind the physician is a man with his left leg bandaged, and behind him stands a dwarf with a large head and a muscular hairy body. This dwarf shows the features now recognized as characteristic of the disease achondroplasia. The rabbit or hare on his back may be the fee for the consultation. Talking to the dwarf is a man who may have an injury to his chest.

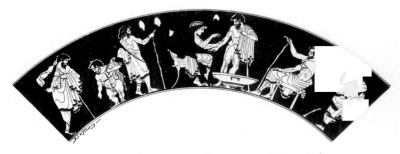

Fig. 17. Greek clinic *c*. 400 B.C., shown on a red-figure Attic vase
(Louvre, Inv. C. A. 2183)

The *Aphorisms* is the most famous book with which the name of Hippocrates is associated. Internal evidence shows the improbability of this collection of short instructions and suggestions having been put together by a single man. The work consists of an unconnected series of brief generalizations, many of which have been confirmed by the clinical experience of later ages. Some have passed into medical commonplaces, others have become popular proverbs. The style of the work suggests an aged physician reflecting on the experience of a lifetime. Among modern medical writings its closest analogue is perhaps the *Commentaries* of the great English physician, William Heberden the Elder (1710–1801), which he commenced after the age of seventy. They occupied the last twenty years of his life, contained a summary of the whole of his vast experience, and were published by his son after his death. A few extracts from the *Aphorisms* of Hippocrates give a good idea of the nature of the book.

Life is short, the Art long, opportunity fleeting, experience fallacious, judgement difficult. Not only must the physician be ready to do his duty, but the patient, the attendants, and external circumstances must conduce to the cure. [This, the most famous of the *Aphorisms*, sums up the ideals of the Hippocratic physician, and emphasizes the clinical and observational approach to the art of medicine.]

Old persons bear fasting most easily, next adults, and young people yet less; least of all children, and of these least again those who are particularly lively. [Metabolism, the rate at which the chemical functions of the body are carried on, is highest in children and lowest in old age.]

If in any illness sleep does harm, it is a symptom of deadly import.

When sleep puts an end to delirium, it is a good sign.

Weariness without [apparent] cause indicates disease. [This possibly refers to pulmonary tuberculosis, common in Ancient Greece, in which an early symptom is often unexplained fatigue.]

If there be a painful affection in any part of the body, and yet no suffering, there is mental disorder.

To eat heartily after a long illness without putting on flesh is a bad portent.

Food or drink slightly inferior in itself, but more palatable, should be preferred to that better itself, but less palatable.

The old have fewer illnesses than the young, but if any become chronic with them they generally carry it with them to the grave.

Those naturally very fat are more liable to sudden death than the thin. [A fat person may have the condition known as fatty heart, in which sudden death is not uncommon.]

The dry seasons are more healthy than the rainy, and attended by less mortality.

Cold sweats in conjunction with an acute fever indicate death, but with a milder fever only prolonged sickness.

A spasm supervening on a wound is fatal. (Tetanus, cf. p. 386.)

Those attacked by tetanus either die within four days, or if they survive these they recover.

Phthisis occurs most commonly between the ages of eighteen and thirty-five years. [This statement is well exemplified by the age incidence of phthisis in modern times.

Diarrhoea supervening in the course of phthisis is mortal. [Some patients suffering from acute or chronic phthisis develop persistent diarrhoea, which is now known to be due to tuberculous ulceration of the bowel. In severe cases the condition is grave.]

It is fatal for a woman in pregnancy to be attacked by one of the acute diseases.

In cases of jaundice, hardening of the liver is a bad sign. [Jaundice as a symptom is in itself comparatively common and unimportant. But persistent jaundice may be due to cancer or cirrhosis of the liver, both of which are marked by a hardening of the liver tissue and an enlargement of the organ. In these cases the lower edge of the liver can be felt to be indurated.]

We should observe the appearance of the eyes in sleep. If any of the white show through the eyelids when closing, this is a bad sign and very dangerous, unless it be due to diarrhoea or to purgation.

Delirium with laughter is less dangerous than with despondency.

Apoplexy is commonest between the ages of forty and sixty.

If you give the same food to a patient in a fever and to a person in health, the patient's disease is aggravated by what gives strength to the healthy man.

The chief clinical achievement of the Hippocratic Collection lies in the descriptions of actual cases. These descriptions are not only without parallel till the late seventeenth century, but they are models of what succinct clinical records should be. They are clear and short, they give all the leading features, yet they show no attempt to prejudge the importance of any particular feature. The records of these cases illustrate the Greek genius for seizing the essential. The writer does not betray the least wish to exalt his own skill. He seeks merely to put the data before the reader for his guidance under like circumstances. It is a reflex of the spirit of honesty in which these men worked that in the great majority of the cases they record that death ensued. Two of these remarkable descriptions may be given:

The woman with sore throat, who lodged with Aristion; her complaint began with indistinct speech; tongue red and grew parched. *First day*, shivered, then felt hot. *Third day*, rigor, acute fever; reddish, hard swelling on both sides of neck and chest; extremities cold and livid; respiration fluttering; drink returned by the nose; she could not swallow; stools and urine suppressed. *Fourth day*, all symptoms exacerbated. *Fifth day*, died.

Although it has been stated that this was a case of diphtheria, this diagnosis seems improbable. (The first clear case of diphtheria in medical literature was described six centuries after Hippocrates.) The condition here appears to have been a very severe quinsy with rapid spread of the septic process to the loose tissues of the neck (septic cellulitis), and thereafter a septic infection of the blood (septicaemia), which was fatal.

In Thasos, the wife of Delearces, who lodged on the plain, through sorrow was seized with an acute fever and shivering. From the beginning she kept on wrapping herself up; kept silent, fumbled, plucked, scratched, and picked hairs [from the clothes]; tears and again laughter; no sleep; bowels irritated but passed nothing; when urged drank a little; urine thin and scanty; to the touch the fever was slight; coldness of the extremities. *Ninth day*, talked much incoherently, and again sank into silence. *Fourteenth day*, breathing rare, large and with long intervals, and again hurried. *Seventeenth day*, after stimulation of the bowels she passed even drinks, nor could retain anything; totally insensible; skin tense and parched. *Twentieth day*, much talk, and again became quiet, then loss of voice; respiration hurried. *Twenty-first day*, died. Her respiration throughout was rare and large; she was completely uninterested; always wrapped up in her bedclothes; throughout either much rambling, or complete silence.

We have here a description of low muttering delirium, a common end of continued fevers, as, for instance, typhoid. It resembles the condition known to physicians as the typhoid state. Incidentally, the case contains a reference to a type of breathing common among the dying. The respiration becomes deep and slow, as it sinks gradually into quietude and becomes rarer and rarer until it seems to cease altogether, and then it slowly becomes more rapid, and so on alternately. This type of breathing is known to physicians as Cheyne–Stokes respiration, in commemoration of two distinguished Irish physicians of the nineteenth century who brought it to the attention of medical men (p. 283). In our own time it has been partially explained on a physiological basis.

We may note that there is another and even better pen-picture of Cheyne–Stokes respiration in the Hippocratic Collection. We read of one Philiscus who lived by the wall and who took to his bed on the first day of acute fever. About the middle of the sixth day he died, and the physician notes that 'the breathing throughout, as though he were remembering to do it, was rare and large'. Cheyne–Stokes breathing is thus admirably described.

In the Hippocratic Collection case-histories of forty-two cases are given, and some of these contain clinical observations which have stood the test of time. For example, in the work *On Diseases* there is a description of a patient with fluid and air in the pleural cavity. The text says: 'You will place the patient on a seat which does not move, an assistant will hold him by the shoulders, and you will shake him, applying the ear to the chest, so as to recognize on which side the sign occurs.' This sign is still considered to be characteristic of the condition and is still used by the physician. It is known as Hippocratic succussion. In another passage in the same work the symptoms of pleurisy are described, and it is said that 'a creak like that of leather may be heard'. This is the pleuritic rub which is heard by the physician in the early stages of pleurisy; it resembles exactly the creaking of leather. Some of the surgical works in the Hippocratic Collection contain masterpieces of compressed description, such as the accounts of the operations for the evacuation of pus from the chest and for trephining the skull.

Immense and, as some may think, overwhelming importance is laid by the Hippocratic writings upon the art of prognosis, that is of predicting the course which the disease will take. The work to which the title *Prognostics* is attached represents a very lofty standard of practice. We quote from it a description of the signs of death to which the name Hippocratic facies has become attached. It is imitated by Shakespeare in his description of the death of Falstaff in *Henry V* (Act ii, Scene iii):

You should observe thus in acute diseases; first the countenance of the patient, if it be like those of persons in health, and especially if it be like its usual self, for this is best of all. But the opposite are the worst, such as these: a sharp nose, hollow eyes, sunken temples; the ears cold, contracted, and their lobes turned outwards; the skin about the forehead rough, stretched and parched; the colour of the face greenish or livid.

If the countenance be such at the beginning of the disease, and if this cannot be accounted for by the symptoms, inquiry must be made whether the patient has been sleepless, whether his bowels have been very loose, or whether he has been starved. If any of these be admitted, the danger is to be reckoned so far the less, and it will become obvious in the course of a day and a night whether or no the appearance is due to these. But if no such cause exist and if the symptoms do not subside in this time, be it known for certain that the end is at hand.

We shall see later the emphasis which the Hippocratic physician placed on the four humours (p. 46); excess or defect of these humours determined the bodily state of the individual. The excess or defect could be counteracted in various ways, but of these the use of drugs was probably the least important. Rest was the most generally applied method of treatment. These Greek physicians also placed great stress on diet, and quite a large proportion of the whole Hippocratic Collection is devoted to this subject. The principle of their diet for fevers is not unlike the principle which determines the choice of such a diet at the present day.

These glimpses will give some idea of rational medicine in the making. In the fourth century B.C. medicine emerges as a definite part of the scientific consciousness. Rational medicine is now in being.

ARISTOTLE

During the fourth century B.C. there lived and worked one whose thought has stamped itself on the whole subsequent course of the biological and medical sciences, and indeed of all science.

Aristotle (384–322 B.C.) was a provincial Greek and son of a Macedonian physician. At seventeen he became a pupil of Plato at Athens. After Plato's death in 347 Aristotle crossed the Aegean to reside in Asia Minor. The main part of his biological observations was made during his stay there. In 342 B.C., at the request of King Philip of Macedon, Aristotle became tutor to Philip's son, Alexander the Great. He remained in Macedon for seven years. About 336, when Alexander departed for the invasion of Asia, Aristotle returned to Athens, where he taught for the rest of his life. He died in 322 B.C., a few months after his pupil Alexander.

Aristotle was the great codifier of ancient science. On him all subsequent biological development, including that of modern times, is based. In his wonderful biological works, which are still read by naturalists, he discusses many problems current to this very day. He laid the basis of the doctrine of organic evolution in his teaching concerning the Ladder of Nature (*scala naturae*) (Fig. 18). He developed coherent theories of generation and heredity. He founded comparative anatomy and he dissected many animals. He did not, however, dissect the human body.

Aristotle gave good descriptions of some organs, regarded from the standpoint of comparative anatomy. These descriptions he sometimes illustrated by drawings, the first anatomical figures of which we have a record. In some cases these drawings can be restored with confidence. Thus, he gave an account of the uterus, his nomenclature of which has been retained in more or less modified form to our time (Fig. 19). Among the best anatomical descriptions given by Aristotle is that of the ruminant stomach, which consists of four distinct chambers. Perhaps his most extraordinary anatomical feat is his account of the development of the dog-fish (*Mustelus laevis*), which he showed was attached to its mother's womb in a way very

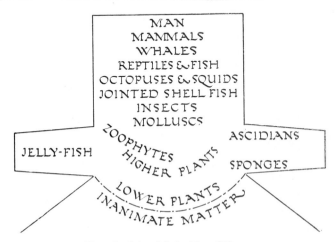

Fig. 18. Aristotle's Ladder of Nature

similar to the attachment of the embryo of a mammal (Fig. 20). This observation was forgotten until well on in the sixteenth century. It raised the admiration of the greatest modern morphologist, Johannes Müller (p. 287), and would in itself be sufficient to establish the claim of Aristotle to a place in the front rank of observing naturalists. Aristotle gave fairly accurate descriptions of the branches of the great veins and of the superficial vessels of the limbs of mammals. He realized that the arteries are usually accompanied by veins. He described the generative and digestive organs of cephalopod molluscs, and many other parts of many other animals.

Something should be said of the errors of Aristotle. Though an excellent naturalist, he was in general much weaker in physiology than in anatomy. Thus, he made no proper distinction between arteries and veins. He failed to trace any adequate relations between the sense organs, the nerves, and the brain. His refusal to attach great importance to the brain is remarkable. Primacy he placed with the heart, which he regarded also as the seat of the intelligence. This was contrary not only to the medical opinion of his day, but also to the popular view, voiced, for instance, by Aristophanes in his play *The Clouds*, written about 400 B.C., where we read of a man who had concussion of the brain. Moreover, Aristotle's teacher Plato placed

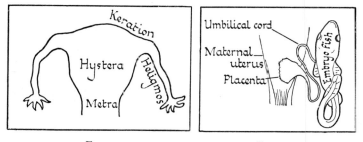

FIG. 19   FIG. 20

FIG. 19. The parts of the uterus according to Aristotle. These names persist in modified form in modern anatomy

FIG. 20. Johannes Müller's diagram of the embryo dogfish, *Mustelus laevis*. The embryo is attached to the uterine wall by an umbilical cord

the seat of thought and feeling in the brain. From all we know of Aristotle, it seems probable that he did not take up this attitude without evidence. It seems likely that he had experimented on the brain and found it devoid of sensation. Hence his view, opposed to current belief, that it is not associated with thought. Aristotle regarded the brain simply as an agent for cooling the heart, and preventing it from being over-heated. This cooling process, he considered, was effected by the secretion of phlegm (*pituita*), an idea still preserved in our anatomical term, the pituitary body.

The views of Aristotle have had a vast influence in determining the direction of medical thought. For more than two thousand years Aristotelian philosophy, in more or less corrupted form, constituted the main intellectual food of mankind. Without some knowledge of the biological work of Aristotle it is impossible to understand the course taken by rational medicine. The influence of Aristotle is specially evident in certain basic biological conceptions.

The problem of the nature of generation is one in which Aristotle never ceased to take an interest. Among the methods by which he sought to solve it was embryological investigation. His most important embryological researches were made upon the chick. His choice was most fortunate, and the chick has remained to this day the classical subject of embryological research. Aristotle asserts that the first signs of life in the hen's egg are noticeable on the third day, the heart being visible as a pulsating spot. As it develops, two meandering blood-vessels extend to the surrounding tunics. A little later, he observes, the body becomes distinguishable, at first very small and white, the head being clearly distinguished and the eyes very large (Fig. 49, p. 126). To follow the main features of the later stages was a comparatively easy task.

Aristotle was greatly impressed by these phenomena. He lays stress on the early appearance of the heart in the embryo. Corresponding to the general gradational view that he had formed of Nature, he held that the most primitive and fundamentally important organs make their appearance before the others. Among the organs all give place to the heart, which he considered the first to live and the last to die. As we have seen, he placed the seat of the intelligence in the heart.

Thus, not only in his account of the Ladder of Nature, but also in his theories of individual development, Aristotle exhibits some approach to evolutionary doctrine. This is somewhat obscured, however, by his peculiar view of the nature of procreation. On this topic his general conclusion is that the material substance of the embryo is contributed by the female, but that this is mere passive formable material, almost as though it were the soil in which the embryo grows. The male, by giving the principle of life, the soul (*psyche*), contributes the essential generative agency. But this soul is not material, and it is not, therefore, theoretically necessary for anything material to pass from male to female. The material which does in fact pass with the semen of the male is, as the older philosophers would have said, an 'accident', not an 'essential'. The essential contribution of the male is not matter but 'form' and 'principle'.

The female, then, only provides the 'material', the male the 'soul', the 'form', the 'principle', that which makes life. Aristotle was thus prepared to accept instances of fertilization without material contact, i.e. in effect, parthenogenesis or virgin birth. In the centuries that came after him such instances were not infrequently adduced, and this doctrine was given a special turn by Christian theologians. Belief in the 'accidental' character of the material contribution of the male was common among men of science till the nineteenth century. The general attitude as to the nature of fertilization set forth, for instance, by William Harvey (p. 120) in his book *De generatione animalium* ('On the Generation of Animals') first published in London in A.D. 1651, is practically identical with the views of Aristotle published in Athens about 350 B.C., just 2,000 years earlier. It is also of great interest to note that recent embryological research goes some way to confirm this view of Aristotle. Without any intervention of the male sexual element, it is possible so to stimulate the egg mechanically as to produce a perfect animal which is thus fatherless from the first. The male element is indeed unnecessary and, in fact, transmits only hereditary characters.

We must say something concerning Aristotle's conceptions of the nature of life itself. He was before all things a vitalist. For him the distinction between living and not-living substance is to be sought not in material constitution, but in the presence or absence of something that he calls *psyche* (soul). His teaching on this topic had profound influence on subsequent anatomical and physiological thought.

Aristotle's theory as to the relation of this *psyche* or soul to material things is difficult and complicated. Its adequate discussion would take us beyond our theme. He holds, however, that the soul is related to the idea of form. In living things the soul is that which gives form. It is the pervasion by the soul that leads to the determinate development of the body and its parts. This activity of the soul, under the Aristotelian term entelechy (which we may perhaps translate roughly as 'the indwelling perfectability' or 'purposiveness'), has an important place in modern biological theory, though at the present time biological opinion seems to be swinging away from the Aristotelian position.

Aristotle defines life, existing in matter, as 'the power of self-nourishment and of independent growth and decay'. Of the soul, the principle of life, he distinguishes three orders or types; lowest, the vegetative soul (nutritive and reproductive), next the animal soul (sensitive), and highest the rational soul (intellectual). The last, he at first held, was peculiar to man, but later he modified this view.

The history of the reception of Aristotle's science by later ages is very strange to modern eyes. Of all Aristotle's scientific teachings, men clung most firmly for many centuries not to his finely thought

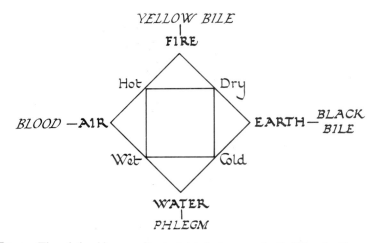

FIG. 21. The relationship, according to Aristotle, between the Qualities, the Elements, and the Humours

out biological conceptions, but to a doctrine of the constitution of matter of which the modern student hears nothing. Aristotle, following more ancient writers, held that there were four primary and opposite fundamental qualities, the 'hot' and the 'cold', the 'wet' and the 'dry'. These met in binary combination to constitute the four 'essences' or 'existences' which entered in varying proportions into the constitution of all matter. The four 'essences', or, to give them their usual name, 'elements', were 'earth', 'air', 'fire', and 'water'. Thus, 'water' was 'wet' and 'cold', fire 'hot' and 'dry', and so forth (Fig. 21). With this theory later writers combined the somewhat similar Hippocratic doctrine which held that the body was composed of the four 'humours' or liquids: blood (*sanguis*), phlegm (*pituita*), yellow bile (*chole*), and black bile (*melanchole*). Some of the Hippocratic physicians had associated excess of the humours with various types of bodily constitution. Their followers made much of the 'temperaments' resulting therefrom, and according to the prevailing humour they distinguished the sanguine, phlegmatic, choleric, or melancholy, temperament (Fig. 38, p. 102).

These conceptions, now departed altogether from our scientific discipline, still persist embedded in our language. Poetry still uses such ideas as the 'raging of the elements' and 'elemental forces'. We may yet speak of a 'fiery nature' or an 'aerial spirit'. We know what is meant by a sanguine or a phlegmatic temperament, and a melancholy or choleric disposition, and such words conjure up real pictures in our minds (Fig. 38). Until it began to be undermined by Robert Boyle (p. 136) and others in the seventeenth century, the doctrine of the four elements persisted in its entirety, while ideas and terms derived from the old humoral pathology can, in fact, be traced in the medicine of the twentieth century.

The biological activity of the School of Aristotle was continued after his death by his pupil Theophrastus (372–287 B.C.). Theophrastus wrote on many subjects, but his writings on plants especially are instinct with a thoroughly scientific spirit, and are rightly regarded as the basic documents of the science of botany. Nevertheless, his works had little effect or influence on his contemporaries and successors. With Theophrastus the purely biological School of Aristotle may be said to come to an end. The biological sciences ceased, for many centuries, to be studied for their own sake and became mere handmaidens of medicine. Neither mistress nor servant was the better for the change.

III

THE HEIRS OF GREECE

THE ALEXANDRIAN SCHOOL

SOON after Aristotle, about 300 B.C., a great medical school was founded at Alexandria in Egypt. That country had been conquered by Alexander the Great, after whom the town was named. On Alexander's death, Egypt came under the rule of one of his generals, Ptolemy, who established a dynasty which became extinct with the famous Queen Cleopatra, thirty years before the Christian era. Alexandria was a favourite residence of this Greek dynasty and became more Greek than Egyptian. Ptolemy and his successors were patrons of learning, and at the Alexandrian School remarkable anatomical and physiological researches were made. These were the work of Greek physicians who, in the tradition of their people, were only too wont to associate their discoveries with sweeping theoretical generalizations, often on very inadequate bases.

The two earliest medical teachers at Alexandria were also the greatest, Herophilus of Chalcedon, who flourished about 300 B.C., and his slightly younger contemporary Erasistratus of Chios. Herophilus may be regarded as the founder of anatomy, Erasistratus as the founder of physiology.

Herophilus was probably the first to dissect the human body in public. He recognized the brain as the central organ of the nervous system and regarded it as the seat of the intelligence, thus reversing the verdict of Aristotle on the primacy of the heart. He was the first to grasp the nature of the nerves, which he distinguished as connected with motion and sensation; nevertheless he did not separate them clearly from tendons and sinews. He greatly extended the knowledge of the parts of the brain. Certain parts of the brain still bear titles which are translations of those which he gave them. He also made the first clear distinction between arteries and veins, and he regarded the pulsation in arteries as due to the activity of their muscular walls.

At the time of the institution of the Medical School at Alexandria, and for long after, there flourished that view of the structure of matter known as 'atomic', propounded by the philosopher Democritus (*c.* 400 B.C.). The chief exponent of the theory was Epicurus (342–270), whose philosophy was of the order which we should now call materialistic. For it the only ultimate realities were atoms and 'the void', and everything was ultimately expressible in these terms. Epicurean philosophy was not without its reactions on medicine at Alexandria, where its leading exponent was Erasistratus of Chios (*c.* 300–250 B.C.)

Erasistratus was essentially a rationalist and professed himself a foe to all mysticism. In the last resort, however, he had to invoke the idea of Nature as a great artist acting as an external power, shaping the body according to the ends to which it must act. This is in direct contrast with Aristotle's view of the soul as an entelechy (p. 45), an innate and inherent factor. Erasistratus sought to express his views in atomic terms, but, to make physiology intelligible, he added a conception, pneumatism, found also among older thinkers. Pneumatism is the belief that the phenomena of life are associated with the existence of a subtle vapour, *pneuma* or spirit, which permeates the organism, and causes its movements. This subtle vapour is held to have some affinities with the air we breathe. Pneumatism is, in fact, a primitive attempt to explain the phenomena of respiration.

Erasistratus observed that every organ is equipped with a three-fold system of 'vessels', vein, artery, and nerve, which divide to the very limits of vision, and he considered that the process of division continues beyond those limits. He thought the minute divisions of these vessels were plaited together and constituted the tissues. Veins, arteries, and nerves were, for him, made of minute tubes of the same nature as themselves, through which they were nourished. Blood and two kinds of pneuma were the essential sources of nourishment and movement. The blood was carried by veins. Air, on the other hand, was taken in by the lungs and passed to the heart, where it became changed into a peculiar *pneuma*, the vital spirit, which was sent to the various parts of the body by the arteries. This spirit was carried to the brain, in the cavities or ventricles of which it was further changed to a second kind of *pneuma*, the animal spirit. The animal spirit was conveyed to different parts of the body by the nerves, which were hollow.

In the brain Erasistratus observed the convolutions, noted that they were more elaborate in man than in animals, and associated this complexity with the higher intelligence of man. He distinguished between the main parts of the brain, the cerebrum and cerebellum, and gave a detailed description of the cerebral ventricles or cavities within the brain, and of the meninges or membranes that cover it. He considered that the cerebral ventricles were filled with animal spirit (cf. Galen's scheme, Fig. 26, p. 64).

Erasistratus attained to a clear view of the action of muscles in producing movement. He regarded the shortening of muscles as due to distension by animal spirit conveyed to the muscles by the nerves. We may note that similar theories as to the nature of muscular action were again set forth, on theoretical grounds, in the seventeenth century by Descartes (p. 138) and by Borelli (p. 140), but that they were rebutted by the experiments of Swammerdam (p. 133). We may recall that we are still in the dark as to the mechanism of contraction of muscle fibre, the structure of which first began to be revealed by Leeuwenhoek (Fig. 53, p. 53).

Erasistratus considered the chief cause of disease to be excess of blood, or plethora. Diseases thus caused differed according to their site. Among them were coughing of blood, epilepsy, pneumonia, and tonsillitis. Most of these diseases could be treated by diminishing the local supply of blood by starvation. Among his contemporaries and successors blood-letting was a habitual practice applied to almost every condition. Erasistratus employed it rarely, and some of his followers banned it altogether. He was consistently opposed to violent remedies. Among the therapeutic measures which he favoured were regulated exercise, diet and the vapour bath.

Erasistratus complained that many physicians of his time were not interested in hygiene. He therefore wrote a treatise on the subject. Though he regarded hygiene as a means of substituting prevention for cure, this did not prevent him from being extremely careful and precise in his treatment of cases.

After the first generation or two, the originality of the Alexandrian School flagged, though the city long remained a great teaching centre, and minor medical advances were made. Surgery (cf. Fig. 15) seems to have languished less than medicine. The stagnation in medical matters at Alexandria is in contrast to the continued activity there in mathematics, astronomy, mechanics and geography.

With the absorption of Egypt into the Roman Empire in 50 B.C. and the extinction of the Ptolemaic dynasty by the death of Cleopatra in 30 B.C., Alexandria ceased to have great scientific importance. The School continued for centuries with restricted activity and devoid of all originality. Intellectually, it had become subordinate to the Metropolis. Rome was now mistress of the world and the future of medicine must be considered from the point of view of the Roman Empire.

MEDICAL TEACHING IN THE ROMAN EMPIRE

The original native Roman medical system was quite devoid of scientific elements and was that of a people of the lower culture. Interwoven, as is all primitive medicine, with ideas that trespass on the domains of religion and magic, it possessed that multitude of specialist deities which was so characteristic of the Roman cults. The entire external aspect of Roman medicine was changed by the advent of Greek science. Yet, notwithstanding the large medical field that the Western Empire provided, and the wide acceptance of Greek medicine by the upper classes, it is remarkable that the Latin-speaking peoples produced no eminent physician.

At first scientific medical education at Rome was entirely a matter of private teaching. The earliest important scientific teacher there was the Greek Asclepiades of Bithynia (c. 124–c. 40 B.C.), a contemporary of the poet Lucretius and, like him, an Epicurean. Asclepiades, like Erasistratus, imported the atomic view of Democritus into medicine. He deeply influenced the course of later medical thought, ridiculed the Hippocratic attitude of relying on the 'healing power of Nature' which he regarded as a mere 'meditation on death', and urged that active measures were needed for the process of cure to be 'seemly, swift and sure'. He founded a regular school at Rome which continued after him.

At first the school was the mere personal following of the physician, who took his pupils and apprentices round with him on his visits. At a later stage such groups combined to form societies or colleges, where problems of the art were debated. A relief on a Roman sarcophagus of the Empire (Fig. 22) represents a physician who is

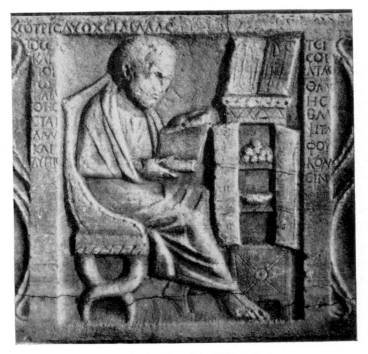

FIG. 22. A physician of the Hellenistic Age
(From a cast in the Wellcome Historical Medical Museum; original, Capitoline Museum, Rome)

perhaps teaching his pupils. He is reading from a scroll, and other scrolls are contained in a small cabinet beside him. A case of surgical instruments stands open on this cabinet. Towards the end of the reign of Augustus (reigned 27 B.C.–A.D. 14) or the beginning of that of Tiberius (reigned A.D. 14–37), these societies constructed for themselves a meeting-place on the Esquiline Hill. Finally the emperors built halls (*auditoria*) for the teaching of medicine. The professors at first received only the pupils' fees. It was not until the time of the Emperor Vespasian (reigned A.D. 70–79) that medical teachers were given a salary at the public expense. The system was extended by later emperors.

Thus Rome became a centre of medical instruction. After a time subsidiary centres were established in other Italian towns. From Italy the custom spread, and we meet traces of such schools at the half-Greek Marseilles as well as at Bordeaux, Arles, Nîmes, Lyons and Saragossa. For the most part these provincial schools produced workaday medical men, few of whose writings have come down to us. They were perhaps largely training-places for the army surgeons. That class seldom had scientific interests, though Pedanios Dioscorides (*fl.* middle of 1st cent A.D.), one of the most eminent physicians of antiquity, and one who deeply influenced the modern pharmacopoeia, served in the army under Nero. His book, usually known as the *De materia medica*, is in fact an extremely useful though ill-arranged compendium of drugs. Dioscorides wrote in Greek, and his work was not translated into Latin until the fifth century.

The earliest scientific medical work in Latin is the *De re medica* of Aulus Cornelius Celsus (*fl.* A.D. 10–37) written about A.D. 30. It is in many ways the most readable of ancient medical books. It is, however, not an original work but a compilation from the Greek, and the sole surviving part of a complete encyclopaedia of knowledge. Many of its phrases are closely reminiscent of the Hippocratic Collection. The ethical tone is high and the general line of treatment sensible and humane. Celsus, though almost forgotten in the Middle Ages, was the first classical medical writer to be printed (A.D. 1478). It is usually held that he was not a professional physician, but an extremely able compiler from the works of others.

The treatise of Celsus opens with an interesting account of the history of medicine. It then passes on to deal with diet and the general principles of therapeutics and pathology; next it discusses internal disease, and then turns to external diseases. The last part of the work is devoted to surgery, and is perhaps the most valuable of the whole.

Celsus professes himself a follower of Asclepiades of Bithynia (p. 51), but, unlike his master, he by no means despises the Hippocratic 'expectant' method of 'waiting on the disease'. He gave a very detailed and accurate description of malaria. His descriptions of the symptoms of phthisis are interesting, and the treatment advocated by him for that condition—including sea voyages, moderate exercise, massage and dietetic measures—would have passed as sound practice until the nineteenth century. Celsus formulated the four

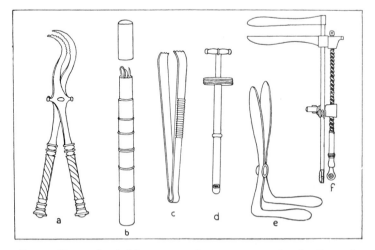

FIG. 23. Roman Surgical Instruments, first century A.D., found at Pompeii
(*a*) Forceps, probably for handling bone.
(*b*) Small pocket-case of instruments; a sharp spoon and a probe can be seen.
(*c*) Fine-toothed forceps.
(*d*) Trocar and cannula for tapping fluids contained in cavities.
(*e*) Vaginal speculum.
(*f*) Wound dilator, used to permit of free examination.
(Drawings, different scales, from originals in the National Museum, Naples)

cardinal signs of inflammation, namely, pain, redness, heat and swelling. A fifth, loss of function, was added about a century later, and these five signs are still regarded as the fundamental signs of inflammation.

In many matters we are struck with the boldness of the surgical practice which he records. Thus he describes plastic operations on the face and mouth, and the removal of polypus from the nose. He tells too of the very dangerous operation for extirpating a goitre, and also of cutting for stone. He gives an excellent account of what might be thought the modern operation for removal of tonsils.

His descriptions of the treatment of various fractures and dislocations are excellent. He was so much in advance of his time that to
prevent loss of function he advocated exercises after the fracture
had healed. He was thus a forerunner of modern rehabilitation
therapy. Noteworthy also is his description of dental practice, which
includes the wiring of loose teeth and an account of a dental mirror.
An idea of the surgical instruments in use in his time can be obtained
from those recovered from Pompeii (Fig. 23).

MEDICAL SERVICES IN THE ROMAN EMPIRE

If, in medicine itself, the Roman achieved but few advances, in the
organization of medical services, and especially in the department
which deals with public health, his position is far more noteworthy.
Latin writers on architecture pay adequate attention to the orienta-
tion, position and drainage of buildings. From an early date sanitation and public health drew the attention of statesmen. Considering
the dread of the neighbourhood of marshes on the part of these
practical sanitarians of ancient Rome, and in view of modern knowledge of the mosquito-borne character of malaria (p. 460), it is
entertaining to find the mosquito net ridiculed by the poets Horace,
Juvenal, and Propertius.

Sanitation was a feature of Roman life. Rome was already provided with subterranean sewers (*cloacae*) in the age of the Tarquins
(6th century B.C.). The Cloaca Maxima itself, the main drain of
Rome, which is still in use, dates back to that period.

The antiquity of hygienic ideas is seen in a law of about 450 B.C.,
which contained an interdict against burials within the city walls, and
also in the instructions issued to the town officials to attend to the
cleanliness of the streets and to the distribution of water. Among
these ancient laws we may note one attributed to the first king of
Rome, which directed the opening of the body in the hope of extracting a living child in the case of a woman dying in pregnancy. It is
the origin of the operation of Caesarean section on the living mother,
the method by which Julius Caesar (102–44 B.C.) himself is said to
have been brought into the world. At the date of these decrees
physicians in Rome were either slaves or in an entirely subordinate
position. Their status was improved by Julius Caesar, who, in order

to induce physicians to settle at Rome, conferred citizenship on all who practised medicine there.

The finest monument to the Roman care for the public health stands yet for all to see in the remains of the fourteen great aqueducts which supplied the city with 300 million gallons of potable water daily (cf. Plate IV). No modern city is better equipped. In the early days of the Empire there were a hundred and fifty public latrines in Rome. Many statutes dealt with the food supply. Wheat was kept in the imperial granaries. The markets in which foods were sold were supervised by special officials to prevent the sale of unsound food.

The early Empire also saw the inauguration of a definite public medical service. Public physicians were appointed to the various towns and institutions. A law of the Emperor Antoninus of about the year A.D. 160 regulated the appointment of these physicians, whose main duty was to attend the poor. In the code of the Emperor Justinian (A.D. 533) is an article urging them to give these services cheerfully rather than the more subservient attendance on the wealthy. Their salaries were fixed by the municipal councillors. They were encouraged to undertake the training of pupils. Inscriptions attest the respect in which these public physicians were held in many towns.

It is in connexion with the army that we see the Roman medical system at its best. There was an adequate supply of military medical attendants who were well organized (Fig. 24). The defects of the Roman army medical system were, however, absence of any elastic scheme for the ranking of medical officers, and complete subordination of the medical to the combatant officer. These facts are of a piece with the general Roman indifference to theoretical science, and explain why the Roman army surgeons made no additions to knowledge. The social status of the medical staff in the Roman military hierarchy was that of the non-commissioned personnel, which included accountants, registrars, and secretaries.

ROMAN HOSPITALS

The great contribution of Rome to medicine—and it is a very great one—is the hospital system. It is a scheme that naturally arose

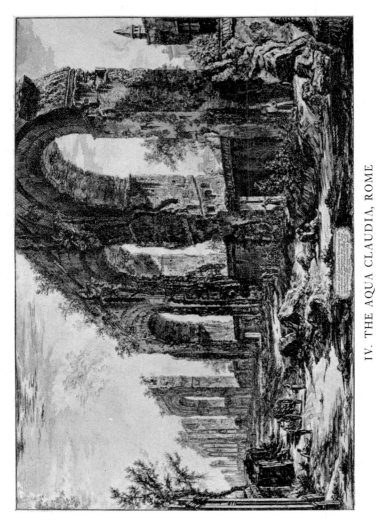

IV. THE AQUA CLAUDIA, ROME

Part of this structure was formerly called the Aqueduct of Nero

(Etching of 1775 by Giovanni Battista Piranesi (1720-1778). From an impression in the British Museum)

(See p. 56)

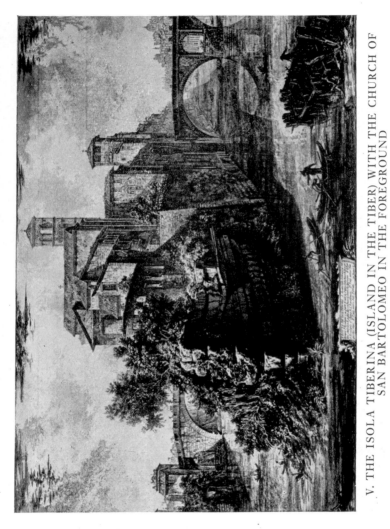

V. THE ISOLA TIBERINA (ISLAND IN THE TIBER) WITH THE CHURCH OF
SAN BARTOLOMEO IN THE FOREGROUND

Etching of 1775 by Giovanni Battista Piranesi (1720–1778). From an impression in the British Museum)

(*See p.* 57)

out of the Roman genius for organization and is connected with the
Roman military system. Among the Greeks surgeries (*iatreia*) were
well known; they were, however, the private property of the medical
man. Larger institutions were connected with Aesculapian temples,
and there is evidence of some degree of scientific medical treatment

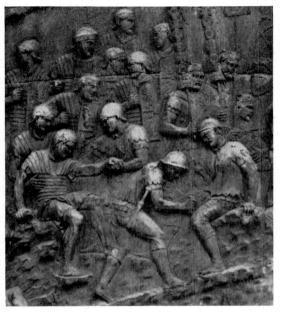

FIG. 24. Roman advanced dressing-station
(Trajan's Column, Rome)

in these places. In the Republican period the Romans were no better
off. Despite the vast numbers of slaves, there was no public provision
for them when sick. A temple to Aesculapius had been established
on the Island of St. Bartholomew in the Tiber in the time of the
Republic (p. 25). This island is built and carved to represent a ship,
and on the port bow there is a sculptured head of Aesculapius with
his staff and serpent (Plate V, directly above right-hand end of the
inscription). It became the custom to expose the sick and worn-out
slaves on this island to avoid the trouble of treating them. The
Emperor Claudius (reigned A.D. 41–54) decreed that these slaves
were free, and that, if they recovered, they need not return to the

control of their masters. Thus, the island became a place of refuge for the sick poor. We may regard it as an early form of public hospital.

Later writers speak of infirmaries (*valetudinaria*) for such persons, and give humane directions for their management. These infirmaries were also used even by Roman citizens. The excavations at Pompeii show that a physician's house might even be built somewhat on the lines of a modern nursing home. It was probably in the provinces that private institutions first developed into subventioned public hospitals.

This development of public hospitals naturally early affected military life. We have reason to believe that in the Roman army first-aid treatment of the wounded in the field was satisfactory. One of the reliefs on Trajan's column shows an advanced dressing station (Fig. 24). In the centre of the relief a military surgeon is seen bandaging the thigh of a man who from his dress is either an allied auxillary or an enemy prisoner. The uniform of the surgeon is very similar to that of the Roman combatants, but he carries a case of instruments and first-aid material slung from his shoulder. On the left two Roman soldiers are bringing in a wounded comrade. After this preliminary treatment sick and wounded soldiers had at first been sent home for treatment. As the Roman frontiers spread ever wider this became impossible, and military valetudinaria were founded at important strategic points. The sites of several of these have been excavated, notably that near Düsseldorf, founded about A.D. 100.

From the military valetudinarium it was no great step to the construction of similar institutions for the numerous Imperial officials and their families in the provincial towns. Motives of benevolence, too, gradually came in, and public hospitals were founded in many localities. The idea passed on to Christian times, and the pious foundation of hospitals for the sick and outcast in the Middle Ages is to be traced back to these Roman valetudinaria. The first charitable institution of this kind concerning which we have clear information was established at Rome in the fourth century by a Christian lady, of whom we learn from St. Jerome. The plan of such a hospital projected at St. Gall in the early years of the ninth century has survived. It reminds us, in many respects, of the early Roman military valetudinaria. These medieval hospitals for the sick must naturally be distinguished from the even more numerous 'spitals' for travellers and pilgrims, the idea of which may perhaps be traced back to the rest-houses along the strategic roads of the Empire.

The Latin culture, as we have seen, did not adapt itself easily to the prosecution of scientific medicine. Long after the decline of Greece medical writings were usually in Greek rather than in Latin. This is true to the end, and the end came, so far as creative science is concerned, with the second half of the second century. The scene is then, and for centuries to come, mainly occupied by the huge over-shadowing figure of Galen.

Galen of Pergamon (A.D. 129–99) devoted himself to medicine from an early age, and in his twenty-first year we hear of him studying anatomy at Smyrna. To extend his knowledge of drugs he made long journeys to Asia Minor. Later he proceeded to Alexandria, where he improved his anatomical equipment, and here, he tells us, he examined a human skeleton. His direct practical acquaintance with human anatomy was perhaps limited, for dissection of the human body was no longer carried on in his time, though there are indications in Galen's writings that he had himself done some human dissection. His physiology and anatomy were derived mainly from animal sources.

The general medical standpoint of the Galenic is not unlike that of the Hippocratic writings, but the noble vision of the lofty-minded, pure-souled physician has utterly passed away. In its place we have an acute, contentious fellow of prodigious industry, who is frequently satisfied with a purely verbal explanation. Yet he is an ingenious physiologist, acquainted with the internal parts (so far as this is possible from a devotion to dissection of animals), equipped with all the learning of the Schools of Pergamon, Smyrna and Alexandria, and rich with the experience of a vast practice at Rome. Galen is essentially an efficient man. He has the grace to acknowledge constantly his indebtedness to the Hippocratic writings.

Some of Galen's works are, however, mere drug lists, little

superior to those of Dioscorides (p. 53). With the depression of the intelligence that corresponded with the break-up of the Roman Empire, it was these that were chiefly studied and distributed in the West. The Greek medical writers after Galen were but his imitators and abstractors, and they usually imitated and abstracted Galen at his worst. Through some of them Galen's works reached the West at a very early period in the Middle Ages.

THE FINAL MEDICAL SYNTHESIS OF ANTIQUITY

We now turn to the theoretical content of the vast mass of Galenic writings. These set forth a medical system of which the substance is based on the Hippocratic Collection and the form derived from Aristotle. This synthesis, in more or less corrupted form, provided the theoretical basis of medical practice for the next fifteen hundred years. Galen's view of the human body may be examined under two aspects, which we describe as (a) philosophical and (b) descriptive.

First as to the philosophical aspect. Galen's voluminous works are saturated with the theory that all structures in the body have been formed by the Creator for a known and intelligible end. In the anatomical works masses of explanation, based on this view, dilute the often imperfect accounts of structures. Thus, following the Aristotelian principle that 'Nature makes nought in vain', Galen seeks to justify the form and structure of every organ—nay, of every part of every organ—with reference to the functions for which he believes it is destined. To do this is to claim that in every work of creation—of which the human body is a type—and in every detail of such work, we can demonstrate God's design along known principles. It is to claim, in fact, a complete knowledge of the Laws of Nature. No modern man of science, however intoxicated with his own achievements, has as yet arrogated such powers to himself. To conceive that such claims could be made by a pious, theistically minded author, the reader must think himself back into a very different philosophical environment from that to which we are nowadays accustomed.

The prevailing philosophy of Galen's world was the Stoic. In the world of the Stoic philosopher all things were determinate, and they were determined by forces acting wholly outside Man. The type and origin of that determination the Stoic sought in the heavens, and found in the majestic and overwhelming procession of the stars. The recurring phenomena of the spheres typified and foreshadowed, nay, exhibited and controlled, the cycle of man's life. Man dwelt in a finite universe, bounded by a definite frontier—the sphere of the fixed stars. Within that spherical frontier all things worked by rule— and that rule was the rule of the heavenly bodies. Astrology had become one of the dogmas of the Stoic creed.

To such a world Galen's determinism was in itself no strange thought. Yet Galen's view was far from being wholly in accord with Stoicism. Though a determinism, it was a determinism of perfection in which all was fixed by a wise and far-seeing God, and was a reflection of His perfection. Such a scheme did not ill fit the new creed, just beginning to raise its head, which was destined to replace Stoicism and all the other pagan schemes. Galen's thought, in fact, made a special appeal to the Christian point of view, and this is, doubtless, the reason why his works have been preserved in larger bulk than those of any other pagan writer. The Galenic standpoint appealed equally to the theological bias of Islam. The medical knowledge of the Muslim writers was based almost entirely on Galen.

We may now turn from the philosophical to the descriptive bases of Galen's medical system, namely to his anatomy and physiology.

We may begin with the bones. These Galen had studied on an actual human skeleton at Alexandria. He divided them into long bones with a central canal and flat bones without such a canal. He had a fairly good idea of the bones of the skull. He regarded the teeth as bones, and he gives a good description of their origin. He recognized twenty-four vertebrae terminated by the sacrum. Galen gives accurate elementary descriptions of the vertebrae, of the ribs, of the breastbone, of the collar-bone, and of the bones of the limbs. He divides joints or junctions of bones into two main orders, those with movement and those without movement, and the titles that he gives to his main divisions have survived in our modern nomenclature.

As regards the muscular system there can be little doubt that Galen's work was in large part of a really pioneer character. Throughout his works the muscles are perhaps the structures that he describes most accurately. His writings contain frequent references to form and function of muscles of various animals. Thus, the dissection of the muscles of the orbit and larynx was performed on the ox, and the muscles of the tongue are described from the ape. Occasionally he indicates that he is aware of the differences between certain of the muscles he is describing and the corresponding human muscles. For his investigation of muscles Galen used particularly the Rhesus monkey (*Macaca mulatta*), a creature anatomically near enough to man for a knowledge of its detailed structure to be applicable to human surgery.

This similarity between the anatomical features of the muscular system of man and of the Rhesus monkey (or an allied species, the Barbary ape, *Macaca inuus*) is clearly shown in dissections of the hand (Fig. 25). The ape's hand shows all the main muscles and tendons present in the human hand, though there are differences in the relative proportions. Apart from these relative differences, the most striking divergence in the anatomical structure of the hand in the two species is shown by the position of the attachment of a small superficial muscle—the Palmaris brevis—in the palm. This is easily seen by comparing the two dissections (Fig. 25), in which this muscle, marked with an asterisk, has been severed in each case.

Galen's description of the brain and of the vascular system is inferior to his account of the bones and muscles. His account of the nervous system, other than the brain, occupies an intermediate position. His account of the origin of nerves from the brain has left its traces even in modern descriptive anatomy.

Finally we may turn to Galen's theory of the working of the human body, his physiology (Fig. 26). The basic principle of life was a spirit (*pneuma*) drawn from the general World-spirit in the act of breathing. It entered the body through the windpipe (*trachea*) and so passed to the lung and thence, through the *arteria venalis* (our pulmonary vein) to the left ventricle, where it encountered the blood.

Galen believed that food-substance from the intestines was carried as chyle by the portal vein to the liver. There it was converted into blood and endowed with a particular *pneuma*, the natural spirit, which bestowed the power of growth and nutrition. This venous blood then entered the vena cava, from which it passed upwards and

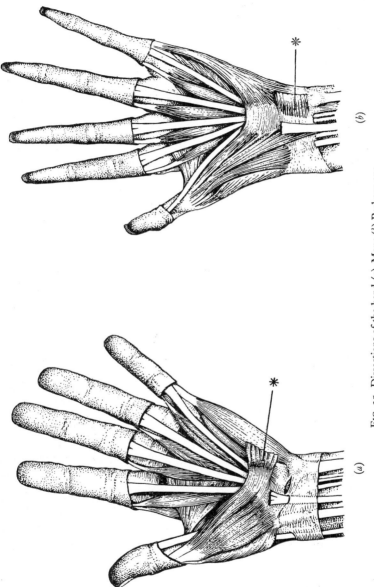

FIG. 25. Dissections of the hand (a) Man; (b) Barbary ape

downwards to the tissues of the body. A portion of this venous blood entered the right ventricle of the heart, from which most of it passed, by way of the *vena arterialis* (our pulmonary artery) and its valve, to the lungs for their nutrition. The small remaining part of the blood in the right ventricle passed by way of invisible pores in the inter-

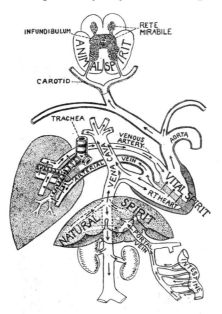

FIG. 26. Galen's physiological system. Diagram to show the source and distribution of the three types of spirits
(After Singer and Rabin, *A Prelude to Modern Science*, Cambridge, 1946)

ventricular septum into the left ventricle. There it mixed with the air, drawn in through the pulmonary vein, to produce arterial blood, which was there charged with a second type of *pneuma*, the vital spirit. Blood containing this *pneuma* passed into the arteries, endowing the various organs with activity. Such arterial blood as reached the brain became there charged with the third and noblest *pneuma*, the animal spirit, which passed through the hollow nerves to initiate motion and sensation in the organism. But the active mingling of the blood and the vital spirit in the left ventricle gave rise to injurious vapours. These passed with the blood from the left ventricle into the arteries. Galen thought, however, that the mitral valve, having only two cusps, was always slightly incompetent; so that blood mixed with vital spirit and injurious vapours passed back into the pulmonary vein and the lungs, by which the vapours were exhaled.

Galen described a network of minute vessels on the under-surface of the brain. This was called the *rete mirabile* (wonderful network). It is found in the brains of many animals, especially those with hooves, but not in that of man. Yet for over thirteen centuries it was believed that this structure was present in the human subject, just as it was believed that the septum of the heart contained the minute pores which had been described by Galen. Both *rete* and pores, though imaginary, were essential to Galen's physiological system.

Galen, like all other authorities in antiquity, had no knowledge of the circulation of the blood. He believed that blood passed from the heart to the tissues both in the arteries and in the veins. New blood was constantly being manufactured in the liver, and it was supposed to be burnt up in the tissues as wood is consumed by fire. The exhalation of the breath, which if sufficiently concentrated was known to be asphyxiating, was compared to the smoke of the fire.

Among Galen's most remarkable efforts are the investigations he made of the physiology of the nervous system. He tells of his experiments on the spinal cord. Injury to the cord between the first and second vertebrae caused, he observed, instantaneous death. Section between the third and forth produced arrest of breathing. Below the sixth vertebra it gave rise to paralysis of the chest muscles, breathing being then carried on only by the diaphragm. If the lesion was lower the paralysis was confined to the lower limbs, bladder, and intestines. He worked out the physiology of the spinal cord most ably and in very considerable detail.

Galen established no School, nor had he any definite followers. His self-satisfaction and love of controversy were not of the kind that would endear him to disciples. On his death in A.D. 199 the active prosecution of anatomical and physiological inquiry ceased absolutely. The curtain descends at once; and, for the subject we are discussing, the Dark Ages have begun.

Rational medicine in the pagan world descends into darkness as surely and even more abruptly than philosophy. The whole system is soon to be overwhelmed. Alexandria has long been in decline. A mob, fanatically Christian, has destroyed her school and library, with all the hoarded wisdom of the pagan past. Men of the new faith fix their eyes on the wrath to come and the glory after it. In the race for salvation, who will pause to consider this miserable tenement of clay? Antiquity is no more. A new age has begun.

IV

THE MIDDLE AGES

(*From about* A.D. 200 *to about* A.D. 1500)

THE observational period of antiquity closed with Galen. He coincided in time with the greatest period of the Roman Empire. After him, the empire gradually disintegrated, and the medical writers became mere compilers from the works of former authors. Few of those who wrote in the Roman Empire of the West need detain us. But we may pause for a moment to mention some of those who, after Constantinople became the capital of the Byzantine Empire on the disintegration of the Western Empire in A.D. 476, strove, though feebly, to keep alight the torch of Greek science. Foremost in this effort were the Church Fathers, who became the guardians of the medical tradition. It is to this period that we can trace the rise of the cult of the healing saints, notable among whom were the brothers Cosmas and Damian. It seems that they were originally practitioners of orthodox medicine who also employed faith-healing. According to the legend they were martyred under Diocletian (A.D. 303), and they later became the patron saints of medicine. Of the legends which are associated with them, the most dramatic relates that a certain man, suffering from gangrene of his left leg, fell down in a coma at the door of the church of Saints Cosmas and Damian at Rome. He dreamt that the saints came and had him removed to a neighbouring hospital. They instructed the surgeons to amputate the gangrenous leg below the knee, and to perform the same operation *post mortem* on a patient who had died in an adjoining bed; this leg they were to graft on the stump of the gangrenous patient. When the comatose patient awoke in the morning he had two sound legs; but as the man who had died was a negro, the resuscitated patient had one white leg and one black. This legend was painted by Fra Angelico; and it is the subject of a very fine panel by the Castillian master, Fernando Gallegos, which, formerly in Barcelona, has for

thirty years been in the Wellcome Historical Medical Museum
(Plate VI). In the Gallegos version it is the saints themselves who
perform the operation. An angel is seen bearing away the amputated
gangrenous leg, while one of the saints—probably Damian—grafts
on the black leg. It is to legends such as this that we owe some of the
finest paintings of the European Renaissance.

At about the same time as the martyrdom of Saints Cosmas and
Damian, the alleged martyrdom of St. Sebastian took place. Sebastian, an officer in the Roman army, was shot to death with arrows
because he refused to denounce his Christian faith. He was one of
the saints invoked against the plague which broke out in Rome in
683. There are innumerable pictures and statues of Cosmas and
Damian, as well as of Sebastian, which were and are held sacred.

During the long decline of the heritage of classical antiquity a few
medical writers were of some importance. Among them was Oribasius (325–403), a native of Galen's birthplace, Pergamon, who wrote
extensively on medical subjects. Perhaps the most interesting of his
writings today are those which deal with diet and with the diseases of
children. Alexander of Tralles (525–605) had a great reputation as a
physician, and his medical writings show that he was a good observer
and a competent practitioner, but that he lacked the scientific knowledge which had become moribund after Galen's death. He was also
extremely superstitious. Alexander practised in Byzantium, where
his brother was the architect of the famous cathedral church of St.
Sophia. Paul of Aegina, who flourished in the seventh century,
practised in Alexandria. He wrote a large work on medicine, the most
important part of which is devoted to surgery and is one of our
principal sources for its practice in the early Middle Ages. Paul is
especially precise in his descriptions of operations on the genital
system.

THE PERIOD OF DEPRESSION IN EUROPE

THE centuries that followed the death of Galen exhibited progressive
deterioration of the intellect. For that deterioration many causes have
been assigned. An important factor was certainly the philosophical
outlook of later paganism. Men lacked a motive for living. Their

view of the world was dreary and without hope. It is sometimes alleged that the advent of Christianity was a factor in the decay of science, but science was, in fact, in headlong decay before Christianity was in a position to have any real effect on pagan thought.

Christianity came to the ancient world as a protest and a revulsion against the prevailing and extremely pessimistic pagan outlook. Christianity brought men something for which to live. It was natural that it should oppose the philosophical basis of pagan thought. In this sense Christianity was certainly anti-scientific. Early Christian thought exhibited an aversion to the view which places the whole of man's fate under the dominion, the inescapable tyranny, of Natural Law. It is, however, essential to remember that the early Church, in developing this opposition, was not dealing with living observational science. The conflict was simply with a philosophical tradition which contained dead, non-progressive and misunderstood scientific elements.

For some eight centuries from the time when Christianity finally replaced paganism in the Roman Empire—from about A.D. 400 to about A.D. 1200—such remains of classical learning and classical science as survived were in monastic keeping. It was only in the monasteries that there were any who cared at all for these things, and it was only in the monasteries that manuscripts could be either written or preserved. Of the many who wrote at this period, the most learned was Bishop Isidore of Seville (570?–636) (Isidorus Hispalensis). His encyclopaedia of etymologies and origins was the favourite medieval textbook, and one part is devoted to medicine. First printed in 1472, the *Etymologiae* went through many editions.

The curse of the science of medicine, as of all sciences, has always been the so-called practical man, who will consider only the immediate end of his art, without regard to the knowledge on which it is based. Monkish medicine had no thought save for the immediate relief of the patient. All theoretical knowledge was permitted to lapse. Anatomy and physiology perished. Prognosis was reduced to an absurd rule of thumb. Botany became a drug-list. Superstitious practices crept in, and medicine deteriorated into a collection of formulae, punctuated by incantations, which became less understood and further removed from their originals at each copying. Medicine

remained surrounded by sacred associations. For example, a seventh-
century fresco of St. Luke (Fig. 27) shows him as an Evangelist

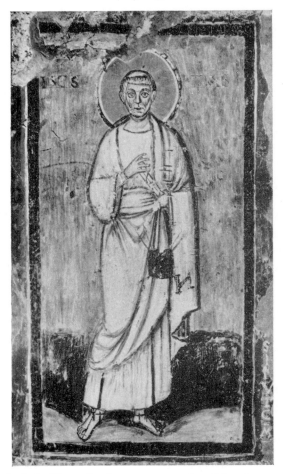

FIG. 27. St. Luke. The earliest known representation of the saint as a physician
Fresco, Church of Saints Felix and Adauctus in the Catacombs, Rome. Painted in the
reign of Constantine IV (Pogonatus), 668–85
(After J. Wilpert, *Die römischen Mosaiken und Malereien der kirchlichen Bauten von IV
bis XIII Jahrhundert*, Freiburg i. B., vol. iv, 1917)

holding a scroll, and as a physician carrying suspended from his left-
hand a bag containing four instruments, one of which is a lancet.
His head is tonsured like that of a monk. Partly because of these

religious associations, the scientific stream, which is the life-blood of Medicine, was dried up at its source.

There was just one area in the Latin West where a slightly higher standard prevailed. In the south of Italy the Greek tongue still continued for centuries to be spoken and written. Though civilization had sadly deteriorated with the disorders of the times, yet there remained here and there in that region a slightly higher intellectual standard than prevailed elsewhere in Europe. Moreover, about the same time as the Norman Conquest of England, there was a Norman conquest of south Italy also. The strong arm of the Norman administrator might wield the weapon of a tyrant, but at least it brought order where there had been anarchy. Learning under the Normans could lift a timid head. Notably at the town of Salerno, not far from Naples, there arose in the ninth century something resembling a medical school. There is a legend that this School was founded by a Greek, a Latin, a Jew, and a Saracen. Though this statement is certainly not literally true, it does indicate that the School of Salerno arose from the coming together, in that cosmopolitan town, of medical practitioners from widely separated parts. At Salerno in the eleventh century there was a certain amount of translation of medical works from Greek into Latin. The physician Gariopontus (died *c.* 1050) wrote his work called *Passionarius*, a compilation made from the works of Galen, Alexander of Tralles, Paul of Aegina, and others. Petroncellus, his contemporary, wrote a work on medical practice which was also a Latin derivative from Greek originals. In general the choice of works for translation was very poor, but it was something that enough mental energy existed for the effort.

Salerno differed too from other centres of learning of the time in that instruction was not entirely under monastic auspices (Fig. 28). Some, at least, of the Salernitan physicians were laymen. At the time of the Norman conquest of Salerno, the School was stimulated by the advent of a wanderer from Arabic-speaking lands, Constantine the African (*c.* 1010–87). He was born in Carthage, and had studied in Jewish circles at Kairouan in Tunisia. On his arrival in Salerno he became oriental secretary to Robert Guiscard, Duke of Apulia. Later he became a monk at the famous monastery of Montecassino,

about sixty miles from Salerno, and the remainder of his life was
spent in study and in translating medical texts into Latin. When he
came to Italy he brought with him medical works in Arabic which

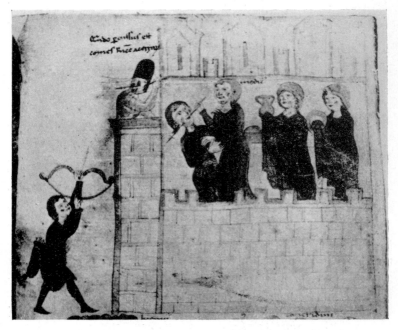

FIG. 28. Richard of Accerra wounded at the Siege of Naples, 1194

He is treated by a *medicus* in lay costume, attended by two nurses who bear salves and
dressings. The miniature provides evidence of the existence of lay physicians at Salerno
at that date

(Peter of Eboli, *De rebus siculis carmen.* South Italian MS., *c.* 1196; Berne, Civic Lib.,
cod. 120. From the facsimile in Muratori, *Rerum Italicarum scriptores*, vol. xxxi (ed.
Rota), 1904, tav. xvi)

he was able to translate into rude Latin. The Latin versions prepared by Constantine, corrupt, confused, barbarous, often almost
incomprehensible, were yet a better intellectual fare than that on
which the torpid mind of Europe had long fed. The Salernitan
medical writings of the eleventh and twelfth centuries exhibit some
faint-hearted attempts to return to Nature. Constantine was but the
harbinger of the great Arabian revival, the further origins of which
we must now seek to trace. Before doing so we may note that the

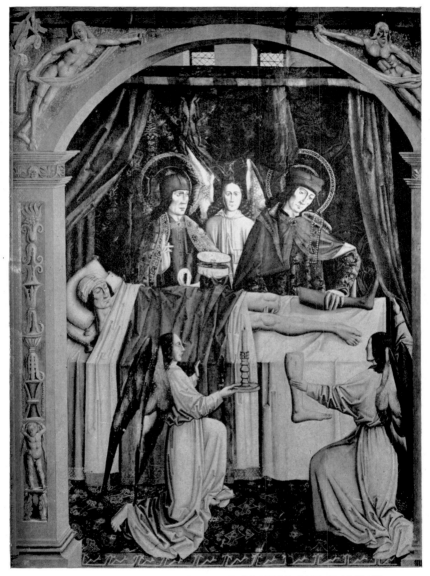

VI. THE MIRACLE OF SAINTS COSMAS AND DAMIAN
(Fernando Gallegos (1475–1550). Picture in the Wellcome Historical Medical Museum.
Panel, 66 in. by 49 in.)

(*See p.* 67)

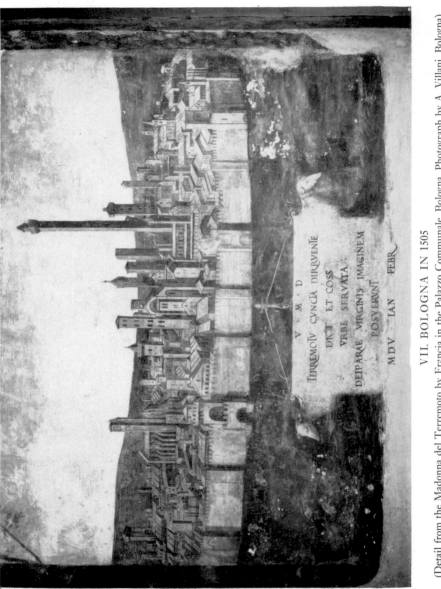

VII. BOLOGNA IN 1505

(Detail from the Madonna del Terremoto by Francia in the Palazzo Communale, Bologna. Photograph by A. Villani, Bologna)

(*See p.* 78)

Regimen sanitatis, a poem on the laws of health, was allegedly written in Salerno. It went through hundreds of editions in its long life, was translated into many languages, and in a late version contains over three hundred stanzas. Even today some might well find its crude counsel not completely useless:

> Use three Physicians still; first Doctor Quiet,
> Next Doctor Merry-man, and Doctor Dyet.
> Rise early in the morne, and straight remember
> With water cold to wash your hands and eyes,
> In gentle fashion retching every member,
> And to refresh your braine when as you rise,
> In heat, in cold, in Iuly and December.
> Both comb your head, and rub your teeth likewise:
> If bled you have, keep coole, if bath'd, keepe warme:
> If din'd, to stand or walke will do no harme.

This is far removed from the stuff medical textbooks are made of; and yet thousands of physicians have been trained on this poem. In the twelfth and thirteenth centuries the School of Salerno reached the peak of its reputation, and it was regarded as the world centre of medical teaching. By the fifteenth century it was declining rapidly in competition with the young universities, and later it became a mere shadow. As a medical school it did not formally cease to exist until 1811, when it was suppressed by a decree of Napoleon I.

ARABIC MEDICINE

Barbarian incursions sapped and finally destroyed the Western Roman Empire. The influence of those incursions on the Eastern Empire was less dramatic. It is true that the intellectual outlook of the East Roman or Byzantine Empire was no less modified, in the course of time, than was that of the West. In the absence, however, of any collapse of the system of government, the ancient Greek learning, or rather the documentary casing in which it was enshrined, was better preserved than were the Latin traditions. Men in the Eastern Empire could still read the ancient Greek medical works in the language in which they had been written, and, if their reading was unintelligent, it was at least persistent. Moreover, heretical Christian sects on the confines of the Eastern Roman Empire prepared for themselves translations of many of the ancient Greek authors. One of these heretical sects, the Nestorians, exhibited great missionary activity. It was perhaps on this account that the Nestorians prepared translations of many Greek medical works into their own language, Syriac.

In the seventh century Islam arose, and soon swept over vast areas that had formerly belonged to the Emperor of the East. The territory occupied by the Nestorians in the Near East came early under Muslim rule. The Muslims, at first indifferent to infidel learning, came gradually to appreciate it. In the ninth century a great and united Muslim Empire was established with its centre at Baghdad. The need for translation of Greek scientific works into Arabic, the common language of Islam, now asserted itself. One after another the medical writings that had been turned into Syriac were translated into Arabic, and Greek science in general and Greek medicine in particular were thus spread far and wide in the Muslim world.

Greek science in the Arabic version came in time to be better understood by Arabic-speaking students than it had been by any since Galen. Nor were the Arabic-speaking peoples content to rest on the texts that had thus descended to them from antiquity. A considerable number of Arabic writers produced works of their own, some not wholly devoid of originality. Unfortunately these men were without effective anatomical or physiological basis for their medical knowledge, though many of them were acute clinical observers, and, even from the modern point of view, some of their works are not wholly contemptible. Thus Rhazes (died *c.* 923), a native of Ray, near Teheran, Persia, wrote a work containing the first known description of measles, which he carefully distinguished from smallpox. His description is classic and shows that he was an acute clinical observer. Like other great Arabians, Rhazes was a prolific writer, and he is said to have written over two hundred books on various subjects. But these individual works were dwarfed by his vast compilation, the 'Kitab al-hāwī', which was the largest encyclopaedia of Graeco-Arabic medicine. The Latin translation of this work by the Jewish translator Faraj ben Salīm (Fig. 29) occupies in manuscript five folio volumes, and the first edition of its printed version (1486) is the largest and heaviest of all incunabula. The

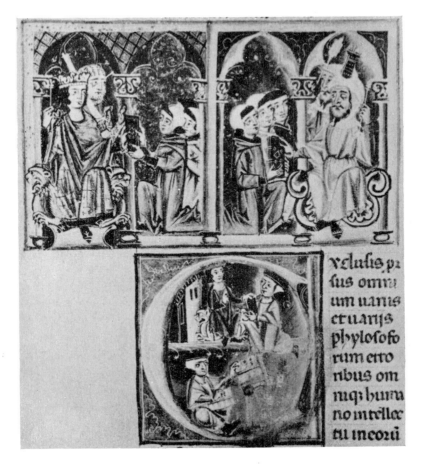

Inside the initial capital, the following text appears:

xelufis pa
fus omni
um uanis
ct uarijs
phylofofo
rum erro
nbus om
mqz hum
no intelle
tu incozu

FIG. 29. Faraj ben Salīm, a great Jewish translator. Charles I of Naples and Sicily had asked the Prince of Tunis for a manuscript of the vast work by Rhazes entitled 'Kitab al-hāwī'. Faraj translated it into Latin with the title *Liber Continens. Top right*: The Prince presents the Arabic manuscript to the Three Neapolitan envoys. *Top left*: the envoys deliver the manuscript to Charles. *Below*: in the upper section of the initial E, Charles is seen giving the manuscript to the translator, Faraj, who is shown in the lower section translating the work into Latin.

(Initial capital from Rhazes, *Liber Continens*, Latin translation; South Italian MS. written in 1282. Paris, Bib. Nat., Lat. 6912, fo. 1ᵛ. After Couderc, *Album de Portraits*, Dept. of MSS., Bib. Nat., Pl. VIII)

Persian Avicenna (980–1037) also composed a great encyclopaedia of medical knowledge, the *Canon*, which served as the main textbook of medicine, both among the Arabic-speaking peoples and in the Latin West, until the seventeenth century. Avicenna was also a very prolific writer on many subjects. On medicine he wrote with the utmost authority, and his clinical histories are still worth reading. Isaac Judaeus (*c.* 832–932) of Kairouan in Tunis composed a treatise on fevers which was the best account of the subject available in Europe during the entire Middle Ages. Abulcasis (died *c.* 1013), of Cordova, left a textbook of surgery which was an important element in the revival of the subject in Italy and France. This textbook is especially valuable because of the many illustrations of surgical instruments which it contains. He was much addicted to the use of the cautery, which he used not only in surgery but also in epilepsy and in apoplexy.

These are only prominent members of a vast school of writers who flourished in Arabic-speaking countries between the ninth and thirteenth centuries. The bulk and number of their writings is portentous. Many of their works were translated into Latin by Gerard of Cremona (1114–87), by Faraj ben Salīm (*fl.* 1280, Fig. 29), and by others. These translations caused a reawakening of the intellect of Europe, and provided the staple reading in the medieval universities.

THE MEDIEVAL AWAKENING

The Iberian peninsula had been inundated by the Islamic tide as early as the eighth century. After a while the waters began to recede. The speech and culture of Islam had become stamped upon the natives of the peninsula, and were only gradually replaced by the Latin civilization and dialect which we now call Spanish. During the centuries of Islamic retreat there was thus a bilingual population in the peninsula, so that access to the Arabic learning became possible. The translations that were to have influence on Europe were always into Latin. To make or to obtain such translations many adventurous spirits journeyed from Christian Europe into Spain, or sometimes into Sicily where conditions were very similar. These men were aided in their work by native Jews or by Mohammedans. The heretical company which they kept, together with the strange and mysterious material which they brought back with them, earned them a reputation as magicians. The memory, for instance, of Michael Scot is connected with the Black Art, and has been presented by Sir Walter Scott in his poem *The Lay of the Last Minstrel.*

The 'wizard' Michael Scot (1175?–1234?) journeyed in both Spain and Sicily, learned Arabic and Hebrew, and had commerce with Mohammedans and Jews. He turned a number of Arabic works into Latin, and, in particular, he prepared versions of the biological works of Aristotle (p. 41) which, though corrupt and second-hand, had much influence in determining the direction of medical thought during the Middle Ages.

There was a large class of such translators and commentators who made Arabic medicine accessible to the West. This Arabic-Latin literature is generally characterized by the qualities most often associated with the words medieval and scholastic. It is extremely verbose and almost wholly devoid of the literary graces. An immense amount of attention is paid to the mere arrangement of the material, which often occupies its authors more than the ideas that are to be conveyed. Great stress is laid on argument, especially in the form of the syllogism, while observation of Nature is entirely in the background. Above all, there is a constant appeal to the authority of the ancient masters, especially Aristotle and Galen. Lip service is often paid to Hippocrates, but his spirit is absent from these windy discussions.

When the Latin translations from the Arabic reached the readers for whom they were intended, they were eagerly studied. The texts were, however, by no means permitted to remain in their pristine state, but were submitted to exactly the same process to which their Arabic authors had themselves subjected their Aristotelian and Galenic models. The Christian writers of the West treated the Latin translations of Rhazes, of Avicenna, of Isaac, and of Abulcasis as subjects for commentary. Their works were expanded, annotated, castigated again and again, and without any new inflow of ideas. The result is a progressive elaboration of form and deterioration of content throughout the centuries. Vast masses of argument, rebuttal, refutation and confirmation drowned again the human spirit, which hardly recovered from its submersion until the sixteenth century.

THE UNIVERSITIES

Nevertheless, when these translations were new to Europe, and especially in the thirteenth century, they caused much stir. In this awakening a large part was played by the universities. These were established in numbers during the thirteenth and the following centuries. University life gradually came to exercise a profound effect on social, political and intellectual conditions. In most of the univercities medical faculties grew up. The medical teaching was entirely theoretical and there was no clinical instruction, though at the beginning of the fourteenth century some advance was made by the introduction of brief and superficial anatomical demonstrations (p. 80).

As a type of medieval university we may take Bologna, which was an important centre of learning from a very early date. (Plate VII is interesting because it shows a view of Bologna as a detail in the fresco by Francesco Francia which he was commissioned by the city fathers to paint as a thankoffering for the safety of the city during the earthquake of 1505 in which many citizens died. The picture, the Madonna del Terremoto, was painted in that year. The detail shows Bologna as a walled medieval city with its numerous tall towers, some of which still stand.) As the universities multiplied, they began to some extent to specialize. Bologna had appeared first as a law school and continued to develop along the same line. In the second half of the thirteenth century it was by far the most important seat of legal learning in Europe.

An organized medical faculty existed at Bologna as far back as 1156. The teaching there, as in other medical schools, consisted entirely of readings of Latin translations from Arabic which were becoming ever more accessible. Yet it was at Bologna that public dissection was first practised. The early advent of dissection has often impressed the historian. There was still no botany worthy of the name, no zoology, hardly any naturalistic art, no experimental science, no systematic record of observation in any department. Yet dissection had become recognized at Bologna by the end of the first quarter of the fourteenth century. The question is why men, so little interested in Nature and Nature's ways, should have lent themselves to so repellent a process as dissection of the human body ? The answer is that the earliest reason for examining the human body was simply the gathering of evidence for legal processes. As time went on, post-mortem examination passed into anatomical study. But still dissection did no more, and was asked to do no more, than verify Avicenna —whom nobody doubted. It was, in fact, little but an aid to the memory of students.

At Bologna we can trace the rise of a surgical school beginning about the end of the twelfth century. Prominent among its early surgeons was William of Saliceto (c. 1210–c. 1280). He wrote a very able treatise on surgery, which contained a section on anatomy. The anatomical portion is borrowed from the current Arabian anatomies, but it contains some evidence of direct access to the dead human body. He includes a long description of the dressings employed after trephination. He also recommended the use of the knife instead of the cautery. Treatment by the cautery was then much employed on the Arabian model (p. 76). All wounds were liable to suppuration, to which those cauterized were specially·prone. Nearly all medieval surgeons had taught that it was good practice to encourage the flow of pus. But William of Saliceto held quite definitely that pus-formation was bad for wound and patient. He recommended simple dressings of white of egg and rose water instead of the usual messy ointments and held that wounds should heal 'by first intention'. We shall hear more of this phrase later. This sound surgical principle was also held by his contemporary Theodoric, Bishop of Cervia (1205–98), who himself fills an important niche in the history of medicine. William of Saliceto and Theodoric stand out like stars in the dark night of medieval surgery.

The surgical opreations performed in the Middle Ages were usually of an emergency nature. The operation for trephining the skull was still being carried out, and contemporary illustrations show the use of another type of drill for that purpose (Fig. 30). This was the thong drill, which is known to have been still widely used in surgery (Fig. 31).

A most interesting contemporary was Thaddeus of Florence (1223–1303) (Taddeo Alderotti), who also taught at Bologna. This man perceived the importance of access to Greek sources, as distinct from

Graeco-Arabic, and he encouraged the preparation of good Latin translations of medical works direct from the Greek. He stamped his personality on the whole development of medicine at Bologna, and he is bound up with the beginning of dissection. But if medicine owed a debt to Thaddeus for introducing better texts and better anatomy, he did grave harm to the subject in another direction. The scholastic and argumentative form assumed by medieval medicine is largely due to him, and it is to the assumption of this form that we owe the almost complete absence of scientific advance between the thirteenth and sixteenth centuries.

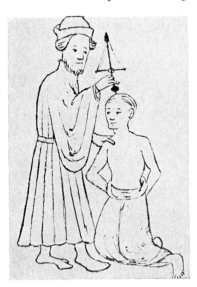

FIG. 30. Trephining the skull in the Middle Ages. The primitive thong drill used is explained in Fig. 31 (After the Laudian Miscellany, 13th cent. Bodleian Lib., Oxford)

MEDIEVAL ANATOMY, SURGERY AND INTERNAL MEDICINE

At the very end of the thirteenth century there came to Bologna a Norman student, Henri de Mondeville (1260?–1325?). In 1301 he settled at the famous medical school at Montpellier in southern France, and thus transplanted to France the medical, surgical and anatomical traditions of Bologna. Those traditions were of Arabic origin, and mainly borrowed from Avicenna.

Contemporary with Henri de Mondeville was one whose method of teaching shines as a good deed in a naughty world. Mondino de' Luzzi (1275?–1326) generally known under the latinized form Mundinus, was a pupil of Thaddeus and a fellow student of Henri. He worked systematically at anatomy and dissected the human body in public. His treatise on anatomy, written in 1316, is the first modern work on the subject. Those who preceded him incorporated their anatomical work in larger treatises on surgery, and do not refer directly to their own anatomical experiences. With Mundinus this is changed. His work is essentially a practical manual of the subject and he is with justice called the Restorer of Anatomy. He had read widely the Arabian anatomists, and had naturally borrowed from them. Nevertheless, his work contains a considerable number of references to actual anatomical procedures. Moreover, he deals not only with anatomy in our modern sense, but he also includes physiology and much discussion of the application of anatomical

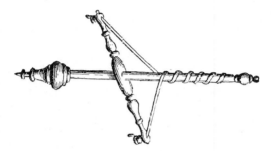

FIG. 31. Thong drill, sixteenth century. The twist of the thong causes rapid rotation of the axis and point of the drill (cf. Fig. 30)

and physiological principles to medicine and surgery. His book thus gives a good deal of insight into the scientific knowledge of the day.

We would emphasize the fact that Mundinus dissected in person. In this respect he was wiser than his successors until the time of Vesalius. As dissection gained formal inclusion in the curriculum, the professor became more haughty, further removed from the object of his study. Leaving his position by the body, where he might demonstrate to his students, he ascended his high professorial chair (*cathedra*), a great elevated structure provided with steps and a reading-desk. From there he read from his textbook, and he and his students, all in academic dress, took no part in the dissection. This was carried out by a menial *demonstrator* under the guidance of the *ostensor*, who pointed out the structures with his wand. A famous illustration (Fig. 32) shows the lecture in progress. All was thus done at third hand according to the written word. We are in the scholastic period, and must not expect any frequent appeal to Nature. Having once got into his chair, it took a good deal to persuade the professor to descend from that dignified position. Thus, it is saying much for

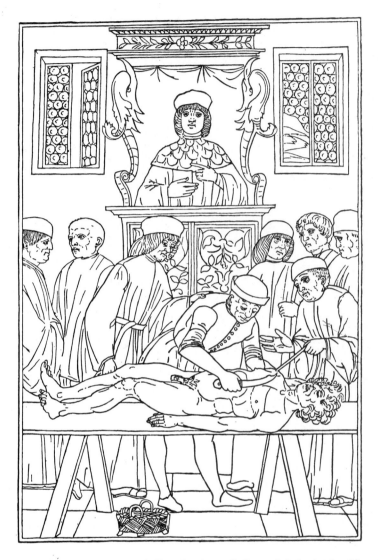

FIG. 32. Anatomical lecture and dissection in an Italian university in the fifteenth
century
(After the Italian *Fasciculo di Medicina*, Venice, 1493)

Mundinus that he was his own demonstrator. He took the first and perhaps the greatest step. It was two centuries and more before the next step was taken.

Typical of medieval surgeons was Guy de Chauliac (1298?–1368), who studied at Montpellier, Paris, and Bologna, and practised at Montpellier and afterwards at Avignon, where he was a member of

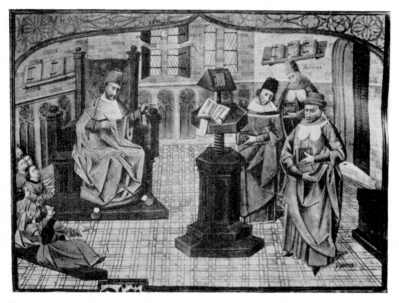

FIG. 33. Bernard de Gourdon (died *c.* 1320), author of the celebrated *Lilium medicinae*, teaching the practice of medicine at Montpellier at the end of the thirteenth century. Before him pass Hippocrates, Galen and Avicenna, each bearing one of his books

(Paris, Bib. Nat., MS. lat. 6966, fo. 1)

the Papal Court. While there he was a victim of the plague, from which he nearly died. He describes his illness and recovery in one of his books. Guy was a man of much learning, and his *Chirurgia magna* ('Great Surgery') became the standard treatise on the subject during the later Middle Ages. It fixed medieval practice. It is to be found in scores of manuscripts and was frequently translated and printed. Among the good points of his practice is his acceptance of responsibility for certain operations, such as those for rupture and for cataract, which at that time were usually left to wandering charlatans, who regarded themselves as specialists. A famous passage in his work describes the use of a narcotic inhalation frequently used during the Middle Ages and into modern times. Of such a narcotic it is written that:

> I'll imitate the pities of old surgeons
> To this lost limb, who, ere they show their art,
> Cast one asleep, then cut the diseased part.
> (Thomas Middleton, *Women beware women*. First acted 1622.)

The general character of internal medicine during the later Middle Ages was below that of surgery. Modern clinical medicine is firmly based on such sciences as physiology, pharmacology, pathology, biochemistry and epidemiology. In the Middle Ages and far beyond physiology was still that of Galen, and had lost in exactness what it had gained in bulk from the Arabic and Latin commentators; pathology was still that of the four humours; the knowledge of drugs was empirical, and the sciences of pharmacology and biochemistry had not yet been conceived; while the medieval conception of the nature of epidemics was the very perversion of reason and common sense. Nevertheless, as we shall see, the Middle Ages ultimately succeeded in instituting a limited number of effective preventive measures.

MEDIEVAL HOSPITALS AND HYGIENE

The development of the medieval hospital system from the Roman military valetudinaria has already been described (p. 58). But it should be remembered that the health conditions of a medieval town were far below those of the same town under the Roman Empire. Water-supply was deficient, drains were absent, streets and houses filthy and overcrowded, rooms unventilated. Nevertheless, there is one important hygienic conception for which our own age owes a considerable debt to that which preceded it. Despite their acumen in many branches of science, it is yet true to say that among the physicians of classical antiquity we find no consistent view of the transmission of infection by contact. Indeed the whole idea of infection was effectively absent from them, so that preventive measures based upon it could not be developed. It was reserved for the Middle Ages to conceive serious official measures against the spread of epidemics. These measures were consciously derived from the leper ritual of the Bible with its fundamental concept of isolation.

From illustrations in manuscripts we have some indication of the

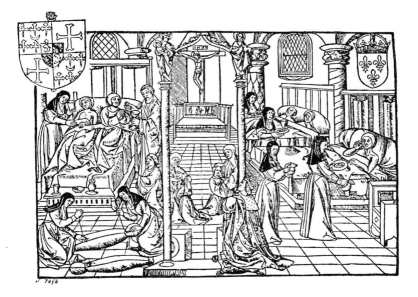

FIG. 34. A ward in the Hôtel-Dieu at Paris in the sixteenth century
(From a contemporary woodcut)

conditions which existed in medieval hospitals. But these illustrations tended to be stylized, and it is probable that the conditions as shown were better than they were in reality. Fig. 34 shows a ward in the Hôtel-Dieu, the great hospital in Paris. On the left there are two patients in the same bed, one being tended by a nun, and the other receiving the sacrament from a priest. In the foreground two nuns are sewing shrouds—an indication perhaps that the patients in the bed are both dying. On the right nuns are taking food to three patients, two of whom are in one bed. In the foreground nuns receive postulants, and a royal donor kneels in prayer. There is reason to believe that the wards in medieval hospitals were much more crowded than this one appears to be.

During the early centuries of the Christian era, leprosy, which had till then been confined to the East, crept along the Mediterranean littoral and thence northward throughout Europe. The disease was from the first regarded as contagious, and various regulations were introduced to isolate and separate the unfortunate sufferers. The medieval treatment of lepers is one of the dark incidents of man's inhumanity to man. The leper was banished from human society. He was declared legally dead. He was even excluded from church or allowed to attend only in special seats where a special basin of holy water was assigned to him. How rigorously this segregation from the ranks of free people was carried out by law is well known. The cruel edicts were, however, effective. In the course of centuries Europe was freed from leprosy, of which it is said there were at one time some 20,000 cases in France alone. On this showing about one person in 200 would have been a leper, and the burden on the community must have been heavy. But modern research has shown that a large proportion of these so-called lepers were suffering from other conditions.

Leper inspection, the regular examination of all suspects and carriers of leprosy, became a most elaborate business. It was entrusted to a special branch of the civil service and was gradually freed from ecclesiastical control.

This preventive method of combating a chronic disease, which as we now know has a very low infectivity, had a peculiar and unlooked-for result. The meticulous system of warding off the contagion of leprosy so occupied the attention of physicians that they came to see allied conditions in the same light. So it was that in the thirteenth century the general concept became current of disease as contagious or infectious. A number of other diseases besides leprosy were recognized as infectious. Among these were plague, fevers with obvious rashes, phthisis, granular conjunctivitis, the itch, and erysipelas. Municipal authorities were from time to time ordered to put patients suffering from one or other such diseases outside the city gates. Such patients were forbidden to traffic in articles of food and drink and were placed under restrictions not unlike those of lepers. The devastating epidemic of the Black Death of 1347–8 brought restrictions of this order into special force. Thus the Black Death had somewhat the same effect on the health administration of the day that the cholera outbreaks of the thirties of the nineteenth century had upon modern Europe. The health service began to be put into more efficient order.

In the later Middle Ages there were actually instances in which the Pest was averted or successfully combated by these means. This seems to have been the case at Milan and Venice between the years 1370 and 1374. At that time plague was again advancing through Europe. The most drastic regulations were invoked to prevent infected persons from entering the cities, and these regulations came into force well in advance of the disease.

There is one incident in this medieval attempt to prevent plague that has left a mark on our language. The Republic of Ragusa, on the eastern side of the Adriatic, adopted and extended the regulations that had been so successful at Venice. A landing-station was established far from the city and the harbour. There incoming suspects had to spend thirty days in the open air and sunlight, and any who had traffic with them were isolated. The period of thirty days was spoken of as the *trentina*. Later this period was found to be too short. The thirty days became forty days, the *quarantina*, whence we have the word quarantine. The system of quarantine gradually spread through Europe. It was accompanied by very drastic destruction by burning of all goods belonging to the infected.

These attempts to arrest epidemic disease were sometimes successful and the elaboration of quarantine measures was among the few advances with which we may credit the Middle Ages. The fact that we can now dispense with quarantine must not blind us to its value in conditions other than our own.

V

THE REBIRTH OF SCIENCE

(From about 1500 *to about* 1700)

THE ANATOMICAL AWAKENING

DURING the Middle Ages beliefs about physiology were always based on Galen. They were frequently confused and often the result of a misunderstanding of his work. The fifteenth century, however, was marked by the Renaissance or Revival of Learning. Greek works which had been trickling in since the thirteenth century began to be recovered more rapidly, and to be more accurately studied. The first step towards any improvement on the views of Galen was naturally a proper understanding of what he had really said. For that there was needed a better knowledge of Greek than had been possessed by the Middle Ages. In the fifteenth century Greek scholarship made great advances and there was enthusiasm for classical learning. Accurate translations of the Greek works of Galen were made. The printing press was invented about the middle of the fifteenth century. Towards its end printed copies of the improved translations began to appear. So it came about that the Revival of Learning produced a revival of the ancient scientific knowledge.

This scientific revival led to a new interest in anatomy. During the Middle Ages the occasional dissections at the universities were merely supposed to illustrate Avicenna and Galen (Fig. 32 and p. 82). Dissection became much more widely practised in the fifteenth century, but it was nearly the middle of the sixteenth before any real and open discussion of Galen's views took place in the universities.

There were, moreover, other influences at work. Along with the revival of learning there was also a renaissance of art. Some of the great artists of the Renaissance—Michelangelo, Raphael, and Dürer among them—began to study the human form very closely. They soon found that to represent it accurately some knowledge of anatomy, and especially of the bones and muscles, was needed. The artists, therefore, began also to dissect. Among these great artists were some

VIII. DRAWINGS OF THE HEART BY LEONARDO DA VINCI
(Royal Library, Windsor Castle. Reproduced from *Quaderni d'anatomia*, II, fol. 3v.)

(*See p.* 89)

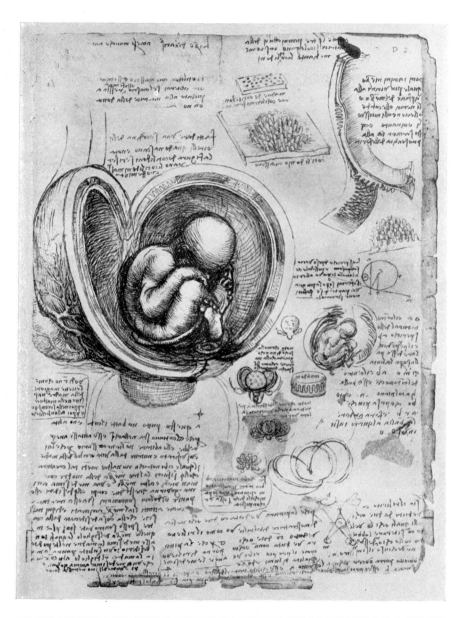

IX. DRAWINGS OF THE FOETUS IN UTERO BY LEONARDO DA VINCI
(Royal Library, Windsor Castle. Reproduced from *Quaderni d'anatomia*, III, fo. 8r.)

(*See p.* 90)

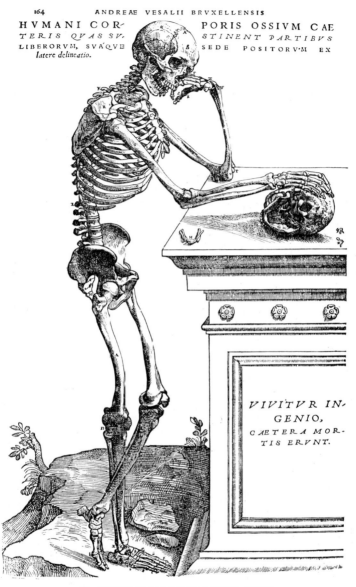

HVMANI COR‑ PORIS OSSIVM C AE
TERIS QVAS SV‑ *STINENT PARTIBVS*
LIBERORVM, SVA'QVE SEDE POSITORV·M EX
latere delineatio.

*VIVITVR IN‑
GENIO,
C AETERA MOR‑
TIS ERVNT.*

X. SKELETON FROM THE SIDE

The inscription on the tomb reads 'The spirit lives on; all else is death's portion'

(Andreas Vesalius, *De humani corporis fabrica*, Basle, 1543. Copy in the Wellcome Historical Medical Library)

(*See p.* 94)

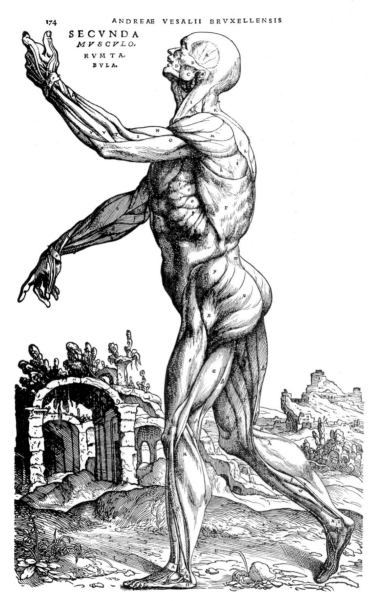

SECVNDA
MVSCVLO.
RVM TA.
BVLA.

XI. SUPERFICIAL MUSCLES FROM THE SIDE

(Andreas Vesalius, *De humani corporis fabrica*, Basle, 1543. Copy in the Wellcome
Historical Medical Library)

(*See p.* 94)

who took more than a purely artistic interest in the structure and
workings of the body. Of these the most important for us was
Leonardo da Vinci (1452–1519). He was a man of enormously
powerful and inquiring mind, and his achievements in science are
at least as remarkable as his works of art. Leonardo had carried out
anatomical dissection for many years, and he later worked on the
preparation of a textbook of anatomy and physiology in collaboration
with a young medical teacher at Padua, Marcantonio della Torre
(1473–1506). Owing to the death of della Torre this work was
never finished, but many of Leonardo's beautifully illustrated notebooks on these subjects have survived.

Leonardo was the first to question the views of Galen. He made
careful first-hand investigations of the bodies of men and animals,
and performed many physiological experiments. Though a man of
the most lofty genius, centuries ahead of his time, yet his outlook is,
in many respects, typical of his age. His interest in anatomical investigation is therefore not surprising, for such inquiries were then
astir. It happened that he was particularly interested in the heart and
blood-vessels. He reached the correct conclusion that, contrary to
Galen, the branches of the air-tubes in the lungs do not come into
direct relation with the blood, but, after branching and gradually
diminishing in size, they finally end blindly. He inflated the lungs
with air and found that, whatever the force used, air could not be
driven from the air-tubes into the heart. He therefore inferred quite
correctly that Galen's *arteria venalis* (our pulmonary vein) did not
convey air to the heart, as the followers of Galen believed.

Leonardo then turned to examine the structure and form of the
heart itself. He prepared more accurate drawings of it than had been
made by any before him, making sections and dissections and examining its valves (Plate VIII). Ultimately he succeeded in grasping
the nature and action of the valves at the root of the great arteries as
they arise from the heart, and he verified his view by remarkable
experiments. He proved that the valves allowed the blood to pass
only in one direction, and prevented its regurgitation. Yet Leonardo
gives no complete or clear description of the action of the heart. He
could not emancipate himself from the old idea of the passage of the
blood from the right ventricle through the septum into the left

ventricle (Fig. 26), though he sometimes seems doubtful about this passage.

Leonardo was also especially interested in the manner in which individual muscles move the bones to which they are attached. He made beautiful drawings to show his dissections of groups of muscles; and in other sketches certain muscles are replaced by wires to illustrate the action of the muscles on the bones during muscular contraction. He was also much interested in the development of the individual during intrauterine life. One of his drawings of a foetus in the uterus is a thing of rare beauty (Plate IX). He even studied the cavities of the brain—which after death is a very soft and friable organ—by injecting them with wax.

It must be remembered that Leonardo did not publish his researches. It is only fairly recently that his notebooks have become fully accessible. But although Leonardo's work remained in manuscript, it must not be assumed that his views were wholly without effect on his contemporaries. At any rate, soon after his time the questions that he had raised concerning the heart and blood-vessels were attracting others and were generally regarded as forming an important problem needing solution.

The task of writing an anatomical textbook based on direct observation, to which Leonardo did but put his hand, was achieved by one who was only four years old at the time when the great artist died. The central place in the unfolding drama is occupied by Andreas Vesalius of Brussels (1514–64). This extraordinary man studied first at the University of Louvain and afterwards at Paris. Since the passing of the Middle Ages anatomical instruction had improved at Paris, for much better texts of Galen's works were being printed there from about 1530. But Vesalius soon tired of hearing long passages of Galen read out by the professor. He therefore resolved to go to northern Italy, where more dissection was being practised. Padua was the place of his choice. He immediately made his mark there, and was himself appointed professor of anatomy and surgery when only twenty-four years of age. He established a scientific tradition at Padua which that university still retains.

No sooner was Vesalius settled at Padua than he applied himself with unparalleled diligence to anatomical research. Students came to see his demonstrations. To aid them he issued, in 1538, a short guide to anatomy and physiology in the form of six anatomical plates (*Tabulae anatomicae sex*). An examination of these plates shows that his physiological views were still those of Galen and Aristotle. After their issue Vesalius found that Galen and Aristotle were by no means always to be trusted. The realization of this led him constantly to doubt any statement by them. His scepticism was sometimes excessive, but it led him to put every statement made by his predecessors to the test of experience. This gives his later work an epoch-making value.

During the next four years Vesalius had ampler opportunities to dissect than he had yet encountered. He devoted a fiery energy to the preparation of his great work entitled *De humani corporis fabrica* ('The Fabric of the Human Body'). By 'fabric' he meant the 'workings' of the human body. For Vesalius anatomy was essentially living anatomy, the structure of a machine which either was, or might at any moment be, in action. The book was printed at Basle in 1543 as a magnificent and beautifully illustrated volume. It is a landmark in the history of science, and a wonderfully full record of a prodigious number of accurately recorded discoveries and investigations made by a single observer.

The title-page to this book (Plate I, Frontispiece), besides being a very fine example of the woodcut, tells us much about Vesalius and his methods. It is designed to show Vesalius dissecting a female subject at Padua about 1540. The view is now held that this idealized anatomical theatre never existed; but, while the lofty columns and architectural decoration in the background may be a product of the artist's expression of the desires of Vesalius, the attentive crowd which fills the foreground may have been drawn from life. The bearded Vesalius is seen standing by the subject's right hand. Beyond the body there is an upright articulated skeleton, presumably to indicate the emphasis which Vesalius placed on osteology. By his hand the various instruments of dissection can be seen on the table. A naked model, looking at the scene from the pillar on the left, indicates the importance which Vesalius attached to the surface markings which indicate the position of underlying structures. The two assistants, who would in earlier times have been carrying out the dissection, are now engaged in such tasks as the sharpening of instruments. Left and right two other attendants lead in an ape and a dog, thus symbolizing the fact that, while Vesalius laid the main emphasis on human dissection, he did not hesitate to dissect animals when there was a shortage of human subjects. These animals perhaps indicate also that he carried out vivisections. The spectators appear to be divided into two groups. Beyond the bar, or we might say in the gallery, are members of the lay public, among whom may be seen gallants, elderly scholars, a monk, and a young man reading a book. The onlookers around Vesalius himself appear to be students and professional men. Though the setting may be idealized, the interest and enthusiasm of the students shown in this woodcut certainly typify Vesalius's aspirations for Padua as a teaching school. The difference in spirit and action from that shown in Fig. 28, drawn fifty years early, is notable.

The masterpiece of Vesalius is not only the foundation of modern medicine as a science, but the first great positive achievement of science itself in modern times. As such it ranks with another work that appeared in the same year, the treatise of Nicholas Copernicus entitled *De revolutionibus orbium coelestium* ('On the Revolutions of the Celestial Spheres'). The work of Copernicus removed the Earth from the centre of the Universe; that of Vesalius revealed the real structure of man's body. Between the two they destroyed for ever the medieval theories on the subjects of which they treat. But the work of Copernicus is one of close and subtle reasoning, still retaining many medieval elements, and is hardly a great exposition of what we now call the experimental method. The work of Vesalius far more nearly resembles a modern scientific monograph than does the treatise of Copernicus.

The achievement of Vesalius was very well received by the scientific world. Nevertheless, soon after its publication, Vesalius resigned his professorship to take up the position of a court physician to the Emperor Charles V, the great monarch of the age. He was then only twenty-nine years old, but his scientific career was closed.

The first edition of the *Fabrica* was soon exhausted, and the demand for more copies was met by imitations of the work by other hands. At last, in 1555, Vesalius was induced to issue a second edition. This contains certain changes in point of view that are important for the subsequent development of physiology. Vesalius now no longer merely hints his doubts as to the character of Galen's physiology; he openly asserts that he had been unable to verify its fundamental bases.

We may take a single instance of this new outspokenness. In his description of the septum of the heart, he had written in the first edition:

> The septum of the ventricles of the heart is very dense. It abounds with pits on both sides. Of these pits none, so far as the senses can perceive, penetrate from the right to the left ventricle. We are thus forced to wonder at the art of the Creator, by which the blood passes from right to left ventricle through pores which elude the sight. (Cf. Fig. 26, p. 64.)

This passage is altered to something quite different in the second edition, where he writes:

> Although sometimes these pits are conspicuous, yet none, so far as the senses can perceive, passes from the right to the left ventricle. I have not come across even the most hidden channels by which the septum of the ventricles is pierced. Yet such channels are described by teachers of anatomy, who have absolutely decided that the blood is taken from the right to the left ventricle. I, however, am in great doubt as to the action of the heart in this part.

In the second edition he further sets forth his whole policy with reference to Galen's view in the following interesting passage:

> In considering the structure of the heart and the use of its parts, I bring my words for the most part into agreement with the teachings of Galen; not because I think these on every point in harmony with the truth, but because, in referring at times to new uses and purposes for the parts, I still distrust myself. Not long ago I would not have dared to diverge a hair's breadth from Galen's opinion. But the septum is as thick, dense and compact as the rest of the heart. I do not, therefore, see how even the smallest particle can be transferred from the right to the left ventricle through it. When these and other facts are considered, many doubtful matters arise concerning the blood-vessels.

The *Fabrica* is divided into seven books, not all of which are equally important. The first, second and seventh books, dealing respectively with the bones, the muscles and the brain, are specially valuable because of their clear and full descriptions, their accuracy, the beauty of their illustrations, and their modern attitude. The three full skeletons which illustrate the first book (one of which is reproduced here as Plate X) are far in advance of any drawings of the skeleton which had appeared previously. In his section on muscles Vesalius continued the usual custom of giving illustrations of the whole body with different layers of muscles dissected away in each case. Anatomy was for him 'living anatomy'. He attempted to describe and illustrate the muscles as if they were actually in action. The second muscle tabula, which illustrates the superficial muscles from the side, is reproduced here as Plate XI, and describes better than words the principles which he had in mind.

The work terminates with a little chapter 'On the dissection of living animals'. We note that this, while dealing skilfully with the methods of physiological experiment, does not exhibit any very marked advance on the work and views of Galen.

Among the experiments on living animals that Vesalius enumerates are excision of the spleen, the loss of which he showed was consistent with life; and the cutting of the nerves that supply the organ of voice, with resultant loss of that faculty. He demonstrated that longitudinal section of a muscle interferes little with its function, but cross section produces disability in proportion to the injury. Such experiments had been performed by Galen, who had also reached the same conclusions as Vesalius, that it is through the spinal cord that the brain acts on the various muscles of the limbs and trunk. Vesalius repeated Galen's experiments on section of the spinal cord (p. 65). The most striking of his experiments were those on respiration. Here he showed that, even though the chest-wall be pierced, the animal may be kept alive if the lungs are continuously aerated by means of a bellows, and that a flagging heart may be revived by similar means.

The work of Vesalius at once placed the knowledge of the human body in a new position. It cannot be said that he completed the task of describing the naked-eye structure of the human body. Yet he went so far towards this that no dramatic improvement has since been made on his methods. It is a fair statement that the whole of modern descriptive anatomy may be treated as a commentary on, and a correction and amplification of, Vesalius. His work moreover stimulated a host of investigators.

THE ANATOMICAL REACTION ON SURGERY

The immediate effect of the new knowledge of anatomy was an improvement in surgery. The wars of religion of the sixteenth and seventeenth centuries were fierce and prolonged, and the army

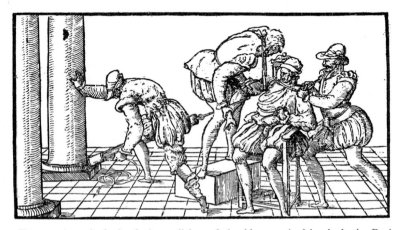

FIG. 35. A method of reducing a dislocated shoulder practised by Ambroise Paré. Three main forces, acting in different directions, are applied to the patient's body; one of these is provided by a sling round the surgeon's neck
(After Ambroise Paré, *Œuvres*, Paris, 1575)

surgeons of the time had much experience of the treatment of wounds. The most prominent of the military practitioners was the Frenchman, Ambroise Paré (1510–90). He began his career as an apprentice to a barber-surgeon, and then served for some years as an assistant-surgeon in the Hôtel-Dieu, a great Paris hospital. From 1536 he was an army surgeon for a period of nine years, and he saw much active service in the wars of religion. After his campaigns he rapidly became the foremost surgeon in France, and indeed in Europe. During his long life he was surgeon-in-chief to four kings of France in succession. Paré perceived the importance of anatomical knowledge and adopted its discoveries to the needs of surgery. He did much to elevate the surgeon's profession from a despised handicraft to a position equal to that of other branches of the healing art. Not the least important of his contributions to surgery and to knowledge was the fact that he wrote in his native French, for he was, not unfortunately, unable to write in Latin. His collected works were later translated into Latin, and into several European languages, including English.

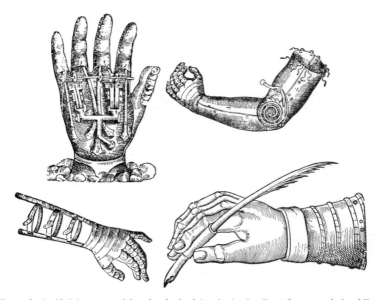

FIG. 36. Artificial arms and hands, devised by Ambroise Paré for wounded soldiers. In use after 1560
(After Ambroise Paré, *Œuvres*, Paris, 1575)

Apart from the introduction of anatomical discipline into surgery, Paré's four contributions to the surgical art were: firstly, his discovery that gunshot wounds are not 'poisonous' as had previously been thought, and that therefore they do not require the application of boiling oil, but are best healed by soothing applications; secondly, the cognate doctrine that bleeding after amputations should be arrested, not by the terrible method of indiscriminate use of the red-hot cautery, but by simple ligature; thirdly, his advocacy of the method of turning the child in its mother's womb before delivery in certain abnormal cases; and fourthly, his ingenious devising of artificial limbs (Fig. 36). None of these four was without precedent. Nevertheless, the eminence, skill and wide experience of Paré were the main factor in the spread of these practices. But the greatest of all Paré's contributions to surgery was the service of his own personality, the example of his steadfast efforts to increase his knowledge of human anatomy and his skill in the art, and his constant emphasis on the surgeon's duty to exert his utmost efforts to avoid or relieve the patient's suffering.

In a famous passage Paré describes how he, a 'fresh-water soldier', on his first campaign, watched the other surgeons following the old rule of treating all gun-shot wounds with boiling oil. At first he formed his practice on theirs. The theory was that gun-shot wounds contained a poison, which the boiling oil was believed to drive out. Paré tells of his agitation when one evening, his supplies having run out, he had to treat men without the boiling oil. Next morning he was astonished to find that every man whose wounds had been treated only with a simple lotion had rested fairly comfortably, while all who had undergone the customary treatment were, as we may well believe, in great pain. 'Then I resolved within myself never so cruelly to burn poor wounded men.' Another saying of the shrewd old surgeon is the famous adage: 'I dressed him and God cured him'. Paré's works exercised the widest influence on surgical craft in the sixteenth and seventeenth centuries. Like Vesalius, he is an example and type of a large class. In every country surgeons arose who made an effort to utilize the new anatomical knowledge.

One of the most important of these was Girolamo Fabrizio, generally called Fabricius ab Aquapendente (c. 1533–1619) after the small Tuscan village where he was born. This famous anatomist taught at Padua for nearly forty years, from 1565, when he was appointed professor of anatomy and surgery, until 1604, when he retired to devote himself entirely to research. He continued to write almost until his death at about eighty-six. He made many contributions to the advancement of anatomy, most of which had physiological bearings. Thus, he was the effective founder of modern embryology and the author of the first illustrated work on that subject, in which he describes the formation of the chick in the egg. He was the first to give accurate figures of the structure of the eye. He developed the mechanics of muscular motion. He added to his qualities as an observer the power of attracting younger men. During his long professorship at Padua he became the foremost anatomist and surgeon in Italy. Some of his operations—such as those for the tying of arteries and for the tapping of the chest—became standard procedure. He also described apparatus for the treatment of spinal curvature and wry neck.

Another Italian surgeon distinguished himself in a limited but difficult field. This was Gaspare Tagliacozzi (1545–99), a pioneer of plastic surgery. Remodelling of the nose had been attempted by Hindu surgeons in ancient times. Tagliacozzi revived the operation and introduced his own methods. He partially cut a strip of flesh from the patient's arm and attached it to the nose. The base of the strip was left attached to the patient's arm, which was itself supported by a harness, so that the graft remained attached to the arm until it had taken root on the nose. Tagliacozzi also performed similar operations for the repair of the ears, lips (Fig. 37) and tongue.

CONCEPTS OF DISEASE

While the anatomical awakening, which was born and reached its climax in the work of Vesalius, had important reactions on surgery, there were mysteries of the living body which were studied neither by anatomists nor surgeons. The old Galenic physiology still held the field; Galen's ideas on the origin and treatment of disease were still current. With the great rebirth of science in the sixteenth century new conceptions of disease were suggested. The contrasted figures of Fernel and Paracelsus must suffice to illustrate the position.

Jean François Fernel (1497–1558), born in Amiens, became professor of medicine at Paris. He wrote a textbook of the whole art of medicine (*Universa medicina*, 1554) which was a standard work for at least a century. Although, as a distinguished classical scholar, Fernel was deeply imbued with the humoral theory and other doctrines of ancient medicine, he had inspired the breath of freedom of thought which was characteristic of the Renaissance. His great work was divided into three parts, the first of which dealt with physiology, and showed quite a new approach to this subject, which

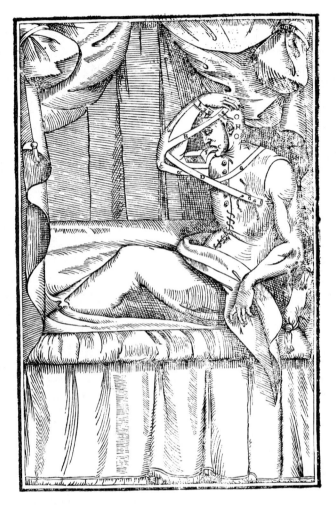

Fig. 37. Method recommended by Tagliacozzi for the repair of an injury to the lower lip. The supporting harness and the flesh graft from arm to lip are shown

(G. Tagliacozzi, *De curtorum chirurgia per insitionem*, Venice, 1597)

with anatomy constitutes the gateway to medicine. The second part dealt with pathology, that is, with the structure of organs in a diseased state. Although the conception of this part was essentially based on the teachings of the ancients, the idea of devoting a book, or even a section of a book, to pathology was new to its time. The third and final section of Fernel's book dealt with treatment. Fernel was thus the first man to write on modern lines a textbook which, apart from anatomy, covered almost the whole field of the practice of medicine.

Very different from Fernel was his Swiss contemporary Philip Bombast von Hohenheim (1493–1541), who assumed the names of Aureolus Theophrastus Paracelsus, by the last of which he is generally known. Paracelsus was born at Einsiedeln, near which is the great monastery which still contains many precious medieval manuscripts. He studied at Basle, and travelled in Italy and Germany, continuing his studies at other universities. Paracelsus was essentially a wanderer, and he practised medicine in various towns. At thirty-four he was invited to return to Basle to become the town physician, and he was also appointed a professor in the university. His relations with the medical faculty at Basle were unfortunate. This ancient university was a centre of the revival of ancient learning, including that of medicine. Into this scholarly environment Paracelsus immediately thrust his heterodox views and his forceful personality. He condemned all medical teaching not based on experience, and is said to have publicly burned the books of Galen and Avicenna to emphasize his position. The faculty repudiated him and he was excluded from all official functions. Another bone of contention was that he lectured in his native German instead of in Latin. After several years he had to leave Basle, and he spent the rest of his life wandering in central Europe. A man of quick passions, Paracelsus was also addicted to alcohol, and it is said that some of his works were written while he was drunk. He died at Salzburg.

It is not easy to assess the importance of Paracelsus to medicine. Some of his ideas were in advance of his time, but their expression is so clouded in mystical language that it is hard to separate the gold from the dross. His philosophy of medicine included the conception of an active force which he called an *archaeus*, supposed to exert an influence over dead matter. What exactly this force was is not very clear. He also emphasized the importance of the three principles, 'salt', 'sulphur', and 'mercury', in the composition of matter. In the field of practical medicine, however, Paracelsus was on much firmer ground. He was one of the earliest to study a disease characteristic of a certain occupation, namely, the fibroid phthisis so common among certain types of miners. He was also one of the first to use chemistry in the service of medicine, and he introduced laudanum, mercury, sulphur, and lead into the Western pharmacopoeia. He also saw the relationship between cretinism and endemic goitre (p. 521). In one respect at least his influence was wholly good, for he taught that the 'healing power of Nature' applies also to wounds, and recommended simple dressings instead of the ointments and plasters of his day.

THE RISE OF INTERNAL MEDICINE

From what has been said about the concepts of disease it will be seen that internal medicine lagged behind surgery at this period. Fernel had merely pointed the way to a scientific physiology, and without this there can be no science of internal medicine. It is unfortunate that the anatomical reforms of Vesalius were unaccompanied by any commensurate advance in physiology. The ruling idea was still that of the four humours, corresponding to the four temperaments. Apart from frequent references to these in general literature, they pervade the whole of medical writings until the late sixteenth century, and pictorial representations of individuals characterized by the predominance in them of one or other of the four temperaments are found not infrequently both in manuscripts and in printed works. One of the most interesting of the manuscript versions is a page in the manuscript Guild Book of the Barber-Surgeons of York. The illustration on this particular page was executed about the year 1500 (Fig. 38, and cf. Fig. 21). When ancient conceptions such as these were still acceptable in the seventeenth century, it is not surprising that the practice of the physicians at this period also remained mainly medieval. We can, however, perceive four distinct lines of advance in the physician's art during the sixteenth and first half of the seventeenth century. Firstly, there was

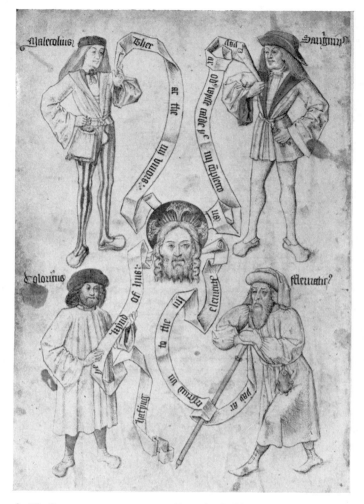

Fig. 38. The four temperaments, *c.* 1500. From the Guild Book of the Barber-Surgeons of York

Top left, the *melancholy* man; top right, the *sanguine*; bottom right, the *phlegmatic*; bottom left, the *choleric*. The phrase on the scroll may be transcribed: 'There are four humours, that are otherwise called the four complexions, that are received into the four elements, having the nature of humours'

(British Museum, Egerton MS. 2572, fo. 51ᵛ)

some improvement in the medical texts that were habitually read. Secondly, the extension of geographical knowledge and the formation of settlements and colonies brought new drugs on the market. Thirdly, there was an advance in botany, and therefore of the sources of vegetable drugs. Fourthly, there was some advance in the knowledge of the natural history of infectious disease.

The improvement in the medical texts was due largely to the fact that more reliable translations were now available. Notably the great Hippocratic and Galenic works, now translated into Latin direct from the original Greek, became more widely disseminated. Very important were the translations of some of Galen's works made by the humanist and physician Thomas Linacre (1460?–1524), who virtually founded the Royal College of Physicians of London (1518).

On the foundation of colonies in the New World many new plants, some dangerous and others useless, were brought home by adventurers. To these men Europe owed valuable new drugs, including ipecacuanha, cinchona, and tobacco. The first part of an important work on such drugs by Nicolas Monardes (1493–1588) of Seville appeared in 1569, and the third and final part (1574) bore the title *Historia medicinal de las cosas que se traen de nuestras Indias Occidentales*. This serial work was translated into English by John Frampton (*fl.* 1577–96) as *Joyfull Newes out of the Newe Founde Worlde* (1577).

It was unfortunate that the advance of botany was cursed with the 'practical' spirit, and only those plants thought to have an application as drugs were figured and described exactly. Nevertheless, the great German writers of herbals in the sixteenth century exercised a profound influence on the observational side of the science of botany. The earliest of these works was the Herbal (1530) of Otto Brunfels (1490?–1534). The text is in Latin, and the work shows many errors, but the drawings are accurate and beautiful. Under the influence of Brunfels, his younger contemporary Hieronymus Bock (1498–1554) published in 1539 a herbal which was at first not illustrated at all. But the text was written in his native German, and showed much first-hand observation. The most beautiful of these early herbals was the *De historia stirpium* of Leonhart Fuchs (1501–66), published at Basle in 1542 with superb figures. Fuchs was himself a professor of medicine in German universities, and he was

well known as a physician and the author of a work on the plague.
Though the descriptions of plants in his Herbal are clear and accurate, the plants themselves are chosen as usual because of their supposed medical uses. The most important aspect of these three great
Herbals was that they encouraged accurate observation of natural

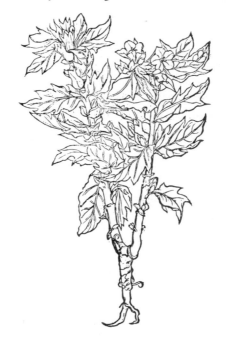

FIG. 39. Hyoscyamus figured by Brunfels
(O. Brunfels, *Herbarum vivae eicones*, Strasburg, 1530)

phenomena and this influence spread far beyond botany and
medicine.

The natural history of infectious disease had been considered by
Hippocrates, Galen, and other ancient physicians, but no progress
had been made towards an explanation of the fact that these diseases
were communicable, either from person to person or by means of
infected articles (fomites). Lucretius in his great poem *De rerum
natura*, written in the first century before our era, had made some
significant observations which can, in the light of what we know today, be interpreted as meaning that he had guessed that infection is

due to the 'seeds' of the disease being passed from a sick to a healthy individual. But these observations of Lucretius were contained in a few lines of his poem. Although the poem was widely read for centuries, it is doubtful whether it had any influence on the progress of science.

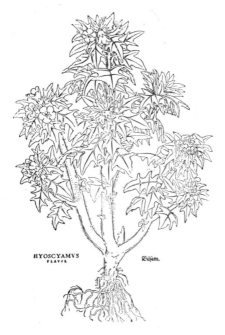

HYOSCYAMVS
FLAVVS   Bilfam.

FIG. 40. Hyoscyamus figured by Leonhart Fuchs
(Fuchs, *De historia stirpium*, Basle, 1542. From an uncoloured copy in the British Museum)

The first rational theory of the nature of infection was placed before the public in 1546 by Girolamo Fracastoro (1478–1553), a physician of Verona. He had studied at Padua and at other Italian universities, and, though steeped in the classical tradition, he preserved an independent outlook. In 1546 he published his celebrated *De contagione et contagiosis morbis* ('On contagion and contagious diseases'), which gave for the first time a logical explanation of the facts. Fracastoro distinguished three forms of contagion, namely, by simple contact; by indirect contact through the agency of infected articles; and by transmission from a distance. He regarded infection as due to the passage of minute bodies from the infector to the person infected. These hypothetical minute bodies had the power of self-multiplication. This conception bore a superficial resemblance to the modern germ theory of disease. An important contribution to the conception of epidemics was also made by the French physician Guillaume de Baillou (1538–1616), who reintroduced the old Hippocratic idea of an 'epidemic constitution', that is, that particular seasons and particular years are of their nature subject to particular diseases. The idea was extended and developed by the English physician Thomas Sydenham (p. 110).

In connexion with their epidemiological work these three men, Fracastoro, de Baillou, and Sydenham, made significant additions to the knowledge of particular infectious conditions. Thus, during the sixteenth and seventeenth centuries there arose an exact body of teaching concerning acute infectious diseases which was the necessary prelude to the introduction of more effective preventive measures at a later date. To one infectious disease we may refer more particularly.

During the Middle Ages there had smouldered in various districts an obscure disease, sometimes more or less dimly distinguished under various specific names, but most frequently confused with leprosy. Towards the end of the fifteenth century this disease, which was still imperfectly distinguished in men's minds from leprosy, broke out in epidemic and virulent form all over Europe. It caused great destruction of life and developed everywhere as a problem of national importance. Various names were given to it, such as pox, the French disease (*morbus Gallicus*), the Spanish disorder. Only slowly was it recognized that the disease was usually of venereal origin. Not till 1530, on the suggestion of Fracastoro, did it receive its modern cognomen syphilis. In that year Fracastoro published a poem entitled *Syphilis sive morbus Gallicus* ('Syphilis or the French disease'). This poem is a fantasy of the adventures of a rich young shepherd, Syphilus, who insulted Apollo. The god in anger inflicted on him a loathsome disease. Fracastoro then described the symptoms of syphilis in polished Latin verses. From the time of its recognition, syphilis has been pursued by a portentous mass of literature, the mere sifting and verification of which is a formidable task. Alarm, misunderstanding, religious feeling, false modesty, wil-

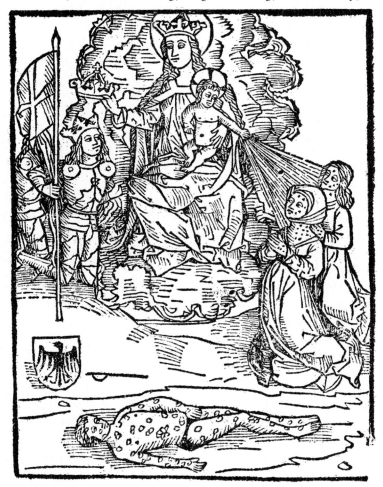

Fig. 41. An allegory of epidemic syphilis. The Virgin crowns a crusader, who kneels by her side. The Holy Child casts forth the scourge of syphilis on mankind. Two suppliant women are covered with the syphilitic rash, as also is the corpse in the foreground (Joseph Grünpeck, *Tractatus de pestilentiali scorra*, Augsburg, 1496)

ful misrepresentation, and change in type of the disease itself have all contributed their quota of obscurantism and fable to a naturally difficult subject (Fig. 41). Fracastoro did something to bring order out of the confusion. To him also we owe the first good scientific descriptions of several other destructive diseases, among which typhus fever, now known to be conveyed by lice (p. 451), takes a prominent place.

In recent times there arose a bitter controversy over the remote origin of syphilis. It was pointed out that a Spanish physician had stated about 1505 that some of the sailors of Columbus were suffering from syphilis on his return from the discovery of America in 1493. Other evidence for the view that these sailors were responsible for introducing syphilis to the Old World soon accumulated. In support of this view is the fact that syphilitic bone lesions are rare and not very definite in European skeletons of the pre-Columbian period. The question is not yet settled; but it seems probable that, perhaps as the result of the introduction from America of a new strain of the organism of syphilis, the disease in Europe changed its character completely during the closing years of the fifteenth century.

This new disease demanded energetic treatment. Almost from its first appearance in epidemic form syphilis was treated with mercury, mainly in the form of mercurial ointment, or of a lotion prepared from corrosive sublimate. Mercury was later strongly advocated by Paracelsus. About 1508 a Spaniard who was suffering from syphilis went to the island of San Domingo and discovered that the natives used for treatment a local product, guaiac wood. He was cured by its use, and he set up as a seller of the wood. Guaiac became at once a favourite remedy, and it was regarded as a specific for syphilis for at least a century. A course of treatment lasted thirty days and consisted largely in confinement to bed, reduction of diet almost to starvation level, and the taking of frequent draughts of a warm decoction of guaiac wood, which produced profuse sweating. One course was supposed to effect a cure. There is an interesting engraving after Jan Van der Straet (Johannes Stradanus) which shows on one side the preparation and weighing of the guaiac chips and the making of the decoction over a wood fire, and on the other the patient taking the warmed decoction (Fig. 42). This print appeared about 1580 in a set of engravings, consisting of an engraved title-page bearing the title *Nova reperta* ('Recent discoveries'), and nine plates; so that the guaiac decoction was still regarded as so important sixty

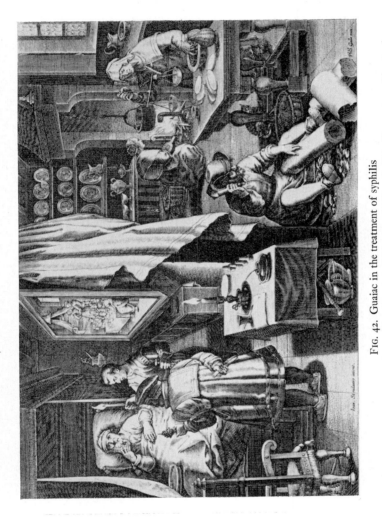

FIG. 42. Guaiac in the treatment of syphilis

(Engraving after J. Van der Straet (Stradanus), published by Philipp Galé in *Nova reperta* [Amsterdam, *c.* 1580]. From an impression in the Wellcome Historical Medical Museum)

years after its first introduction to Europe as to be hailed as a 'recent discovery'.

De Baillou (p. 106) first described whooping cough, and was the first to use the word rheumatism in the modern sense. He was, moreover, the first since Hippocratic times to distinguish between rheumatism and gout. De Baillou's works deeply influenced Sydenham, who held very similar epidemiological views and used a somewhat similar vocabulary (p. 728).

We have seen how the knowledge of anatomy forwarded surgery, while, with the lag in physiology, internal medicine remained in a backward state. It is well to recall however that a knowledge of anatomy and physiology will not, of themselves, make a man a scientific physician. The object which presents itself to a physician is neither a living anatomy nor a physiological model. It is a sick and suffering patient. The physician's first task is to examine exactly the phenomena of sickness and suffering, and in doing this the first demand on his knowledge will be the history and fate of others who have endured like sickness and suffering. When he has ranged these instances in his mind he may turn, for explanation and relief, to the resources suggested by other sciences, anatomy and physiology among them. But all the anatomy and physiology in the world will not aid the practitioner who is unacquainted with the natural history of disease. This is the truth that was firmly seized by Thomas Sydenham (1624–89) of London.

Sydenham dominated the field of clinical medicine in the seventeenth century as no other man did at that time. The credit due to him is all the greater when we consider that he never taught in a university, that he founded no school, and that he had no pupils in the usual sense. He had completed some of his medical studies at Oxford when the Civil War broke out, and he became an officer in the Parliamentary cavalry. After the Second Civil War Sydenham commenced to build up in London the practice which became famous all over Europe, although it was not until 1663 that he obtained the Licence of the Royal College of Physicians.

The Natural History of Disease was a subject which Sydenham pursued with lifelong devotion. Before his time the phenomena of disease had been classified, subdivided, discussed, and treated with all the subtlety and skill of scholastic thought. Men had now and again shaken themselves free from the shackles of the medieval system, and had here and there corrected the views of Galen or amplified the limited achievements of their predecessors. Yet none before Sydenham had set himself to consider all the actual cases of disease that lay before him as a subject of scientific description and analysis. That was the great achievement of the 'English Hippocrates'. We should not find it easy to point to any important discovery to associate with his name. But he did more than discover. He initiated a new mode of approach. He was the founder of modern clinical medicine.

In 1666 Sydenham published his classic work, *Methodus curandi febres* ('The method of treating fevers'), dedicated to his friend Robert Boyle (pp. 136–7). The book opens with the almost Hippocratic phrase 'A disease, in my opinion, how prejudicial soever its causes may be to the body, is no more than a vigorous effort of Nature to destroy (*exterminare*) the morbific matter, and thus recover the patient'. We have here the 'healing power of Nature' of Hippocrates (p. 35), which had been obscured and overlaid in the twenty centuries which lay between the two great physicians. The works of Sydenham may be regarded as the first great clinical commentary on the Hippocratic theme. Sydenham set well on its way the conception of infectious conditions as specific entities, a conception which has since been illuminated by the germ theory of disease (pp. 326 ff.).

THE FIRST PHYSICAL SYNTHESIS

Manifestations of the human spirit are not accustomed to confine themselves exactly within the convenient limits of the centuries. Nevertheless, it happens that in the history of science the year 1600 does, in fact, correspond to something of the character of a real change in the current attitude to Nature. That year really ushers in the era of physical experiment. The last of the great transitional thinkers who mark the waning of Renaissance philosophy was Giordano Bruno, the martyr of science.

Giordano Bruno (1548–1600), who was no practical scientist, had eagerly incorporated into his often fantastic philosophy his ill-worked-out conclusions from Copernicus (p. 92). Nominally adopting the Copernican theory, he modified it fundamentally. Copernicus, having placed the Sun at the centre of the Universe, and made the Earth and other planets circle round it, had still left the stars at a fixed and definite distance, as had the ancient astronomers. The limitation of the sphere of the fixed stars was obnoxious to Giordano, and he removed the boundaries of the Universe to an infinite distance, in accordance with the principles of his philosophy. The change may seem unimportant save for astronomy, but, in fact, it came to influence every department of scientific thought, for the endlessness of Nature is implicit in the modern scientific attitude.

Giordano was burned at the stake at Rome, after seven years' imprisonment, in 1600. In the same year the experimental era was ushered in with the work *De magnete, magneticisque corporibus, et de magno magnete tellure* ('On the magnet, magnetic bodies, and on the great magnet, the Earth') by William Gilbert (p. 185), in which he not only demonstrates experimentally the properties of magnets but also shows that the Earth itself is a magnet. In the same year, too, Tycho Brahé (1546–1601) handed over the torch to Johannes Kepler (1571–1630). Tycho was the last of the older astronomers who worked on the Aristotelian view of circular and uniform movements of heavenly bodies. Kepler was the real founder of the modern astronomical system. The period from 1600 onward lies with new men, Galileo (pp. 113–15) and Kepler among astronomers and physicists, Harvey (pp. 120–3) among biologists, and Descartes (pp. 138–40) among philosophers.

The seventeenth century opened with an extraordinary wealth of scientific discovery. As we glance at the mass of fundamental work produced during that period, we perceive the major departments of science, as we know them today, becoming clearly differentiated. The acceptance of observation and experiment as the only method of eliciting the laws of Nature reaches an ever-widening circle. Even to enumerate the names of the seventeenth-century pioneers would be a formidable task. The sciences penetrated to the universities and influenced the curricula. The number of scientific men became so large and so influential that separate organizations were formed by them in the interests of their studies. It is the age of the foundation of the Academies, of which the Royal Society of London is a type.

From the multitude of workers on these subjects we can but select a few names. In the first half of the century Galileo and Kepler are the main exponents of natural law. Descartes takes his place here as the first since antiquity who sought to explain the phenomenal universe on a unitary basis. In the second half of the period comes the mighty figure of Newton (pp. 145 ff.), whose researches ushered in the modern phase in our story.

The early training of Galileo Galilei (1564–1642) had been scholastic and Aristotelian. By 1590, however, he had begun to doubt, and was making experiments on the rate of acceleration of falling bodies. By 1591 he had reached his conclusions, though the legend of his dropping weights from the leaning tower of Pisa in that year must be abandoned. He did, however, succeed in demonstrating that, contrary to the Aristotelian view, the rate of fall was a function not of the weight of the object but of the period of fall. Revolutionary also was Galileo's work of 1604. In that year a new star appeared in the constellation Serpentarius. He demonstrated that this star was situated beyond the planets and among the remote heavenly bodies. Now this remote region was regarded in the Aristotelian scheme as absolutely changeless. Although new stars had been previously noticed, they had been considered to belong to the lower and less perfect regions nearer to the Earth. To the same lower region, according to the then current theory, belonged such temporary and rapidly changing bodies as meteors and comets. But Galileo had attacked the incorruptible and unchangeable heavens.

In 1609 Galileo made accessible two instruments that were to have a deep influence on the subsequent development of science, the telescope and microscope. It is with the former instrument that his name is most frequently associated. His first discoveries made by means of the telescope were published in 1610. That year was crowded with important observations, especially on the inner planets and notably on Venus. It had been rightly claimed in criticizing the Copernican hypothesis that, if the planets resemble the Earth in revolving round the Sun, only such parts of them should be luminous as are exposed to the Sun's rays. In other words, they should exhibit phases like the Moon. Such phases in Venus were now actually observed by Galileo. In the following year he described sun-spots and traced them round the Sun's disk.

We need not follow the further astronomical observations of Galileo, nor need we discuss the contest with the older school on which he embarked. It is sufficient to remind ourselves that the appearance of a new star, the behaviour of the rings of Saturn, the observations of the phases of Venus and of the Sun's spots, struck a blow at Aristotelian astronomy comparable to that delivered against Aristotelian physics by Galileo's conclusions on the acceleration of falling bodies. Aristotelian astronomy demanded heavens eternally changeless. Here were changes and new appearances in the heavens, clearly visible to all who would see.

During these years, too, Galileo was laying the foundations of the science of mechanics. Out of his mechanical researches came a new way of looking at the objects of Nature which has profoundly influenced the entire subsequent course of science. That way is best expressed in Galileo's own words, which place him among the philosophers whose thought influences all those who deal with scientific themes.

As soon as I form a conception of a material or corporeal substance, I simultaneously feel the necessity of conceiving that it has boundaries and is of some shape or other; that relatively to others it is great or small; that it is in this or that place, in this or that time; that it is in motion or at rest; that it touches, or does not touch, another body; that it is unique, rare, or common; nor can I, by any act of imagination, disjoin it from these qualities. But I do not find myself absolutely compelled to apprehend it as necessarily accompanied by such conditions as that it must be white or red, bitter or sweet, sonorous or silent, smelling sweetly or disagreeably; ... and if the senses had not pointed out these qualities discourse and imagination alone could probably never have arrived at them. Hence I think that these tastes, smells, colours, etc., with regard to the object in which they appear to reside, are nothing more than mere names, and exist only in the sensitive body; so that when the living creature is removed all these qualities are carried off and annihilated, although we have imposed particular names upon them, and would fain persuade ourselves that they truly and in fact exist. . . . But I do not believe that there exists anything in external bodies for exciting tastes, smells and sounds, except size, shape, quantity, and motion, swift or slow, and if ears, tongues, and noses were removed, I am of opinion that shape, quantity, and motion would remain, but there would be an end of smells, tastes, and sounds, which, abstractedly from the living creature, I take to be mere words.

This passage is a veritable charter of science. From Galileo's day to ours, men of science have occupied themselves in measuring size, shape, quantity, and motion, the primary qualities, and expressing their knowledge in that measured form. They have relegated colours, smells, tastes, sounds, and other sense-impressions to the position of secondary qualities, and have tried to express them, when they express them at all, in terms of the primary qualities. We need not enter on the philosophical discussion as to how far the primary qualities are in truth more real than the secondary, but it is a fact that, since the time of Galileo, science has come to be regarded more and more widely as an exact process. Science is measurement. It is a conception that has affected the medical no less than the other sciences, and it is a conception that medicine owes to Galileo. The writings of Giordano Bruno and of Galileo made nonsense of the idea of the Macrocosm and Microcosm which had pervaded the Middle Ages.

THE REVIVAL OF PHYSIOLOGY

The first to apply Galilean principles of measurement to biological matters was Santorio Santorio (1561–1636), called Sanctorius. He studied medicine at Padua, and then spent fourteen years in practice in Poland. At the age of fifty Sanctorius returned to Padua to fill the chair of medicine, and during the remainder of his life he experimented unceasingly. While he was still in Poland he published a small book (1602) which deals essentially with differential diagnosis. In it he makes brief mention of an instrument which he called a 'pulsilogium'; this was intended to help him to remember the relative rates of the pulse in different individuals. Many years later he gave a description of this instrument. It consisted of a simple pendulum, the length of the suspending string of which was adjusted until the beat of the pendulum coincided with that of the pulse. The measurement which Sanctorius observed was the length of the pendulum (Fig. 43 *d*). In his time physicians examined the quality of the pulse carefully, but they had no means of measuring its rate. Sanctorius thus broke new ground not only in putting the emphasis on the rate, but also in devising an instrument to compare rates. In 1612 Sanctorius published another work in which he described a thermometer to measure body temperature, and thirteen years

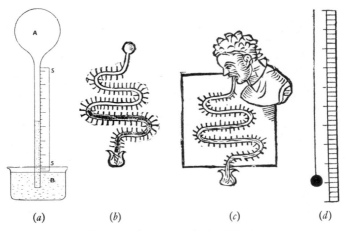

(*a*)   (*b*)   (*c*)   (*d*)

Fig. 43. Thermometer and pulsimeter

(*a*) The principle of Galileo's thermometer. The bulb *A* is inverted over the mercury bath *B*. A rise in air temperature causes expansion of the air in *A* and a fall in the mercury level in the tube, and vice versa. The readings are inaccurate since the instrument acts both as a thermometer and a barometer, and the atmospheric pressure therefore influences the result.

(*b*) Galileo's thermometer as adapted by Sanctorius.

(*c*) The Sanctorius instrument used as a clinical thermometer.

(*d*) The pulsimeter of Sanctorius.

later he explained how the thermometer was to be used in studying diseases in human patients (Fig. 43). It is an indication of the transitional character of the science of the time that the 1612 work was a commentary on Galen's *Art of Medicine*, and that the 1625 work was a commentary on a medieval translation of the *Canon* of Avicenna.

Sanctorius is perhaps best remembered because of the famous illustration which shows him seated in a chair suspended from the arm of a steelyard (Fig. 44). Galen had assumed that a certain amount of 'respiration' takes place through the skin as well as that which occurs through the lungs with condensation of the breath.

That which took place through the skin was known as the 'insensible perspiration'. Sanctorius estimated its amount under different conditions, such as when the individual was awake or asleep, eating or resting, and even under different emotional conditions. The

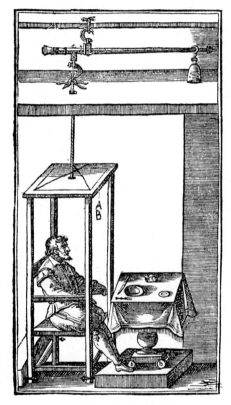

FIG. 44. Sanctorius in his balance
(Sanctorius, *Commentaria in primam fen . . . Canonis Avicennae*, Venice, 1626)

subject which he used for all his experiments was himself, and he often ate and slept in his balance-chair. His experiments lasted over thirty years, and in 1614 he gave his results to the world in a series of aphorisms, published in his *De medicina statica*. This famous book went through many editions and was translated into several languages. By these experiments Sanctorius laid the foundations of the modern study of metabolism (pp. 578 ff.).

While Sanctorius was engaged in this pioneer work at Padua, the movement that Vesalius had inaugurated there was making further conquests in the purely biological line. Vesalius had been succeeded at Padua by a series of anatomists of great eminence. Perhaps the most prominent among these was Fabricius ab Aquapendente

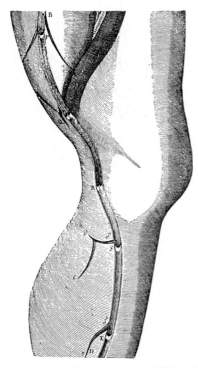

(p. 97). But, in spite of all his powers, Fabricius never shook himself free from ancient views, and especially he was steeped in the theories of Aristotle and Galen. This backward-looking habit prevented his work from being as important as it might otherwise have been. In connexion with the circulation, for instance, he made a striking discovery, but wholly failed to appreciate its most important lesson.

In 1603 he published his book *De venarum ostiolis* ('On the valves ['little doors'] of the veins'). In it he says that these structures are so placed that their mouths are always directed *towards* the heart (Fig. 45). Yet in

FIG. 45. An illustration by Fabricius of valves in a vein. The valves are shown at *P, Q, R, S, T*
(H. Fabricius, *De venarum ostiolis*, Padua, 1603)

his explanation he missed the true function of the valves in the veins. In the leg, for example, the veins are long, and if much blood flowed back in them towards the foot, the veins would be liable to burst. Fabricius thought that the purpose of the valves was to prevent too much blood from flowing downwards. If he had appreciated the point he would have seen that their true function was to prevent absolutely any flow of the blood away from the heart. The theory of the circulation of venous blood depends on this fact, but Fabricius was too set on the old Galenic physiology to permit such a revolutionary thought.

The crucial demonstration that the whole of the blood circulates through the body was made by Harvey. But a few men had already known of the lesser circulation through the lungs. The first to question Galen's views was probably Ibn an-Nafis (1210–88) of Damascus and Cairo. His opinion, unearthed in 1924, was that the interventricular septum is solid, and that that part of the blood which passes from the right to the left ventricle does so by way of the pulmonary artery, the lungs, and the pulmonary vein.

These views seem to have been lost until the sixteenth century. In 1553 a theological work, *Christianismi restitutio*, was published by the Spanish theologian and medical practitioner Miguel Serveto (1511–53), usually known as Servetus, who had studied medicine in France. For the heretical doctrines expressed in it Calvin had Servetus burned at the stake a few months later, and most copies of the book were thereafter destroyed, though three escaped and still survive. A century and a half later, long after the publication of Harvey's work, it was noticed that the book contained a passage expressing views very similar to those of Ibn an-Nafis.

In 1559 the *De re anatomica* of Realdo Colombo was published posthumously. In it he gave reasons, based on clinical observations, anatomical dissections, and experiments on animals, for the existence of the lesser circulation. Colombo was possibly teaching these views as early as 1546. His work is superior to that of Servetus, which may have been an inspired guess. Both may have had the same idea; or either may have been influenced by the ideas of the other; or either or both may have heard of the views of Ibn an-Nafis. For over twenty years it has been known that Colombo may have had indirect contact with a translator of the works of Ibn an-Nafis.

Another contestant for honours is Andrea Cesalpino (1524–1603), Italian physician and botanist. The Italians base their claim that he 'discovered' the circulation of the blood on his use of the word 'circulatio'. But by this word he meant flux and reflux, circulation in the chemical and not in the Harveian sense. He has no place in the demonstration of the circulation of the blood.

The Englishman William Harvey (1578–1657), after education

at Cambridge, went to Padua in 1598 when Fabricius was at the height of his powers. Returning to England in 1602, he set up in practice in London. During the years which followed, he was dissecting and experimenting very industriously. In 1616 Harvey gave lectures on anatomy and physiology which included a brief mention of the circulation of the blood. Nearly three centuries later the manuscript notes which he made for this course of lectures were discovered. These notes demonstrate that he had reached by 1615 a clear conception of the circulation (Fig. 47). It is characteristic of Harvey's caution that he continued to experiment but published nothing until thirteen years later. Then, in 1628, there appeared his *Exercitatio anatomica de motu cordis et sanguinis* ('An anatomical disquisition concerning the motion of the heart and blood'). This small book—usually called *De motu cordis*—is certainly one of the greatest works ever written in the medical field. In it Harvey laid the foundations of the sciences of experimental physiology and experimental medicine.

To discuss the actual steps by which Harvey made his discovery would be beyond our scope. He had, however, been well trained in experimenting on living animals by Fabricius, and had read widely in anatomical literature. He was of a contemplative turn of mind and his quiet and cautious temper, united with his enthusiasm and skill as an experimenter, provided a superb mental equipment for a life of scientific investigation.

Harvey, early in his work, reached two fundamental conceptions concerning the vascular system. He perceived that the valves in the veins would permit the blood to pass only towards the heart (Fig. 46), while those in the great arteries arising from the heart would permit the blood to pass only away from the heart. In connexion with the movement of the blood, Harvey's crucial point is that it must be *continuous*, and *always in one direction*. This really clinches the matter, for consider the capacity of the heart. Let us suppose that either ventricle holds but 2 ounces of blood. The heart beats 72 times a minute and 4,320 times an hour. In the course of one hour, therefore, the left ventricle will throw into the aorta, or the right ventricle into the pulmonary artery, no less than 8,640 ounces (38 st. 8 lb.) of blood. In other words, in one hour the ventricle will

throw into the great artery more than three times the body weight
of a heavy man. Where can all this blood come from? Whither can it
all go? It cannot come from the ingested food and drink, for no one
could consume so much in one hour. It cannot reach and remain in
the tissues, for they would soon all burst and ooze with blood. The
solution of the problem, Harvey came to see, is that it is the same

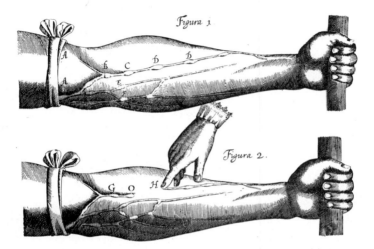

FIG. 46. Harvey's illustration to show the action of the valves in the veins in the
living subject. If the upper arm is bandaged, the valves are shown as nodes on the
swollen veins. If the finger is pressed along a vein, in a direction away from the heart,
from one node to the next (e.g. *O* to *H*), the section *OH* will be emptied of blood. It will
remain empty, since the valve at *O* does not permit blood to flow away from the heart
(W. Harvey, *De motu cordis*, Frankfort, 1628)

blood that is always being pumped into the arteries, and the same
blood that is always coming back through the veins. In other words
the blood *circulates*, a fact which Harvey proceeded to demonstrate
with convincing thoroughness (Fig. 46).

We may note that, though Harvey demonstrated the existence of
the circulation, he was never able to follow it throughout, for he did
not see the capillary vessels by which the blood is conveyed from the
terminal branches of the arteries to the smallest tributaries of the
veins. These were first demonstrated by Malpighi (p. 124).

The knowledge of the circulation of the blood has been the basis of the whole of modern physiology and with it of the whole of modern rational medicine. The attitude of Galen and Aristotle towards the heart and the great vessels passed into the shadow. The

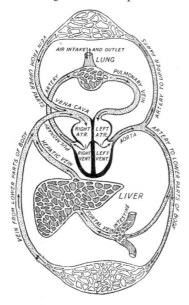

FIG. 47. Diagram to illustrate the nature of the circulation of the blood. Leaving the left ventricle, when the walls of that cavity contract, the blood is forced through the valves into the great artery known as the aorta. From the aorta it passes into smaller and ever smaller arteries, finally reaching the systemic capillaries or the portal capillaries. After travelling through one or other capillary network it enters a vein. Thence it passes into larger and ever larger veins, until it ultimately enters the great vein known as the vena cava that opens into the right atrium. It has now completed the Greater Circulation. As the right atrium contracts the blood passes through the valves between the right atrium and right ventricle into the right ventricle. From there it enters the Lesser Circulation, passing into the great pulmonary artery, which conducts it to the lung. In the lung the pulmonary artery breaks up into branches and finally into capillaries. Through these the blood travels until it reaches a tributary of the pulmonary vein and finally the pulmonary vein itself. The pulmonary vein empties its blood into the left atrium. From the left atrium the blood passes at last into the left ventricle from which it started, having traversed both the Greater and the Lesser Circulation.

To understand the change which Harvey wrought in the conception of the workings of the body, this description and diagram should be compared with Fig. 26 and the accompanying text (pp. 62–65).

blood, it was seen, is a carrier always going round and round on the same course. What it carries, and why, how, and where it takes up and parts with its loads, are questions which have become the main problems of physiology in the centuries that have followed. As each of the questions has obtained a more and more rational answer, so clinical medicine has always made a step forward, and has come to approach more nearly to a true science. Thus it is that the work of Harvey lies at the back of almost every important medical advance.

Before we leave the circulation, mention should be made of two highly significant discoveries related to it. The practically colourless body fluid called lymph also circulates throughout the body in special vessels known as lymphatics. A particular type of lymphatic vessels, called the lacteals, is found in relation to the intestines. These convey the chyle, the fluid containing nutriment derived from the process of digestion, from the intestines to the blood-stream. The lacteals, containing the milky-white chyle, were discovered by Gaspare Aselli (1581–1626) of Cremona. His posthumous book was published in 1627. If Harvey had known about the lacteals, they would have added weight to his argument, but probably he had not seen Aselli's book. Aselli thought that the lacteals passed to the liver. The thoracic duct was discovered in the dog by Jean Pecquet (1622–74) in 1647. The connexion of the intestinal lymphatics with the thoracic duct was discovered in 1651 by Olaf Rudbeck (1630–1702), a Swede who was then studying at Padua. Thomas Bartholin (p. 627) later disputed the priority of this discovery.

A significant development in the physiology of the seventeenth century was made by Francis Glisson (1597–1677). Glisson graduated at Cambridge, was an original Fellow of the Royal Society, and president of the Royal College of Physicians. Though he held the regius chair of physic at Cambridge for over forty years, he was almost never there, but practised as a physician in London. Glisson wrote what was in effect the first account of the disease rickets, and gave a good description of the anatomy of the liver, containing several noteworthy discoveries. During the last years of his life he wrote two books in which he set forth his important views on the 'irritability' of tissues, and especially of muscle fibres. These views had a great influence on Albrecht von Haller (p. 153).

MICROSCOPICAL EXAMINATION OF THE ANIMAL BODY

The compound microscope was first made into an effective instrument by Galileo. It was, as it were, a by-product of his invention of the telescope. With that instrument he had seen enough to convince himself that the movement of the Sun round the Earth was but an appearance. At the very time that Harvey was giving his first course of lectures securely in London, Galileo's teaching was attracting the unwelcome attention of the Inquisition in Rome.

Galileo's microscopes, however, were far less satisfactory than his telescopes. For optical reasons, which we need not discuss, these early compound microscopes failed to give a clear picture. With any high degree of magnification the image was always blurred and distorted. More than three centuries were to pass before a better compound system was introduced. But about 1650 a way was found of constructing and mounting simple lenses of very high power. Many of the most important microscopical discoveries of the second half of the seventeenth century were, therefore, made with a simple lens. This was notably the case with much of the work of the great investigators Malpighi and Leeuwenhoek.

Marcello Malpighi (1628–94) was born in the year in which Harvey's work was published. He became a professor at Bologna, having early developed great skill in minute investigation. His first work, which appeared in 1661, supplied the element missing in the investigations of Harvey, for he describes the actual passage of blood from the arteries to the veins through the capillary blood-vessels (Fig. 48). Harvey, who did not use a microscope, had no definite knowledge of the existence of capillaries, though he knew very well that there must be some sort of channel between the smallest arteries and the smallest veins. The object which yielded up the secret was the lung of the frog. This organ in the frog happens to be almost transparent, is very simple in structure, and is furnished on its surface with particularly conspicuous capillary vessels. Malpighi could hardly have selected an object better suited for this particular research. This important discovery of his drew the attention of scientific men in England. The Royal Society soon entered into

correspondence with him, and during the remainder of his life undertook the publication of his researches.

The contributions of Malpighi to biological knowledge were very
numerous and important. The study of early development, now
included in embryology, was greatly extended by him. The later
stages of embryological development had been investigated by
Fabricius (p. 97), and some additions to the subject had been made
by Harvey in his work *De generatione animalium* ('On the generation

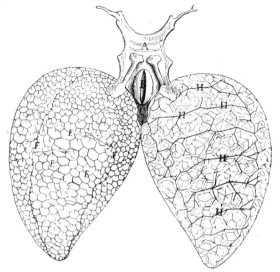

Fig. 48. Lungs of a frog, showing capillaries. The left lung (on right of illustration) has
been laid open, and between the veins, *HHH*, capillary vessels are seen
(M. Malpighi, *De pulmonibus*, Bologna, 1661)

of animals'), published in 1651 (p. 45). Malpighi, applying his
microscope to the earlier germ of the animal body, described in
detail the development of the organs, notably of the heart and the
nervous system. He also demonstrated the minute structure of the
skin, spleen and liver, in all of which there are anatomical structures
that still bear his name. He investigated microscopically the structure
and physiology of insects and plants. A few figures are reproduced
from Malpighi's two works on the embryology of the chick. In
Fig. 49a the whole embryonic area, with the embryo in the centre, is
shown at about the end of the second day of incubation. Vessels

passing from the body of the embryo branch and form a network over the vascular area. In Fig. 49b the embryo is shown at a slightly greater magnification. The head shows the rudimentary brain, consisting of three cerebral vesicles, and one of the large eyes is shown. The segmented tissue (somites) which will later form the body muscles is shown further enlarged in Fig. 49c. The heart (Fig. 49d) is in the form of a loosely coiled tube. The part marked D will later

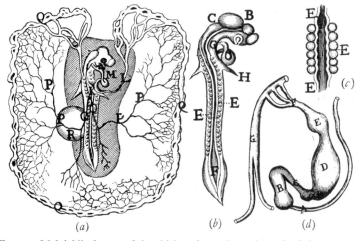

FIG. 49. Malpighi's figures of the chick embryo about the end of the second day (a), (b), (c) from M. Malpighi, *De ovo incubato*, London, 1686; (d) from his *De formatione pulli in ovo*, London, 1673)

form the ventricle, and the part B the atrium. At F the aorta divides into three branches which are soon reunited. Later researches by other embryologists showed that these branches represent the vessels which in fishes form the blood supply to the gills. All Malpighi's figures are careful and accurate.

A most remarkable contemporary microscopist was the Dutchman, Antoni van Leeuwenhoek (1632–1723). Without medical or scientific training, desultory and secretive in his mode of working, he was withal an observer of genius and a very shrewd investigator. During his long and industrious life he made a series of disconnected discoveries which for originality and importance have been surpassed by no other microscopist. Leeuwenhoek did not use a compound microscope; he used a simple microscope of his own design—

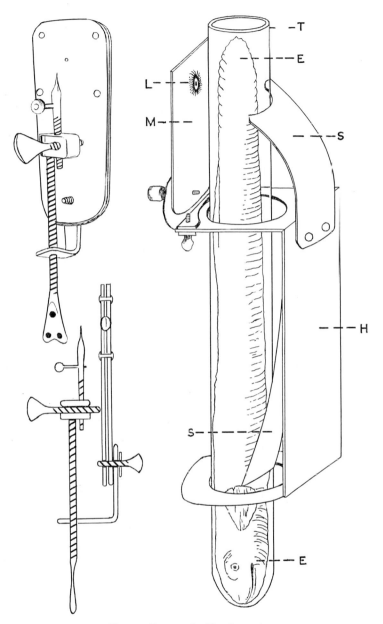

FIG. 50. Leeuwenhoek's microscopes

(a) The normal form of instrument: a composite drawing made from several examples (after Dobell);

(b) The instrument adapted for examining a living animal (after B. W. Richardson).

really a magnifying glass. A typical example of a Leeuwenhoek microscope is shown in Fig. 50a. The whole instrument is only 3 inches
tall. The body of the instrument consists of two thin rectangular
metal plates rivetted together. Towards their upper end an aperture
passes through both plates, and the sides of this aperture support a
tiny biconvex lens of very small focal length. Approximately opposite
the lens a needle-pointed rod is supported vertically behind the body
and the object to be examined was fixed to this point. By means of
the adjusting screws shown, this object could be brought exactly
opposite the lens, and could also be focused, that is, have its distance
from the lens varied. In use the observer's eye was brought close up
to the lens, and the object was viewed through it. Leeuwenhoek
made all his own microscopes. He was a master of the art of lens-
grinding. He made a new instrument for each new object which he
examined, and thereafter he kept the instrument with the object
attached to it. When he died several hundred microscopes in various
metals, some gold and many silver, were among his possessions.
With his best instruments Leeuwenhoek was probably able to obtain
a magnification of nearly 300 diameters.

Leeuwenhoek adapted one of his instruments in order to study the
circulation of the blood in the tail of a young eel. Though he does
not give an illustration of the complete apparatus assembled, he does
provide in one of his papers detailed drawings of the various parts.
Fig. 50b is a composite modern drawing of the apparatus, as he described it. An instrument of this type which he is supposed to have
made and used is preserved at Leyden; in principle and design it
differs slightly from the type illustrated by Leeuwenhoek and in
Fig. 50b. Referring to the modern drawing it is seen that the essential
part of the instrument is the body of the microscope (M), bearing
the lens (L) towards the top. The body of the microscope is
attached to a metal tube-holder (H), which carries a glass tube (T).
The tube is held firm by two rectangular springs (S, S). The eel (E)
was placed head-downwards in the tube, and the tube was adjusted
so that the tail of the eel was opposite the lens. Adjusting screws were
provided so that the object could be focused.

Leeuwenhoek's success was due to his patience as an observer, to
the excellence of the lenses which he ground, and probably also to

the fact that he had wonderful near-sight. He studied in some detail in man and certain animals the red blood corpuscles previously seen by Swammerdam (p. 133); he estimated their size, and figured them

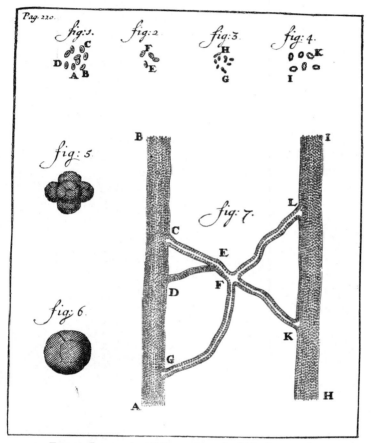

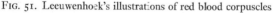

FIG. 51. Leeuwenhoek's illustrations of red blood corpuscles

(1) In a salmon; (2)–(4) in an eel; (5), (6) aggregations of several eel corpuscles, forming globes; (7) the capillaries between an artery (HI) and a vein (BA) in an eel

(A. van Leeuwenhoek, *Arcana Naturae Detecta*, Leyden, 1719)

(Fig. 51). He was the first to illustrate spermatozoa, and to describe and illustrate a protozoon (an animal consisting of a single cell, in this case Vorticella). In the eel and the frog he observed the circulation in the capillaries, and studied the walls of the small vessels (Figs. 51 (7)

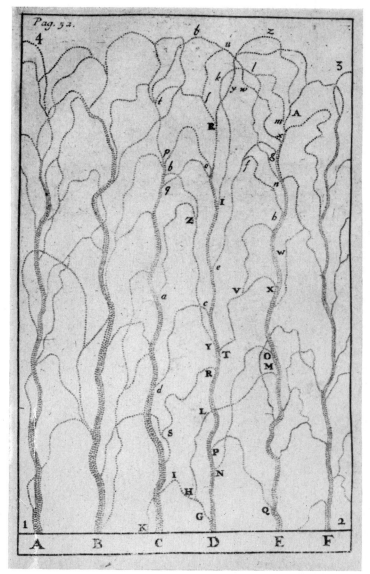

FIG. 52. Leeuwenhoek's illustration of the capillary network in the web of the frog's foot
A, C, E, arterioles; B, D, F, venules

(A. van Leeuwenhoek, *Arcana Naturae Detecta*, Leyden, 1719)

and 52). He was the first to demonstrate that voluntary muscles are made up of bundles of muscle fibres, and that indivdual fibres show

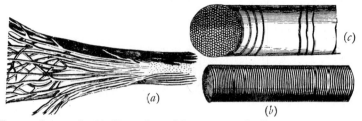

FIG. 53. Leeuwenhoek's illustrations of the structure of voluntary muscle

(*a*) A muscle teased into bundles of fibres.

(*b*) Further enlargement of a bundle of fibres; on the left the cut ends of the fibres are seen.

(*c*) A single fibre highly magnified, showing the characteristic striation.

(A. van Leeuwenhoek, *Arcana Naturae Detecta*, Leyden, 1708)

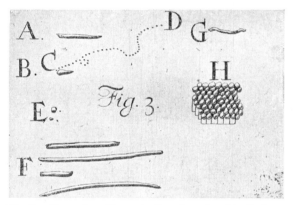

FIG. 54. The first illustration of bacteria. Organisms found in the human mouth by Leeuwenhoek. The modern idertification of the organisms shown is as follows (Dobell):

A, a motile bacillus.

B, *Selenomonas sputigena*. The figure shows (C . . . D) the path of its motion.

E, micrococci.

F, *Leptothrix buccalis*.

G, a spirochaete, probably *Spirochaeta buccalis*.

H, a sarcina.

(A. van Leeuwenhoek, *Phil. Trans. Roy. Soc.*, 1683)

a characteristic striated appearance (Fig. 53). Of his other discoveries certainly the most important is the fact that as early as 1683 he described and illustrated bacteria (Fig. 54).

An outstanding investigator was the English scientist Robert Hooke (1635–1703), distinguished not only as a scientist and inventor, but also as an architect. As a young man Hooke caught the attention of Robert Boyle (p. 136) at Oxford. He became Boyle's

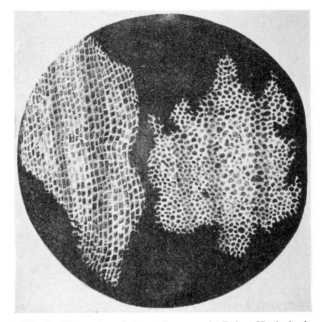

Fig. 55. The first illustration of plant cells as seen by Robert Hooke in the structure of cork. On left in longitudinal section, on right in transverse section
(R. Hooke, *Micrographia*, London, 1665)

assistant, and later he was appointed the first Curator of Experiments to the infant Royal Society. In 1665 Hooke published his great book, entitled *Micrographia*, the first important work to contain figures of microscopical objects. In it he gives drawings and a description of the structure of a piece of cork. These showed that the cork was made up of compartments which he called 'cells' (pp. 320 ff.). This is the first mention in scientific literature of the microscopic plant or animal cell, and the first use in the English language of the word 'cell' with this meaning. (Fig. 55). The *Micrographia* was also noteworthy because of the fact that the text was published in English and not in Latin.

The short life of a second Dutch microscopist of the seventeenth century, Jan Swammerdam (1637–80), was abbreviated yet farther, as regards scientific achievement, by his insanity. In his brief working period he developed a marvellous technique of fine dissection of small animals carried out under the microscope, and acquired great skill in making injection preparations. His first work, the *Historia insectorum generalis* ('General history of insects', 1669) embodies illustrations of his dissections. In 1675 he published his *Ephemeri vita* ('The life-history of the may-fly'), a very detailed and complete treatise on the anatomy of this insect. Swammerdam extended our knowledge of embryology, and made two other discoveries important in medicine. One of these was his discovery of the red blood corpuscles—in the frog. This observation was made years earlier than Leeuwenhoek's more complete study of these corpuscles in the blood of various species of animals. By his other discovery Swammerdam first introduced the very modern use of the nerve-muscle preparation in physiological research. Until his time it was held that when a muscle contracts something passes down the nerve into it and that the muscle increases in volume. Some of Swammerdam's figures illustrating his experiments on this subject are shown in Fig. 56. He used a large muscle from the leg of a frog dissected out, with its nerve left attached, immediately after the death of the animal. Fig. 56*a* shows the muscle held at each end by the operator; when an assistant stimulated the nerve by pinching it, the muscle contracted and tended to pull the hands together. Fig. 56*b* shows the muscle contained in a glass tube, each end of the muscle being transfixed by a pin. On stimulation of the nerve the pins were drawn towards each other, and the contracted muscle filled up the middle of the tube. In Fig. 56*c* the muscle is seen suspended in a glass cylinder which is tightly closed below by a stopper; the upper end of the cylinder is drawn out to a capillary tube. The nerve to the muscle is arranged over a loop of wire. A thread is attached to the nerve, then passes through the loop and down between the stopper and the cylinder wall. By pulling the end of the thread the operator can squeeze the nerve in the wire loop, so that it is stimulated. The apparatus above the stopper is filled with water, and the water in the capillary tube contains a bubble of air (*e*). Any change in the volume of the muscle is shown by a movement of the air bubble. Using this apparatus Swammerdam showed that contraction of the muscle was not accompanied by any change of volume, thus refuting the old theory. He also applied the method to the recently dissected and still beating heart of a frog (Fig. 56*d*). In this case no mechanical stimulus had to be applied. The upper mark (*c*) in the figure indicates

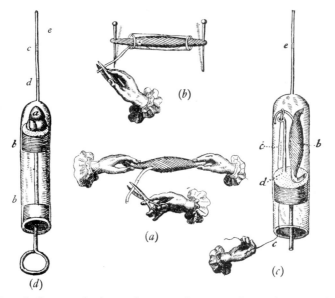

FIG. 56. Swammerdam's experiments on the nature of muscular contraction (J. Swammerdam, *Biblia Naturae*, ed. Boerhaave and Gaubius, Leyden, 1737–8, Tab. xlix)

the position of the air bubble with the heart in diastole, and the lower mark (*d*) its position in systole. The difference in volume between the two positions indicates the change in volume of the heart's chambers caused by its contraction.

Swammerdam left at his death a mass of unpublished manuscripts and drawings of dissections. Many years later these were purchased by Boerhaave (p. 149), who, jointly with Hieronymus David Gaubius (1705–80), professor of chemistry at Leyden, published them at Boerhaave's expense, with the two earlier books, in a Dutch-Latin edition with the title *Biblia Naturae* ('Bible of Nature', 1737–8).

This work is still consulted for the great beauty and accuracy of its illustrations.

These microscopists and several others in the seventeenth century did much to explore the minute structure of the animal body. Their revelations showed at once an unexpected complexity of all the parts, and an unexpected resemblance of some of those parts which appear diverse to the naked eye. Thus, the structure of the body came to be subjected to a process of microscopical examination. For long after the time of these classical microscopists no effective improvements were made in the microscope, and these studies made no progress. With the improvements of the microscope in the nineteenth century, the method was taken up again with triumphant results.

FROM ALCHEMY TO CHEMISTRY

During the sixteenth and the first part of the seventeenth century the basic science of mechanics had been placed on a firm footing by Galileo. Astronomy, with Galileo and Kepler, had made the great break with the past. Anatomy and physiology had put on their modern dress. Chemical knowledge, however, remained peculiarly backward. Many advances, it is true, had been made in technical processes, but investigations designed to throw light on theory were mostly prosecuted by the band of dupes and charlatans who, since the Middle Ages, had been seeking the philosopher's stone. The old theory of the four elements, earth, air, fire, and water (p. 46), formed an ill basis for experiment. Some philosophers, it is true, had put forward crude atomic theories, but they had little experimental evidence to adduce. Nevertheless even the alchemists had made some advance and had, for instance, perfected a system of weighing.

The great defect of the ancient view of matter was that it contained no definite conception of the nature of a pure substance. Metals, for instance, were regarded, like other substances, as a mixture in certain proportions of the four elements of Aristotle (p. 46). Thus, the transmutation of one metal or one substance into another by distillation did not seem an absurdity, or even a task of special theoretical difficulty.

The main agent in changing the chemical outlook was the Honourable Robert Boyle (1627–91), known as the Father of Chemistry. He was a member of a small body of men which met first in London, then in Oxford, and at the Restoration returned to London, and in 1662 was incorporated by Charles II as the Royal Society of London. These men were satisfied that the only way to learn anything effective about Nature was by observation and experiment. From their discussions all purely speculative views were excluded. They agreed to meet together solely to compare experiences, to demonstrate experiments, and to draw immediate deductions. None of them was more active in these matters than Boyle.

The actual chemical and physical discoveries of Boyle were very numerous, but his great achievement, the real service he rendered to learning in general and to medicine in particular, was his introduction of a new spirit into chemistry. Under him that study was no longer prosecuted for purely practical ends; it was set free from the mystic factor in alchemy and it was loosed from the chains which bound it to medicine, to the disadvantage of both. Chemistry thus became an independent science, the principles of which were to be ascertained by experiment, and its truths pursued for their own sake.

Boyle demonstrated that the air is a material substance and has weight. By means of his air-pump he proved clearly that this substance is necessary for the support of respiration (Fig. 57). The law of the compressibility of gases is still known by his name. Most important of all Boyle's contributions to chemical theory was his adumbration of the conception of a chemical element in our modern sense, and his view of the atomic structure of matter, derived ultimately from the Greek atomistic philosophers. Boyle's best-known work is *The Sceptical Chymist*, first published in 1661.

Under the inspiration of Boyle and his colleagues, chemical works of the second half of the seventeenth century exhibit in general a positive, cautious, experimental spirit, and show a great contrast to the mystical and obscure writings of the first half of the century, which have much affinity with alchemy. A fine exponent of this new spirit was John Mayow (1641–79), who was prevented by an early death from fulfilling all his promise. He was the first to recognize clearly that there is a substance or principle in air which is concerned at once with combustion, respiration, and the conversion of venous into arterial blood (Fig. 66). These experiments of Mayow were long misunderstood.

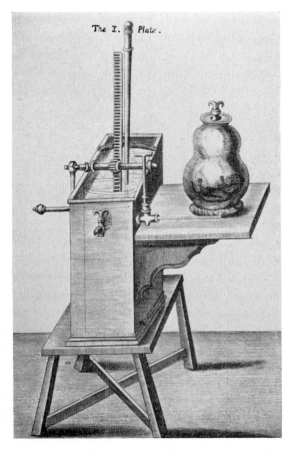

FIG. 57. Robert Boyle's second air-pump. A cat in the receiver shows signs of asphyxia as soon as the air is exhausted by the pump

(R. Boyle, *A continuation of new experiments physico-mechanical, touching the spring and weight of the air*, Oxford, 1669)

THE MEDICAL THEORISTS

The great advances in the physical and biological sciences, instituted during the sixteenth and seventeenth centuries, left the old medical theories derelict. We have already traced the wrecking of the Galenic physiology. With its destruction the old ideas concerning the three types of spirit, natural, vital, and animal, went by the board. The doctrine of the circulation of the blood (pp. 119 ff.) and the investigations of the new chemistry accorded ill with the old humoral pathology, which ascribed all disease to excess or defect of one of the four humours, blood, phlegm, bile, and black bile (p. 46). Numerous fresh theories arose, of which the more important can be classed under the three headings Iatrophysics, Iatrochemistry, and Vitalism.

(a) Iatrophysics

The physical discoveries of Galileo (p. 113) and the demonstrations of Sanctorius (p. 117) and of Harvey (p. 120) gave a great impetus to the attempt to explain the workings of the animal body on purely mechanical grounds. The writers who took this point of view are known as the Iatrophysicists. One of the earliest and most impressive exponents of physiological theory along these lines was the French philosopher René Descartes (1596–1650). His work on the subject appeared posthumously in 1662. It is important as the first modern book entirely devoted to the subject of physiology.

Descartes had not himself any extensive practical knowledge of the subject with which he was dealing. On theoretical grounds he set forth a very complicated apparatus which he believed to be a model of animal structure. Subsequent investigation failed to confirm his findings, and his work soon passed into oblivion. For a time, however, it attracted much attention and many followers. A strong point in his theory is the great stress laid upon the nervous system, and its power of co-ordinating the different bodily activities. Thus stated, his view may seem not far from the modern standpoint, though in fact he was grotesquely wrong in detail. An important part of his theory is the complete separation of Man from all the other animals. Man, according to him, differs from all other animals by his possession of a soul, which is situated in a structure in the brain known to physiologists as the pineal body. Animals, he held, have no soul, and all their actions and movements, even those which seem to express pain or fear, are purely automatic. It is the modern theory of behaviourism with man excluded. These views of Descartes are exemplified by his theory of the relation between a sensory impression and a motor impulse (Fig. 58). The image of the object ABC passes to the eye and is formed on the retina. Owing to the optical properties of the eye, it is there inverted. The image is inverted yet again within the brain, where it passes to the pineal gland H at the

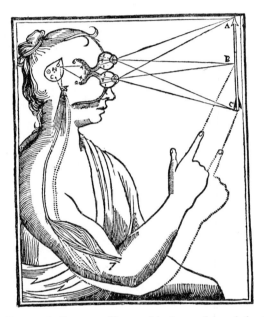

FIG. 58. Descartes's diagram to illustrate his theory of the relation between
a sensory impression and a motor impulse
(R. Descartes, *De homine*, Leyden, 1662)

point *b*. The position and character of the image formed on the retina determines the nature and distribution of its effect on the pineal body. According to the nature and distribution of that effect is the result on the nerve, and through it, by the passage of nervous fluid, on the muscles. The movement in the nerve is initiated at the point *c*. The relation between *b* and *c* is an insoluble mystery in which is wrapped up the very nature of the soul.

In Descartes's diagram to illustrate his theory of nervous action (Fig. 59), P R and *q s* are nerves which supply the muscles of the eye T and V V. Descartes held that these nerves were hollow and provided with valves, which can be seen at the point at which the P R and *q s* first branch. These valves were partly controlled by little fibrils in the main stems and in certain of their branches. These valves control the movement of the fluid within the hollow spaces of the nerves. Additional complication is lent to the scheme by the fact that P R and *q s* intercommunicate at certain points. The view of Descartes, and all such theories of nervous fluid, were destroyed by the experiment

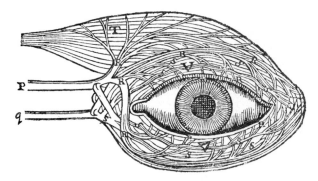

FIG. 59. Descartes's diagram to illustrate his theory of nervous action
(R. Descartes, *L'homme*, Paris, 1664)

of Swammerdam (Fig. 56), which, however, long remained unpublished.

More lasting was the achievement of Giovanni Alfonso Borelli (1608–79), an eminent mathematician who was professor at several Italian universities and the friend of Galileo and Malpighi. Stirred, like Descartes, by the success of Galileo in giving a mathematical expression to mechanical events, Borelli attempted to do the same with the animal body. In this undertaking he was, in fact, very successful. That branch of physiology which treats of muscular movement on mechanical principles was effectively founded and largely developed by him (Figs. 60 and 61). Here his mathematical and physical training was specially useful. He endeavoured, with some success, to extend mechanical principles to such movements as the flight of birds and the swimming of fish. When he came to an analysis of some of the other activities of the body, such as the action of the heart or the movements of the intestines, he was less successful, and he naturally failed altogether in his attempt to introduce mechanical ideas in explanation of what we now know to be chemical processes, such as digestion in the stomach.

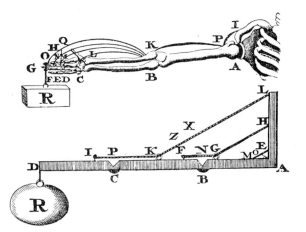

FIG. 60. Borelli on the contraction of muscles. Two of his figures analysing arm movements (cf. Fig. 61)

(G. A. Borelli, *De motu musculorum*, Rome, 1680)

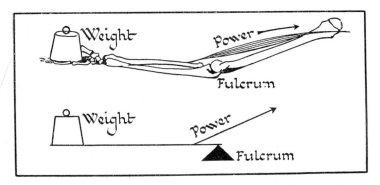

FIG. 61. Diagrammatic resolution of a simple arm movement in terms of the lever (cf. Fig. 60). As Borelli perceived, however, natural movements of the body are rarely as simple as that illustrated

Undeterred by Borelli's failure, other writers sought to find mechanical explanations of physiological processes. As is usual in such cases, the amount of theory was inversely proportional to the amount of knowledge. The views of some of the later iatrophysicists became very fantastic. Belated representatives of the school are some of the writers of the French *Encyclopédie* (1751–72), and notably its main author, the man of letters Denis Diderot (1713–84).

(b) Iatrochemistry

Just as there were some who thought to explain all animal activity on a mechanical basis, so others resorted to chemical interpretation. These may be termed Iatrochemists. One of the earliest of these men, who followed in the footsteps of Paracelsus (p. 100), was Jean Baptiste van Helmont (1577–1644) of Brussels, who may be said to have discovered carbon dioxide (though he did not recognize it as such), and who invented the term 'gas'. Though some of his chemical work is valuable, his physiological ideas were mystical. His mysterious forces (*archaei*), which were supposed to govern the workings of the body, led nowhere; and the six ferments which he postulated to explain digestion in the stomach and intestine and certain other physiological processes were equally imaginary. Yet his conception that his 'sixth digestion' takes place in the tissues themselves, though based on no chemical or physiological experiments, was in the right direction. Van Helmont was important in guiding physiological thought into chemical channels, and from that aspect he may be regarded as the founder of chemical physiology.

The most prominent and influential of the iatrochemists was Franz De le Boë (1614–72), generally known as Franciscus Sylvius, who was professor of medicine at Leyden. That university had become, in the second half of the seventeenth century, the most progressive scientific centre north of the Alps. It was the seat of the first university laboratory, built at the instigation of Sylvius.

Sylvius devoted much attention to the study of salts. He recognized that they were the result of the union of acids and bases, and he attained to the idea of chemical affinity—an important advance. He looked at the phenomena of life also from the chemical point of view. Well abreast of the anatomical knowledge of his day, and accepting the broader lines of mechanistic advance in biology, such as the circulation of the blood and the mechanics of muscular motion, Sylvius sought to interpret other activities in chemical terms. His position and abilities as a teacher gave his views wide currency and he and his pupils occupy a large part of the field of medical theory until well into the eighteenth century.

Under the influence of this school, almost all forms of vital activity were expressed in terms of acid and alkali and of fermentation. The latter process was assumed to be of a chemical order, and no clear distinction was made between changes that are brought about by chemical ferments, such as gastric juice or rennet, and changes that are brought about by the action of micro-organisms, such as alcoholic fermentation or leavening by yeast. Nevertheless, the School of Sylvius and its immediate successors added considerably to our knowledge of physiological processes, notably by their examination of the body fluids, especially the digestive fluids such as the saliva, and the secretions of the stomach and of the pancreas.

(c) Vitalism

Yet another school of medical theorists arose under the leadership of the German chemist and physician Georg Ernst Stahl (1660–1734). Stahl popularized the theory of Johann Joachim Becher (1635–82), extended it, and renamed Becher's *terra pinguis* 'phlogiston', a hypothetical substance with which bodies were supposed to part while burning. Stahl is thus the effective founder of the phlogiston theory; he grouped chemical phenomena and systematized the study of chemistry. Stahl stands as the protagonist of that view of the nature of the organism which now goes under the term Vitalism. Though expressed by him in obscure and mystical language, it is, in effect, a return to the Aristotelian position and a denial of the view of Descartes. To Descartes the animal body was a machine. To Stahl the word machine expressed exactly what the animal body was not. The phenomena characteristic of the living body are, he considered, not governed by physical and chemical laws, but by laws of a wholly different kind. These laws are the laws of the sensitive soul. The 'sensitive soul' of Stahl is, in its ultimate analysis, not dissimilar to the *psyche* of Aristotle (p. 45). Stahl held that the immediate instruments, the natural slaves of this sensitive soul, were chemical processes, and his physiology develops along lines of which Aristotle could know nothing. This does not, however, alter the fact of his hypothesis being an essentially vitalistic one of Aristotelian origin.

The language and the theories of the iatrophysicists, the iatro-chemists, and the vitalists of the seventeenth and eighteenth centuries have long been discarded by men of science in the form in which they were originally propounded. Nevertheless, they represent three attitudes to the activities of living things which have present and current meaning. Each seems to present some aspect of truth. Whether some physiological thinker will combine all three aspects into one coherent whole is for the future to decide. Yet it is certain that all three lines of approach remain of value, and the stimulus provided by each of the three inspires investigation at the present day. In this sense we enter on the period of modern medicine in the seventeenth century. In this sense too the foundations of modern rational medicine may be said to have been laid by Borelli, Sylvius and Stahl, with Galileo, Boyle and Harvey standing behind them.

VI

THE PERIOD OF CONSOLIDATION

(from about 1700 to about 1825)

THE REIGN OF LAW

DURING the sixteenth and seventeenth centuries the European mind cast off its medieval vestments and, having refreshed itself at the spring of antiquity, turned to array itself in the garments of the New Philosophy. The advent of new ideas and new knowledge had been very rapid. The method of research had been determined by Galileo at the beginning of the seventeenth century. The meaning of research was determined by a second great investigator, Sir Isaac Newton (1642–1727), at the end of the same century.

The change wrought in the thought of their time by Vesalius, Galileo, Harvey, and their like, was quantitative rather than qualitative. They discovered new laws of Nature, but the discovery of such new laws was hardly unprecedented. Law had been traced in the heavens from of old. The rules of planetary and stellar motion had been gradually developed from the simple astronomical theories of the ancients. The great astronomers of the sixteenth and seventeenth centuries did not hesitate to appeal to the records and doctrines of medieval writers, for new mathematical relationships of the heavenly bodies had been elicited even during the Middle Ages. In the sixteenth century astronomy under Tycho Brahe prepared herself for the Great Instauration of the coming age. And then Galileo (pp. 113–15) startled the world with that new star of his, among the most remote heavenly bodies in the very region held by the Aristotelian and Platonic schemes to be utterly changeless. The revolution in thought had begun, though no new order had been established.

By 1618 Kepler had enunciated his three laws of planetary motion. Then the experimental philosophers set forth to establish terrestrial mechanics. They determined the mode of action of gravitation, and Galileo came near to the three laws of motion which we call Newton's. But it was Newton who first stated them clearly

L

and succeeded in linking them with Kepler's laws of planetary motion. Before Newton no man had perceived or demonstrated that the earthly and heavenly bodies are directed by the same physical laws. Nay, faith and reason alike would have been against such a view. It was Newton's unique achievement to prove that the relationship amounted to identity, to move men's minds to see that the force that causes the stone to fall is that which keeps the planets in their path. It was Newton who first enunciated a law whose writ ran alike in the Heavens and on the Earth. With Newton the Universe acquired an independent rationality, and the whole cosmology of Aristotle, of Galen, and of the Middle Ages lay in the dust.

When Newton had completed his work, the gravitation of the Earth and of the Heavens was seen to be one, and all the mechanism of the Universe lay spread before him. The vision was set forth in his *Philosophiae naturalis principia mathematica* ('The Mathematical Principles of Natural Philosophy'), 1687. It established a view of the structure and working of the Universe which has survived to our own century.

But now as to the change wrought in men's minds. It was something more than a revolution. It was the establishment of a new order. Newton conceived a working universe wholly independent of the spiritual order. How far his vision is philosophically tenable and how far he realized its revolutionary nature are matters which we need not discuss here. There can, however, be no doubt that Newton utterly destroyed the very foundations of medieval thought. With Newton there sets in the last stage of scientific determinism.

During the almost three centuries since the *Principia* appeared, science has developed prodigiously along the lines into which Newton led her. In reliance on the universality of natural law, the stars in their courses have been paced, weighed, measured, analysed. The same process, directed to our own planet, has traced its history, determined its composition, and demonstrated its relation to other bodies. Physicist and chemist have suggested a structure in terrestrial matter similar to that of the stars and suns. The Universe has been reduced to a unitary system. Wherever men have sought law, they have found law. With search skilful enough and patient enough, law has ever emerged. It has been the Age of the Reign of Law.

It is true that in our own time philosophers in general have come to see that these laws of nature are within us as much as without; that they are, in part at least, the result of the structure of our minds. This is a point of view, however, which has not affected, and perhaps will not affect, the working man of science. His constant occupation, since the days of Newton, has been the pursuit of law, and he has usually been satisfied that law has only to be sought in order to be found. This conception has affected the medical and biological sciences very deeply. Thus the influence of the Newtonian philosophy is as traceable in them as it is in the astronomical and physical sciences. Galileo showed men of science that weighing and measuring are worth while. Newton convinced a large proportion of them that weighing and measuring are the *only* investigations that are worth while. The question as to whether this view is ultimately true or philosophically justifiable does not need discussion at the moment. The point, for our immediate purpose, is that the view has been very widely held.

THE RISE OF CLINICAL TEACHING

The eighteenth century dawned with the refreshing breeze of Newtonian philosophy blowing through it. During the previous 200 years there had been an immense amount of new and fruitful research along diverse lines. Chemistry, mechanics, botany, comparative anatomy, descriptive anatomy, experimental physiology, epidemiology, and microscopical investigation, had all yielded startling results. The new generation was bewildered with the very mass and novelty of the material. When the biologists of the time contemplated the beauty and symmetry of the mathematical relations that Newton and his followers had introduced into cosmic conceptions, they must have been wellnigh hopeless of reducing their vast accumulations to order. Thus the eighteenth century was for biology a period of pause and consolidation, during which attempts were made to introduce unitary conceptions into the mass of accumulated material. It was, moreover, a period of consolidation not only of ideas but also of teaching. These tasks at first turned men's minds away from the immediate accumulation of further knowledge. There was an urge to apply philosophical principles to the practice of medicine. This led to the invention of various medical systems to explain the phenomena of disease and the principles of treatment. One example is the Vitalism of Stahl (p. 143). Another system was that of Friedrich Hoffmann (1660–1742), a chemist and physicist who sought to apply mechanistic principles to treatment. He regarded the body as made up of individual fibres. Each fibre was able to dilate and contract by virtue of a property called tonus, regulated by a 'nervous ether' which had its seat in the brain. This 'ether' was sent to all parts of the body by imaginary contractions of the meninges, the membranous coats of the brain and spinal cord. Every modification in tonus brings an alteration in health. Hoffmann aimed to regulate tonus, and hence a number of drugs used by him were called 'tonics'.

Several systems were based on the physiological views of Hoffmann. One was that of William Cullen (1710–90), who held important chairs in the Universities of Edinburgh and of Glasgow. In Cullen's theory the normal state of the body was determined by 'nervous energy', derived from the nervous system and affected by external stimuli. A pupil of Cullen, John Brown (1735–88), created the Brunonian theory which had a long and eventful life. On this theory health was due to a correct balance of stimuli. Some diseases are due to excessive stimuli and are treated by sedatives; others are caused by defect of stimuli, and are treated by stimulants.

Such conflicting theories absorbed much of the interest of inquiring physicians during the early eighteenth century, and there was a gap in the progress of research. But during this period a new method of teaching medicine was evolved. The reforms in medical education were largely due to the efforts of Boerhaave and Haller, both of whom added greatly to the respect with which the medical profession was regarded.

Until the seventeenth century there was no systematic clinical teaching. The universities gave medical degrees on the basis of a spoken disputation. No contact with the patient was demanded. The first effective attempt to change this was at Leyden, where about 1636 clinical teaching was instituted. Owing to this, and to the fact that, as at Padua, students of every religious denomination were accepted, Leyden became much frequented by foreign and especially by Protestant students. Its attractions were increased by Franciscus Sylvius (pp. 142-3), who in the second half of the seventeenth century added laboratory instruction to his clinical teaching. Leyden had several eminent anatomists, while its botanic garden and museums added to the practical character of the medical instruction that it offered.

Hermann Boerhaave (1668-1738) was first appointed as a teacher at Leyden in 1701. At once the medical school attained a front-rank reputation which rapidly came to surpass even that of Padua. Boerhaave had only twelve beds at his disposal, but never did man make better use of his opportunities. Besides clinical, chemical, botanical, and anatomical instruction he followed such of his patients as died into the post-mortem room and there demonstrated to his students the relation of lesions to symptoms. He is thus the introducer of the method of medical instruction still in vogue in our modern medical schools.

Boerhaave was a man of wide culture. He purchased and published at his own expense the plates of the priceless *Bybel der Natuure* (*Biblia Naturae*) of Swammerdam (p. 134). Apart altogether from his clinical ability and acumen Boerhaave was a skilled chemist, botanist, and anatomist. He wrote a textbook of chemistry which was used throughout Europe. No epoch-making discovery in the medical field can be credited to him, but his *Institutiones medicae* ('The institutes of medicine'), one of the earliest textbooks of physiology, was used in every medical school. Much of his ripe clinical wisdom is enshrined in his *Aphorisms*, which, like those in the Hippocratic Collection, consist of short, pithy sentences. Several commentaries on these aphorisms were published by later writers.

With all these accomplishments Boerhaave was better able than any man of his time to achieve something like a medical synthesis, to bring all the sciences to the service of the patient. Taking one thing with another, considering his influence as a teacher, his clinical acumen, his power of inspiring younger workers, his wide learning, his balanced vision, his eagerness for new knowledge, his sanity, his humanity, his generosity, and his prophetic power, Boerhaave must be regarded as the greatest physician of modern times. To him the debt of British medicine, and through it of British well-being, is quite incalculable. Through his pupils he is the real founder of the Edinburgh Medical School, and through it of the best medical teaching in the English-speaking countries of the world.

Students at Leyden at this period also had the benefit of instruction in anatomy from the greatest anatomist of his time. This was Bernhard Siegfried Albinus (1697–1770). Appointed to the chair of anatomy and surgery at Leyden at the age of twenty-four, he introduced a new standard of accuracy into practical anatomy, and of accuracy and beauty into anatomical illustration. In collaboration with Boerhaave, Albinus produced in 1725 a superb edition of the collected works of Vesalius (p. 90), which exhibits remarkable prevision of the needs of scientific scholarship today. Of the anatomical works of Albinus, the greatest is the *Tabulae sceleti et musculorum corporis humani* ('Plates of the skeleton and muscles of the human body', 1747). The illustrations (Plates XII and XIII) for this work were prepared under the constant and direct supervision of the author. The intention was not merely to depict the parts as they were seen by artist and anatomist, but to select suitable examples from a large number of bodies, so that the resulting illustration would be fully representative. In order to show the parts in their true proportions, the bodies were frequently viewed from a distance of forty feet; and to preserve the perspective two nets with meshes of appropriate sizes were interposed between artist and subject. The ornamental backgrounds seen in these plates were inserted not merely for decoration, but in order to give the object drawn its proper tone value. These illustrations were intended for physicians and also for artists, and no finer work of their type has ever been executed.

ANATOMY AND THE EDINBURGH SCHOOL

The success of the Edinburgh School, founded while Boerhaave was still in his prime, can be ascribed directly to his inspiration. The enthusiasm of the early Edinburgh teachers, and the concentration of all the medical teaching, both clinical and subsidiary, in one great university school can both be traced to Leyden.

Anatomy affords a familiar example of the success of the Edinburgh School. Alexander Monro (1697–1767), known as Monro *primus*, was appointed professor of anatomy there in 1720, and for nearly forty years he continued to teach. At the start of his career he had only 57 students, but at the end the number in his classes ran to several hundreds. He trained his son, Alexander Monro *secundus* (1733–1817), to succeed him. Monro *secundus*, in addition to being a very famous teacher of anatomy, was also a distinguished physician. When he finally took over the chair from his father there were about 190 students in the class; and when he handed over the chair to his own son, Alexander Monro *tertius* (1773–1859), the class numbered about 400 students. The third Monro did not maintain the prestige of his two predecessors. Though an able man, he was somewhat indifferent to the success of his teaching. When he finally resigned the chair in 1846, it had been held by grandfather, father, and son for a period of over 120 years.

William Cullen (p. 148), another pillar of the Edinburgh School, became professor of medicine at Glasgow in 1751, and he was the effective founder of the Glasgow School. He returned to Edinburgh, where he filled with distinction the chairs of chemistry, materia medica, and finally of the practice of physic. He drew students from all over Europe. His textbooks on materia medica and the practice of medicine were very widely used.

In London a most distinguished anatomist was William Cheselden (1688–1752), a surgeon to St. Thomas's Hospital. He was famed for the rapidity of his operations, especially that for stone in the bladder. His textbook of anatomy went into many editions, and his superb work entitled *Osteographia* (1733) contained many accurate and beautiful engravings of skeletons and of individual bones (Plate XIV).

PHYSIOLOGY PASSES TO THE MODERN STAGE

The only figure in the eighteenth century whose influence is comparable to that of Boerhaave is his pupil, the Swiss Albrecht von Haller (1708–77), one of the most accomplished men of all time. In actual scientific achievement Haller stands, indeed, far above his master. He achieved distinction as poet, botanist, anatomist, and novelist, carried on a prodigious correspondence, was an exceedingly learned bibliographer, and perhaps the most voluminous of all scientific authors. His special distinction, however, is as a physiologist.

Haller was known throughout western Europe for his *Primae lineae physiologiae* ('First lines of physiology'), a short textbook for students first published in Latin in 1747 and translated into several languages. His greatest work, *Elementa physiologiae corporis humani* ('The elements of the physiology of the human body'), which appeared in eight volumes between 1757 and 1766, was a comprehensive and critical treatise embracing the whole of the physiological knowledge of his time. It marks the modernization of the subject of which it treats. Of the highest importance were Haller's researches on the mechanics of respiration, on the formation of bone, and on the development of the embryo. He did good work on the action of the digestive juices. His most important contributions, however, are his conceptions of the nature of living substance and of the action of the nervous system. These conceptions formed the main background of biological thinking for a hundred years, and are still integral parts of physiological doctrine.

All branches of medicine must be influenced by the views we may hold on the nature and action of the nervous system, just as all parts of the body are influenced and indeed are linked together by that system. Thus the growth in knowledge of the physiology of the nervous system is extremely important to us if we would gain a true idea of the progress of rational medicine.

When we look into the history of nervous physiology before Haller, we are struck by the smallness of the observational foundation of a vast speculative structure. That we may be the more charitable in our judgement of such fanciful developments, we may recall that the mind is so constructed that it can take little interest in the accumulation of instances unless it can adduce general laws therefrom. Theory is thus as necessary to practice as practice to theory. The earlier doctrines of the nature of nervous action are, however, so unlike those we now hold that we can afford to pass over them lightly. They consist of speculations on the topic of the seat of the soul, together with explanations which suppose the passage down the nerves either of the nervous fluid or of some chemical

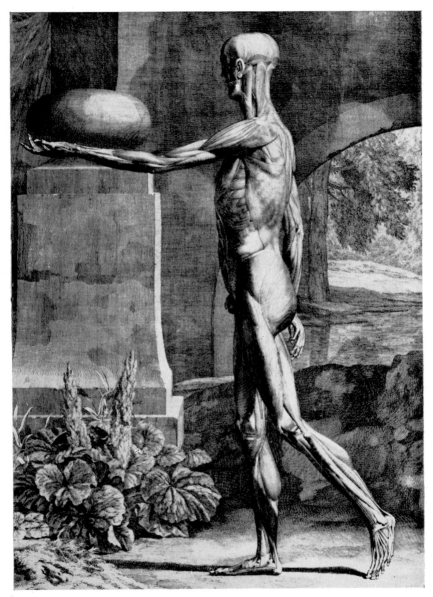

XII. SUPERFICIAL MUSCLES FROM THE SIDE

(B. S. Albinus, *Tabulae sceleti et musculorum corporis humani*, Leyden, 1747. Copy in the
Wellcome Historical Medical Library)

(*See p.* 150)

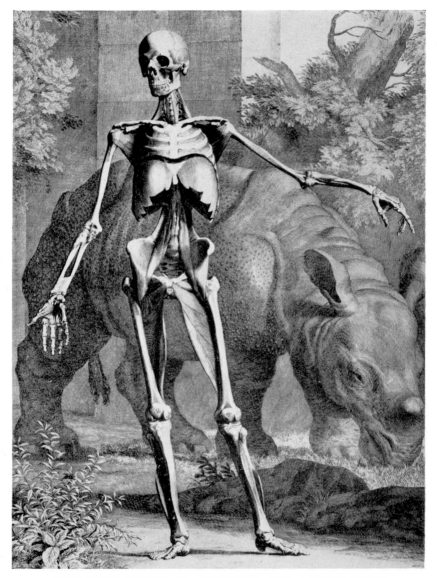

XIII. DEEP MUSCLES OF TRUNK AND LOWER LIMBS

(B. S. Albinus, *Tabulae sceleti et musculorum corporis humani*, Leyden, 1747. Copy in the
Wellcome Historical Medical Library)

(*See p.* 150)

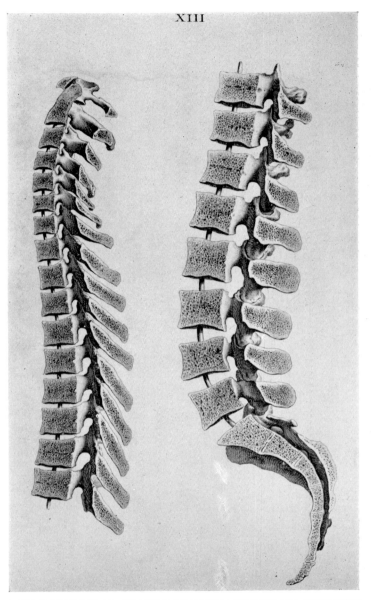

XIV. VERTEBRAL COLUMN IN LONGITUDINAL SECTION
(W. Cheselden, *Osteographia*, London, 1733. Copy in the Wellcome
Historical Medical Library)

(*See p.* 151)

change. Haller was the first to construct a theory of the nervous system that has an appearance of modernity.

During the seventeenth century the favourite doctrine of nervous action supposed the existence of a nervous fluid. This, it was held, passed down the nerves to inflate or extend the muscle fibres. Inflation was supposed to shorten the fibres and so the muscle came to contract. An exquisite experiment by Swammerdam with his nerve-muscle preparation had disproved this (p. 133). But Swammerdam's work was unknown till published by Boerhaave in 1737, and so the matter stood till Haller's time.

Haller concentrated the problem on an investigation of the fibres. A muscle-fibre, he pointed out, had in itself a tendency to shorten with any stimulus, and afterwards to expand again to its normal length. This capacity for contraction Haller, following in the footsteps of Francis Glisson (p. 123), called irritability. He recognized the existence of irritability as an element in the movement of the viscera, notably of the heart and of the intestines. The characteristic of irritability is that a very slight stimulus produces a movement altogether out of proportion to itself, and that it would continue to do this repeatedly so long as the fibre remains alive.

But besides the force inherent in a muscle-fibre Haller showed that there was another force which is carried to the fibre from the central nervous system by the nerves, and is the power by which muscles are normally called into action. This force, like that of irritability, is independent of the will, and like it can be called into action after the death of the animal. Haller thus distinguished the 'inherent muscular force' from the 'nerve force'. Both these forces he further distinguished from the natural tendency to contraction and expansion, under changing conditions of humidity, pressure, and so on, of all tissues, living or dead.

Haller, having dealt with the question of movement, turned to that of feeling. He was able to show that the tissues are not themselves capable of sensation, but that the nerves are the sole channels or instruments of this process. He showed how all the nerves are gathered together into the brain, and he believed that they tended to its central part. These views he supported by experiments and observations involving injuries or stimulation to the nerves and different parts of the brain. He ascribed special importance to the cortex, but the central parts of the brain he regarded as the essential seat of the living principle, the soul.

Throughout his discussion Haller never falters in his display of the rational spirit. He develops no mystical or obscure themes, and, although his view of the nature of soul may lack clarity, he separates such conceptions sharply from those which he is able to deduce from actual experience. He is essentially a modern physiological thinker, and certain of his themes were developed by writers who come on the frontiers of what we have called the 'period of consolidation'.

Among these writers we would select the Scottish surgeon Sir Charles Bell (1774–1842), who spent most of his professional life as a teacher and operator in London. In 1811 he published a small work in which he showed that the nerve fibre conveys either motor or sensory stimuli, but not both, and therefore transmits impulses in one direction only. Bell also showed that stimulation of the anterior of the two roots (Fig. 82, p. 253) by which all spinal nerves arise from the spinal cord produces convulsions of the muscles; on the other hand, stimulation of the posterior root produces no motor effect. By these discoveries Bell not only completed the views of Haller on the central nervous system, but also brought them within the range of practical medicine.

It is unfortunate that Bell's phraseology in this small work lacks precision. Ten years later the question of the functions of the two spinal roots again came to the fore, especially in the light of the further experiments of François Magendie (1783–1855), a great French physiologist. In 1822 Magendie showed quite definitely that the anterior root is motor, while the posterior root is sensory. He made other important observations on the nervous system, and he was also the founder of the science of toxicology.

SOME PHYSIOLOGICAL ADVANCES

Haller provided a philosophical basis to physiological conceptions. There were, however, other workers of the time who added to the knowledge of the actual workings of the animal body. First among these, both in time and eminence, stands the Rev. Stephen Hales,

Perpetual Curate of the parish of Teddington in the county of Middlesex.

Stephen Hales (1677–1761) was by inclination a biologist, but he had received a training in mathematics and physics. With this ideal equipment he proceeded to investigate the dynamics of the circulation. His method consisted in applying the principle of the pressure gauge or manometer to living things. By tying tubes into the arteries and veins of animals he was able to record and measure the blood-pressure. He thus laid the foundation of an important mode of studying and diagnosing disease. He extended his exact investigations into most of the mechanical aspects of the circulation. He computed the circulation rate, and he estimated the actual velocity of the blood in veins, arteries, and capillary vessels. He made a very important contribution by showing that the capillary vessels are liable to constriction and dilatation, a knowledge that has since become not only important for physiological theory but of primary significance to the practising physician (p. 559). He began to explore the wonderful mechanism of the heart, by which that organ adjusts itself to its output needs. He exhibited his versatility by important contributions to many other subjects, as for instance his discoveries on respiration, his campaign for temperance, and his improvements in ventilation in ships and prisons. The old prison of Newgate was about to be demolished because of the high incidence in it of jail-fever (typhus). Hales attempted to save the prison from destruction by designing for it a roof-ventilator of the windmill type, with a ventilating shaft and ducts (Fig. 62). This experiment, however, was only partially successful. The work of Hales on the circulation is contained in the second volume (1733) of his *Statical Essays*.

In the meantime considerable progress was made in the knowledge of the digestive processes. The naturalist René Antoine Ferchault de Réaumur (1683–1757), best remembered for his thermometer (1731) and for his superb work on insects (1734–42), made a series of experiments on gastric digestion in birds (1752). By an ingenious contrivance he succeeded in obtaining gastric juice in a pure state. He was able to demonstrate its power to dissolve food substances in a test-tube kept at body temperature. This was important, since many believed that the process of solution was the result of a churning action induced mechanically by the muscles of the stomach-wall. Réaumur thus gave the death-blow to the iatrophysical conception of digestion (p. 141).

The investigation of gastric digestion was further pursued by a versatile Italian, the Abbate Lazaro Spallanzani (1729–99), who

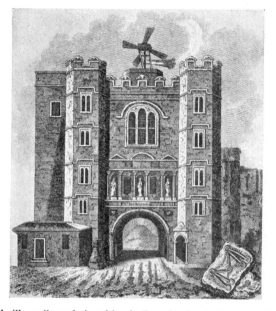

FIG. 62. Windmill ventilator designed by the Rev. Stephen Hales. Erected in 1752, by order of the Aldermen of the City of London on the roof of Dick Whittington's Gate at Newgate Prison
(From a line-engraving in the British Museum)

showed that the churning action is an aid, but not an essential, to the process of digestion (1782). He proved that digestion was not of the nature of putrefaction and differed essentially from the fermentation of wine. Spallanzani thus improved on the view of Sylvius (p. 143), and took a step towards that solution of the natures of putrefaction, fermentation, and digestion which was finally provided by Pasteur (p. 330). He showed that the gastric juice was secreted by the stomach itself, and not introduced into it from other organs. A suspicion that the gastric juice contained a free acid crossed his mind. He observed that it curdled milk and so began our knowledge of a separate ferment, that of rennet. Spallanzani's results may be summarized by saying that he showed that gastric juice had a solvent power *sui generis*, and that this power or faculty was of a different order from putrefaction or vinous fermentation. The phase of digestive physiology represented by Réaumur and

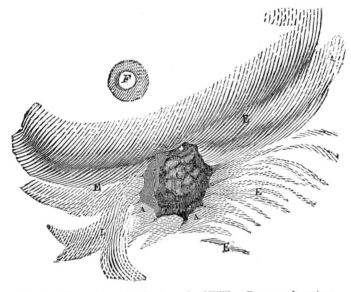

FIG. 63. The opening into the stomach of William Beaumont's patient (W. Beaumont, *Experiments and Observations on the Gastric Juice*, Plattsburg, U.S.A., 1833)

Spallanzani was brought to a close by the English physician William Prout (1785–1850), who demonstrated in 1824 the existence of free hydrochloric acid in the stomach. He showed that the presence of this acid was necessary for gastric digestion, but that the actual process of digestion of food was the work of another agent. The matter was at last brought into the range of medical practice by an American army surgeon, William Beaumont (1785–1853), who, in the ten years ending 1833, had the opportunity to investigate gastric juice in a man who, having been shot in the stomach, had a permanent fistula. Through this the juice could be obtained and the lining membrane of the stomach examined at will. In this way

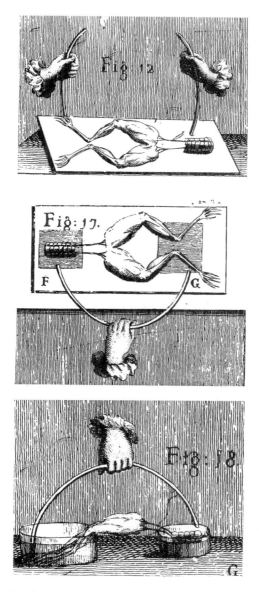

FIG. 64. Galvani's experiments on 'animal electricity'
(Galvani, *De viribus electricitatis*, Modena, 1792)

Beaumont studied the movements of the stomach, and the variations in the flow of gastric juice under various conditions (Fig. 63).

An important new branch of physiology was initiated by the
extension of the knowledge of electric phenomena to the living
body. Static electricity had been studied since the beginning of the
seventeenth century. Luigi Galvani (1737–98) of Bologna, while
investigating the susceptibility of nerves to irritation, showed that
nervous action could be induced by electrical phenomena (1791).
He was, as a matter of fact, producing an electric current. Galvani
discovered the phenomenon while working with a frog nerve-muscle
preparation, and three of his experiments are shown in Fig. 64. The
upper drawing (12) shows two rods of brass and silver respectively,
one of which is in contact with the frog's foot and the other with its
spinal cord. When the free ends of the rods are brought together,
contraction of the leg muscles results. In the middle and lower drawings a single bent rod is used to complete the circuit. In the middle
drawing (17) spinal cord and legs rest respectively on squares of
brass and copper foil. In order to produce a contraction it is only
necessary for the ends of the rod to touch these pieces of foil simultaneously. In the lower drawing (18) a similar result is obtained by
using two liquids in which the legs and cord are respectively immersed. In these experiments he generally obtained stronger contractions when two different metals were used. Many thought at the
time that a new kind of 'animal electricity' had been produced and
they dubbed it 'galvanism'. But this view was disproved by Alessandro Volta (1745–1827) of Pavia, deviser of the voltaic pile, who
had for long been experimenting with electricity. He was able to
demonstrate (1800) that galvanism is without any essential animal
relationship, and showed that a muscle can be thrown into continuous contraction by repeated electrical stimulation. Some of his apparatus, by which he established the principle of the voltaic pile, are
illustrated here. In the top row of Fig. 65 is seen the *couronne de
tasses*. A series of vessels contain salt water, and each contains also
a plate of silver A and of zinc Z. Strips of metal *aaaa* connect the
zinc and silver plates as shown. If the first and the last vessels are
similarly connected, a current flows from one to the other. The left
figure in the middle row of Fig. 65 shows a simple pile, consisting

of alternate disks of silver and zinc, adjoining pairs being separated
by disks of wet leather. The lowest disk is connected by a metal

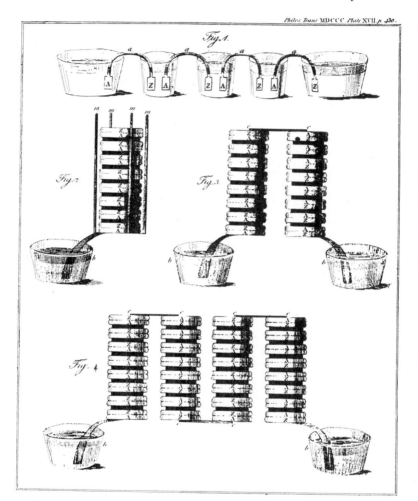

FIG. 65. The origin of the voltaic pile. Four of Volta's experiments
(A. Volta, *Phil. Trans. Roy. Soc.*, 1800)

strip to a vessel containing salt water. If the upper disk is then connected to the vessel, a current flows from disk to vessel. The right
figure in the middle row shows a similar arrangement consisting of

two piles connected by a metal plate *cc*. If the vessels *bb* are connected, a current will flow from one to the other. The bottom row shows a further extension of the principle of connecting cells in series. These simple experiments were the origin of voltaic electricity.

Humbug and misunderstanding in connexion with the electrical relations of living tissues were rife, and it was not till after the period we are now considering that electricity came to take a place in rational medicine. The change came with Emil Du Bois Reymond (p. 289), who in 1843 and the following years took the matter up scientifically. He showed that the nervous impulse is accompanied by local differences in electrical potential, and that this effect passes along the nerve from segment to segment in the form of a wave, the velocity of which was subsequently measured by Helmholtz (p. 289). It should be added that, despite all the work since done upon the nervous system, this is still the only physical accompaniment of a nerve impulse that has been detected.

DISCOVERY OF THE NATURE OF THE AIR

The seventeenth century saw advances in our knowledge of the air. In 1654 Boyle (p. 136) had shown by means of his air-pump that air was a material substance and could be weighed. By exhausting the air from a vessel in which an animal had been placed, he showed that it was this material substance and no ether, spirit, or other mysterious entity which supported respiration. In 1668 Mayow (p. 136) demonstrated clearly that a part only of the air was necessary for life, and later that this same part was removed both by respiration and combustion. The apparatus used by Mayow for two of his experiments on combustion is illustrated in Fig. 66a. In one of these experiments a lighted candle was fixed to the bottom of the outer vessel containing water. A large cupping-glass (i.e. a small flask) was then inverted over the candle and was pushed down into the water. In order that the water levels inside and outside the flask should be the same, one limb of a glass U-tube was inserted into the flask, and was pushed down with the flask into the water; air escaped from the outside limb of the U-tube, the water-levels were equalized, and the tube was at once withdrawn. The U-tube was not used to withdraw air for testing, and Mayow has no claim to be the discoverer of the methods of 'pneumatic chemistry'. After the withdrawal of the U-tube the candle continued to burn, and as it burned the water slowly rose inside the flask. But after a time the candle went out. Mayow showed that the water-level at which the candle ceased to burn was always approximately the same.

The same apparatus also served for an experiment in which combustible material (tinder, sulphur, and camphor) supported on a

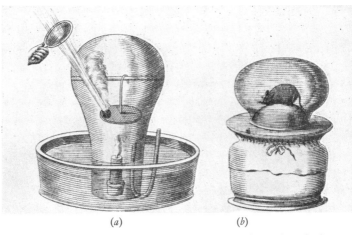

(a)   (b)

FIG. 66. Two of Mayow's experiments on combustion and respiration
(J. Mayow, *Tractatus quinque*, London, 1674)

shelf in the inverted flask was ignited by a burning-glass outside the flask. In this case there was an initial expansion of the air in the flask owing to the heat produced by the combustion. But the flame in due course burned itself out, and, when the apparatus had cooled, a rise in the water-level was observed similar to that in the candle experiment.

One of Mayow's experiments on respiration is shown in Fig. 66b. A moistened bladder was stretched over the mouth of a glass jar and tied tightly to it. A smaller jar, containing a mouse, was then inverted over the bladder. As the animal breathed the upper jar adhered to the bladder; and as more of the contained air was used up by the animal, the bladder was gradually sucked up into the upper vessel. Although Mayow appreciated that some essential constituent of the air was used up in combustion and respiration, he thought it consisted of hypothetical particles which he termed 'nitro-aerial'. He had no idea that it was a gas and that it could be isolated. The great theorists, Stahl, Boerhaave, and Haller, did not appreciate the signifiance of Mayow's experiments, and Stahl's doctrine of phlogiston put the clock back. No advance was made till the work of Joseph Black (1728–99), which appeared soon after the middle of the eighteenth century.

Black was a cautious investigator and his success was due to the accuracy of his measurements. He was aware of the fact that chalk, when heated, is transformed into quicklime (equation 1, below), thereby losing its power of effervescing with acids, but gaining the power of absorbing water (equation 2). In modern nomenclature, the changes are:

$$(1) \quad CaCO_3 = CaO + CO_2$$
$$(2) \quad CaO + H_2O = Ca(OH)_2$$

The first achievement of Black was to show that in the process of heating the chalk lost weight (equation 1). Black now showed that if slaked lime is treated with a mild alkali, such as the carbonate of sodium, it is changed back to the state in which it was before heating, in fact into chalk, while the mild alkali is converted into a caustic alkali. As we now express it:

$$(3) \quad Ca(OH)_2 + Na_2CO_3 = CaCO_3 + 2NaOH$$

Black's triumph consisted essentially in showing that the reactions were reversible, and that thus the same amount of $CaCO_3$ could always be extracted from (3) as was put into (1). Moreover, he showed that a definite amount of chalk, whether or not heated to produce quicklime, neutralized the same weight of acid; the only difference was that the neutralization took place with effervescence and loss of weight if the chalk was unheated, and without effervescence or loss of weight if the chalk was first heated into quicklime. Thus:

$$(4) \quad \textit{Unheated} \quad CaCO_3 + 2HCl = CaCl_2 + H_2O + CO_2$$
$$(5) \quad \textit{Heated} \quad CaO + 2HCl = CaCl_2 + H_2O$$

The substance given off by the chalk in (1), absorbed by it in (3), and produced by the reaction (4), he named 'fixed air'. We now call it carbon dioxide. The conversion of caustic lime into ordinary chalk by exposure, $CaO + CO_2 = CaCO_3$, proves that carbon dioxide is a normal constituent of the atmosphere. Black learned something of its properties, and his work is also of very great importance as the first detailed quantitative study of a chemical reaction and its reversal. The properties of carbon dioxide were further investigated in 1766 by Henry Cavendish (1731–1810).

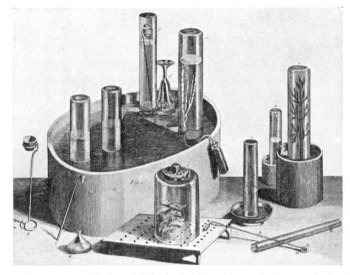

FIG. 67. Apparatus used by Joseph Priestley in his experiments in 'pneumatic chemistry' (Priestley, *Experiments and Observations on Different Kinds of Air*, vol. i, Birmingham, 1774)

The next advance in the chemistry of the air was made by the English Unitarian divine, Joseph Priestley (1733–1804). A series of important observations was made by him in the seventies and eighties of the eighteenth century. Priestley was the first to make full use of the methods of 'pneumatic chemistry', by which individual gases could be collected in vessels over water or mercury. In his illustration (Fig. 67) he shows the 'pneumatic trough'; it contained the water which provided the seal. At one end of the trough a shelf was fixed slightly below the surface of the water, so that a tube leading from a generating bottle could be passed into a cylinder of water standing on the shelf. In the illustration bubbles of a gas are seen ascending into a cylinder of water so placed and displacing the water from it. A combustible substance could be burned in a limited amount of a gas by placing it in a pot supported on a wire stand (5); this apparatus is shown inserted into a cylinder at *f*. Also standing on the shelf is an inverted beer-glass (*d*) in which there is a mouse. Priestley used mice for respiratory experiments, and he kept them in a special bell-jar with a perforated top (3). When the gas in one of his cylinders had to be kept for some time, he plunged a pot into the trough and slid the lower end of the cylinder into it; he then removed cylinder and pot together (2) from the trough.

When Priestley began his researches the number of known gases was three, namely, atmospheric ('common') air, 'fixed air', and 'inflammable air' (hydrogen). He discovered ten new gases, among which were ammonia, sulphur dioxide, carbon monoxide, hydrochloric acid gas, nitric and nitrous oxides, and sulphur dioxide. He showed that air which has been vitiated by the burning of substances or the respiration of animals can be restored by growing green plants in it. In 1771 he obtained from the heating of nitre a gas which he thought was common air, but which we now know was oxygen. In August 1774 Priestley prepared the gas again by heating *mercurius calcinatus per se* (mercuric oxide) and other substances, and he recognized that it differed from common air in that it was a much better supporter of combustion. He did not think that it could be breathed. It was not until 1 March 1775 that Priestley realized that his new 'air' ought to prove in respiration at least as good as common air. He realized also that he had isolated a new gas, and he subsequently regarded this date as that of the discovery of oxygen. Shortly afterwards he tried the gas on two mice and himself, and found that it was much better than common air. Misled by the phlogiston theory he then called it 'dephlogisticated air'. He suggested its use in medicine. Priestley showed that the difference between arterial and venous blood was due to this gas, but these conclusions were also negatived by the phlogiston theory.

Meanwhile the Swede Carl Wilhelm Scheele (1742–86) had been carrying out similar experiments quite independently. He had certainly discovered oxygen in 1771. He called it 'fire air'. But the book containing his account of the discovery was not sent to the printer until 1775, and was published two years later. Priestley's account of his independent discovery of oxygen, and of its great respirability, was communicated to the Royal Society in March 1775, and the credit for the discovery is his by priority of publication. Like Priestley, Scheele was unable, because of his allegiance to the phlogiston theory, to appreciate the true implications of his discovery.

The real passage to the modern point of view in our knowledge of the air was made by the brilliant French chemist Antoine Laurent Lavoisier (1743–94). While Priestley was making his brilliant discoveries of new gases, Lavoisier was carrying out an extensive planned quantitative study of the mechanism of combustion and calcination. By 1773 he had shown that calcination does not continue indefinitely in a closed vessel, and that the process consists essentially of a union between the metal and the air. He had also shown that in the combustion of phosphorus a combination takes place between the phosphorus and the air, or with some gas contained in a certain proportion in ordinary air, and he suspected that this gas might be 'fixed air'. In October 1774 Priestley himself told Lavoisier of his preparation of the gas which he later named 'dephlogisticated air', and Lavoisier at once appreciated that this was the clue which he needed. He repeated Priestley's experiments, and by 1777 he was convinced that common air consists of 'eminently respirable air' and an inert gas. On the basis of his theory of combustion and calcination Lavoisier now proceeded to transform the science of chemistry. In 1887 he revolutionized chemical nomenclature, and two years later he published his *Traité élémentaire de chemie* ('Elementary treatise on chemistry'), in which the approach and the treatment are completely modern.

Lavoisier has no place in the actual discovery of oxygen; but, once he had learned of its discovery, he was able, by brilliant theory and inspired practical work, to explain its properties and to cast off the dead hand of the phlogiston theory. Twelve years after its discovery he called the new gas 'oxygen'.

Soon after the discovery of oxygen Lavoisier adopted the hypothesis that in the lungs there takes place a process of slow combustion. By a series of ingenious experiments, in which an ice calorimeter devised in collaboration with Pierre Simon Laplace (1749–1827)

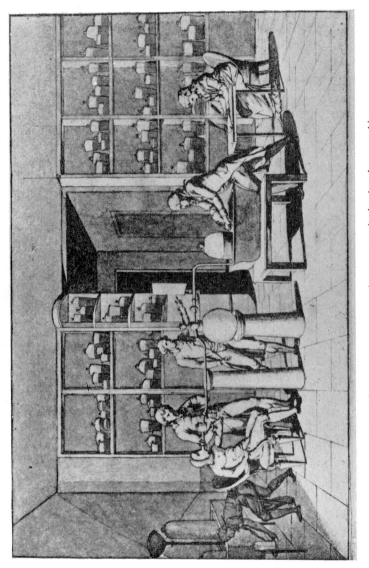

FIG. 68. Lavoisier carrying out an experiment on respiration in a human subject

(After Madame Lavoisier's original drawing in the Bibliothèque de l'Arsenal, Paris)

played an important part, he showed that in a small animal there is a quantitative relation between the amounts of heat and of carbon dioxide produced in its body. He later applied similar methods to a study of respiration in the human subject. One of these experiments is shown in Fig. 68 from a drawing by Mme Lavoisier. The subject is seen breathing oxygen through a mask which is fixed to his face, and his pulse-rate is being counted. Lavoisier himself directs the experiment, and Mme Lavoisier is seen taking notes. As a result of these experiments Lavoisier ascertained the amount of oxygen used per hour by a fasting man at rest. He showed that this amount was increased when the atmospheric temperature was lowered, and increased still further when the subject was digesting food. When heavy muscular work was done during the process of digestion, the subject's oxygen consumption was multiplied several times. Lavoisier therefore recognized very clearly that the amount of oxygen absorbed depends on the three factors, temperature, digestion, and work. He was the pioneer of all quantitative studies of human metabolism.

Lavoisier concluded that water and carbon dioxide are produced by the process of oxidation in the lungs, and that this slow combustion maintains, and is the cause of, body heat. We now know that the oxidation takes place in the blood and tissues, and not only in the lungs, and later research has shown that the processes involved are not as simple as Lavoisier imagined.

MORBID ANATOMY BECOMES A SCIENCE

The main intellectual movement of the seventeenth and eighteenth centuries had been focused, so far as medicine was concerned, on the manner of working of the animal body, the science that we now term physiology. It was necessary to obtain clear concepts of the action of the body in health before venturing into discussion of its action in disease. In 1679 Théophile Bonet (1620–89) had published a work in which he included descriptions of about 3,000 post-mortem examinations drawn from the writings of physicians from the earliest times, together with some personal observations. During the first part of the eighteenth century many practitioners in

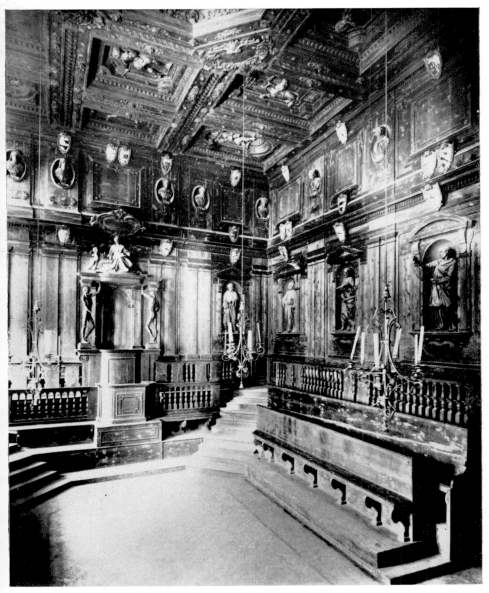

XV. ANATOMICAL THEATRE AT BOLOGNA

Constructed *c*. 1650, this theatre was extensively damaged during the Second World War, and is now being restored.

(Photograph by Emilia, Bologna, *c*. 1910)

(*See p.* 169)

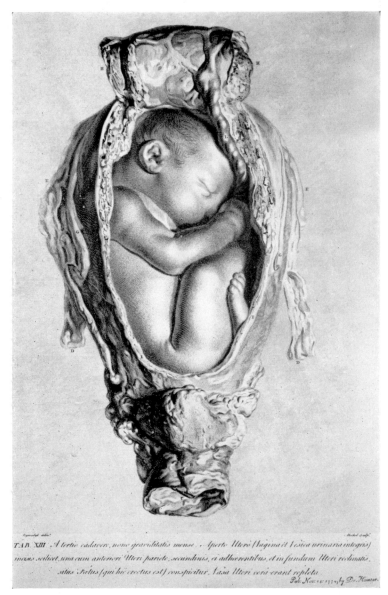

TAB. XIII. A tertio cadavere, nono graviditatis mense. Aperto Utero (Vagina et Vesica urinaria integris) meatus scilicet, una cum anteriori Uteri pariete, secundinis, ei adhaerentibus, et in fundum Uteri reclinatis, situs Foetus (qui hic erectus est) conspicitur. Vasa Uteri cera erant repleta.

Pub. Nov. 1, 1774, by Dr. Hunter.

XVI. THE GRAVID UTERUS IN THE NINTH MONTH
(William Hunter, *The Anatomy of the Human Gravid Uterus*, Birmingham, 1774.
Copy in the Wellcome Historical Medical Library)
(*See p.* 177)

physic and in surgery published isolated cases or groups of cases connected with particular diseases. Boerhaave regularly attended post-mortem examinations (p. 149). No general pathological principles had, however, yet been elicited on a scientific basis. The theories of disease, such as those of Boerhaave, were perforce still mainly speculative, for there were no extensive records of the correlation of symptoms during life with the appearances of the organs of the body after death, the subject we now call morbid anatomy. This gap was first effectively bridged by Giovanni Battista Morgagni (1682–1771) who studied and taught anatomy in the magnificent anatomical theatre at Bologna (Plate XV).

Morgagni was appointed professor of anatomy at Padua in 1715, and he held that chair for fifty-six years. During this time he performed an enormous number of post-mortem examinations, and made important contributions to descriptive anatomy. In his seventy-ninth year, eleven years before his death, there emerged from his vast experience his work *De sedibus et causis morborum* ('On the sites and causes of diseases'). This classical treatise may still be read with profit. Its leading feature is the very careful way in which actual cases are recorded. The life-history of the patient, the history of his disease, the events in connexion with his final illness and death, are all recounted with detail and care. The condition of the organs at the post-mortem examination is minutely described, and an attempt is made to explain how the symptoms were the result of the lesions. Morgagni is justly said to have introduced the anatomical concept into the practice of medicine. This concept is one of the main elements in modern diagnosis, and a modern physician, in reflecting on a case, considers first whether he is able to express the symptoms in terms of the lesion. There are many lesions of great importance and frequent occurrence which Morgagni was the first to describe. Such, for example, are syphilitic tumours of the brain and tuberculosis of the kidney. Morgagni recognized that pneumonia is a type of solidification of the lung, and that where paralysis affects one side of the body only, the lesion is in the opposite side of the brain.

The task which Morgagni had undertaken was worthily continued by the Scot, Matthew Baillie (1761–1823), nephew, pupil, and heir of William Hunter (p. 176). Baillie was a successful London practitioner. He followed a new and convenient method in arranging his work according to organs instead of by symptoms, as Morgagni had done. Baillie performed post-mortem examinations on several men

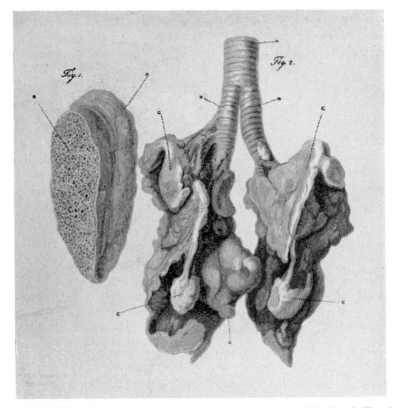

FIG. 69. Baillie's figures of emphysema (Fig. 1), and 'ossification of the lungs' (Fig. 2) (M. Baillie, Atlas to *The Morbid Anatomy* . . . *of the Human Body*, London, 1799–1802)

of eminence, among them Dr. Samuel Johnson, the lexicographer, who suffered from chronic emphysema, in which the air-cells in the lungs run together to form numerous tiny cavities, so that, as Baillie says, they come 'to resemble the air-cells of the lungs in amphibious animals' (cf. Fig. 48). The left-hand portion of Fig. 69 shows the cut surface of a lung from a case of emphysema in Baillie's own collection, and it may be the lung of Dr. Johnson. The 77 plates in the Atlas of Baillie's book (p. 629) were drawn by William Clift (1775–1849), John Hunter's loyal assistant who later became the first conservator of the Hunterian Museum.

The task of naked-eye pathological anatomy, brilliantly begun by Morgagni, was effectively completed by Karl von Rokitansky (1804–78) of Vienna. His most important book (1842–6) was based on an experience extending over 30,000 post-mortem examinations. Though disfigured by a bizarre theory, it left but few gaps for subsequent workers. From now on, the science of pathology was to be prosecuted in a new spirit and with new instruments. Even in his own day Rokitansky was something of an anachronism, with his pure naked-eye anatomy hardly ever involving experimental evidence on the one hand or the findings of the microscope on the other.

CLINICAL METHODS AND INSTRUMENTS

The great teachers of the earlier eighteenth century, though better equipped as regards knowledge than their predecessors, had hardly any better means of diagnosis. Pulse-measurers and thermo-meters, such as those of Sanctorius and Galileo (p. 116), had proved impracticable at the bedside. The microscope had not yet been used in clinical medicine. Chemical analysis as applied to disease had proved as yet of little value.

The first efficient instrument of precision to merit clinical adop-tion was invented by Sir John Floyer (1649–1734), an English provincial physician. It was introduced as early as 1707 as the 'Physician's Pulse Watch' and was an instrument constructed to go for exactly one minute. At that time the making of a twenty-four hours watch with a seconds-hand presented great mechanical difficulties. Floyer's invention was not widely adopted at the time. Attempts were also made to introduce a thermometer into practice, but again the construction of suitable instruments proved impossible.

Effective pulse watches and clinical thermometers did not pene-trate into the general practice of medicine till well into the nine-teenth century. Two instrumental advances of first-class importance to medicine were, however, introduced during the later eighteenth century. These were the methods of percussion, and of auscultation by means of the stethoscope.

Percussion of the surface of the body yields notes of varying degrees of resonance. Its application has proved of great value to the physician in outlining the position of the organs and of lesions, especially those of the chest. It was invented by Leopold Auenbrugger (1722–1809), a Viennese physician who first introduced it in 1761 in his small work *Inventum novum* ('A new invention'). Auenbrugger here described his method of direct percussion of the chest, and the conditions in which the 'morbid sound'—what the physician now calls dullness—was elicited. He confirmed his conclusions by post-mortem examination. Like the thermometer, his method was very slow in entering the general practice of medicine. His work was translated from the original Latin into French nine years after its first appearance, but it still attracted little attention. It was not until after 1808, when the *baron* Jean Nicolas Corvisart (1755–1821), physician to Napoleon I, made a new French translation with an extensive commentary based on his own experience, that the method came into common use.

Auenbrugger deserves great credit for his invention, but he did not work out its application with anything like the completeness that the Breton physician, René Théophile Hyacinthe Laennec (1781–1826), applied to his stethoscope (1819). Laennec's instrument was of the uni-tubular type that is now seldom seen. At first, indeed, he used a mere roll of paper. From this he evolved a wooden tube, about 9 inches long and 1½ inches in diameter. For convenience it was divided into two portions, one of which screwed into the other, and at one end there was also a removable chest-piece (Fig. 70). During the next sixty years many experiments were made on the design of the monaural stethoscope, and the tendency was to enlarge the diameter of the circular ear-piece, and to thin down the stem. Although some of these modifications improved the efficiency of the instrument, the monaural stethoscope always remained a personal tool, dependent for its results on the experience of the user. Towards the close of the nineteenth century the binaural stethoscope, with a rubber tube leading to each ear, came into general use.

But Laennec did far more than introduce a useful and convenient device into medicine. He explored with extraordinary skill the physical signs in the chest which correspond to a large number of diseases. Much of the technique of chest examination and of the

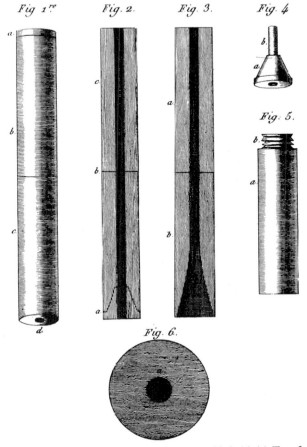

FIG. 70. Laennec's Stethoscope. (1) Instrument assembled. (2) (3) Two forms of the instrument in longitudinal section. (4) Detachable chest piece. (5) Ear piece unscrewed. (6) Transverse section.

(R. T. H. Laennec, *De l'auscultation médiate*, Paris, 1819)

terminology applied to the signs elicited come direct from him Despite continual bad health and the shortness of his life, Laennec's brilliance and devotion to duty at a hospital in Paris enabled him to transmit his views and methods to many other physicians, both

French and foreign. He is unquestionably among the greatest physicians of all time. Clinical medicine assumes with him a completely modern aspect. In reading his work one feels that, had he been called in consultation by a medical man of our own day, the two would have been able to understand each other perfectly, after only a little adjustment and explanation.

SURGERY AND OBSTETRICS

During the eighteenth century the improved knowledge of normal and pathological anatomy was a great aid to the surgeon. The technique of surgery was certainly improved. Operations were now being performed with success that could not before have been attempted. Nevertheless few important new principles were introduced until long after the nineteenth century had dawned. It is indeed probable that as a means of life-saving surgery had an almost inappreciable effect on vital statistics until the advent of anaesthesia and antiseptics. Even the greatest surgeon of the eighteenth century, John Hunter, introduced no fundamentally new surgical principles. True, the names of many surgeons of the period have become associated with operations invented or introduced by them, but it was not till after the advent of antiseptic methods that these were practised with full success. There are but two surgical matters in which advances of great significance can be said to have been made. These were obstetrics and the treatment of venereal disease, both of which were then dealt with by surgeons.

Syphilis, which existed in Europe in the later Middle Ages, had usually been confused with leprosy and other conditions (p. 106). Its treatment by mercury had been practised at least as early as the fifteenth century, perhaps as an inheritance from the Arabic-speaking physicians. During the sixteenth and seventeenth centuries various other remedies were tried (Fig. 42); much quackery arose around them. In the eighteenth century the accumulated experience of generations returned again to mercury. Satisfactory methods of administration were evolved and the treatment became standardized. It hardly changed until the twentieth century.

The treatment and care of women in labour made considerable progress during the period of which we are treating. We have seen how there were advances even during the sixteenth century (p. 96) by, among others, Ambroise Paré. Works on obstetrics intended for women were often printed in the sixteenth century in France, England, and Germany. Scientific obstetric works were produced

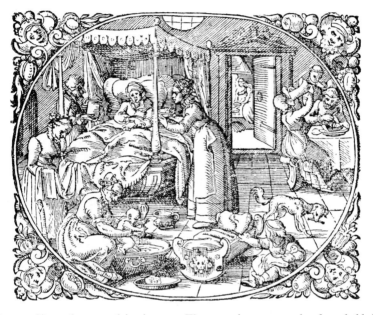

FIG. 71. Sixteenth-century lying-in scene. The room, in an upper-class household, is overcrowded, and the illustration suggests carousal, disorder, dirt, and ignorance of the principles of hygiene

(From a woodcut on the title-pages of early seventeenth-century Dutch editions of Jacob Rueff, *De conceptu et generatione hominis*)

especially in France in the second half of the seventeenth. But in the sixteenth century and much later these works contained little that was likely to influence the hygiene of labour. Even in well-to-do households the labour often took place in a room containing useless well-wishers (Fig. 71), and it was allowed to interfere as little as possible with the normal routine of the household. The obstetric instruments used were crude and cruel (Fig. 72), and some had been employed from ancient times. In a difficult labour the aim always was to save the mother, and infants were mercilessly sacrificed. The obstetric forceps were invented by Peter Chamberlen (died 1631) early in the seventeenth century. They remained a secret instrument in his family until about 1700. After that period 'men midwives' began to replace the ignorant female midwives, with a consequent decrease in mortality. William Smellie (1697–1763) was a very

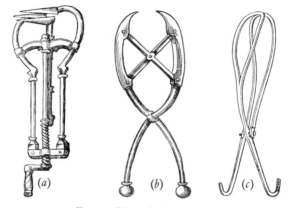

FIG. 72. Obstetric instruments

(a) *Speculum matricis*, to force open the mouth of the uterus in difficult labour (cf. Fig. 23).

(b) Apertorium, with sharp edges which tore open the mouth of the uterus.

(c) Obstetric forceps, seventeenth century, found in 1813 hidden under the floor of a house formerly occupied by one of the Chamberlen family.

successful London obstetrician and teacher. He introduced effective forceps, and practised efficient measures in placenta praevia and other abnormalities. Smellie's *Treatise on the Theory and Practice of Midwifery* (1752) was the first work to include satisfactory rules for the use of forceps and for distinguishing a contracted pelvis by measurement. It was followed by his *Anatomical Tables* (1754) which deal only with obstetrics. Smellie's pupil William Hunter (1718-83), brother of John Hunter, was the most successful obstetrician and the greatest anatomical teacher of his time in London. His private medical school in Great Windmill Street attracted students for years after his death. He also made a magnificent collection of books and manuscripts, coins, pictures, and anatomical and pathological specimens, which formed the nucleus of the Hunterian Museum and Library at Glasgow University. The preparation of his *Anatomy of the Gravid Uterus* (1774) occupied him for twenty-five years, and with its beautiful plates it remains one of the classics of book production (Plate XVI).

Two Continental obstetricians of this period are worthy of mention. François Mauriceau (1637–1709) of Paris published in 1668 his *Traité des maladies des femmes grosses et de celles qui sont accouchées* ('Treatise on the diseases of pregnant and lying-in women'), which was beautifully illustrated and remained a standard work for many years. Mauriceau overthrew the idea that the pelvic bones are separated in normal labour; he was the first to describe tubal pregnancy and epidemic puerperal fever. Important also was his Dutch contemporary Hendrik van Deventer (1651–1724), who wrote on the mechanics of child-birth and on deformities of the pelvis.

Despite the absence of any great new principle in the surgery of the period, there can be no doubt that a new spirit was introduced by John Hunter (1728–93). Ten years younger than his brother William, John had neither William's education nor his culture. Yet he had a driving force which carried him over many obstacles. At twenty he migrated from his native Lanarkshire to London to assist William in his dissections. Soon he was teaching anatomy, and this was followed by a distinguished career as a surgeon. Hunter did most of his operating and teaching in London, but a great deal of his research on comparative anatomy was carried out at his country house at Earl's Court (Fig. 73). Here he had a menagerie, and also a laboratory in which he was at work most mornings by 6 a.m.

John Hunter's complex and interesting character demands better treatment than it has yet received. As an investigator his powers were superb, but, like Leonardo, he was handicapped at every turn by literary incoherence. Nevertheless, with him surgery begins to appear at last as a real science and not as a mere applied art. Hunter brought to bear on the subject a mind stored with ideas drawn from comparative anatomy and pathology. Quick to detect analogy, shrewd in his scientific judgements, tireless and unsparing of himself in his pursuit of truth, a victim of disease self-inflicted in the service of science, to which he was tragically a martyr in his death, he shows as a heroic figure, rendered no less heroic by some very human failings. Fully to appreciate so incoherent a writer it is unfortunately necessary to wade through many works written in his own clumsy and ill-arranged manner. To gain any real idea of this great personality we must consult the writings of his contemporary colleagues.

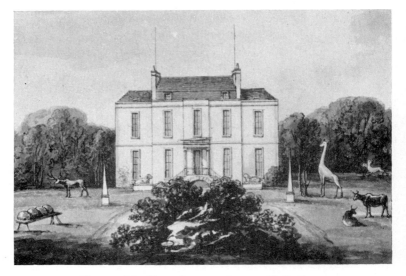

FIG. 73. John Hunter's country house at Earl's Court
(From the grangerized copy of Jesse Foot's *Life of John Hunter* in the
Wellcome Historical Medical Library)

So far as actual advances are concerned, two may be connected with Hunter's name. Firstly, in the treatment of the deadly condition known as aneurysm he introduced a method of operation which is still in vogue. Secondly, he enormously improved the method of making a medical museum. His monument is the Hunterian Museum at the Royal College of Surgeons in London, which was founded to display his 13,000 specimens. Unlike his brother's specimens which dealt mainly with human anatomy, John's collection of dissections covered much of the animal kingdom on a comparative basis. They were chosen and dissected by himself to illustrate the physiological processes of animals and man. Despite the irreparable losses which the College suffered as a result of enemy action in 1941, many of Hunter's original specimens can still be seen there. The museums of natural history, as now constituted in all civilized countries, have been influenced by, if they have not been derived from, that which he literally gave his life's blood to found. He was right when he said musingly in an illness, 'You will not easily find another John Hunter.'

One other British surgeon of this period should be mentioned. Percivall Pott (1714–88) was a surgeon to St. Bartholomew's Hospital in London. He was a brilliant operator and a prolific writer. He described a fracture-dislocation of both leg bones at the ankle (Pott's fracture, 1765), and it is said that a broken leg which he suffered as a result of a fall from his horse was of this type. Among the other conditions by which his name is perpetuated is the partial paralysis of the legs due to disease and curvature of the spine (Pott's disease, 1779). Three years later he recognized that the disease is associated with pulmonary tuberculosis, and we now know that it is essentially a tuberculous abscess affecting one or more vertebrae. Pott gave the first description of congenital hernia (1756), and of an occupational cancer—the cancer of the genital organs which occurred in chimney sweeps (1775).

THE BEGINNINGS OF THE SCIENCE OF VITAL STATISTICS

Attempts to combat widespread disease and to improve the public health are to be found in the history of all civilizations, both ancient and modern. Nevertheless, the rational method cannot come into operation until it has exact data upon which to work. Such data may be numerically expressed, a fact first appreciated by John Graunt (1620–74), the founder of vital statistics. The son of a London haberdasher, Graunt was at first an apprentice to his father, and by the time he was thirty he had much influence in the City of London. His help was then sought by Dr. (later Sir) William Petty (1623–87), who is known as the author of *Political Arithmetick* (1683) and as the father of the science of political economy. Petty had had an adventurous career in his youth, and he became deputy to the professor of anatomy at Oxford, whom he succeeded about the time when he first became associated with Graunt. Petty flourished and became the owner of estates in Ireland, while Graunt later fell on hard times. Perhaps for this reason Graunt's great work was long attributed to Petty, but this legend has now been exploded. They probably discussed the book together while it was being written, and Petty possibly himself believed that it was partly his own.

Graunt's book, *Natural and Political Observations upon the Bills of Mortality*, appeared in 1662. It was based on a series of weekly Bills, the records of individual deaths and their causes in the London area extending back to 1603. Graunt showed arithmetically that life in the country was more healthy than in the city. He also showed that, though there is a slight excess of male births, this is automatically balanced by a relatively higher mortality among male infants. He was fully aware of the imperfection of his materials, and on this account he urged the necessity of providing a system and a government department for the collection of accurate statistics.

Graunt was a Fellow of the Royal Society and other Fellows now began to take an interest in statistics. Chief among these was Edmund Halley (1656–1742), the astronomer. Towards the end of the century Halley produced a mass of statistics on the chances of death at various ages, designed for the estimation of the price of annuities (1693). During the eighteenth century numerous writers devoted themselves to similar investigations. An important contributor to the mathematical basis of vital statistics was the French Huguenot and friend of Newton, Abraham de Moivre (1667–1754). His *Doctrine of Chances* (1715) and his *Annuities upon Lives* (1725) are important contributions to the subject. His celebrated hypothesis that among a body of persons over a certain age the successive annual decreases by death may be considered as nearly equal (that is, that 'the decrements of life are in arithmetical progression') was under discussion for a century.

In 1761 Johann Peter Süssmilch (1707–67), produced an extraordinary theological work, *The Divine Ordinance manifested in the Human Race through Birth, Death, and Propagation*. Its object was to exhibit God's design in the constancy of the numerical relationships of vital statistics. Despite the motive—somewhat unpromising for a scientific treatise—the work is of great historic and scientific importance, for it was based upon a vast mass of statistics and showed a great advance in method. It stressed the importance of accurate data and the necessity for numerous observations if reliable conclusions were to be drawn. From the time of the publication of the work of Süssmilch the statistical study of population advanced rapidly. The basis of statistics was greatly improved by the introduction of the census system which was put into action in Great Britain in 1801 (pp. 712 ff.).

The science of vital statistics was founded by the Belgian astronomer Lambert Adolphe Jacques Quetelet (1796–1874). His early work, *On Man and the Development of his Faculties, or an Essay on Social Physics* (1835), contains an account of his statistical researches on the development of the physical and intellectual qualities of man and on the 'average man' both physically and intellectually considered. He followed this in 1846 by his *Letters on the Theory of Probabilities*, which is considered more fully later (p. 725). His conception, elaborated and further analysed, has formed the basis of all subsequent researches in vital statistics.

MILITARY, NAVAL, AND PRISON MEDICINE

The eighteenth century saw some of these principles put into practice. There was, as yet, but one section of public life in which scientific principles of preventive medicine could be applied. Only in the Army and the Navy were sufferers from disease under adequate control and observation, and only there were proper statistics of sickness and health available. Thus, some of the most important movements in preventive medicine during the eighteenth century, both in Great Britain and other countries, were initiated by naval and military surgeons.

Military surgeons had been known since ancient times, but it was only after the advent of firearms that wound surgery diverged from civil surgery and merited special treatises. The first vague mention of gun-shot wounds appears in a work on military surgery by Heinrich von Pfolspeundt (1460), a Bavarian surgeon. As his book remained in manuscript until it was published in the nineteenth century, its influence must have been limited. The first real treatise on the subject was the *Buch der Wund-Artzney* ('Book of wound surgery') by Hieronymus Brunschwig (1450–1533), published in

Strasbourg in 1497. This book was heavily illustrated with pictures of instruments and operations. Brunschwig took the view that all gun-shot wounds are poisoned, and he therefore advised the use of a seton—a silk cord pulled through the sinus in order to remove the powder—and the promotion of suppuration. Another famous work on the subject was the *Feldtbuch der Wundartzney* ('Field book of wound surgery', Strasbourg, 1517), by Hans von Gersdorff (*fl.* 1490–1520), who for forty years had been active mainly as a military surgeon. While he still advocated the cautery on occasion, his methods were more humane than those of his predecessors; he was inclined to use warm, not boiling, oil as a dressing, and to cover an amputation stump with a flap of skin and muscle. The great popularity of the cautery and the use of boiling oil in the treatment of wounds was really due to Giovanni da Vigo (John of Vigo) (1460–1520), whose surgical treatise entitled *Practica copiosa in arte chirurgica* ('A compendious practice of the art of surgery') was first published at Rome in 1514, went through more than forty editions in many languages, and had a very wide influence in its time.

The earliest work dealing exclusively with gun-shot wounds was that published in 1552 by Alfonso Ferri (1515–95). He favoured the conservative treatment of such wounds. Ferri noted correctly that pieces of clothing and armour left in the depths of the wound led to suppuration, and he advised their removal. The work of Ambroise Paré in this field (p. 97) was set out in his treatise on wounds made by arquebuses and other firearms (1545). Paré's counterpart in the English army of Henry VIII was Thomas Gale (1507–87), who wrote a book on gun-shot wounds (1563) which was not based largely on his own cases. Like Paré he considered that gunpowder was not poisonous, but his dressings were not as bland as those used by Paré. More notable among English surgeons was William Clowes (1544–1604) who served not only in the Army but also in the Navy. He was with Warwick's expedition to France and Leicester's to the Low Countries, and he served as a surgeon in the fleet which defeated the Spanish Armada. He was for many years a surgeon to St. Bartholomew's Hospital in London. Clowes's work on gun-shot wounds (*A Prooued Practise for all Young Chirurgians*, 1588) shows him to have been a careful and humane surgeon, well read in the surgical litera-

ture of his day. His Surgery contains the first description and illus-
tration of a military medical chest. The *Discourse of the whole Art of
Chyrurgerie* (1596) of the Scot Peter Lowe (1560–1610) contains the
first reference in English to ligation of the arteries in amputation.
Lowe founded the Royal Faculty of Physicians and Surgeons of
Glasgow (1599). On the Continent Wilhelm Fabry of Hilden
(Fabricius Hildanus) (1560–1634) introduced the now universal
method of amputation above the gangrenous area in a limb.

In the seventeenth century the best-known writers in this field
were Wiseman, Purmann, and Le Dran. Richard Wiseman (1622–76),
the greatest British surgeon of his time, served with the Royalist army
during the Civil War. He amputated the limb in the case of gun-shot
wounds of joints, and he gave the first description of the 'white
swellings' of joints caused by tuberculous disease. In his *Severall
Chirurgicall Treatises* (1676) he set out the fruits of his experience of
military as well as civil surgery. Matthäus Gottfried Purmann (1648–
1721) served for nine years in the army of the Elector of Brandenburg
and took part in two battles and many sieges. His numerous surgical
writings contain accounts of his daring operations, such as the removal of a bullet from the brain. The French representative, Henri
François Le Dran (1685–1770), saw service in the military hospitals
in Flanders, wrote a well-known book on military surgery (1737), and
became famous for his operation for the stone. Although he was not a
military surgeon, John Hunter (p. 177) used the experience gained
during his service in the army in the expedition to Belle Isle as a
basis for his *Treatise on the Blood, Inflammation, and Gun-shot
Wounds* (1794).

About this time it was appreciated that campaigns can be won by
preventing disease and by greater care for the health and welfare of
the common soldiers. Frederick William (1620–88), the Great
Elector of Brandenburg, improved the sanitary organization of his
armies, and also the pay and status of their medical personnel. Although van Swieten (p. 280) had no actual experience of military
matters, he wrote a work on the diseases met with in camps (1758); it
was translated into many languages and had much influence. From
these and other signs it is obvious that quiet reforms were in progress.

Among military medical reformers an important place is taken by a Scottish pupil of Boerhaave, Sir John Pringle (1707-82). He had a large military experience in the British Army, occupied a position of great influence, and was able to get many of his views and reforms generally accepted. Pringle was among the first to see the importance of ordinary putrefactive processes in the production of disease, and certainly the first to apply these principles in hospitals and camps. Important conclusions on these matters were published in his 'Experiments upon septic and antiseptic substances, with remarks relating to their use in the theory of medicine', which appeared in the *Philosophical Transactions* of the Royal Society in 1750. He identified jail-fever (typhus) with hospital fever. He laid down important rules for the hygiene of camps which involved the provision of adequate latrines and proper drainage, and the avoidance of marshes. His most permanent service was probably his suggestion that army hospitals should be regarded as neutral, and be mutually protected by belligerents. This great physician is a precursor of the 'new humanity' which came into public life in the early nineteenth century. In much of that movement one may feel the influence of that most humane of physicians, Hermann Boerhaave (p. 149). Pringle's observations on these subjects were collected and extended in his *Observations on the Diseases of the Army* (1752). This work is the beginning of modern military medicine. In the United States Benjamin Rush (p. 190) followed in Pringle's footsteps with a book entitled *Directions for preserving the Health of Soldiers* (1778) which was published officially.

Perhaps the greatest of all military surgeons was the *baron* Dominique Jean Larrey (1766-1842), who spent much of his life in the service of France and was Napoleon's personal surgeon. He was wounded three times in battle. Larrey tried refrigeration to dull the pain of amputations, and he introduced the 'flying ambulance', a light one-horse vehicle which could remove casualties quickly from quite near the fighting-line. Larrey's British counterpart is George James Guthrie (1785-1856), whose book *On Gun-shot Wounds of the Extremities* (1815) is based on his great experience in the Napoleonic Wars. The most outstanding general surgeon in France in the early nineteenth century was the *baron* Guillaume Dupuytren (1777-1835), whose work on the surgical treatment of aneurysm was outstanding,

and whose name is still remembered in connexion with a fracture of
the lower end of the arm, and with a peculiar contracture of the
fascia covering the palm of the hand. Dupuytren also wrote an ex-
haustive work (1834) on war wounds. In Germany the leading writer
on military surgery was Georg Friedrich Ludwig Stromeyer (p. 658);
his book on this subject was published in 1855. Stromeyer introduced the operation of cutting the tendon of Achilles for the cure of
club-foot, and he was one of the founders of orthopaedics as a
speciality. In the United States the most important work in the field
of military medicine was the book on gun-shot wounds of nerves
(1864) by Silas Weir Mitchell (1829–1914), who had served in the
Civil War; he became the greatest American neurologist of his time,
the author of important publications both in the physiological and
the clinical fields.

The first field dressing for use on the battlefield was introduced by
Johann Friedrich August von Esmarch (1823–1908) in 1869. The
work of Pringle and Larrey for the non-surgical welfare of the
wounded was carried to the end of its first stage by Jean Henri
Dunant (1828–1910). He was present at the battle of Solferino, and
his account of the sufferings of the wounded in that battle, *Un
souvenir de Solferino* (1862), led to the Geneva Convention of 1864
and the foundation of the Red Cross.

Naval medicine as a speciality became necessary as a result of the
change in the design of ships and the fact that long voyages became
possible. In the Mediterranean oared galley it was possible to mount
guns only fore and aft, and voyages lasted only a short time. With
the abolition of slavery in Europe, and the advent of sail and heavy
artillery, the aim of ship design was to mount as many guns as
possible on the sides of the ship. Hence the living quarters for the
crews became constricted, and the evils of lack of ventilation resulted.
The mariner's compass became a practical proposition about 1420,
and, mainly due to the efforts and encouragement of Prince Henry of
Portugal, the Navigator (1394–1460), it made possible the era of the
long voyages of exploration. Thus began also the era of the sea
diseases, scurvy, fevers, and fluxes (dysentery).

The first notable figure in naval medicine was William Gilbert
(1544–1603) of Colchester, the author of the celebrated work *De*

magnete (p. 112). When England was expecting the attack of the Spanish Armada Queen Elizabeth appointed a small commission of four well-known physicians, of whom Gilbert was one, to supervise the health of the men.

The first work dealing specifically with sea diseases and the cure of diseases and injuries at sea was *The Surgions Mate* (1617) by John Woodall (1556?–1643). Woodall was at first a military surgeon, and later he became Master of the Company of Barber-Surgeons, and surgeon to St. Bartholomew's Hospital. It is probable that he never served in the Royal Navy, but he made several long voyages with the ships of the East India Company. In 1612 he was appointed surgeon-general to that company, and in this capacity he was concerned with the appointment of the surgeons and surgeons' mates of the fleet. His book, a manual for the latter, deals with their duties, their instruments, and their drugs. The book treats not only of surgical conditions and operations, but also of the medical diseases of seamen.

The first work to deal exclusively with the medical aspects of sea diseases was *Nature and Cure of Distempers of Seafaring People* (1696) by William Cockburn (1669–1739). Cockburn was Physician to the Fleet of Sir Clowdisley Shovell in the Mediterranean (1704), and he spent much of his life as a professional medical officer in the Navy. His book was translated into several languages, and went through three editions. (In the third edition the alternative title *Sea Diseases* was prefixed to the title.) Although so widely used, Cockburn's book was not very sound, his comments on scurvy being especially uninspired.

Hardly less important than the work of Pringle for the Army was that of his brother Scot, James Lind (1716–94), for the Navy. Lind was a pupil's pupil of Boerhaave, and after serving his apprenticeship he became a naval surgeon. In a cruise which lasted ten weeks in 1746, no less than 80 men of the complement of 350 in Lind's ship suffered from scurvy. This disease was then a very grave problem at sea. Lind then spent ten years in civilian practice, during which period his first two books appeared. In 1758 he returned to the Navy as physician to Haslar Hospital, a post which he held for the rest of his life. In 1753 he published *A Treatise of the Scurvy*. In this important work he demonstrated how scurvy might be prevented by the adequate use of fresh fruit or, when this was not available, of lemon juice. Fresh water had always been a difficulty on sea voyages. Lind arranged for sea-water to be distilled for the purpose. He introduced rules for the prevention of typhus on ships, and made great improvements in naval hygiene. His *An Essay on the most effectual Means, of preserving the Health of Seamen* (1757) is a classic. He also wrote an important *Essay on Diseases incidental to Europeans in Hot Climates* (1768), which opened the campaign for the conquest of the tropics (p. 452).

Lind, like Pringle, is one of a type that is very fully represented in the eighteenth century. An excellent example of that school was Captain James Cook (1728–79), the explorer, who adopted Lind's principles. He established a record in one of his voyages to the South Seas. The voyage lasted three and a half years, and many hardships had to be endured, but out of 118 men only one died, and he was consumptive when he embarked in England.

Lind's work on the prevention of scurvy was never officially endorsed by the Admiralty during his lifetime. That reform was due to another Scotsman, Sir Gilbert Blane (1749–1834). Blane came to London and when he was thirty-one he was appointed Physician to Rodney's fleet. The result was his *Observations on the Diseases incident to Seamen* (1785). After twelve years as a physician to St. Thomas's Hospital, Blane was appointed Commissioner on the Board of Sick and Wounded Seamen. He then induced the Board of Admiralty to order the use of lemon juice and other fruits and vegetables as antiscorbutics in ships at sea (1796). The reforms jointly introduced by Lind and Blane included improvements in the hygiene and ventilation of the men's living quarters, the regular provision of clean clothing, and suitable measures to prevent newly pressed men from introducing typhus into ships' companies, together with a more rational diet.

Another Scot, Thomas Trotter (1761–1832), did much for the welfare of both officers and men. He was especially sound on the question of diet; he deplored the practice of reducing the purchases of the essential antiscorbutics in the seasons when they were expensive, and he took official action in this matter. Trotter's *Observations on the Scurvy* (1786) was a work of considerable importance which went into a third edition. His most comprehensive work was his *Medicina nautica*, published in three volumes (1797–1803), in which he reviewed the health of the Fleet during four critical years. Trotter was probably the first to introduce vaccination into the Navy. This was in 1798, the year in which Jenner (p. 202) published his discovery, and sixty years before the practice was made compulsory by the Admiralty.

The prevalence of scurvy was much reduced by the shortening of the duration of voyages on the advent of steam. After the Admiralty had officially endorsed the reforms of Lind and Blane, it was customary to depend on vinegar, sauerkraut, and other supposed antiscorbutics for prevention, and to reserve the supply of the 'rob' of lemons for actual cases. But during the nineteenth century outbreaks of scurvy in ships were still not infrequent. In some cases lime juice, which was more easily obtained, had been substituted for lemon juice. In 1918 it was shown by guinea-pig experiments that lime juice has no antiscorbutic effect, and its use in the Navy was discontinued. As a result of these outbreaks of scurvy in ships it was shown that the keeping powers of different samples of lemon juice vary. The causal factors involved in scurvy are complex.

Naval hospitals for sick and wounded seamen were first proposed by John Evelyn (1620–1706), the diarist, in 1666; he had Chatham especially in view, but the proposal did not receive the royal assent. In 1705 by a patent of William and Mary the partly rebuilt but still unfinished Greenwich Palace was granted for conversion into a hospital for seamen and naval pensioners. In 1869 the inmates were legally compelled to leave and the Hospital became the Royal Naval College. Assent was finally given to an Admiralty proposal of 1744 that three hospitals should be erected—at Chatham, Portsmouth, and Plymouth. The Royal Hospital at Haslar (Portsmouth) was built between 1754 and 1762. The Plymouth hospital, at Stonehouse, was erected between 1758 and 1762. James Lind was the physician to Haslar Hospital from 1758 to 1783, and he established there a great tradition of skilled treatment.

Comparable with the reforms effected by these men were the individual efforts of certain physicians to improve the towns in which they practised. As an example we select Manchester, which was greatly changed for the worse by the Industrial Revolution. Thomas Percival (1740–1804), a physician to the Manchester Infirmary, effected improvements in the Bills of Mortality for that city, and he attempted to have its population counted. He also campaigned for legislation to improve the working and living conditions of the cotton operatives. In 1792 Percival drew up a comprehensive scheme of medical conduct, part of which was designed especially for the medical staff of the Infirmary. It was distributed to his medical colleagues and discussed for ten years. In 1803 the revised work was published with the title *Medical Ethics*, and later there were two further editions. It remains a standard work on the subject.

A contemporary of Percival, John Ferriar (1761–1815), was also a physician to the Manchester Infirmary. He was active in attempts to improve the condition of the lodging-houses in which many of the cotton operatives lived. In 1789–90, and again in 1794, there were very severe outbreaks of typhus in Manchester, and Ferriar showed how the disease was kept alive because the patients were not removed from their surroundings. With the help of Percival and others he was able to have a number of fever wards ('houses of recovery' as they were euphemistically called) erected on ground belonging to the Infirmary. Forecasts that the disease would be further spread by these measures proved quite erroneous. It is interesting to note that, in order to enable steps to be taken to remove the patient to the fever ward, a notification fee of 'one or two shillings' was to be paid by the Infirmary physicians to the person who first gave information of the occurrence of typhus fever in a house situated in the Infirmary district. Rewards were also paid to the head of the family if he disinfected his house and the patient's clothes after the fever had subsided.

The eighteenth century was essentially a period of individual effort. The time was not yet ripe for public action on a large scale in matters of hygiene. Pringle, Lind, and Percival had, however, their humanitarian parallels among prison reformers. Scientific attempts to improve the ventilation and sanitation of prisons had been instituted by the Rev. Stephen Hales (pp. 155, 156). None brought greater devotion to the task than John Howard (1726–90), a native of London who spent his vigorous powers in investigating the prison system. His researches extended to the hospital, quarantine, and prison systems of France, Flanders, Holland, Germany, Italy (Fig. 77), Greece, and Turkey. His reports were directly instrumental in the improvement of the hygiene both of prisons and hospitals, as well as in the institution of special fever hospitals in many countries. Some aspects of Howard's work were carried on by the great Quaker philanthropist, Elizabeth Fry (1780–1845).

In his work Howard was helped by two celebrated physicians. John Fothergill (1712–80), a Quaker, made a large fortune as a London physician, and he used it in philanthropical works and to maintain a great garden at Upton in Essex. Here he cultivated all sorts of rare and valuable plants. Fothergill gave the first description of tic douloureux, and the first really accurate description of megrim (sick headache). His most important medical work was his *An Account of the Sore Throat attended with Ulcers* (1748). This work is a model of clinical description. Although there is some doubt regarding the actual condition described, it was probably what we now know as malignant scarlatina. Fothergill worked with Howard in the prisons, and the two men gave evidence before the House of Commons which led to the passing of the Act for preserving the health of prisoners in jail. They were also associated in an experiment designed to produce two penitentiary houses on a better system. John Coakley Lettsom (1744–1815), another Quaker physician, was also associated with Howard. As a young physician he became interested in the prevalence of typhus in debtors' prisons, and in the lack of medical treatment for sick prisoners. He was later a prominent supporter of vaccination. He is now best remembered as the virtual founder of the Medical Society of London.

The eighteenth-century humanitarian movement was active and had many able representatives in the United States. Foremost among them was Benjamin Franklin (1706–90), while in the ranks of medicine none takes a higher place than Benjamin Rush (1745–1813) of Philadelphia. Rush was particularly revolted by public punishments, to the abolition of which he devoted much energy. In matters of hygiene Rush was ahead of his time. He wrote on the hygiene of troops and laid special stress on fresh air and cleanliness of body and mind as an aid to health. He was peculiarly horrified and repelled by alcoholic intemperance, and he was responsible for the first systematic work on insanity published in America. He left a fine account of a yellow fever epidemic at Philadelphia, and he approached the truth in his view that the disease arose in Philadelphia itself and was not brought in as an infection from without.

THE INDUSTRIAL REVOLUTION

During the eighteenth century the character of British civilization became modified by a factor which has since profoundly influenced all civilized countries. There was a rapid increase in the number and size of towns. The main cause of this was the transformation of industry by the use of mechanical power. The change that resulted in the life and outlook of the people was very profound. These changes and the causes that gave rise to them are usually spoken of as the Industrial Revolution. That revolution had effects that were both wider and deeper than followed any other such single upheaval in history. With the mechanical elements that were behind the Industrial Revolution, such as the improvements in transport, the invention of many industrial machines, the enclosure of common land, and the new position of agriculture, we are nor here directly concerned. What does affect our story is the increasing urbanization of the population, which began early in the century, increased rapidly soon after its middle, and has progressed continuously ever since. Together with this change in the distribution of the inhabitants, there occurred a progressive increase in the size of the population as a whole (Fig. 74). This increase showed itself clearly after 1740, and early in the nineteenth century the rate of increase was accelerated. These great changes in the population are discussed more fully later. In this matter Great Britain is but a type, for all other civilized countries followed in her wake, though at a somewhat later date.

Along with the growth of towns and the increased population there was an increased demand for food. The country became better cultivated and better drained, and there were many improvements in agriculture. Thus, certain diseases began to diminish, notably malaria, essentially a disease of undrained and ill-cultivated lands.

The conquest of this disease, as of typhus, was the work of the nineteenth century (pp. 454 ff.).

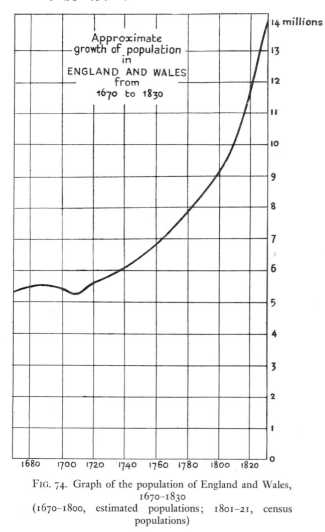

FIG. 74. Graph of the population of England and Wales,
1670–1830
(1670–1800, estimated populations; 1801–21, census
populations)

It is often assumed that the physical evils of life became accen-
tuated by the rise of the great towns. Nevertheless, investigation
shows that the opposite has been the case. During the eighteenth
century men and women began to crowd into the great towns from

the country. They were, in fact, right in their choice, for their chances of life there were greater than upon the land. In the rural districts infamous housing conditions, an overcrowding beyond anything which we now encounter, exposure to weather, uncertainty and fluctuation in the prices of commodities, low wages, inaccessibility of medical aids, and the fact that in winter the roads were impassable combined to render life, and especially child life, more precarious than in urban areas.

The improvement of hygienic conditions in the towns began in England soon after the middle of the eighteenth century. Westminster obtained an Improvement Act in 1762, Birmingham in 1765, the City of London in 1766, Manchester in 1776, and most of the other provincial towns soon followed. As a result of such Acts noisome streams which were but open drains were covered in, the streets were paved and lighted, and the sewers were improved. There were still many glaring defects of sanitation which have occupied and still occupy reformers, but certainly by the end of the century the general appearance of a street in one of the more advanced cities was much what it now is. The change from the primitive conditions of the century before was at least as great as the changes that have since taken place.

But if the streets had improved there was much under and around them which would horrify us now. Water-supply, as in London, was usually drawn mainly from surface wells and rivers. In most towns a continuous water-supply was unknown. Even when water mains existed, the supply to the houses was limited. Thus, even in the early nineteenth century London houses had a water-supply only three times a week, and then only for a few hours at a time. The water mains were often defective, and there was not always that clear distinction between a water main and a sewer that we now regard as desirable. Floods were a constant trouble in all riverside towns. Even in London cesspools were in use as late as the middle of the nineteenth century, and water-closets did not become general, even in the better houses, until about 1830. The methods of disposal of sewage hardly bear relation. In London the sewage simply polluted the rivers.

The improvement of such conditions as these could be made only by action on the part of the Central Government. The eighteenth century did well where individual activity was concerned. It was reserved for Southwood Smith (pp. 210 ff.) and Chadwick (pp. 209 ff.) to introduce into the sphere of practical political action the truth, set forth by Bentham (p. 208), that all factors which influence the health of the country must be the concern of the legislature.

We pass from this dark picture of urban life to the hospital and dispensary movement which took its rise about the middle of the century. Many of the great hospitals, both in England and in Continental countries, were either founded or rebuilt about this time. The London Hospital was rebuilt in 1752, St. Bartholomew's (Fig. 75) in 1730–53. Between 1700 and 1825 no less than 154 hospitals and dispensaries were founded in the British Isles. Though defective from the modern point of view, yet under the influence of the sanitary reformers, Hales (p. 155), Pringle (p. 184), Lind (p. 186), and Percival (p. 189), these were incomparably better equipped, better ventilated and better heated than such institutions would have been at the beginning of the eighteenth century. The notes of the industrious Howard (p. 189) give us a very complete picture of them, and one that is more favourable than might, perhaps, have been expected.

A defect of the hospitals of the time was certainly the nursing. This, however, did not apply to the lying-in hospitals, where the services of a better type of woman were available, and where ladies served on the committee of management. The general state of the hospitals remained much the same until transformed by the changes in surgery and nursing in the second half of the nineteenth century, though a number of special fever hospitals and pest-houses were established (Fig. 76).

Something must be said of the more prevalent diseases of the Industrial Revolution. Stress is often laid on the effect of urban conditions on child life. Yet there can be little doubt that historically the movement has been beneficial to it. This comes out well in the death-rates. Thus, in England, in the period around 1740, before the Industrial Revolution had begun, about 75 per cent. of children born died before the age of five. In the period around 1800, when the Industrial Revolution had set in, the percentage of deaths had

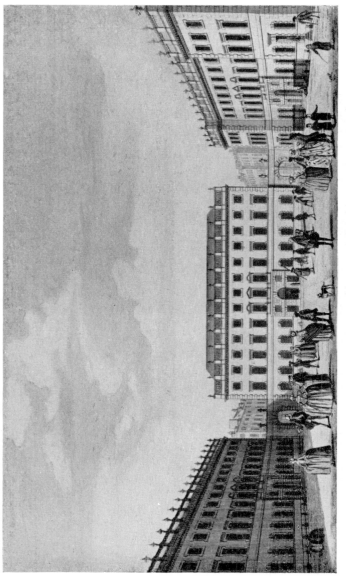

Fig. 75. St. Bartholomew's Hospital, Smithfield, towards the end of the rebuilding
(Line engraving published by T. Jefferys, 1752)

fallen to about 41. In the period 1950–5 it was about 3. Among the most characteristic diseases of children is rickets. It is very difficult to trace the early history of this disease, but its incidence seems to have been very high about 1700, and to have fallen progressively throughout the eighteenth century. This fall, it has been suggested,

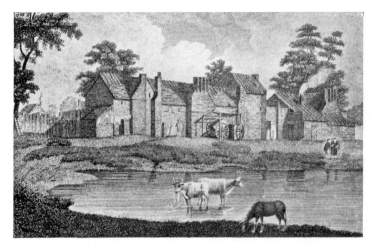

FIG. 76. The pest-house, Tothill Fields, London, in 1796
(From a print in the British Museum)

was due to agricultural improvements which led to better supplies of better-fed meat. It was these improvements and better supplies that, in their turn, made the big towns possible.

We have already spoken of scurvy in ships. It was, however, well known on land, especially in winter when green vegetables were not to be had. Lind (p. 186) found it common in the land population in the mid-eighteenth century. The advances in agriculture removed it altogether from the land diseases during the eighteenth century.

COMMUNAL DISEASE AND HYGIENE

In the eighteenth and early nineteenth centuries a few enlightened physicians were thinking of the diseases prevalent in certain places, or among certain groups of persons, with a view to their prevention. Giovanni Maria Lancisi (1654–1720), physician to the Pope and professor at the Sapienzia in Rome, had studied several outbreaks of malaria there. Then in 1717 he published a book entitled *De noxiis paludum effluviis* ('On the noxious effluvia of marshes'). The title stakes out his belief in the miasmatic theory; but despite this he already believed that malaria is transmitted, and he suggested the role of mosquitoes in transmitting. His book on sudden deaths (*De subitaneis mortibus*, 1707) is a careful pathological study in which he described the part played by cardiac dilatation and by vegetations on the valves. His work on aneurysms (1728) is also important.

A contemporary of Lancisi, Bernardino Ramazzini (1633–1714) of Modena, wrote the first treatise on occupational diseases. His *De morbis artificum diatriba* (1700) deals with about forty different trades, and many more were added in the supplement to the second edition. In the United Kingdom the mantle of Ramazzini was assumed after a long interval by Charles Turner Thackrah (1795–1833), the founder of the Leeds Medical School. His small book, *The Effects of Arts, Trades and Professions . . . on Health and Longevity*, was published in 1831. It caused sufficient interest to stimulate the author to produce a greatly enlarged second edition in the following year.

In the field of communal hygiene one name stands out above all others. This was Johann Peter Frank (1745–1821), who practised medicine in ten different cities in Germany, Austria, and Russia, besides holding chairs in five universities. From his student days he was determined to investigate the causes of diseases which act collectively on the general population. During much of his life he held appointments at the courts of German princes, and was thus able to influence the local regulations which governed the training and practice of doctors and midwives, and also the construction and administration of hospitals. He was for ten years professor of practical medicine at Pavia, where he reorganized the medical curriculum. At a later date he became head of the great General Hospital in Vienna, and professor in the University. Again he improved the hospital administration and extended the teaching.

Frank's greatest book is his *System einer vollständigen medicinischen Polizei*, the first volume of which was published in 1779 and the sixth in 1817. The translation 'A complete system of medical polity' probably expresses the meaning as well as any other. The phrase 'medical police' has often been used; but Frank had something broader in mind. It might be expressed as the enforcement of health by regulations derived from the state. He covers the whole life and activities of man from the cradle to the grave. The first volume dealt with reproduction, marriage, pregnancy, and childbirth; and he argued that persons suffering from dangerous hereditary diseases should be medically examined before being allowed to marry. The second volume dealt with child hygiene and with venereal disease and foundling hospitals. The third volume dealt with food, clothing, and housing; the fourth and fifth with accidents, crimes, and the disposal of the dead. The sixth volume discussed medical education and the influence of the practice of medicine on the welfare of the state.

Frank wrote in one volume that he had been in a position to test out many of his recommendations. Despite this, there is much in this vast work which is probably still untested. Frank lived before his time, and his book remains an inspiration for the future.

CONTROL AND RECOGNITION OF EPIDEMIC DISEASES

Over one branch of public health there was some state supervision during the eighteenth century. The ports were guarded against the introduction of epidemic diseases, and especially against plague. Throughout the eighteenth and early nineteenth centuries there was plague in the Near East, which extended at times to various parts of Europe. It was epidemic in Russia in 1709 and about 150,000 died of it. In 1719 it spread to eastern central Europe. One historic outbreak was at Marseilles and Toulon in 1720, when 90,000 died. The outbreak caused great alarm in Britain, but the disease did not reach this country, nor has there since been any outbreak here. Quarantine is now regarded as antiquated, vexatious, inhumane, expensive, and ineffectual. It seems probable, however, that during the eighteenth century, when drastically enforced, as in France during the Marseilles epidemic, it had indeed the effect of keeping the disease within bounds. Incidentally, it led to the foundation of many plague hospitals and lazarettos, of the conduct of some of which Howard (p. 189 and Fig. 77) speaks well.

During the eighteenth century smallpox was never absent from this country. From time to time the disease became epidemic, and there were many serious outbreaks. Thus, in 1774 there was an outbreak of smallpox at Chester. In 1775 an investigation was made of the degree to which the population had suffered. It was then

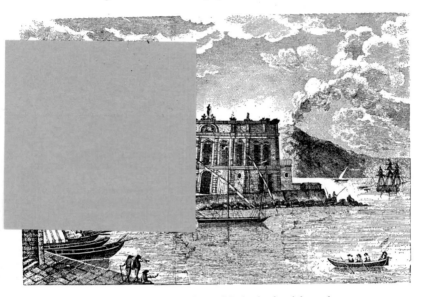

FIG. 77. The quarantine station at Naples in the eighteenth century
(J. Howard, *An Account of the Principal Lazarettos in Europe*, Warrington, 1789)

found that before the outbreak there were in Chester only 15 per cent. who had not already had the disease. The incidence on those unprotected by a previous attack was 53 per cent., with a death-rate of about 17 per cent. of those actually infected and of about 9 per cent. of the entire unprotected population.

With the likelihood of contracting smallpox before their eyes, men sought a way of getting it in a mild form. Outbreaks of smallpox varied greatly in virulence, and infection with a mild form would lead to protection from a graver one. In the East a method of direct inoculation of the disease from a patient suffering from a slight attack was widely in vogue from an early date. In the years 1713–16 two papers describing personal knowledge of the practice at

Constantinople were read before the Royal Society by Emmanuel Timoni (*fl.* 1713–21) and Giacomo Pylarini (1659–1718). The practice attracted little attention in Europe until Lady Mary Wortley Montagu (1689–1762) studied it at Constantinople. It was then soon taken up in England, and became recognized on the Continent.

The efforts of Lady Mary in England were reflected on the other side of the Atlantic. The famous Puritan leaders, Increase Mather (1639–1723) and Cotton Mather (1663–1728), turning from their exploits against the witches, ardently urged the operation. In England the learned Richard Mead (1673–1754), an eminent and far-seeing physician who exercised very great influence on the medical world in his day, published in 1747 a work in which he supported the practice of inoculation with all the weight of his authority. During the subsequent half-century the practice spread widely. The trifling operation was not without risk, for not infrequently it conveyed a grave form of smallpox which was sometimes fatal. To avoid these accidents some inoculators devised methods of still further reducing the severity of the inoculated disease. As a result it sometimes happened that a person who had been inoculated was exposed to infection from a smallpox patient and developed the natural disease. The operation was largely in the hands of specialists who were not always medical men.

Such was the state of affairs when the country practitioner Edward Jenner (1749–1823) came upon the scene. Jenner was born in the village of Berkeley in Gloucestershire, but he had been for three years the favourite house-pupil of John Hunter in London. There is no doubt that a successful career as a London physician or surgeon was open to him had he desired it. Instead he chose to return to practise in his native village. In certain country districts there was at that time a belief that those who had had cow-pox—a naturally occurring disease of the udders of cows—were protected against smallpox. About 1771 Jenner heard of this belief from a patient, while he was apprenticed to a country surgeon. He determined to put the matter to the test. The reasons which caused him to delay so long are beyond the scope of this book. It is sufficient to say that on 14 May 1796 he vaccinated a boy named James Phipps with lymph taken from the cow-pox vesicles on the finger of a dairymaid,

Sarah Nelmes (Fig. 78). Phipps developed a typical cow-pox pustule, familiar nowadays to most persons who have been vaccinated. On 1 July Jenner inoculated the boy with smallpox matter in the usual way. He did not develop smallpox. So far as it went, the evidence in this single case was complete. But many further experiments were necessary. After an interval Jenner proceeded to inoculate other persons with cow-pox matter taken from infected cows.

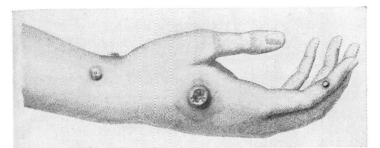

FIG. 78. Cow-pox contracted naturally from the udder of an infected cow. The hand of the dairy-maid, Sarah Nelmes, from which Jenner made his first vaccination (E. Jenner, *An Inquiry into the Causes and Effects of the Variolæ Vaccinæ*, London, 1798)

It is sometimes said that Jenner was not the discoverer of vaccination, since other persons had previously inoculated individuals with cow-pox matter taken from infected cows. This statement shows a complete misunderstanding of what constitutes 'vaccination' in the sense in which Jenner envisaged the procedure. It is a fact that a farmer had, years previously, inoculated his wife and sons in this way, and that they were subsequently shown to be protected against smallpox. There was nothing very original in such a procedure, and about that time others carried it out quite independently. But what Jenner had constantly desired was to stamp out smallpox everywhere, all over the world. But cow-pox is a disease which occurs only in certain districts and at intervals. It is in fact something of a rare disease. To serve his purpose Jenner had to have available, at any time and in any place, a stock of fresh cow-pox matter. If he could show that, when an individual had been inoculated with cow-pox matter taken from a cow, matter from this inoculated person could be used successfully to inoculate another individual, then part of his difficulty would be solved. But he then had to show that this matter could be passed in series through other individuals indefinitely, without the disease becoming so mild as to lose its power of protecting against smallpox.

After an interval Jenner proceeded in this manner, and he found that the disease *could* be passed on to other individuals. His experiments were limited by circumstances, but so far as they went they were conclusive. In July 1798 Jenner published his results in his famous book, *An Inquiry into the Causes and Effects of the Variolæ Vaccinæ*. Cow-pox is now technically known as 'vaccinia', and the process of inoculating it as *vaccination*. Within two years from its discovery the practice was spreading widely, and before Jenner's death it was known and practised in all civilized communities throughout the world. But from the start he also met with opposition in certain quarters, and this, though unfounded, persisted despite the fact that official investigations showed beyond doubt the great value of the procedure. Vaccination was introduced into the United States by Benjamin Waterhouse (1754–1846), the first professor of medicine at the new medical school at Harvard College. It was introduced to Italy and some other European countries by Luigi Sacco (1769–1836) of Milan, one of Jenner's staunchest supporters.

It so happened that the genius and persistence of Jenner triumphed in the case of a disease in which the action of the immunizing agents is so complex that even today it is not completely understood. Jenner has been unjustly criticized for his slowness; but the difficulties are perhaps most easily appreciated from the fact that it was over sixty years before any new work was done on the lines which he had so clearly indicated. Then commenced a vast train of new researches and new conceptions which ultimately established immunology as an dependent science.

Besides plague and smallpox many other epidemic diseases became more clearly understood during the period we are considering. Among these was scarlet fever, the history of which is particularly interesting for the variations which it has shown in virulence. The first clear description of a disease showing a rash resembling scarlet fever was given by Giovanni Filippo Ingrassia (1510–80) of

Palermo in 1553; in the same book he gave the first description of varicella (chicken-pox). Daniel Sennert (1572–1637), professor of medicine at Wittenberg, described an outbreak which occurred in that city in 1619; he was the first writer to mention the desquamation which follows the rash. The outbreak was severe, with a high mortality. Sennert's son-in-law, Michael Doering (?–1644), saw an epidemic of this disease in Warsaw in 1625, and his observations were published by Sennert. Doering was one of the first to notice complications in the joints and dropsy of the abdomen and limbs in scarlet fever. Forty years later there was another outbreak with a high mortality in Poland.

Up to the year 1683 scarlet fever was therefore well known in certain areas, but it was often confused with measles, and it still had no name. In that year Sydenham (p. 110) gave a not very adequate description of it in London, and he called it scarlatina, or scarlet fever. By then the disease was very mild, and Sydenham made no mention of the sore throat. Sydenham's younger contemporary Richard Morton (1637–98) published about this time his *Phthisiologia* (1689), in which he dealt comprehensively with pulmonary tuberculosis and showed that the formation of tubercles is a necessary part of the development of this lung disease, and also that the tubercles often heal spontaneously. Morton also noted the enlargement of the tracheal and bronchial glands in cases of pulmonary tuberculosis, but these observations remained for long unheeded. Morton now turned to scarlet fever (1694), and he described a malignant as well as a mild form of the disease; he also described the acute inflammation of the throat and complications which remained well known until recent times. But Morton erred in holding that scarlet fever was the same disease as measles, the only difference being in the type of the eruption.

There is evidence that in the first half of the eighteenth century sore throats accompanied by scarlatiniform rashes were becoming a serious medical problem. In such outbreaks as that described by Fothergill (p. 190) in 1748 it is probable that both scarlet fever and diphtheria were present. Then the severity of the outbreaks diminished until the end of the eighteenth century, when many outbreaks were of the virulent type. These outbreaks, and scarlatina itself, were carefully studied and described by Robert Willan (1757–1812), the founder of British dermatology, in his great work *On Cutaneous Diseases* (1808). His pupil Thomas Bateman (1778–1821), who was also an important writer on dermatology, kept records of the diseases prevalent in London between 1804 and 1816. By this time, although scarlatina was very prevalent, it was of a mild type. In Dublin there were large and very fatal outbreaks from 1801 to 1804, after which the disease was of a mild type until 1831. After 1837 scarlatina was of a severe and very grave type in Great Britain up to about 1875. A very high peak mortality was reached in 1863. Whole families were sometimes wiped out by it. About this time a future Archbishop of Canterbury lost five of his six children from it within a month. Since 1885 the virulence, though not necessarily the prevalence, of scarlet fever has steadily declined.

During the greatest part of its history scarlet fever has been very liable to be confused with diphtheria. The clinical distinction was first clearly made in 1826 by Pierre Bretonneau (1771–1862) of Tours, who gave diphtheria its present name. The same French physician performed the first successful tracheotomy in a case of diphtheria. He is also known for pioneer work in the recognition of typhoid fever.

Previous to Bretonneau the Devonshire physician John Huxham (1692–1768) published *A Dissertation on the malignant ulcerous Sore-throat* (1757), in which he clearly described diphtheria, including palatal paralysis, although he did not differentiate it from scarlet fever. In 1750 Huxham recognized in his *Essay on Fevers* that the lymphoid patches in the small intestine—first described by Johann Conrad Peyer (1653–1712) of Schaffhausen in 1677—were specially affected in typhoid fever. But neither Huxham nor Bretonneau clearly differentiated typhoid from typhus. In 1739 Huxham described Devonshire colic and associated it with the drinking of cider. Sir George Baker (1722–1809) asserted that the colic was due to lead poisoning caused by the lead then used in the cider-vats peculiar to Devon (1767). He proved the point by extracting lead from Devonshire cider and showed that it could not be extracted from cider made in other counties.

VII

PERIOD OF SCIENTIFIC SUBDIVISION

(from about 1825 onwards)

ORIGINS AND IMPLICATIONS OF SCIENTIFIC
SPECIALIZATION

WE have seen how the philosophy of Newton, with its implication, the Reign of Law, which is the Uniformity of Nature, has come to pervade scientific thought (pp. 145 ff.). Now, before Newton as after him, there were certain broad groups of scientific activity corresponding in some degree to the types and faculties of men. Since science first began there have been mathematicians, biologists, physical experimenters, because in fact the particular powers which enable a man to reach distinction in one of these sciences are of less value in the others. Until the period with which we will now deal, investigators were accustomed to explore at large within these great fields of knowledge. Such specialist professions as actuarial calculators, economic entomologists, physical chemists, or, in the field of medicine itself, medical statisticians, aural surgeons, immunologists—familiar to us now—were unknown and undreamt of then. This subdivision is a new thing, and is a characteristic product of the period of which we have now to treat. The subdivisions, unlike those of old, are largely artificial. Thus, the aural surgeon who deals with the organ of hearing cannot be separated clearly by his training, his powers and faculties, his operative skill, nor even perhaps by his field of work, from the stomatologist who deals with the mouth, or the rhinologist who deals with the nose. Nevertheless, these minute subdivisions are convenient and beneficent in medical as in other fields. The question of scientific specialization is so important and characteristic that we must examine it a little farther.

It is often thought that, since no man can compass all knowledge, this scientific subdivision is merely an attempt to master a part of that growing mass of knowledge which is becoming progressively less compassable in its entirety. The movement, however, both in origin and development, is less simple than this, for there never was a time when a man could know all that was known about his world. In this respect our own age is even as other ages. Were the view philosophically tenable—which it is not—that science becomes yearly less comprehensible, our outlook would be gloomy indeed. For since there is no evidence of any increase in the mental capacity of the human race—at least in historic time—such a view would imply a progressive diminution in the number of those competent to treat any wide scientific area, and a corresponding progressive separation from each other of minds with scientific insight. Fortunately such conditions do not prevail; the view that they do is simply due to a gross, yet widespread, misconception of the nature of science.

Equally fallacious is the idea, which has become diffused by the existence of scientific specialization itself, that the progress of any science is to be measured by the mass of observations that its followers have succeeded in accumulating. This is far from being the case. The advance of a science is measured by the degree with which it succeeds in bringing a multiplicity of observations under general laws. Judged by this standard, we should probably rate very highly, for example, the present state of what is called demography, the study of the life conditions of communities, while we should rank much less highly, for example, the present state of the study of aural surgery. Yet, for one publication on demography there must be many on aural surgery. In the one case, however, the accumulation of knowledge follows a well-directed and rational scheme. In the other it is prompted and occasioned by the immediate needs of individual sufferers. This must not be considered as derogatory to those whose task it is to treat the patients. The point is that the one activity, of its nature, exhibits the rational spirit better than does the other.

Since rational medicine is the subject that we treat here, we shall select for discussion those branches which best illustrate its spirit. This does not imply, and is not meant to imply, any belittlement of the less fortunate subjects. On the contrary, the less any branch of scientific activity has succeeded in eliciting general laws, the more necessary it is that those most capable of making such an advance should devote their attention to that field of work. It may, indeed, reasonably be urged that a leading defect in our scientific organization is that men of scientific insight crowd to just those studies where their special powers have already been best exhibited.

In previous chapters, dealing with more remote times, we have been able to place our facts in historic perspective. Despite the enormous mass of scientific literature dating from the seventeenth, eighteenth, and early nineteenth centuries, there is no real obstacle to selecting what is most important in it. True, it is beyond the power of any one student to examine all this literature at first hand, but it has been arranged and indexed, posterity has passed its verdict, and the historian can find his way through the thicket.

The face of affairs changes, however, when we pass into a period which differs for different topics, but may be roughly defined as beginning somewhere between about 1820 and about 1870. We then begin to encounter the very questions with which men of science are occupied in our own time. Since many of these questions still remain unsettled, it is impossible for the historian to say with certainty which are the most fruitful lines of work. The most he can hope to do is to distinguish the more influential and stimulating thinkers and observers from those who have been less so, and to say something about the ideas with which the more important schools of thought were instinct.

When we look into the origin of the system of specialization, whether in medicine or in any other branch of science, we shall find at work certain philosophical tendencies of which the modern man of science is the heir, though often the unconscious and sometimes the ungrateful and even the misunderstanding heir. Neither men of science nor medical men are always philosophers, or at least not always consciously so. Nevertheless, they are as surely influenced by the streams of thought of their time as they are by their heredity and their physical environment. The general tendencies of medicine in this or in any other age cannot be interpreted without some reference to the intellectual atmosphere in which it has arisen and in which it has flourished.

The intellectual atmosphere in which scientific specialism arose was that of the Utilitarian Philosophy. Many of the dicta of that school, which came into prominence toward the end of the eighteenth century, are still used as part of the language of men of science and others. 'The greatest happiness of the greatest number' is a formula launched upon our common speech by Joseph Priestley (p. 164). The pursuit of such idealized happiness as the main object of human activity is taught by the Utilitarian Philosophy, a phrase coined by the English political and social thinker, Jeremy Bentham (1748–1832). To Bentham, the founder of that philosophy, we owe such useful additions to our language as 'codification' and 'international', and these, together with 'utilitarian', give us some clue to the character and mode of his thought. It is probable that no thinker had a larger share than Bentham in ushering in the era of the subdivision of the sciences.

Bentham made a sustained attempt to draw a parallel between the physical and the social sciences, and this gave him a special influence over medical thinkers and especially over those who dealt with the public health. His pupil John Stuart Mill (1806–73) speaks of his master's mode of working as 'the chemical method'. It is thus not remarkable that Bentham should exert a great influence on medicine, both directly and indirectly. The peculiarly logical, uncompromising and perhaps un-English character of his mind, while it prevented him, fortunately for himself, from taking an active share in the task of government, did not prevent him from influencing those who did.

THE REVOLUTION IN PREVENTIVE MEDICINE

Of all the many changes in medicine and medical thought that the Period of Scientific Subdivision has witnessed, none have been more revolutionary than those in the field which deals with preventive medicine. Great and important reforms were introduced during the course of the eighteenth century. These, however, even when the result of legislation, were the outcome of the effort of individuals, or were concerned with the Army and the Navy In the period that follows, the public health becomes a general political, legislative, and administrative matter, and prevention becomes its watchword. The public consciousness—moralists will call it the public conscience—had been aroused, and has never again entirely slept. The chief agent in the awakening process, the intellectual force at its back, was Jeremy Bentham. If Bentham was the harbinger the alarm was sounded by the epidemic of cholera which reached these shores in 1831, and attained its peak in 1832, the year in which Bentham died. Cholera is a virulent infectious disease, often epidemic in the Orient. It had not previously been seen in western Europe. Before the epidemic subsided it had left a train of death in some of the large cities of the United Kingdom, and many small towns had also been affected. It was to return to these shores on three subsequent occasions.

Rational medicine has, in general, no national frontiers. To it men of all the national units have made important contributions. But the care of the public health in the period on which we now enter, being an affair of legislation and administration, has developed along national lines and it is difficult to discuss it save on a national basis. It is a source of justifiable national pride that the United Kingdom has, from the first and throughout, been the leader of the public health movement. But while we lose little and gain much by dealing with the British and American points of view, it has still to be remembered that, just as rational medicine has, fortunately, no spiritual frontiers, so, unfortunately, sickness and suffering have no physical frontiers. Epidemics pass the most scientifically constructed boundaries upon the surface of the map. In our time, this evident proposition has obtained, at least, formal recognition. International health legislation has now been established for over thirty years.

(a) Preventive Medicine in Great Britain

It is significant that the great public health movement which transformed the health of the inhabitants of this country in the second half of the nineteenth century, and the environment in which they lived, was associated in its beginnings with a reform of the Poor Law. It was due especially to the perspicacity, the administrative drive, and the meticulous collection of evidence on the part of a great civil servant, Sir Edwin Chadwick (1800–90).

Chadwick was a barrister and journalist by profession (though he never actually practised in court), and when he was reading for the bar he came within Bentham's circle and met Neil Arnott and

Southwood Smith, with both of whom he was to have much contact in later life. Neil Arnott (1788–1874) was an Aberdeen graduate in medicine who had travelled widely and, settling in London, became a successful physician. He was a popular lecturer on physics, the author of a well-known book on that subject, and the inventor of many devices for ameliorating the physical condition of humanity. Of these inventions the best known are his smokeless grate and the Arnott valve, an appliance for ventilating rooms. Arnott had wide interests, and he was one of the founders of the University of London.

Thomas Southwood Smith (1788–1861) long combined the office of Unitarian minister with that of physician. He settled in London in 1820 and came under the influence of Bentham. By his essay on *The Use of the Dead to the Living* (1824) he did something to remove the odium attached to dissection. The scandals of the time and the common sense of the Utilitarians (p. 207) led to the passing of the Anatomy Act of 1832. Thus by a proper legal process bodies became available for dissection by medical students. Bentham died just before this Act became law, and by his will he left his body to Southwood Smith to be the subject of dissection and of an anatomical lecture.

Southwood Smith's services to the spread of interest in public health were numerous. He published a simple and popular work entitled *The Philosophy of Health* (1835). He served on a central board of inquiry into the condition of children in factories (1832), and he was especially useful to the Poor Law Commissioners by reason of his exceptional knowledge of fevers. He was the founder of a Health of Towns Association (1840), and of another association for 'improving the Dwellings of the Industrial Classes' (1842). In 1848 he became a member of a new government department, the General Board of Health (p. 218). His official reports on quarantine (1845), cholera (1850), yellow fever (1852), and on the results of sanitary improvements (1854), were of world-wide utility.

Chadwick—who never held any medical qualification—was to be prominently associated with one other medical man. This was James Phillips Kay (later Sir James Phillips Kay-Shuttleworth) (1804–77), who graduated at Edinburgh and then became the medical officer to the Ancoats and Ardwick Dispensary in Manchester, an institution which he had been instrumental in founding. He was painfully aware of the insanitary conditions in which the poor of that city existed, and of the horrors which were brought to light by the cholera epidemic of 1832. In that year he published *The Moral and Physical Condition of the Working Classes employed in the Cotton Manufacture in Manchester*. His experiences in this slum area burned into him the conviction that it was futile to look to charity and medical skill alone to deal with social evils. As an Assistant Commissioner for the Poor Law Kay-Shuttleworth gave invaluable assistance in providing Chadwick with the fuel which he needed for his reports. Kay-Shuttleworth was appointed in 1839 as Assistant Secretary of the Education Committee of the Privy Council, and he became the pioneer in the training of teachers and was responsible for many other developments in education.

When Chadwick was twenty-eight he contributed, by invitation, to the *Westminster Review* an article which bore as an uninspiring title 'The Means of Insurance against Accidents'. In it he argued convincingly that the length of life had increased, and that by appropriate sanitation and hygiene it might be improved still more. It contained the germ of what Chadwick later called 'the sanitary idea'. The Benthamites were delighted. In the following year his article 'On a Preventive Police' embodied many of the doctrines which Bentham was advocating. Two years later Bentham invited Chadwick to make his house in Queen Square his home, and to act as his secretary and literary assistant. Chadwick accepted, but characteristically he turned down Bentham's offer of an annuity for life if he would devote himself solely to the propagation of Bentham's doctrines. As we have noted Bentham died in the following year, and at thirty-two Chadwick was still without a real profession.

At this time there was much dissatisfaction about the administration of the Poor Laws, and about the different standards on which relief was granted in the 15,000 virtually autonomous parishes which had the power of granting it. The Government appointed a Royal Commission to inquire into the problem, and Chadwick was asked to act as one of the Assistant Commissioners, who carried out the field investigations, and to examine the administration of the Acts in London. A preliminary report issued by the Commissioners (1833) showed that Chadwick was already master of the subject; and when the full *Report* of the Royal Commission was published (1834) that portion of Chadwick's evidence which was printed filled a folio volume. It was probably intentional on Chadwick's part that the portion which was printed did not show his knowledge and sympathies in their true light, and as a result his name has long been held in opprobrium in Poor Law circles, although he was the chief architect of a system which was unchanged for a century. But the recent examination—for the first time—of the vast mass of his un-published evidence has shown that even in 1834 he had a much deeper sense of the causes of pauperism than the later full report would lead us to suppose. He was obviously the only investigator in the inquiry to take account of the health of the pauper population. He understood the relationship between insanitary housing and excessive sickness, and significantly he considered that it might ultimately be a public economy to spend money on the dwellings of the poor.

As a result of the publication of the Report of the Royal Com-mission, a definitive Poor Law Commission, consisting of three paid Commissioners, was appointed. Chadwick, the one man who had really investigated the whole subject, both in the field and through reports from his delegates, was thunderstruck to find that he was not offered an appointment as a Commissioner. In a belated effort to rectify the harm which had been done by this omission, the Chan-cellor of the Exchequer appointed him Secretary to the Commission, with a private understanding that Chadwick would act as a 'fourth Commissioner'. This private arrangement does not seem to have been known to the other three, and years of friction ensued. During this period the Bill which became the Registration Act of 1836 was brought forward. It gave rise to great opposition from the Churches and other bodies. Chadwick was erroneously supposed to have been its author, and he was bitterly attacked. He did in fact support the Bill on every occasion, and it was mainly due to him that the Registration Districts were made coincident with the Poor Law Unions, and that not only the occurrence of a death but also its cause had to be registered. It was intended to make the post of Registrar General a political appointment, but it was Chadwick who ensured that the Registrar General would be assisted by someone who had genius and professional training—in other words, William Farr (p. 717).

As Secretary of the Poor Law Commission Chadwick was receiving reports from the unions which suggested that much of the poor relief actually granted was bound up with the prevalence of 'fever'—meaning mainly typhus fever—and that the incidence of this condition might be reduced by abating nuisances and improving dwellings. In fact, some unions had prosecuted landlords for failing to abate nuisances, and had charged the costs of prosecution to the poor rates; but the Government auditor had refused to sanction the charge on the ground that the Act only allowed expenditure on poor relief. In 1838 the typhus cases rose to a disgraceful peak, and Chadwick pointed out to the Commission that there was no limit to the amount of money which might be spent in relieving individual cases of fever unless the basic cause of the disease was removed. He therefore recommended a special investigation by Arnott, Kay(-Shuttleworth), and Southwood Smith into the causes of fever in certain areas of the metropolis.

The Commissioners agreed to these suggestions, and in May 1838 Kay and Arnott began their investigation among the poor of Wapping and Stepney, and Southwood Smith his in Whitechapel and Bethnal Green. Their reports were published in the Annual Report of the Commissioners for the same year. They suggested very definitely that the current view that pauperism was due to 'voluntary' causes—such as idleness, improvidence, and drunkenness—was wrong. On the contrary, much of it was probably due to causes which were beyond the control of the individuals concerned, such as ill health brought about by foul environmental conditions. Southwood Smith had investigated 27,000 pauper cases; of these 14,000 had been rendered destitute by fever and 13,000 had died. The Poor Law Commissioners, urged by Chadwick, made a recommendation to the Home Secretary that as a temporary measure the Boards of Guardians should be allowed to prosecute for the abatement of nuisances. But these powers would have widened the activities of the Poor Law Commission, which had already assumed responsibility for registration, and which was shortly to draw vaccination and education into its orbit. The Government appreciated the wide implications of any further powers which they might grant, and they hesitated. But in August 1839 the Bishop of London moved in the House of Lords that an inquiry should be made into the extent to which the causes of disease, which had been found by the three special investigators to prevail in the metropolis, prevailed also among the labouring population of the country as a whole. The Poor Law Commissioners were commanded to carry out this investigation, which resulted in Chadwick's masterly report on the subject.

Chadwick spent two years on his inquiries in the Provinces. At the beginning of this period he thought that the solution lay in improving the houses; but by the end of his inquiries he had placed the emphasis on external sanitation and on drainage. Before his report was finished an energetic member of parliament caused a Health of Towns Commission to be founded. Chadwick was not officially connected with this Commission, but he was its inspiration, and he had already examined most of the witnesses called before it. Chadwick's own document, the *Report on the Sanitary Conditions of the Labouring Population*, was to have been published under the name of the Poor Law Commissioners; but when they had perused it and seen how far he had gone in his advocacy of coercive measures—which would certainly conflict with many vested interests—in his attempt to stamp out the insanitary living conditions of the poor, they decided that they would indeed publish it, but that it would come out under Chadwick's own name. The report was published in 1842, and had an immediate and unprecedented success.

It is convenient to summarise at this point Chadwick's attitude to the problem of excessive disease among the poor. His consuming interest in the problem was, at this stage of his career, not humanitarian but practical. Could the cruel drain on the funds available for poor relief be diminished by preventing certain diseases, and if so, how? All the enlightened medical opinion of the time—the views, for example, of Arnott and Southwood Smith—favoured the 'pythogenic theory' of fevers. According to this theory a 'fever' was caused by the action of an unknown 'influence' (cf. influenza) in the atmosphere, present only at the time of the epidemic, upon the noxious exhalations given off by putrid animal or vegetable matter in ditches, stagnant drains, cesspools, middens, and in the houses themselves. We refer later (p. 729) to the long struggle between the miasmatists and the contagionists. At the time of the Sanitary Report the best medical opinion was in favour of this 'pythogenic' or miasmatic theory. Southwood Smith, one of the greatest authorities on fevers in the country and the author of a standard *Treatise on Fever* (1830), supported it whole-heartedly and discounted the theory of contagion. Under his influence Chadwick virtually discarded quarantine. It is easy to scoff today at these theories; but there are mitigating factors which are easily overlooked. Although some pathogenic organisms had been seen, none had been shown to be the cause of a specific disease. Further, the killing diseases with which Southwood Smith and his colleagues had to contend were frequently typhus fever or enteric fever, and in neither case was there any direct transmission by contact from the patient to the newly infected person. Holding these theories, Chadwick not only acted as if all 'smell' was disease, but even as if all disease was 'smell'.

The main recommendations made by Chadwick in the Sanitary Report and in the years immediately after 1842 were the following. Accummulations of refuse should be removed compulsorily. Night soil should be flushed into the drains and hence into sewers, and cesspools should be abolished. The sewers at that time were badly constructed and inadequately designed, so that noxious matter stagnated in them. The levels were sometimes such that, if much water was introduced into them, the contents flowed in the wrong direction back into the houses. Chadwick inspired revolutionary experiments on the design of sewers, and John Roe (1795–1874), the civil engineer who helped Chadwick much throughout his campaign, eventually devised a sewer which was egg-shaped in cross-section. Given a sufficient supply of water this sewer enabled its contents to be thoroughly flushed towards their destination. In these investigations Chadwick came into conflict with the Commissioners of Sewers, who were responsible for such matters. Further, the proper functioning of such sewers depended entirely on a constant supply of water for flushing. So also did the cleansing of the streets. During the cholera epidemic of 1832 in Exeter and other cities very special arrangements for the supply of water for short periods had to be made to flush the streets. In all towns during the mid-nineteenth century the water-supply of a large group of houses would be one well, or one stand-pipe, in the yard. The 'intermittent' system of supply was universal; the water was turned on for a few stated hours each day and was then cut off. For the efficient functioning of water-

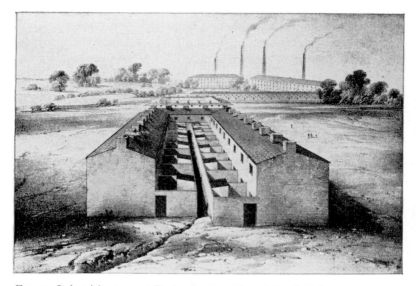

Fig. 79. Industrial cottages at Preston in 1844. The privies of all the cottages empty into the common open gully which runs between the two rows of cottages along the whole length of the block

(Evidence of the Rev. John Clay, *Health of Towns Commission, First Report*, vol. i, London, 1844)

closets, drains, and sewers, an adequate constant supply of water was necessary. Water was supplied by privately owned water companies, and Chadwick inevitably came into conflict with these. Further, consideration had to be given to the best means of disposing of the sewage and of the large quantities of water employed. This might affect an administrative area far removed from the area in which the sewage was generated. Apart altogether from the scientific and technical considerations involved, the administrative difficulties were very great. Chadwick appreciated that, in order to cut through the tangled web of local, private, and commercial interests, *all* matters affecting the health of the people would have to be controlled by one central authority. He was indeed a bold man who could launch such a revolution in early Victorian England. Chadwick also inaugurated action against the evils of common lodging-houses and similar dwellings. Not the least important section of his great report was his insistence on the appointment of medical officers of health by local authorities. On this action he considered that the success of his scheme rested.

In three related fields Chadwick had also done valuable pioneer work. In 1833 he was appointed one of the three commissioners who constituted the Royal Commission on the State of the Children in Factories, and he was largely responsible for the soundness of the subsequent Factory Act, and for the system of inspection which limited children's hours of work in factories. He wrote most of the First Report of the Royal Commission on the best means of establishing an efficient Constabulary Force (1839), and was one of the founders of the modern police force. After the publication of his Sanitary Report he became active in connexion with the gross overcrowding of burial grounds in urban areas. His report of 1843 on this subject led to great improvements. It may be mentioned also that the current system of pensions and the instruction of discharged soldiers and sailors in various trades is the descendant of a scheme of Chadwick's devising. An item in the evidence attached to one of the reports is the public provision of open spaces for recreation, a topic which is still of current interest.

The first official reaction to the Sanitary Report was the appointment of a Royal Commission, known as the Health of Towns Commission, the function of which was virtually to ascertain the means whereby the principles set out in the Sanitary Report could be applied. Although Chadwick was not a member of this Commission, he had great influence in the choice of members. He did most of the detailed work for it, drew up the questions to witnesses, and two-thirds of the First Report of the Commission (1844) was in his own handwriting. The Second Report was published in 1845. These very authoritative reports had a great influence on public opinion, which was changing rapidly in favour of the sanitary reformers. Out of the First Report sprang the Health of Towns Association, a voluntary body which was founded largely by Southwood Smith. This body, with its branches in the Provinces, gave a further impetus to public feeling.

Despite the activities of the sanitary reformers Parliament could not be induced to pass a Public Health Act until 1848. During nearly all the intervening period Chadwick had been the nominal Secretary of the Poor Law Commission. But relations between him and the Commissioners were now so bad that he had no access to them, and he had practically nothing to do with the work of the office. His time indeed was spent almost entirely on sanitary affairs. Matters might have gone on long enough in this fashion but for a squabble in Parliament over the poor food given to the inmates of a certain provincial workhouse. As a result Chadwick was virtually removed from his post, with the promise that he would be found other work in the public health field.

The passing of the Public Health Act and the Nuisances Removal Act in 1848 led to the appointment by the Government of a General Board of Health in the same year. The Board was appointed for a period of five years. It consisted of three members, of whom Chadwick was the paid member: Southwood Smith was appointed as Medical Assistant. One of the other two members of the Board was Antony Ashley Cooper (1801–85), at that time Lord Ashley, but later the seventh Earl of Shaftesbury, known for his philanthropic work among the poor, for his knowledge of the social conditions of factory workers, and for his efforts on behalf of the 'climbing boys'. Despite his humility, Shaftesbury could on occasion be an imperious fighter, and he and Chadwick had much in common.

The activities of the Board of Health during its statutory five years of existence are too complicated for summary here. But it may be said that it was the period in which, owing to Chadwick's insistence, large authorities were appointing medical officers of health, and field work in public health was becoming an established fact. The Board itself was much concerned with the establishment of water-supplies and of sewerage systems. There was great opposition to the Board's engineers on the part of the engineers of local sewerage boards, and a general rear-guard action was fought by numerous small authorities who felt that their powers were being abrogated by the bureaucratic General Board. With some difficulty the life of the Board was prolonged for another year. But when efforts were made in Parliament in 1854 to reconstitute it in a different form, a storm of opposition broke out, and Chadwick was made the scapegoat. One member said in the debate that England wanted to be clean, but not to be cleaned by Mr. Chadwick. The Board had been particularly hard on vested interests in London, and it was largely because of these interests that it was not given continuing powers. It ceased to exist, and at the age of fifty-four Chadwick had to retire on pension. Though his official career was ended, he continued for over thirty years to influence the course of public health by his speeches and writings.

We have dealt in some detail with Chadwick's career because it is in itself the history of the foundations of the public health movement in Great Britain. Though inspired originally by Bentham, Chadwick's practical and administrative abilities owed nothing to his former master, least of all, as Chadwick himself said, on sanitary matters. Without Chadwick British public health would have been something different. When he retired into private life the future of public health lay with the new men, such as John Simon, who had developed under his aegis.

Just as the Board of Health came into action in 1848 there was an explosive outbreak of cholera in England, of which 54,000 persons died. The statistics available under the new system made possible the deduction that the infection is conveyed by drinking-water and led to suitable precautions. These important conclusions were due almost entirely to the epidemiological work of John Snow (p. 345), who at that time was better known as our first professional anaesthetist. This is one of the many instances in which the practice of prevention of a germ-borne disease preceded any knowledge of its cause, or indeed any direct knowledge of disease germs at all.

The first town to appoint a medical officer of health was Liverpool, and in 1847 William Henry Duncan (1805–63) became the first such officer in the United Kingdom. At the same time Liverpool appointed an inspector of nuisances—an officer who was responsible to the medical officer of health, and who was later to be designated the sanitary inspector. The Corporation of London followed in 1848 and Sir John Simon (1816–1904) was appointed to that post. After Southwood Smith and Chadwick, Simon was the foremost figure in the history of the public health of this country. He later became medical officer to the General Board of Health. The work of this Board—together with its medical officer—was taken over, for political and administrative reasons, by the Privy Council. The Medical Department of the Privy Council became in 1871 part of the Local Government Board, the functions of which were included in those of the Ministry of Health on its creation in 1919.

During the eight years when Simon was responsible for the health of the City of London he completely transformed the general amenities of the area. Under his direction the sanitary inspectors carried out routine inspections of houses, underground dwellings, workshops, and industrial premises. In this short period cesspools were completely abolished, for rich and poor, throughout the square mile of the City, although for long afterwards they were common in the residential areas of the rich in other parts of the metropolis. Simon also effected a great improvement in the sewerage and water-supply of the City, and many offensive trades were eliminated. He also instituted a working arrangement with the Registrar General whereby the latter provided Simon each Monday afternoon with particulars of all persons who had died in the City during the previous week. Simon was thereby enabled to have the residences of the deceased persons visited at once; action was taken in the case of infectious disease, and advice was given. The eight annual reports which Simon presented to the Corporation of London during his years of office are the most famous health reports ever written. They embody an incredible record of success, and years later legislation was based on them which culminated in the great Public Health Act of 1875.

One important result of these measures was that it became possible to abandon the cruel and wasteful system of quarantine that had been of value in the eighteenth century. Simon's plan, which was gradually adopted, was to trust to the same preventive methods for foreign as for native infections. This was, of course, only possible with an efficient sanitary service such as that which he succeeded in instituting. These measures were aided by laboratory investigations, begun by a small staff. At first largely occupied with examinations in connexion with actual outbreaks, its scientific functions rapidly grew. Working on a wider basis, these functions have been performed for the nation since 1911 under the direction of the Medical Research Council.

One result of the improved measures for the treatment and prevention of indigenous fevers was an increasing interest in diseases

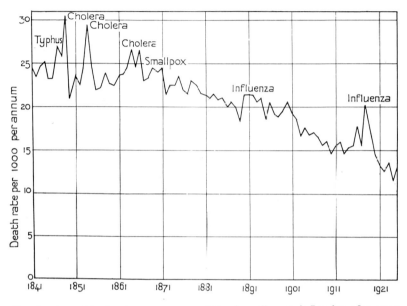

FIG. 80. Annual death-rates per 1,000 population from all causes in London, 1841–1924
The continuing fall in the death-rate began about 1870. Typhus disappeared as an important cause of death in the forties, and cholera and smallpox in the sixties. Influenza continued to cause isolated peaks

which were not common in the United Kingdom, but which were sometimes introduced by persons returning from the tropics, such as seamen. A Seamen's Hospital Society was founded in England in 1817. Its first hospital was the *Grampus*, an old 50-gun ship moored off Greenwich. This was succeeded in 1830 by the *Dreadnought*, 104 guns (Fig. 81), and this in 1857 by the *Caledonia*, 120 guns, renamed the *Dreadnought*. In 1870 this last wooden *Dreadnought* was broken up and the patients were transferred to a building on shore close by. The darkness, damp, ill-ventilation, noisiness, and septic character of a wooden ship made it thoroughly unsuitable for hospital purposes.

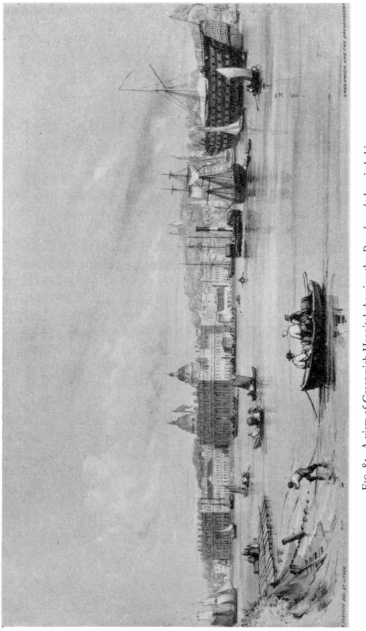

FIG. 81. A view of Greenwich Hospital showing the *Dreadnought* hospital ship
(Lithograph of *c.* 1848 by W. Parrott)

In 1899 the Seamen's Hospital Society established a special Hospital and School for Tropical Diseases, such as are peculiarly common among seamen.

The Public Health Act 1875 remained the charter of English public health for sixty years. During the rest of the nineteenth century great advances in environmental conditions and in the combating of infectious diseases was made under it. But early in the twentieth century attention was gradually turned to the health of the individual, and several new services were officially initiated. These services are dealt with briefly below. With the passing of the National Health Insurance Act of 1911 the State assumed greater responsibility for the treatment of the individual than it had ever done previously.

The growth of the work of the Medical Department of the Local Government Board led to a great increase in its administrative functions. The professional administrators of the Board came more and more to guide its medical policy, and in 1876 Simon resigned his post of Chief Medical Officer in protest. His successors under the Board and, from 1919, under the Ministry of Health, have been: Edward Cator Seaton (1815–80); Sir George Buchanan (1831–95); Sir Richard Thorne-Thorne (1841–99); Sir William Henry Power (1842–1916); Sir Arthur Newsholme (1857–1943); Sir George Newman (1870–1948); Sir Arthur Salusbury MacNalty (1880–); Sir William Wilson Jameson (1885–). Each of these men is known especially for his work in certain branches of preventive medicine. Seaton was an authority on vaccination, and was mainly responsible for the Compulsory Vaccination Act of 1853. Buchanan and Thorne-Thorne were known for their field work in infectious diseases, and the latter was mainly responsible for the wide establishment of isolation hospitals and for the abolition of quarantine. Power was known for his work on the segregation of smallpox hospitals, on lead poisoning arising from drinking-water, and for the establishment of the food section of the Local Government Board. Newsholme exercised a very wide influence on public-health administration, on the control of certain infectious diseases and of tuberculosis, on infant mortality, and he was active in the creation of the Ministry of Health. Newman was the architect of the school medical service and is known also for his work connected with the provision of a pure milk supply.

MacNalty is known especially for his work on tuberculosis and on infectious diseases of the central nervous system; since 1940 he has been Editor-in-Chief of the Medical History of the Second World War. Jameson is a distinguished teacher of preventive medicine and has been active in the development of hospitals and in the improvement of medical services in the colonies.

The school medical service. The most clear-cut example of the foundation of a new service connected with the health of the people during this century is the school medical service. It was recognized in the closing years of the nineteenth century that ill health in adult life was often determined by malnutrition, poor physique, and minor defects in childhood. The extent of the problem was not clearly understood, and accurate information was required. In 1890 the London School Board voluntarily appointed a medical officer to examine children in their elementary schools, and Bradford, Salford, and Halifax took similar action. By the Education Act of 1902 the School Boards were abolished and greatly improved educational powers were granted to their successors, the Local Education Authorities. The provision of meals at schools was empowered by an Act of 1906. In the following year the Education (Administrative Provisions) Act made it compulsory for each Local Education Authority to arrange for the medical inspection of all children on beginning their school career ('entrants') and at such other times during it as the Board of Education might direct. It was left to the discretion of each Authority whether or not it made arrangements for the treatment of any defects discovered.

The President of the Board of Education at once established a medical department under a Chief Medical Officer (Newman). Local authorities now appointed school medical officers to perform the inspections, and in most authorities the medical officer of health was appointed chief school medical officer of the area. In this way the health of the school children was linked to the health of the community as a whole, and the machinery of the public health department was available in the abatement of disease in schools. The Board directed that each child should be inspected as an entrant, at the age of seven or eight years, at ten years, and preferably also on leaving school.

In 1908 the Board suggested to local authorities that they should appoint school nurses, establish school clinics, provide hospital treatment for sick children, and spectacles for those who required them. School clinics were intended to treat diseases of the eyes, ears, nose and throat, teeth, and minor ailments which could be dealt with effectively in such clinics. As a result of the suggestion about fifty authorities arranged to provide school nurses and about twelve school clinics. Since then these facilities have been provided by all local authorities. School dental clinics were an early addition to this list.

Special schools for children suffering from incapacitating conditions, such as blindness, deaf-mutism, and crippling conditions were started by the Board of Education in 1908. Schools for mental defectives and open-air schools soon followed. Although a nursery school had been established philanthropically at New Lanark in Scotland in 1816, no State grants for such schools were payable to local authorities until 1919.

On the formation of the Ministry of Health in 1919 the Chief Medical Officer of the Board of Education became also its Chief Medical Officer. Further co-ordination of the medical work of the two ministries was thus effected. As a result of the work of the school medical service since its inception fifty years ago there has been vast improvement in the health of school children. Dental caries has been much reduced in extent and incidence, and as a result diseases in which it plays a causative role have been diminished. Skin diseases have also been much diminished, especially conditions such as ringworm which are now very effectively treated. Nutrition has improved, and diseases such as rickets are in most areas now never seen.

Maternity and child welfare. Measures to reduce the great wastage of child life during infancy came into operation more gradually and were at first largely dependent on voluntary efforts. In certain countries the death-rates of infants admitted to foundling hospitals were very high. Of over 10,000 infants admitted to the Dublin Foundling Hospital in the twenty-one years ending in 1796, only forty-five survived—a death-rate of over 99 per cent. About this period ten books were published dealing with the high infant mortality. About this time, too, important books were beginning to appear on paediatrics, of which the most influential was *A Treatise on the Diseases of Children* by Michael Underwood (1737–1820), first published in 1784 and often subsequently revised. When official statistics for infant mortality first became available in 1841, the infantile mortality rate was about 155 deaths under one year per 1,000 live births. The succeeding sixty years saw no significant reduction, and the highest figure recorded was noted in 1899.

At the turn of the new century the time was ripe for action. So far as the infants were concerned it developed on three lines—the appearance of health visitors, the institution of birth notification, and the establishment of child welfare centres.

At the start the health visitors' movement was purely voluntary. In 1862 the Ladies' Sanitary Reform Association of Manchester and Salford was founded. The idea was that voluntary members of the Association should visit mothers in their homes and give them advice on the management of their children. The area was divided into districts, and a paid visitor was in charge of each of the districts. The Association carried on its work without any official assistance or supervision until 1890, when the Manchester visitors were placed under the supervision of the City Health Authority; the Salford visitors later came under the Salford Authority. None of these visitors—paid or voluntary—had any specialized training.

Florence Nightingale (p. 704) now arranged for a course of training to be started in Buckinghamshire, and in 1892 the Bucks. County Council appointed three of those who had taken the course. Very soon local authorites were appointing whole-time health visitors to superintend the work of voluntary visitors. These professional health visitors had usually been trained either as nurses or as sanitary inspectors. In health visiting knowledge and experience of both subjects is required, and few of these early visitors had such knowledge. A standard of training was first enforced by the London County Council in 1908, and this became virtually a national standard in 1918.

One difficulty which soon confronted health visitors was the fact that they too frequently heard about births only when much valuable time had already been lost. The institution of the system of notifica-

tion of births was virtually the work of the mayor of Huddersfield, and of its medical officer of health, Samson George Haydock
Moore (1866–1940). In 1904 Moore showed that nearly half the
babies who died in Huddersfield did so from preventable causes. In
the following year he instituted a system of visits to young babies by
two assistant medical officers, followed by visits by voluntary visitors.
The scheme was handicapped by the fact that the health authority
often did not get to know of the birth until it was too late to save the
child. In 1906 the Huddersfield Corporation Act required every
birth occurring in the borough to be notified to the medical officer of
health within forty-eight hours of its occurrence. The success of this
Huddersfield scheme led to the adoptive Notification of Births Act
of 1907, and later to the 1915 Act which made notification obligatory
throughout the country.

The third arm in the fight against infant mortality was the establishment of child welfare centres. The first infant consultation centre
(*consultation de nourrissons*) was established at the Charité Hospital,
Paris, in 1892 by Pierre Constant Budin (1846–1907), professor of
obstetrics in the University of Paris. Budin aimed to keep the infants
under his personal supervision until they attained the age of two
years. A centre for the distribution of milk was first opened at
Fécamp in France in 1894, and in the United Kingdom a similar
centre was opened at St. Helens in 1899. There was, however, this
difference that, within four years, a doctor was certainly holding
weekly consultations at this St. Helens centre. In 1905 the medical
officer of health of Battersea in London, George Frederick McCleary
(1867–), established infant consultations there, and consultation
centres in other areas soon followed.

Associated with these great improvements in the management of
infants were the concurrent improvements in the management of
pregnancy and labour. The Midwives Act of 1902 created the Central
Midwives Board and made it an offence for any woman to attend,
habitually and for gain, women during their confinements except
under the supervision of a doctor, unless she was registered as a
midwife under the Act. The Board issued stringent regulations, and
later Acts have further extended the training and regulation of midwives.

As a result of these measures there has been a very great improvement in the health and welfare of infants. The infant mortality rate per 1,000 live births, which reached its peak (163) in 1899, fell gradually to 27 during the five-year period 1951–5. There was not only a great saving of life during the first year, but numerous ailments, minor and major, have been prevented in the pre-school period. There has been a general improvement of nutrition, and crippling conditions have been much reduced. Newsholme, as a result of a series of important reports to the Local Government Board, played a large part in determining the legislative and administrative action which has produced these rusults.

Tuberculosis. In the treatment, control, and prevention of tuberculosis the State and local authorities have played an equally important role. These measures may be briefly considered under the following heads: the provision of sanatoria and special hospitals; the establishment of tuberculosis dispensaries; notification; and measures to prevent the spread of the disease.

The first institution for the treatment of pulmonary tuberculosis on open-air lines was that established by George Bodington (1799–1882) at Sutton Coldfield in Warwickshire. In 1840 Bodington published *On the Treatment and Cure of Pulmonary Consumption, on Principles Natural, Rational, and Successful.* The institution was not very successful, though it embodied the basic points in the sanatorium treatment of the disease. The first successful sanatorium for treatment on open-air lines was opened in 1859 by Hermann Brehmer (1826–1889) at Goerbersdorf in Silesia.

Sanatorium treatment really involves, in addition to open-air treatment, the principle of subjecting the patient to absolute rest until his fever has subsided, and then to exercising the body very gradually until he can go through a day involving light work without adverse reaction. The first to introduce these methods successfully was Otto Walther (1853–1919), who established his sanatorium at Nordrach-in-Baden in 1888. In this country the method was later modified by Marcus Paterson (1870–1932), who explained the beneficial effects as due to 'autoinoculation' of the patient with small doses of toxins produced by the graduated exercise. Paterson's principles, though now discredited, had a wide influence. Before the end of the nineteenth century several hospitals for diseases of the chest had been established in London and elsewhere, and some of these now built sanatoria in the country as annexes.

The tuberculosis dispensary system was founded in Edinburgh in 1887 by Sir Robert William Philip (1857–1939). He found that tuberculous patients who had been discharged from hospitals and sanatoria often had relapses on return to their homes. Under the scheme which he inaugurated these discharged patients were invited to attend at the tuberculosis dispensary, where he examined them, gave them minor treatment when necessary, and advised them regarding the conduct of their lives. Nurses were trained to visit the homes of these patients, and to give them practical advice regarding their living conditions. Inquiries were also made regarding the health of house-contacts of the patient. A few other areas followed, a long time afterwards, the lead given by Edinburgh, notably Oxfordshire (1910) and Sheffield (1911).

Notification to the medical officer of health of patients suffering from tuberculosis had been advocated by many persons, but there were practical difficulties. In New York it had been introduced voluntarily in 1893, and made compulsory in 1897. In that year voluntary notification was introduced in Oldham, Lancs., and other towns followed. By private Acts Sheffield (1903) and Bolton (1905) had obtained compulsory notification. In 1911 tuberculosis of the lungs became compulsorily notifiable throughout England and Wales.

When the National Health Insurance Act came into operation in 1911, the duty was imposed on local authorities to provide sanatoria and other forms of treatment. At that time only a few sanatoria, and still fewer dispensary schemes, existed. A departmental committee, known as the Astor Committee from its chairman, Lord Astor, was appointed, and from its important recommendations sprang rapidly a comprehensive tuberculosis service. The appointment of tuberculosis officers, the establishment of tuberculosis dispensaries, and the provision of sanatorium and hospital beds for tuberculosis was made obligatory for the major authorities. Twenty-five years later there were nearly 500 tuberculosis dispensaries in England and Wales, and in this period the sanatoria and hospital beds had increased fivefold.

A peculiarly British contribution to the tuberculosis problem, with its many clinical, social, financial, and industrial facets, was made in 1914 by (Sir) Pendrill Charles Varrier-Jones (1883–1941), with the support of Clifford Allbutt (pp. 625–6). This took the form of a colony or village settlement, to which selected tuberculous patients were admitted with their families on a semi-permanent basis. Cottages were available for the settlers, together with workshops in which they did work according to their physical ability at the time, and a sanatorium and a hospital in which they were treated when they were ill. Four years later the colony moved to Papworth, where it was much expanded. Although much copied elsewhere, it remains one of the few, if not the only, institution of its type which enables the moderately fit tuberculous patient to maintain himself by his own efforts.

Although the general principles of rest and fresh air are still important in sanatoria, special methods of treatment were introduced quite early. Of these the induction of artificial pneumothorax (p. 372) is best known. Between the wars there was a great increase in this practice, often with very satisfactory results. The very significant advances in chest surgery during and since the Second World War have tended to substitute permanent collapse of a diseased lung by the operation of thoracoplasty for the temporary collapse afforded by artificial pneumothorax. Such major operations, together with the excision of the whole or part of a diseased lung (pneumonectomy), have recently made the practice of artificial pneumothorax obsolete.

In the field of prevention, much valuable work has been done in the supervision of contacts of tuberculous cases. In this work valuable information is obtained from tuberculin and similar tests, which are now more scientifically applied. Reference is made later to the use of B.C.G. vaccine (p. 426). In the inter-war years the importance of the bovine tubercle bacillus in causing non-pulmonary tuberculosis was increasingly recognized. Even as late as 1932 between 2 and 13 per cent. of all samples of raw milk showed the presence of live tubercle bacilli. In studies on the bacteriology of milk and in the campaign for clean milk supplies Sir William George Savage (1872–) played an important part. Tubercle-free herds were gradually built up, but there was for long considerable discussion regarding the desirability of general pasteurization of the milk supplies. Pasteurization is now very widely used.

Although these measures have had a very beneficial effect in reducing the incidence of clinical tuberculosis, it is not generally agreed that they account for the whole of the marked reduction which has taken place since the late War.

Infectious disease and water-supplies. During the middle of the nineteenth century public health was dominated by the urge to save the country from the ravages of serious outbreaks of epidemic diseases. At this time the conception was held that most infectious diseases were caused by filth. The science of bacteriology (pp. 379 ff.) had not yet been born. This erroneous conception led to an unparalleled war against dirt and nuisances, great improvements in the conveyance and disposal of sewage, and to a gradual substitution of pure water-supplies for the numerous public and private wells which were a blot on all large cities. Although the conception was wrong, the 'sanitary revolution' which it caused was undoubtedly right. When a case of infectious disease occurred in any house, the testing of the drains was almost the first administrative action taken, and the belief that diphtheria was caused by 'bad smells' died especially hard. In the case of cholera (p. 730) and typhoid (p. 731) a miasmatic conception was at first almost universal. Of this belief Max von Pettenkofer (1818–1901) was the greatest champion. Pettenkofer made many early contributions to biochemistry, and at Munich he founded a world-famous institute of hygiene. That city suffered severely from cholera and typhoid, and he was led, from results obtained on the sinking of numerous test wells, to conclude that the incidence of these diseases was correlated with the height of the ground water. Even as late as 1866 Simon was still interested in these theories, and Pettenkofer himself never wavered in his beliefs, even long after the discovery of the cholera and typhoid bacilli.

The second half of the nineteenth century saw the completion of large storage-reservoirs for the water-supplies of the great cities of England and Scotland. The Metropolitan Water Board was founded in 1902. In this period efficient slow and rapid methods of purification by filtration and other processes were perfected. In London valuable research was carried out on the bacteriology and purification of water by Sir Alexander Cruikshank Houston (1865–1933).

The first London medical officers. We conclude this brief sketch of the development of the public health movement in Great Britain with some remarks about the medical administrators who in large local authorities not only implemented the recommendations of the Privy Council and the Local Government Board, but by their research and administrative methods were often responsible for new recommendations. Apart from Liverpool and London, the first medical officers of health were appointed in the London area, which was that now covered by the present London County Council. It then contained forty-six sanitary districts excluding the City of London. The Metropolitan Management Act of 1855 required each district to appoint a medical officer of health, and by the following year all these men had been appointed. Viewed collectively, there has probably never been anywhere such a distinguished body of medical men engaged in the practice of public health. There were among them several Fellows of the Royal Society. Some were physicians to famous London teaching hospitals, and others had distinguished themselves in microscopical and chemical work. Of these men the most brilliant was (Sir) John Scott Burdon Sanderson (1828–1905), who was medical officer of health of Paddington for ten years (1856–66). He was later professor of physiology at University College, London, and at Oxford, and finally he occupied the regius chair of medicine at Oxford. Sir George Buchanan (p. 223) was for twelve years a London medical officer of health, and Frederick William Pavy (1829–1911) was a physician to Guy's Hospital and was known for his chemical investigations, especially on diabetes.

(b) Preventive Medicine in the United States and Canada

In the United States the history of public health is different from that of British public health, the national service having been associated with the mercantile marine and the navy in a manner foreign to British traditions. The Federal health service had its origin in the old Marine Hospital Service, first authorized by an Act of Congress in 1798. This Act enabled the President to appoint medical officers at ports for the purpose of giving relief and medical treatment to sick and disabled merchant seamen. The funds for this work were to be obtained by a levy on the pay of seamen in American merchant vessels. By an amending Act of the following year the levy and the benefits were extended to officers and men of the United States Navy.

The first marine hospital to be owned by the Federal government was at Washington Point, Norfolk County, Virginia. This was purchased, still incomplete, from the State of Virginia in 1801 and occupied by patients soon after. At Boston the sick had been accommodated in temporary premises since 1800, and in 1804 they were transferred to a newly completed building. In 1807 the Marine Hospital at Boston became the teaching hospital of the Harvard Medical School. Other marine hospitals were built or acquired at important seaports; and in 1837 Congress authorized the extension of the Service for the relief of seamen on inland waters, and further hospitals were established accordingly.

The evolution of public health functions from this service was along natural lines. The medical officers, in providing medical treatment for the American merchant marine, were often the first to diagnose such diseases as cholera, yellow fever, and smallpox, which were being imported into the United States. In the epidemics of cholera which occurred in certain of the ports, the marine hospitals and their medical officers were used for the treatment of the patients. During the Civil War the marine hospitals and their staffs were used by the military authorities, both of the north and the south, for the treatment of soldiers.

In 1870 the Service was reorganized and provided with a titular head, responsible to the Secretary of the Treasury. He was to be known as the Surgeon General, and should not be confused with the Surgeon General to the Armed Forces. The first Surgeon General of the Marine Hospital Service was John Maynard Woodworth (1837–79), who reorganized the Service from an aggregation of local appointed officials into a homogeneous mobile medical corps the members of which were available for duty as required in any part of the country. He also established cordial relations with the State and local health authorities. In 1875 he revived the old Quarantine Act of 1799, which had become a dead letter, by issuing instructions to his medical officers detailing their duties in respect of quarantine.

Largely as a result of Woodworth's advocacy the first of the national quarantine Acts was passed in 1878.

Just before Woodworth's death Congress authorized, for four years only, a National Board of Health with powers to report direct to the President. Its activities, however, overlapped those of the Marine Hospital Service, and some of the measures of Woodworth's successor were effectively blocked. When the powers of the Board expired by limitation, the Service took charge of all Federal quarantine and public health measures, and in 1890 it was given further authority to deal with interstate quarantine regulations. The Act setting up the Board was expressly repealed by the second of the national quarantine Acts, passed in 1893.

In a second reorganization of 1902 the name of the Service was changed to the Public Health and Marine Hospital Service, and six administrative divisions were established. In the same year the Biologics Control Law was passed authorizing the Service to control the sale and transportation of all sera, vaccines, antitoxins, and similar products throughout the country. New divisions of the Service were authorized by later Acts, and in the third reorganization of 1912 the present name, the United States Public Health Service, was adopted, and the existing divisions were retained. Authorization was also given for field studies on human diseases and on the pollution of navigable streams. In the fourth reorganization of 1943 the divisions were grouped into four Bureaux, each under a bureau chief responsible directly to the Surgeon General.

In the meantime, in 1887, Joseph James Kinyoun (1869–1946), who had studied in Europe under Koch, had set up in one room of the Marine Hospital at Staten Island, New York, a laboratory which later received official recognition as the Hygienic Laboratory. Kinyoun remained as director till 1899, and the Laboratory was further expanded into an organization of five separate divisions by his successor Milton Joseph Rosenau (1869–1946), an outstanding laboratory worker and also a first-rate administrator. Much work in connexion with the Biologics Control Law was undertaken by the Laboratory, and in the First World War its activities increased still further. In 1930 it was reorganized as the National Institute of Health, and seven years later it was merged with the Division of

Scientific Research of the Public Health Service. About this time an estate at Bethesda, Maryland, was presented for the accommodation of the separate institutes, now seven in number with a clinical centre and laboratories serving them all. In the reorganization of 1943 the whole was grouped as one of the four Bureaux, the Institutes of Bethesda retaining their titles, and the headquarters of the Bureaux being called the National Institute of Health.

During the course of Federal development the separate States of the Union were not devoid of advocates of State action in matters of public health. Among these Lemuel Shattuck (1793–1859), like Chadwick, was not a medical man but a student of social problems. Under the influence of Chadwick he was mainly responsible for the drafting in 1850 of the report of the Sanitary Commission of the State of Massachusetts. This report reviewed the history of public health in various countries and ages, suggested a scheme of public health measures, and recommended the formation of a Board of Health. But Shattuck's own state, Massachusetts, did not establish its health department until 1869, and meanwhile two other states had established health departments. During the seventies and eighties twenty-seven state health departments were established, and at the beginning of the twentieth century there were still eight states that had not taken similar action. The last of these, the state of Texas, established its department in 1909. The cities, however, were earlier in the field, and Philadelphia, New York City, and Boston had established health departments before the close of the eighteenth century. The first three-quarters of the nineteenth century saw more cities following suit; but, as with the states, it was in the seventies and eighties that most of the city health departments were established. This was the period in which the general principles suggested by the work of Pasteur (p. 330) and Koch (p. 336) were put into effect. In America, as in Europe, the working hypothesis of the sanitarians was that filth and bad drainage were direct factors in the production of epidemic disease, and the improved environmental conditions, such as housing, drainage, and water-supply, undoubtedly led to a great improvement in the general comfort and health. The first diagnostic laboratory to be established under municipal auspices was in New York City, where it was obtained through the action of Herman

Michael Biggs (1859–1923) in 1892, and he became its first director. Biggs was active in public health spheres. In 1902 he became Medical Officer of Health of New York City, and later Commissioner of Health for the State of New York. It was largely through his efforts that other cities followed New York's example.

In Canada quarantine for plague was introduced at Quebec in 1721. As a result of the great English Public Health Act of 1875, a similar Act was passed in the Province of Ontario in 1882. The Province of Quebec followed in 1886, and the other provinces later. A Dominion Department of Health was not established until 1919.

THE TRANSITION TO A PHYSIOLOGICAL SYNTHESIS

Modern developments in physiological knowledge introduce an important period in the history of medicine, for the study of the functions of the body is a natural portal of entry to the study of the perversions and suspensions of those functions that we call disease. The general character of physiological thought during the modern period may perhaps be described as the synthetic study of the animal body. The study has become synthetic because organs have been studied not so much in and for themselves as in relation to other organs. There has been, in fact, during the period an increasing consciousness of the integration of the organs into one organic whole, the entire process being under the control of the nervous system, the various parts of which are themselves integrated (pp. 263 ff.), and of the endocrine system (pp. 515 ff.). This movement has, to some extent, mitigated the ever-growing evils of scientific specialization.

(a) *Anatomy and Embryology in the Earlier Nineteenth Century*

Let us first glance at the state of anatomical knowledge in the early and middle nineteenth century. The general structure of the animal body was well known. Descriptive anatomy was not far from where it now is. Comparative anatomy, which had made good progress, was given a fresh impetus by the researches and by the authority of a brilliant group of French investigators, headed by the *baron* Georges Cuvier (1769–1832), whose influence spread to

Britain, Germany, and America, where the leading exponents were Sir Richard Owen (1804–92), Karl Gegenbaur (1826–1903), and Edward Drinker Cope (1840–97). Cuvier was a biological dictator whose opinion did much to encourage investigation, and something to discourage some important investigators. His services to comparative anatomy can hardly be overrated. There was, however, still no effective knowledge of the anatomical differences between the races of man, while the species of man and of allied forms, whose skeletons palaeontologists have since described, were quite unknown.

As regards knowledge of the process of development of the animal body, the broad lines of embryology were being put on a firm basis by Karl Ernst von Baer (1792–1876), whose work was finished in 1837, though he lived another forty years. The subject was to be given a new meaning by the evolutionary school, which applied the work of Charles Robert Darwin (1809–82) to new details and particular instances. Foremost of this school was Francis Maitland Balfour (1851–82), whose work entitled *A Treatise on Comparative Embryology* (1880–81) is a classic of science. Balfour's untimely death in the Alps robbed Europe of one of its most promising young scientists.

(b) Chemical Physiology in the Earlier Nineteenth Century

The analysis of the functions and workings of the body had advanced far less than the knowledge of its structure. The study of respiration was perhaps in the best position. The elementary conception of respiration attained by Lavoisier at the end of the eighteenth century (p. 168) was hardly extended till Eduard Friedrich Wilhelm Pflüger (1829–1910) of Bonn, in the sixties and seventies of the nineteenth century, showed that the essential chemical changes of respiration do not occur in the blood or in the lungs but in the tissues, a fact already suggested by Mayow.

A very important figure in the scientific world of the thirties and forties of the nineteenth century was the German Justus von Liebig (1803–73), who studied chemistry at Bonn and at Erlangen. As there was no practical teaching in this subject at these universities, he then worked in Gay-Lussac's laboratory at Paris. At the age of twenty-one Liebig was appointed professor of chemistry at Giessen, where he remained for twenty-eight years. He did much to introduce laboratory teaching, and certain apparatus which he invented is still in constant use.

Liebig greatly improved the methods of organic analysis and notably he introduced a method for determining the amount of urea in a solution. Urea is of great importance because it is regularly formed in the body in the process of breaking down the characteristic nitrogenous substances known as proteins. With Friedrich Wöhler (1800–82), Liebig wrote a famous paper (1832) in which he showed, for the first time, that a small organic group of atoms—or radicle as it was called—is capable of forming an unchanging constituent through a long series of compounds, behaving throughout as though it was an element. The discovery of the benzoyl radicle—the first of many radicles to be recognized—is of primary importance for our conceptions of the chemical changes in the living body.

From 1838 onwards Liebig devoted himself to attempting a chemical elucidation of living processes. In the course of his investigations he did pioneer work along many lines that have since become well recognized. He taught the true doctrine, then little understood, that animal heat is the result of combustion, and is not 'innate'. He also classified articles of food with reference to the functions that he conceived they fulfilled in the animal economy. An outcome of this was his food for infants and his extract of meat. Very important was his teaching that plants derive the constituents of their food, their carbon and nitrogen, from the carbon dioxide and ammonia in the atmosphere, and that these compounds are returned by the plants to the atmosphere in the process of putrefaction. This discovery made possible a philosophical conception of a sort of 'circulation' in Nature. That which is broken down is constantly built up, to be later broken down again. Thus the wheel of life goes on, the motor power being energy from without, derived ultimately from the heat of the sun.

It was very unfortunate that Liebig conceived and adhered to a view of the nature of putrefaction and fermentation, which, in the light of the knowledge at that time, was becoming untenable.

THE NERVOUS SYSTEM AND NEUROLOGY

We now turn to a summary of the manner in which our present considerable knowledge of the nervous system and its disorders has been built up, leaving certain basic physiological principles of the action of nerve for later discussion.

The Hippocratic physicians knew a little of the anatomy of the brain, of the eye, and of the bony labyrinth. They held that the brain, or some part of it, is a gland which cools the blood and secretes the mucus (*pituita*) which flows from the nose. It was then also known that wounds of the brain produced convulsions or paralysis on the opposite side to the lesion. By Alexandrian times more attention was being given to the nervous system. As we have seen (pp. 48 ff.) both Herophilus and Erasistratus extended our concept of the functions of the brain, and Herophilus especially described new points in its anatomy. Of organic nervous lesions the best known were paralysis and epilepsy. From experiments on animals Galen learned that transection of the spinal cord at the level of the fourth cervical vertebra or above immediately causes death; whereas, if the section is made between the sixth and seventh vertebrae, the thoracic muscles are paralysed and the animal breathes only by means of its diaphragm. He thus gained some preliminary knowledge of the function of the phrenic nerve.

Aretaeus of Cappadocia (A.D. 81–? 138) clearly differentiated between mental and nervous diseases about the early second century A.D. He considered apoplexy as a paralysis of the whole body. Paraplegia is a loss of movement and sensation in an arm or leg; whereas paresis or paralysis is a loss only of movement. He knew the condition of ptosis, caused by paralysis of the levator palpebrae muscle, and that it is often associated with dilatation of the pupil. He described the aura and hallucinations that precede an attack of epilepsy.

Soranus of Ephesus (A.D. 98–138) was acknowledged to be the greatest writer on obstetrics and gynaecology in antiquity, and his packing of the uterus for post-partum haemorrhage sounds very modern, though septic complications must have been common. For prolapse of the uterus he recommended hysterectomy. His most important contribution to the practice of obstetrics was his use of podalic version. It is possible that there was no real advance in obstetrics after Soranus until the work of Paré (p. 95). The book on obstetrics by Soranus also contains a section on paediatrics, the first treatise on that subject. Although this treatise deals mainly with the handling, care, and feeding of the new-born child, it also has chapters applicable to older children, such as those on rashes, cough, and looseness of the bowels. It contains the first account by a medical writer of the age-old custom of salting the new-born infant, and a reference to a condition which was very probably rickets. Soranus was a prolific writer in Greek, and many of his other works have been lost, including his books on acute diseases and on chronic diseases, which contained his observations on nervous conditions. Fortunately we possess the Latin translation of these books which was made by Caelius Aurelianus (fifth century A.D.).

Soranus seems to have been the soundest of ancient physicians in his treatment of insanity (p. 494). He devoted over one book of his work on acute diseases to the discussion of phrenitis and of lethargy. The sections on apoplexy and paralysis are surprisingly detailed, and the accuracy of the clinical picture shows that Soranus must have been a very acute observer. The excellence of his account is really hardly vitiated by the fact that he regards apoplexy as an acute disease, accompanied by a 'seizure of the mind', whereas paralysis is a chronic disease. What he means in effect is that paralysis is a chronic condition supervening on the acute—that is, sudden—seizure, apoplexy. Soranus gives a long account of epilepsy. He also describes 'scotoma', from the description of which he obviously refers to scotoma scintillans, one type of which he correctly describes as a precursor of an epileptic attack.

The works of the Byzantine writers contain some new observations, but those on nervous diseases are generally inferior to those of Soranus. Oribasius (p. 68) mentions abscess and erysipelas of the brain, conditions which are also referred to by later writers. He has sections also on hydrophobia, heatstroke, and migraine. His descriptions of diseases at different levels of the spinal cord are good. Alexander of Tralles (p. 68) has long sections on hemicrania and epilepsy. Paul of Aegina (p. 68) deals especially with apoplexy and epilepsy. His descriptions of the symptoms and signs are much shorter than those of Soranus, and his sections on these conditions are devoted largely to treatment.

(a) *Anatomy and physiology of the nervous system.* Two errors in our knowledge of the nervous system which had been accepted by Galen proved to be remarkably persistent. One was that the base of the human brain shows a plexus of anastomosing vessels known as the *rete mirabile.* This structure is found in ungulates, but is absent in man. The other error was that the pituitary body (infundibulum) secretes the pituita, which passes through the cribiform plate of the ethmoid to the nose.

No advance of any kind was made during the medieval period. The first of the Renaissance anatomists to take an interest was Leonardo (p. 89). By making wax casts of the ventricles of the brain he was able to obtain a very accurate idea of their shape. We remind the reader that Leonardo's work was unpublished for centuries, and therefore had no direct influence. In 1518 Laurentius Phryesen (d. *c.* 1532) of Colmar published his *Spiegel der Artzny.* In this book is an anatomical sheet which includes six illustrations showing dissections of the brain at different stages. From these it is evident that the convolutions and the optic chiasma were well recognized.

Jacopo Berengario da Carpi (?–1550) was a noted anatomist and physician. One of his early works was a treatise on fractures of the skull (1518). Three years later he published a very large and important commentary on the anatomy of Mundinus, and in 1522 there appeared his *Isagogae breves* ('Elementary treatises'). Berengar was the first to describe the vermiform appendix, the thymus, the arytenoid cartilages, and the valves of the heart. In the brain he described the ventricles (especially the fourth), the choroid plexus, and the pineal gland. He gives a diagram which clearly shows the ventricles and the infundibulum. In his earlier work he asserted that the *rete mirabile* was present in man, but in his last book he denied it.

A slightly later contemporary, Johannes Dryander (1500–60) of Marburg, published in 1536 his *Anatomia capitis humani* ('Anatomy of the human head'), which contains rather crude diagrams probably made from dissections. These drawings show that the brain was dissected in an orderly manner, but that Dryander's knowledge of the structure of the brain was very limited.

Charles Estienne (1503–64), a member of the famous publishing house of that name in Paris, was dissecting for some time before 1530, the year in which he began to prepare his work on anatomy. The first (Latin) edition of his book, *De dissectione partium corporis humani* ('On the dissection of the parts of the human body'), was not published until 1545, so that it appeared after the *Fabrica* of Vesalius. It is, however, pre-Vesalian in preparation and approach. For unknown reasons Estienne borrowed certain illustrations of nudes which were well known in his day. Into the block of each figure he inset another block of the dissection of that particular part. The result is that his drawings of dissected areas are small, and the parts are difficult to make out. Nevertheless, one of his figures shows the vermiform appendix; and in his text he described the thymus, the parotid gland, and lymphatic glands in the mesentery. Estienne gives eight diagrams showing the dissection of the brain. He was familiar with the ventricles and some of their communications, with the choroid plexus, the fornix, the optic chiasma, the pituitary, the pineal organ, and he had a fair knowledge of the origins of most of the cranial nerves. In his text he describes the condition known as syringomyelia (p. 276)—an observation which was forgotten for hundreds of years.

With Vesalius (p. 90) the anatomy of the brain became modern at one bound. The seventh book of the *Fabrica* contains fifteen diagrams of the brain and its vessels which are excellent, together with some others which are less inspired. His descriptions of the blood-vessels are in general good, but, as injection of the arteries was not then practised, he missed the circulus arteriosus, the ring of communicating vessels under the base of the brain. This structure was first injected and seen by Thomas Willis, who described it in his *Cerebri anatome* (1664). It is strange that Vesalius should have missed such a prominent structure as the pons, but his diagram of the base of the brain shows no sign of it. Of the two errors which were so dogmatically followed by the ancients, Vesalius only just succeeds in clearing himself of one, but in the case of the other he does not even make an attempt. In the *Tabulae anatomicae sex* (p. 91) he had shown the *rete mirabile* at the base of the brain; in the *Fabrica* he takes nearly a page to prove that everything Galen had said about

this structure in the human is wrong, and he gives a diagram showing the structure according to Galen; but at the same time Vesalius
says that it is 'almost non-existent' in the human body. He not only
accepts the erroneous doctrine that the infundibulum secretes pituita
which is passed out through the nose, but he gives a long account of
the passages by which this hypothetical secretion makes its exit
through the base of the skull.

Having said this, it must be admitted that Vesalius's account of
the brain is far in advance of anything which had appeared up to
that time. He describes the sinuses and the ventricles well, as also
the falx cerebri, the tentorium cerebelli, and the choroid plexuses. He
gives a good account of the corpus callosum (the name is probably
his) and of the fornix. He also explains the septum lucidum and
gives a clear account of the corpora quadrigemina and of the pineal
body. He naturally devotes much attention to the infundibulum. The
description of the cerebellum is generally accurate but less detailed,
and that of the medulla is good. It is, however, in his illustrations
that Vesalius shows his advanced knowledge. In these the following
structures, not mentioned in his text, are clearly seen: thalamus,
caudate nucleus, lenticular nucleus, globus pallidus, putamen, pulvinar, and the cerebral peduncles. He notes that the cerebral sulci
are deeper in man than in animals, in order that the human brain
substance may be the richer. Characteristically he then proceeds to
explain these deep sulci by saying that they make the brain firmer for
the arteries and veins to be distributed through it. Vesalius's account
of the cranial nerves shows deficiencies and inaccuracies.

A contemporary of Vesalius, Bartolommeo Eustachi [Eustachius]
(1520–74), who worked at Rome, wrote a book on anatomy, the text
of which was lost. He had prepared for it a fine series of plates, but
these were not published until 1714 (*Tabulae anatomicae*, ed. B.
Lancisi). They include a very fine illustration of the base of the brain
and the whole of the sympathetic nervous system, in which there are
unfortunately some errors in the cervical part. The five drawings of
the base of the brain given by Eustachius show quite clearly that he
had a sound knowledge of the pons as a separate part of the brain. In
his *Opuscula anatomica* (1564) Eustachius gave descriptions of the
tensor tympani muscle and of the chorda tympani nerve. He also

gave the first modern description of the Eustachian tube, a structure which was certainly described by Alcmaeon of Croton (*c.* 500 B.C.) The discovery of the pons is often credited to Constanzo Varolio (1543–78), who gave a crude illustration of it in a figure of the base of the brain, which appeared in his work *De nervis opticis* ('On the optic nerves', 1573). After him the structure is usually called the pons Varolii, but his illustration is manifestly inferior to that of Eustachius.

In the second half of the sixteenth century attention began to be paid to the cranial nerves and the special sense organs. Vesalius had blundered lamentably in following the medieval tradition that the lens is situated in the centre of the globe of the eye. It was first placed in its correct position in the front of the eye by Matteo Realdo Colombo (1516?–59) in his *De re anatomica* ('On anatomy', 1559). This not-overlong work is more like a modern textbook than anything which had appeared until then. It is not illustrated, but the text is excellent; and the accounts of the pleura, the mediastinum, and the peritoneum are advanced and accurate. Colombo was a pupil of, and assistant to, Vesalius at Padua, and when Vesalius resigned his chair to become an Imperial physician (1544), Colombo was appointed to succeed him and held the chair for a short time before migrating to Pisa and Rome. Colombo has long been a subject of controversy on the subject of the circulation of the blood. It is usually held that he had no idea of the greater circulation, but that he gave the first clear demonstration of the lesser circulation through the lungs. The question whether or not he had previously read the account by Servetus—which was merely a hypothesis and not a demonstration—has been briefly discussed previously (p. 119).

Gabriele Fallopio (1523–62), another pupil and successor of Vesalius at Padua, published in 1561 his *Observationes anatomicae* ('Anatomical observations'), in which he described the tubes named after him, the round ligaments, and other features of the female genital organs. He also described the aqueduct named after him, the cochlea and labyrinth of the ear, and the chorda tympani. His work on the cranial nerves is important, especially the fourth, fifth, eighth, and ninth nerves. The discovery of the stapes (1603) is credited to Ingrassia (p. 202).

In the seventeenth century there were two outstanding works on the nervous system. The first was the *Cerebri anatome* of Thomas Willis (1621–75), which also contains his much improved classification of the cranial nerves, and his account of the hitherto undescribed eleventh (spinal accessory) nerve. In other works Willis, who was also an outstanding physician, described the sweet taste of diabetic urine, an important factor in the diagnosis of diabetes mellitus; and he was the first to describe myasthenia gravis and puerperal fever. Raymond Vieussens (1641–1715) of Montpellier published in 1685 his *Neurographia universalis*, which dealt in an outstanding manner with the central and peripheral nervous systems. In other works Vieussens wrote on the ear, on the structure of the left ventricle, and on the course of the coronary vessels. In his book on the human vascular system (1705) he was the first to describe mitral stenosis. He was also the first to describe aortic insufficiency, and the characteristic 'water-hammer pulse' of that disease which is now associated with the name of Corrigan (p. 283).

In the eighteenth century one of the most celebrated anatomists was the Dane, Jakob Benignus Winslow (1669–1760). In 1733 he published his four-volume *Exposition anatomique de la structure du corps humain* ('Anatomical exposition of the structure of the human body'), which remained the standard work for nearly a century. Winslow divided the sympathetic system into the greater sympathetic with its ganglia, and the lesser sympathetic. He described the foramen leading from the greater to the lesser sac of the peritoneum, which still bears his name. Another great anatomist, Samuel Thomas von Soemmering (1755–1830), published in 1778 a Latin work on the base of the brain and the origins of the cranial nerves, his classification of which superseded that of Willis. Soemmering is also known for a series of treatises on the organs of special sense, and for a textbook of anatomy, in German (1791–6), which contained only observations which he had himself made. In 1753 Monro *secundus* described definitively the interventricular foramen between the lateral ventricles of the brain. Antonio Scarpa (1747?–1832), one of the greatest of Italian anatomists, studied the nerves of the heart, and his work on this subject, *Tabulae nevrologicae* (1794), is brilliantly illustrated by himself. Scarpa was also a pioneer in otology (he described the membranous labyrinth) and in operations for hernia, and several structures in the body are named after him. The mechanism of the ear had already been very thoroughly studied by Antonio Maria Valsalva (p. 628).

In the nineteenth century perhaps the most important work on the gross anatomy of the brain was *Das Menschenhirn* ('The human brain', 1896) of the Swede, Magnus Gustav Retzius (1842–1919), in which he described a gyrus and other structures named after him. Probably the most stimulating of twentieth-century writings on the morphology of the brain are those of Sir Grafton Elliot Smith (1871–1937), whose comparative studies led to new conceptions of the evolutionary development of the cerebral hemispheres. Elliot Smith also carried out intensive work on the anatomy and pathology of Egyptian mummies, and his anthropological writings on the diffusions of culture and the migrations of races were of great importance.

Our knowledge of the microscopic structure of the nervous system was obtained mainly in the nineteenth century, and was inaugurated largely by Remak and by Purkinje. Robert Remak (1815–65), a Pole who studied and worked in Berlin, was writing on the microscopic structure of the nervous system in 1836, and two years later he published his discovery that sympathetic nerve-fibres were grey because they were non-medullated. He noted that the axons of nerves were continuous with nerve-cells in the spinal cord. He was the first to mention the neurolemma (myelin-sheath of nerve-fibres), which was described by Schwann (p. 322) a year later. Remak recognized microscopically the six cortical cell layers of the cerebrum. He was also a pioneer in the embryology of the nervous system, and in the use of electrotherapy in the treatment of nervous diseases.

Contemporaneous with Remak was the Czech physiologist, Johannes Evangelista Purkinje (1787–1869), professor at Breslau and later at Prague. In 1837 he presented at a conference in Prague a paper in which he described nerve-cells, with their nuclei and dendrites, and also described and illustrated myelinated nerve-fibres and the large flask-like 'cells of Purkinje' which are characteristic of the cerebellar cortex. Purkinje also described the germinal vesicle in the embryo and other histological features; he wrote on cutaneous sensation and various subjective phenomena; and he was the first histologist to use the term protoplasm.

The neuroglia, in which the nervous elements of the nervous system are embedded, was so named by Virchow (p. 325) in 1854; he showed that it consisted of a peculiar type of cells. An outstanding histologist who took a great interest in the nervous system was Rudolf Albert von Kölliker (1817–1905), a Swiss who studied under Johannes Müller (p. 287) and Jakob Henle (p. 321). At the age of thirty he was appointed to a chair at Würzburg and he continued to hold the highest anatomical posts in that university for fifty-five years. Kölliker wrote the first comprehensive treatise on histology (1852), and likewise the first on comparative embryology (1861). He was the first to state that hereditary characters are transmitted by the cell nucleus. In 1845 Kölliker showed that nerve-fibres are secondary to nerve-cells, and that at least some of them are processes of nerve-cells. He thus anticipated the neuron theory, which was definitely formulated in 1891 by Heinrich Wilhelm Gottfried Waldeyer-Hartz (1836–1921), usually referred to as Waldeyer. He also discovered the germinal epithelium. Another great histologist who was also interested in the nervous system was the Swiss, Wilhelm His (1831–1904), who held the anatomy chairs at Basle and Leipzig for forty-seven years. In 1887 he showed that axons are outgrowths of primitive nerve-cells, and he later demonstrated that the neuroglia is derived from the ectoderm.

These histological studies were greatly stimulated by new staining methods for nerve-cells and their fibres. The pioneer in this work was Camillo Golgi (1843–1926), who in 1873 described his method of using chromate of silver to impregnate the nerve elements with that metal, as a result of which they appear black when examined microscopically. Golgi used the method both on normal and pathological material. His numerous observations on the histology of the nervous system were collected in his work *Sulla fina anatomia degli organi centrali del sistema nervoso* ('On the microscopic anatomy of the central nervous system', 1885–6). In 1898 he described the Golgi apparatus in animal cells; the function of this interesting part of the cell has not yet been definitely settled.

Even greater than Golgi as a histologist of the nervous system was the Spaniard, Santiago Ramon y Cajal (1852–1934). Golgi's silver method was liable to be rather unreliable. Cajal modified it and used it to elucidate the finer structure of the brain as no one had done previously. On many important points Golgi and Cajal were not in agreement. Golgi, for example, persistently rejected the neuron doctrine, whereas Cajal upheld it stoutly. The award of a Nobel Prize jointly to these two men in 1926 epitomizes the vast importance of their work in the field of neurology. Vittorio Marchi (1851–1908) also holds an important place because of his discovery of the osmic acid stain for the degenerating myelin sheaths of nerve-fibres.

The detailed study of the arrangement of the cells and fibres in the cerebral cortex was due to two pioneers, Alfred Walter Campbell (1868–1937) and Korbinian Brodmann (1868–1918). Campbell's work, *Histological Studies on the Localization of Cerebral Function* (1905), is a classic and is based on function rather than on structure. Brodmann, on the other hand, thought along the lines of comparative morphology, and his book *Vergleichende Lokalisationslehre der Grosshirnrinde* ('Comparative studies on localization in the cerebral cortex', 1909) is also a classic. Jean Nageotte (1866–1948) of Paris worked on the structure of the nerve-fibre and on nerve regeneration.

Detailed mention of the work which led to an understanding of the many pathways for nerve impulses in the central nervous system is much too complex to be dealt with here. Some reference may, however, be made to that part which is simplest and most generally known, viz. the nerve tracts in the spinal cord. It was early realized that the nerve-fibres in the cord which ultimately passed from it in the roots of the spinal nerves were probably grouped in bundles or tracts in the white matter. The first of these tracts to be definitely delimited was the fasciculus cuneatus, lying in the postero-medial column of the white matter, and consisting of ascending sensory fibres from the mid-thoracic region upwards. This tract was described about 1820 by Karl Friedrich Burdach (1776–1847) of Königsberg, a well-known writer on anatomy and physiology.

Although the name of Ludwig Türck (1810–68) of Vienna is usually associated with the anterior corticospinal tract, he was the discoverer of five other tracts in the cord (1849–53). He was also responsible for the important generalization that the direction of degeneration in a nerve tract corresponds to the direction in which it conducts nerve impulses; and hence in the case of transverse section of the spinal cord the ascending (sensory) tracts degenerate above the lesion and the descending (motor) tracts degenerate below it. Türck's work, ignored for ten years, later inspired others. With Johann Nepomuk Czermak (1828–73) he popularized the clinical use of the laryngoscope, which had been invented in 1854 by the London singing teacher Manuel Garcia (1805–1906).

A great stimulus was given to these studies by the discovery in 1850 that if a bundle of nerve-fibres is cut, those parts of the fibres which are then separated from their cells rapidly degenerate. This discovery was made by Augustus Volney Waller (1816–70), the English physiologist who held posts in Great Britain and in Europe. As a result of sections of nerve roots and of the cord, the areas of the degenerated fibres in the cord could be delimited. At a later date it was found possible to group the nerve-fibres in the cord according to the dates at which they acquire their medullary sheaths (the embryological method of Flechsig); and the staining methods of Golgi (p. 247) enabled individual fibres to be followed throughout much of their course. By these methods other tracts in the cord were demarcated. For example, the other main ascending sensory tract, the fasciculus gracilis, lying medial to the fasciculus cuneatus, was described by Friedrich Goll (1829–1903) in 1860; the superficial anterolateral (anterior spinocerebellar) tract by Sir William Gowers (p. 278) in 1880; and the important rubrospinal tract by Constantin von Monakow (1853–1930) in 1909. Ludwig Edinger (1855–1918) of Frankfort-on-Main described the ventral and dorsal spinocerebellar tracts before 1885; and Paul Emil Flechsig (1847–1929) of Leipzig did further work on the dorsal spinocerebellar tract, which is usually named after him. In 1876 Flechsig published important work on the pyramidal tracts. The nucleus dorsalis (Clarke's column) in the grey matter was described by Jacob Augustus Lockhart Clarke (1817–80) in 1851.

The cerebrospinal fluid was discovered by Domenico Cotugno (1736–1822) in 1774, and its examination was greatly facilitated by the introduction of the minor operation of lumbar puncture by Heinrich Quincke (1842–1922) in 1895.

In the field of sensory end-organs, the structure of the retina was worked out very carefully by Cajal, and that of the cochlea by Afonso Corti (1829–88) in 1851.

The modern physiology of the nervous system starts with Sir Charles Bell's *Idea of a New Anatomy of the Brain* (1811) (p. 154), and with the experiments later carried out under its influence by Magendie. Since then there have been enormous developments in our knowledge and we can deal only with a few of these. We therefore select mainly reflex action, cerebral localization, and nervous integration as giving a representative idea of the progress made.

(*b*) *Reflex action.* Even in a state of absolute rest our bodies are constantly subject to reflex actions, of which that of breathing is the most continuous and most essential. The contraction of the pupil on exposure to light is automatically effected without the individual being in the least conscious that the contraction has taken place. There is a difference between these two types of reflex. That of breathing can be consciously inhibited for a time, but the will has no power over the contraction of the pupil on exposure to light. It was noticed quite early that in certain nervous diseases reflexes of the limbs were increased, diminished, or lost, so that from a clinical aspect study of reflex action was important, apart from its great interest in the sphere of physiology.

The fundamental ideas in the conception of reflex action had already been adumbrated by Descartes. In the view of that philosopher any stimulus is transmitted along nerve-fibres to the central nervous system. There, on account of existing nervous connexions, it gives rise to a fresh impulse which passes along outgoing nerve-fibres to the active organ, muscle, or gland, which is thereby excited to activity (p. 139). Thus, every action of the organism, and its life as a whole, conforms to definite laws. These laws must be directed to its preservation, or organisms would cease to exist. It is thus possible to look on organisms simply as elaborate mechanisms. Except that we know that we ourselves think and feel, we might eliminate mind from our consideration of the action of beings other than ourselves. Such was the view taken by the mechanists and other members of the iatrophysical school (pp. 138–42), which followed broadly the teaching of Descartes. The course of physiological advance may be described, briefly, as the expulsion of the mental element from process after process associated with the activity of nerve.

The conceptions of Descartes and his successors were assumptions and were not based on any experimental evidence. The fundamental experiment was performed by Stephen Hales (p. 155), who about 1730 decapitated a frog and found that reflex movements of the legs could still be produced by pricking the skin. He then found that these reflex movements were abolished if the spinal cord was destroyed. Hales did not publish this experiment, but it is quoted by Robert Whytt (1714–66), the predecessor of Cullen in the chair of the Institutes of Medicine at Edinburgh. Whytt's *An Essay on the Vital and other Involuntary Motions of Animals* (1751) is one of the classics of neurophysiology. Whytt thought that the purpose of any involuntary action is to remove anything that irritates or hurts the body. He established the fact that the spinal cord is essential for its completion, and put forward the theory that the reflex is due to a stimulus acting on an unconscious sentient principle, situated in the brain and cord, which reflects the stimulus back to the muscles. He demonstrated that reflex action does not depend on the integrity of the cord as a whole, since stimulation of the skin will produce a reflex if only a small segment of the cord is intact. Whytt also described cases in which certain reflexes were abolished because swellings in the brain substance interrupted the path of the stimulus. Georgius Prochaska (1749–1820) of Vienna thought that there was a special region in the brain—the 'sensorium commune'—which reflected the stimuli back to the muscles (c. 1782). Prochaska's work has probably been overrated. He assumed that there are motor and sensory fibres, but he had no idea of motor and sensory roots. The demonstration of the latter by Bell and by Magendie has already been mentioned (p. 154).

Herbert Mayo (1796–1852), physiologist to the Middlesex Hospital in London, carried the problem a step farther in his *Anatomical and Physiological Commentaries* (1822, 1833). In the first part of this work (1822) he described the functions of the nerves of the face, especially the trigeminal and the facial nerves. In the second part (1833) he showed that a certain small segment of the brain-stem was necessary to produce reflexes in the pupils. Marshall Hall (1790–1857) in a series of inspired experiments illuminated the position. In 1833 he showed that, if the spinal cord of a frog was cut through between the anterior and the posterior limbs, that part of the body anterior to the injury was moved volitionally; the legs, on the other hand, were drawn up and motionless. But on a stimulus being applied to the legs, they moved energetically, but only once for each stimulus. Pain stimuli applied to the legs were not felt by the animal. From these and other experiments Hall deduced that the nervous system is made up of a series of segmental reflex arcs. In the intact spinal cord stimuli passing round these arcs are co-ordinated by the ascending and descending pathways in the cord to form movement patterns. Marshall Hall appreciated that a stimulus cannot be put into the spinal cord through a sensory nerve without it producing effects beyond the anatomical segment to which that nerve belongs. He showed that the spinal cord is more than a great nerve trunk. It has a life of its own, just as the cerebrum has.

The knee-jerk, that well-known reflex which is much used in the clinical examination of the nervous system, was described independently in 1875 by Wilhelm Heinrich Erb (1840–1921) and by Carl Friedrich Otto Westphal (1833–90).

These studies on spinal reflexes were stimulated by the discovery of a centre in the brain which originates and co-ordinates the action of the respiratory muscles. The respiratory movements are involuntary under ordinary conditions. The first to carry out experiments (1812) on this centre was Julien Jean César Legallois (1770–1814). They were confirmed and extended in 1824 by Marie Jean Pierre Flourens (p. 255), a very brilliant French experimental physiologist. By these experiments it was shown that the respiratory centre is situated in the brain-stem, the medulla oblongata.

Since Hall's time there has been a great extension of the conception of reflexes. The following description of a simple spinal reflex is based on Hall's work, but incorporates knowledge available since his time (Fig. 83). An afferent impression from a sense organ to the spinal cord may give rise to an efferent impulse by a purely intra-spinal process. The result of this impulse may be of the nature of a complex and balanced muscular act involving a whole system of muscles, some of which may be mutually antagonistic. All this may take place not only unconsciously, without any intervention from the higher nerve centres in the brain, but even in a decerebrate animal, that is one from which the brain has been removed. On the other

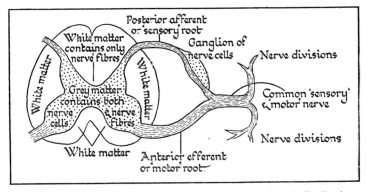

FIG. 82. Transverse section of the spinal cord, and origin and distribution of a spinal nerve.

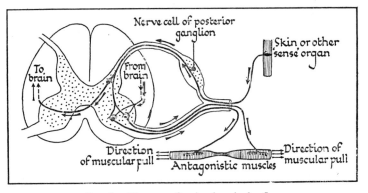

FIG. 83. Diagram of a simple spinal reflex.

hand, paths—indicated in Fig. 83—exist for the passage of impressions to and impulses from higher centres. These higher centres in many cases control or modify the resulting muscular or other action.

It has been shown that, besides the simple reflex arc (Fig. 83), there are more complex reflex arcs which depend for their action on the integrity of an elaborate mechanism. The important researches of Sherrington (p. 263) especially showed that the nervous system is integrated at higher and higher levels, till at last the highest centres of the brain are reached. Many of the ordinary acts of life, sneezing, coughing, standing, walking, and breathing, are expressible as reflex actions. The attempt has also been made to press the 'instincts' into the same category. But it is difficult to separate the instinctive from the volitional elements or define either.

(c) *Cerebral localization.* The localization of specific functions to different parts of the brain itself has a long and interesting history. In his *Cerebri anatome* (1664) Thomas Willis (p. 245) suggested that the cerebrum is responsible for voluntary movements whereas the cerebellum controls those which are involuntary. This was merely a guess, but the observation set others thinking. Then in 1691 Robert Boyle (p. 136) mentioned the case of a knight who had suffered a depressed fracture of his skull; thereafter he developed loss of sensation and of muscular movements in an arm and a leg. At operation the surgeon removed a spicule of bone from the surface of the patient's brain, and all the symptoms of paralysis disappeared within a few hours. This observation suggested that there might be a motor area on the surface of the brain.

An important, though later misguided, worker in this field was Franz Joseph Gall (1758–1828), who devoted much of his life to the anatomy and physiology of the nervous system. While living in Vienna he started to lecture (1796) on the localization of mental faculties in the brain, and on the effects produced by these 'localizations' on the surface of the brain and of the skull. This materialistic approach was distasteful to his contemporaries, and in 1805 Gall left Vienna and began a triumphant tour through various countries before settling in Paris two years later. With him went his pupil, Johann Caspar Spurzheim (1776–1832), and between them they founded the pseudo-science of phrenology. Their theory that the outstanding traits in an individual's character could be ascertained by comparing the 'bumps' on his head with those indicated on a phrenological chart or model long had a popular following. Gall and Spurzheim listed over thirty human faculties, such as acquisitiveness, amativeness, combativeness, and they claimed that the possession by an individual of any of these faculties led to an increased development of certain localized parts of the brain. Even until the early years of the twentieth century 'phrenological heads', in ivory or porcelain, and phrenological charts could be purchased in shops. Their theory was devoid of any scientific foundation, and this fact has tended to the complete discredit of Gall and Spurzheim. Nevertheless, these men were important in the study of other aspects of the nervous system. Their work in four volumes, *Anatomie et physiologie du système nerveux en général, et du cerveau en particulier* ('Anatomy and physiology of the nervous system in general, and of the brain in particular', 1810–19) was a serious scientific work in which they showed that the white matter of the brain consists of nerve-fibres, and that within the brain-stem there is a partial crossing of the pyramidal tracts. The work of Gall and Spurzheim was a stimulus to that of others.

Among these was Luigi Rolando (1773–1831) of Sardinia, who removed the cerebellum and the cerebral hemispheres separately in different animals and observed the effects. He described his observations in his book *Saggio sopra la vera struttura del cervello dell'uomo, degl'animali e sopra le funzioni del sistema nervoso* ('Monograph on the true structure of the brain of man and animals, and on the functions of the nervous system', 1809). Rolando illustrated this work himself, and he also engraved the illustrations, set the type, and printed and bound the copies of the book with his own hands. In this classic work he also concluded that the cerebellum presides over involuntary movements and the cerebrum over volitional acts.

In 1822 Marie Jean Pierre Flourens (1794–1867) began to present memoirs to the Academy of Sciences in Paris on his experiments on the central nervous system. In 1824 he collected these in his important book, *Recherches expérimentales sur les propriétés et les fonctions du système nerveux dans les animaux vertébrés* ('Experimental researches on the properties and functions of the nervous system in vertebrates'), and in 1842 he published a much enlarged edition. Flourens gave a classic description of a pigeon from which he had removed the cerebral hemispheres; one result was that the animal was blind. When only one cerebral hemisphere was removed, the bird lost the sight of the eye on the opposite side. Flourens therefore demonstrated that vision depends on the integrity of the cerebral cortex. He then described the condition of a pigeon from which he had removed only the cerebellum; the bird saw and heard well, but it stood, walked, and flew in an indecisive manner; equilibrium was almost entirely abolished. Two years later Flourens repeated these experiments on a dog, and gave a classic description of the behaviour of a mammal deprived of its cerebellum. He was the first to show that injury to the cerebellum causes inco-ordination of movement, and he thus formally introduced into physiology the idea of nervous co-ordination. He also did important work on the action of the semicircular canals of the inner ear in regulating movements. The work of Flourens on removal of the cerebral hemispheres was confirmed by Magendie (1841) and others.

Flourens made no attempt to remove, or to stimulate, localized areas of the cerebral hemispheres. He was opposed to the ideas of functional localization, carried to excess by Gall and Spurzheim, and his *Examen de la phrénologie* ('Examination of phrenology', 1842) was a serious blow to that theory. About the middle of the nineteenth century it was almost universally considered that there was no localization of function in the cerebrum. It is true that Bartolomeo Panizza (1785–1867) examined the brains of two patients in 1855 and concluded that the parieto-occipital (lateral and posterior) area of the cerebral cortex is necessary for vision. He also removed the occipital area of the cortex of dogs and showed that blindness resulted. But Panizza's experiments passed virtually unnoticed, and they were soon forgotten. In 1861, however, Pierre Paul Broca (1824–80) published a paper in which he claimed that the inferior frontal gyrus in the left cerebral hemisphere (Broca's convolution) was more developed than that on the right side, and that it was the centre for articulate speech.

The next step was made by the clinicians, especially John Hughlings Jackson (1835–1911), physician to the London Hospital, the father of English neurology, whose ideas are still of importance in stimulating new advances. From 1864 onwards Hughlings Jackson studied cases of epilepsy in which convulsions arose unilaterally, sometimes remaining confined to a restricted group of muscles (for example, those moving the digits of one hand), and sometimes spreading from the site of their first appearance to the remaining muscles on the side of onset, and even passing the middle line to

involve those of the opposite side. From these and other observations, including the movements in chorea and the forms of paralysis
ensuing upon local destroying lesions of the cerebral hemisphere,
he concluded that movements were represented, or co-ordinated, in
some special region of the cerebral cortex. The convulsions arising
unilaterally he attributed to 'discharge of energy' from a focus of
cortical cells, usually due to some gross local lesion. Jackson's contemporary, Henry Charlton Bastian (1837–1915) put forward comparable, but less comprehensive, ideas.

Almost at once Jackson's views of a local representation of movements in the cortex received experimental confirmation at the hands
of Gustav Theodor Fritsch (1838–91) and Eduard Hitzig (1838–
1907), who reported in 1870 that in the dog they had found that
electrical stimulation of certain points of the cerebral cortex lying in
front of the central sulcus (fissure of Rolando) produced movements
of certain parts of the opposite side of the body. They also showed
that excitation of similar points in different animals, or upon opposite
sides of the brain in the same animal, produced similar results. In the
case of many other areas of the cerebral cortex excitation produced
movement. The area which could thus be stimulated artificially was
known as the motor area, and Hitzig defined it accurately in the dog
and the monkey in his important monograph, *Untersuchungen über
das Gehirn* ('Experiments on the brain', 1874). The human cortex
was first stimulated artificially in the same year by Roberts Bartholow
(1831–1904), and similar human experiments were later made by Sir
Victor Horsley (p. 368) and others.

The work of these two observers was carried farther by (Sir)
David Ferrier (1843–1928), a young graduate of Aberdeen and
Edinburgh who early settled in London and was appointed to the
staff of King's College Hospital, where Lister was later his colleague.
Ferrier's early experimental work was carried out largely at the West
Riding Asylum in Yorkshire, and at the age of thirty he published
a valuable report on his experiments on the brain of the dog and the
monkey. Three years later his very important book on *The Functions
of the Brain* (1876) appeared. Ferrier removed portions of the
cerebral cortex and noted the results, and he also investigated the
results of electro-stimulation of various areas of the cortex. By

removal of the hand-area of the motor cortex in monkeys he caused paralysis of the hand. Continental workers were not then eager to accept the implications of these experiments. But at the International Medical Congress in 1881 Ferrier showed one of these paralytic monkeys; its attitude was so striking that the great French neurologist Charcot (p. 274) exclaimed 'C'est un malade' (It is a patient). In 1899 the American physiologist George Addison Talbert (1865–1947) stimulated electrically the cortex of conscious dogs by electrodes implanted in their substance; the result was local seizures which resembled those of Jacksonian epilepsy.

It should be emphasized, however, that Jackson's concept of the plan of organization of movements by the cerebral cortex was from the outset different from that adopted then and later by Ferrier and the experimental workers on this problem. Jackson did not believe that individual muscles were represented in the cortex. He conceived that movements were represented, and this was expressed in his aphorism, 'the cerebral cortex knows nothing of muscles, it knows only of movements'. Moreover, he did not believe in contiguous foci of fixed representation of movements, but in an overlapping plan in which the movements of face and hand were largely represented.

Clinical observation has long since confirmed Jackson's views, and the concept of fixed foci of representation of muscles or of movements ('the cortical mosaic') has at last ceased to command the wide acceptance it enjoyed for so long.

At this same meeting of the International Medical Congress Friedrich Leopold Goltz (1834–1902) showed dogs from which the cerebrum had been almost totally removed by a series of operations. Such a dog showed a condition of complete idiocy. It was incapable of understanding, memory, recognition of friends or enemies, of sexual impulses, or desire for food. All its actions were reflex.

With Horsley and other collaborators Schäfer investigated the effects of faradic stimulation of the cerebral cortex and spinal cord in primates. (Edward Albert Schäfer, later Sir Edward Sharpey-Schafer (1850–1935), was pupil of and successor to Sharpey at University College, London, and he afterwards held the chair of physiology at Edinburgh.) It was not then realized that the fissure of Rolando demarcates clearly the motor (anterior) from the sensory (posterior) areas. In monkeys a new plane of accuracy was reached by Sherrington (p. 263) and his collaborators, especially Albert Sidney Grünbaum (later, Leyton) (1869–1921) and Thomas Graham Brown (1882–).

In earlier work Sherrington showed that, when in the chimpanzee paralysis of an arm had been produced by destruction of the arm

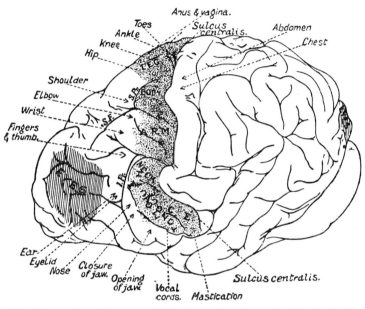

FIG. 84. Diagram by Grünbaum and Sherrington showing cerebral localization in the chimpanzee (C. S. Sherrington, *Integrative Action*, New Haven, 1923)

area in the motor cortex, complete recovery of function took place within four and a half months, and it was shown by another operation later that the destroyed area had not been regenerated. There had been throughout the literature of the motor cortex a tacit assumption that its area was the same as that of the huge Betz cells which are found in it. But the paper by Leyton and Sherrington (1917) is the most careful delimitation of the motor area in the anthropoid apes which has yet appeared. The motor area as defined by them is not co-extensive with that of the Betz cells; and the same observation applies to the human cortex, which had been investigated at operation especially by Wilder Graves Penfield (1891–) and his colleagues. There has therefore been much controversy over the relations between the cytoarchitecture and the functions of the motor cortex. It may be said that the ideas formed by Sherrington and his co-workers regarding the plan of organization of movements in the cortex approximate more closely to those of Hughlings Jackson than they do to those of other experimental workers in this field.

Sir Frederick Walker Mott (1853–1926) worked with Schäfer about 1890 on the effects of stimulating the cerebral cortex, and he did important work on the cerebral localization of vision. Mott later added much to our knowledge of brain structure, especially in organic mental disease. He was the first in Great Britain to demonstrate the *Treponema pallidum* in the brains of general paralytics (p. 507), and he was largely responsible for the foundation of the Maudsley Hospital.

In the United States a flourishing school of neurophysiology was built up at Yale University by John Farquhar Fulton (1899–) between 1930 and 1952. He himself worked in many branches of the subject, especially in that of cerebral localization in the higher apes. At the time when he relinquished active work in this field he was bound to the doctrine of the representation of individual muscles in the cortex.

The work of Flourens on the cerebellum was much extended by the Italian physiologist, Luigi Luciani (1840–1919), who held chairs at the universities of Siena, Florence, and Rome. His early work on the cerebellum was published in 1882, and in 1891 there appeared his great monograph on this organ. Modern work on the cerebellum owes much to his experiments and deductions.

(*d*) *The autonomic nervous system*. An early anatomical observation on this system was that of Willis (p. 245), who described the thoracic chain of ganglia as the 'intercostal nerve'. Reference has already been made to the observations of Eustachius and Winslow. Another important anatomical observation was the discovery of the myenteric plexus in the bowel wall in 1862 by Leopold Auerbach (1828–97).

The discovery that section of the 'intercostal nerve', that is, the cervical sympathetic chain, is followed by ptosis of the eyelid, constriction of the pupils, and enophthalmos (a withdrawing of the eyeball into the orbit) was published by François Pourfour du Petit (1664–1741) in 1710. He described a series of cases of gun-shot wounds of the head and neck which showed these signs, and he endeavoured to reproduce the signs experimentally in animals. His conclusion was that Eustachius and succeeding writers were wrong, and that the 'intercostal nerve' is not a cranial nerve but that it originates from the spinal cord. The syndrome of Pourfour du Petit mentioned above was later described independently by Edward Selleck Hare (1812–38), by Claude Bernard (p. 294), and by Johann Friedrich Horner (1831–86) in 1869, and the syndrome is now known by Horner's name.

The discovery that the sympathetic system consists of small medullated nerve-fibres was announced in 1842 by Friedrich Heinrich Bidder (p. 582) and Alfred Wilhelm Volkmann (1800–77).

It had long been known that paralysis was often accompanied by changes in the temperature of the paralysed parts. The first crucial explanation of this phenomenon was made by Claude Bernard (p. 294) in 1851. In the rabbit the cervical sympathetic is quite separate from the vagus. Bernard cut the cervical sympathetic in a rabbit and found that the temperature of that side of the head was appreciably increased. This was a point which Pourfour du Petit had missed. Later in the same year he repeated this experiment in the dog and showed that the section was followed by the signs which constitute Horner's syndrome and also by appreciable increase in temperature. The next logical step was taken in 1852 by Charles Édouard Brown-Séquard (1817–94), who at that time was giving lectures on Bernard's work. Brown-Séquard stimulated the cut end of the cervical sympathetic by galvanism, and found that the overheated skin became paler and cooler. This work was unknown to Bernard when he himself carried out the stimulation and obtained the same result. The explanation of these phenomena was at first obscured by Bernard's belief that he was dealing with an effect upon arteries and veins; but it later became clear to him that the action was really on the capillaries. The cervical sympathetic is a vasoconstrictor nerve, and its stimulation produces contraction of the capillaries. In 1857 he first discovered that there are also vasodilator fibres, for example, in the nerve supply to the submaxillary gland, stimulation of which produced dilatation of the capillaries. To Bernard therefore belongs the credit for the discovery of vasomotor nerves, constrictor and dilator, and the possibility of control of the blood flow by the action of the nervous system.

Our modern knowledge of the autonomic nervous system is due very largely to the work of the two Cambridge physiologists, Gaskell and Langley. Walter Holbrook Gaskell (1847–1914) published a paper on the vasomotor nerves of striated muscle in 1874. Eight years later he published his important work on the innervation of the heart. Gaskell next worked on the central sympathetic proper, which he showed was not a separate nervous system, but was made up of efferent fibres given off by the thoracic and upper two lumbar segments of the spinal cord. This was the thoracolumbar outflow; and in 1886 Gaskell demonstrated two further outflows, the bulbar from the cervical region, and the sacral. He included all three outflows under the term 'involuntary nervous system'.

John Newport Langley (1852–1925) was assistant to Sir Michael Foster (1836–1907) whom he eventually succeeded in the chair of physiology at Cambridge. He worked for many years on similar lines to Gaskell, but introduced many new concepts. In 1898 he applied the name autonomic nervous system—instead of involuntary nervous system—to cover the nervous system of the glands and the involuntary muscles; it includes the sympathetic system. In 1889 Langley showed that if a sympathetic ganglion is painted with nicotine, the passage of a nervous impulse across it is blocked. He demonstrated (with Sir Hugh Kerr Anderson, 1865–1928) the unity of postganglionic neurons, and did important work on the segmental distribution of sympathetic fibres and on vasomotor reflexes and the control of the capillaries. The early decades of the twentieth century saw the publication of two great works in this field, Gaskell's *The Involuntary Nervous System* (1916) and Langley's *The Autonomic Nervous System* (1921). Our conceptions of the autonomic nervous system today are still much dependent on these two works. Mention may also be made of Gustave Roussy (1874–1948) of Paris and his work on the nervous mechanism for the control of the functions of the bladder and rectum; of knowledge gained from clinical sources, such as *The Automatic Bladder* (1918) of Sir Henry Head (p. 270) and

George Riddoch (1889–1947); and of experimental work on the control of micturition by Frederick James Fitzmaurice Barrington (1884–1956), urologist to University College Hospital, London.

(e) *Sherrington and nervous integration.* The supreme illumination of the physiology of the nervous system was effected as a result of fifty years of experiments by Sir Charles Scott Sherrington (1857–1952), professor of physiology at Liverpool and later at Oxford. It is convenient to consider briefly his work as belonging to three periods, of which the middle period is that covered by his masterpiece on *The Integrative Action of the Nervous System* (1906).

Sherrington's first important work was to show that in general the muscles do not receive their motor nerve supply from only one segment of the spinal cord. In the limbs especially many muscles receive their motor fibres from three consecutive spinal roots. Hence in the case of these regions no injury to the cord at a certain level could cause paralysis of a single muscle without others being involved. In later investigations he showed that the sensory nerves to areas of skin did not correspond segmentally to the motor nerves of the muscles which were situated under these areas; whereas afferent fibres in the nerves to the muscles themselves corresponded in origin with the motor fibres. These latter were proprioceptive fibres, conveying the 'muscle sense' to the consciousness.

Sherrington then began his studies of reflex action, a subject which had been neglected for over thirty years. As experimental animals he used not only cats and dogs, but also monkeys and later anthropoid apes. He first elucidated the phenomenon known as spinal shock, which occurs dramatically when the spinal cord of the animal is transected. For a period lasting up to hours no reflexes at all can be elicited by the ordinary methods of stimulation, but later the condition passes off and the reflexes return. He showed that the common flexion reflex is essentially a 'nociceptive reaction', designed to remove the limb rapidly from a source of injury, and he demonstrated that the spinal reflexes of this type are not limited by the segments to which the pain stimuli pass. A sensory stimulus passing to one segment of the cord causes motor stimuli to be discharged from all the segments which innervate the flexor muscles of the limb. About the same time he published the first of his many papers on inhibition and reciprocal innervation. If, when a flexion reflex is about to operate, the extensors of the limb are in a state of tension or even of contraction, the flexion will be produced only with difficulty. Descartes and later observers thought that the extensors either relaxed or remained dormant. Sherrington showed that there was an active relaxation of the antagonistic muscles, produced by the mechanism of reciprocal innervation, which made possible the first quantitative estimation of inhibition as an active nervous process. He demonstrated that the inhibition produced is inversely proportional to the degree to which the antagonistic muscles are stimulated. Inco-ordination of movements is due to a failure of the correct relationship between the action of the effectors and their antagonists.

In 1896 Sherrington described the phenomenon of decerebrate rigidity occurring in animals from which the cerebral hemispheres had been removed. He showed that such an animal took up a characteristic attitude, and that when, for example, the left fore paw of such an animal was stimulated, this leg was flexed and drawn forward, as also was the right hind leg. The result of such stimulation was always to couple diagonal limbs in harmonious movements of similar direction.

In his *Integrative Action* (1906) Sherrington summarized his experiments, added many more experimental observations, developed new theories, and built up a conception of the activity of the nervous system which has had far-reaching results. The reflexes which he studied experimentally were especially the flexion reflex, the extensor reflex, and the scratch reflex. Nine years earlier he had postulated that no reflex arc consisted of one single neuron only, but of at least two neurons. There must therefore not only be intracellular, but also intercellular conduction of the nerve impulse. Hence he conceived that there was a transverse barrier between one cell and the next, a barrier which permitted the impulse to pass with varying ease under different conditions. This connexion between neuron and neuron he named the synapse. Sherrington also postulated the theory of the final common path for efferent impulses. The path of the impulse from any receptor point in the skin is a private path. But if it connects through a reflex arc with any muscle it must do so through the motor nerve to that muscle. As many receptor points may be thus connected with that muscle, impulses from all of them must reach it by the same motor nerve.

Sherrington's analysis of these reflexes showed that there was a latent period before the reflex was produced. There was also a refractory phase, so that the rate of the movement produced could not be accelerated beyond a certain point by increasing the rhythm of the stimulus. On the other hand, repeated mild stimuli, each in itself insufficient to produce a response, were summed in the reflex arc to produce a response. These phenomenon do not occur when we are dealing with a single neuron, and the suggestion is that they are produced at the synapse. Inhibition of a reflex also occurs at the synapse.

The reflex is the simplest expression of the integrative action of the nervous system, to enable the body as a whole to function to one definite end at a time. Like reflexes, arriving simultaneously at the common path, are allowed to pass and reinforce each other. Unlike reflexes have successive but not simultaneous use of the common path. This principle of co-ordination is applicable to the nervous system as a whole, so that singleness of action results despite the conflicting sensory impulses which may be received by the surface receptors at the same time.

Where, as in the human body, the nervous system is built up from a series of segments, short reflexes involving only a few segments are integrated so as to give local reactions of the same type. In long reflexes the nervous connexion may extend through many segments, and yet these are integrated so as to give orderly responses. The action of integration is shown very clearly by the attitude adopted by the resting body. It is seldom that this is the attitude which would result were the body subject only to gravity. For long periods the tone shown by certain groups of muscles enables the body to adopt a certain position without conscious effort, and it is likely that the tone is produced by some form of reflex activity, effected by stimuli from the labyrinth, the cerebellum, and the muscles themselves.

Subsequent to 1906 Sherrington continued to elaborate his theories, and of his observations we will mention only those relating to the maintenance of posture. He showed that throughout the muscular frame of an animal all those muscles, and only those, are in action, the activity of which counteracts gravity in the erect attitude. With Edward George Tandy Liddell (1895–) he demonstrated that if the cutaneous and muscular nerves to the limb of an animal were severed with the exception of the nerve arising from a single isolated muscle in it, stretching of the muscle produced a very large increase of tension in it. It was at once shown also that this effect was a reflex due to impulses arising from the nerves in the muscle itself. This stretch-reflex, as it was named, has been fruitful in elucidating muscle tone and posture in the individual.

Of Sherrington's many gifted pupils and co-workers one of the most important was Rudolf Magnus (1873–1927), a German who became professor of pharmacology at Utrecht. While working with Sherrington in 1908 he made an observation—also noticed independently by Sherrington—that rotation of the head in a decerebrate animal alters the muscle tone in the limbs. This was the first of many observations by Magnus on muscle tone and posture which were published in his book entitled *Körperstellung* ('Body posture', 1924). In a lecture in 1926 he announced an important experiment which illuminated the function of the otoliths and the semicircular canals of the inner ear in regulating the position and balance of the body. Another associate of Sherrington was Johannes Gregorius Dusser de Barenne (1885–1940), a Dutchman who worked at Utrecht, Oxford, and at Yale. He did important work on the sensory cortex and on subcortical regions of the brain.

(*f*) *Pavlov and conditioned reflexes.* The particular type of reflexes on which Sherrington built up his theory of nervous integration were those which are inborn and which are characteristic of the central nervous system of any class of animals. They are hereditary and stable, their strength may vary, and they are only slightly dependent on surrounding conditions. About the end of the nineteenth century the Russian physiologist Ivan Petrovitch Pavlov (1849–1936) was investigating the secretion of gastric juice, and he devised an ingenious operation (p. 302) as a result of which a sample of a dog's gastric juice could be collected easily at any time after the ingestion of food. The relation of the amount and quality of the juice to the type of food ingested could thus be ascertained. He found that the secretion of the juice was controlled by a nervous mechanism.

If food is placed in the dog's mouth the stomach secretes juice. This is a simple reflex of the same nature as those dealt with by Sherrington, and is due to a nervous reaction of the same type as that involved when the scorched hand is suddenly withdrawn from the flame. Such reflexes Pavlov called unconditioned. He now found that the dog's stomach would secrete juice if the dog was merely allowed to smell or to see the food. Here the reflexes involved were different. They were conditioned by the animal's previous experience, and they were acquired and not inherited. Pavlov next showed that, if a bell was rung every time the dog was given food, after a short time the stomach would secrete juice when the bell was rung, even though this event was not followed by the giving of food.

This was a new and more important example of a conditioned reflex. Pavlov proceeded to study more and more complex examples, and he built up theories which helped greatly to elucidate the functions of the cerebrum and to develop psychological theories.

In these experiments on conditioned reflexes Pavlov also used the secretory activity of other glands as an indication of the occurrence of such reflexes. The salivary glands were very frequently employed. By a surgical operation a dog's salivary duct was made to open to the skin surface instead of into the mouth. The saliva was collected in a small glass bulb stuck to the skin surrounding the new opening of the duct, and it was measured in drops by an electrical method.

It was soon found that during such an experiment elaborate precautions had to be taken to prevent the dog from being subjected to adventitious stimuli. During the actual experiment it was therefore found necessary to keep the animal in a sound-proof room so that it should not be disturbed by footsteps or voices. At first the experimenter was in the room with the animal; but it became clear that he was a constant source of stimuli to it. Even the blinking of his eyelids might be sufficient to upset the experiment. Pavlov therefore had constructed a laboratory building specially designed for this work. In the accommodation provided for each experiment the experimenter was in a separate room from the dog. He could watch the dog's reactions through a periscope, but the dog could not see him (Fig. 85). All the controls which determined the stimuli received by the dog were situated in the experimenter's room.

By the use of these methods Pavlov demonstrated that different conditioned reflexes showed the property of summation. For example, if a reflex had been set up by giving food and by blowing a whistle, and at the same time another reflex had been established by giving food and scratching the dog's back, when the two stimuli were given together the number of drops of saliva produced was the sum of those produced in each separate experiment. If a conditioned reflex which has been established is not repeated for several months, decay sets in. But the strength of the reflex is reinforced, that is, brought back to its normal level, by a few applications of the conditioning factors. It is possible to use these conditioned reflexes for

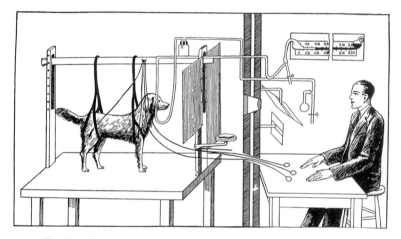

FIG. 85. Pavlov's apparatus for experiments on conditioned reflexes. (Pavlov, *Lectures on Conditioned Reflexes*, trans. W. H. Gantt, London, 1928).

other purposes. For example, two organ pipes of different pitch may be sounded; when one is sounded food is given, but when the other is sounded no food is given. By varying the pitch of the second pipe until it approximates more and more closely to the pitch of the first pipe, the dog's ability to distinguish between notes of different pitch can be estimated.

In the experiment shown in Fig. 85 the skin of the fore and hind limbs of the dog was stimulated mechanically, and immediately after that some weak acid was introduced into its mouth. An ordinary reflex flow of saliva resulted. This procedure was repeated for many days, until ultimately a flow of saliva was produced as soon as the skin stimulation started, and before the acid was introduced into the dog's mouth.

(g) *Sensory perception and sensory disturbances.* Despite the fact that the study of sensory disturbances is an important part of a neurological examination, cutaneous sensibility was not seriously investigated until the second half of the nineteenth century, apart from the work of Müller (p. 287) to which reference is made later.

Histological studies on the skin showed that the cutaneous nerves ended freely in the dermis or communicated with various types of organized bodies, which were assumed to be responsible for the different kinds of cutaneous sensation. Towards the close of the nineteenth century physiological testing of the skin surface showed that it was covered with numerous spots, each of which responded to at least one of the four types of stimuli, touch, cold, warmth, and cutaneous pain. These phenomena were first investigated independantly in 1884 by Magnus Gustav Blix (1849–1904) and by Johannes Karl Goldscheider (1858–1935), who showed that, for example, a pressure spot gave only a sensation of pressure even though the stimulus applied was sufficiently violent to produce pain. The distribution of tactile spots in various regions of the skin was worked out by them; and the strength of the stimulus necessary to evoke a sensation of touch was studied especially by Max von Frey (1852–1932), who introduced his method of testing sensation by means of small bristles mounted in handles.

The correlation of the physiological results with the histological findings proved remarkably difficult. Of many sensory structures described as present in the skin, the more important are Meissner's corpuscles, Merkel's disks, Krause's end-bulbs, and the Golgi-Mazzoni corpuscles. The segmental distribution of the skin areas of hyperalgesia was discovered by Head in 1893. Towards the close of the nineteenth century it was held that the adequate stimulus for a touch spot was deformation of the skin surface; and that the pain produced by heat is probably due to the stimulation of pain spots and not warmth spots. It was also realized that the pain produced from pain spots can be evoked not only by mechanical stimuli, but probably also by thermal, chemical, and electrical stimuli. At that period Sherrington discarded the supposition that there are separate efferent nerve fibres the function of which is to carry pain impressions to a 'pain centre'.

About the same period advances were made in knowledge of the proprioceptive receptors in muscles. Sir Charles Bell (p. 154) was the first to state the theory that there is a muscle sense which may be compared to the other senses, and his view led this muscle sense to be often referred to as the sixth sense. Elongated bodies had been noted in 1851 lying between the muscle fibres, and a decade later they were more fully described by Kölliker. The best early description of these proprioceptive receptors was given (1863) by Willy Kühne (1837–1900), who called them muscle spindles. No particular function was attributed to them until Angelo Ruffini (1864–1929) made a histological study of their nerve endings in 1892, and in the following year Sherrington traced to the spinal ganglia the nervefibres which arose from them. The organs of Golgi were first described by J. P. M. Rollett in 1876 and more fully by Golgi in 1880 and the Pacinian corpuscles had long been known to occur in tendons.

These anatomical and physiological findings were of no great assistance to the clinical neurologists, who found that they did not explain sensory disturbances frequently met with in patients suffering from organic nervous lesions. In these circumstances the clinical aspect was investigated by (Sir) Henry Head (1861–1940). With his collaborators, William Halse Rivers Rivers (1864–1922) and James Sherren (1872–1945), Head published in 1905 an important paper entitled 'The afferent nervous system from a new aspect'. Head had the radial nerve divided in his own arm, and thereafter he and his colleagues analysed the disorders of sensory function which resulted, and the restoration of sensation as the nerve regenerated. In order to explain these different types of cutaneous sensations Head postulated the existence of a double system of cutaneous sensory nerves and end-organs (receptors) which he named respectively 'protopathic' and 'epicritic'. Wilfred Batten Lewis Trotter (1872–1939), who was responsible for many advances in neurological surgery and as the author of *The Herd Instinct in Peace and War* (1916) has claims to be a founder of social psychology, had a similar but more extensive experiment carried out on himself. His results differed from those of Head in certain important ways, as also did those of Edwin Garrigues Boring (1886–). Nevertheless, Head's hypothesis of the existence of protopathic and epicritic nerve-fibres in the skin continued to influence neurological thought, despite the absence of any anatomical evidence of their existence, for nearly forty years.

One of the difficulties of linking up clinical findings with histological evidence was the fact that the accuracy of the microscope preparations was under suspicion. It was thought that some at least of the receptors and fibres described might be artifacts produced by aberrant properties in the stains used. A method of staining nerve-fibres *in vivo* in the skin by methylene blue was devised by Herbert Henry Woollard (1889–1939) and his results were published posthumously in 1940. Since then Woollard's former colleagues and pupils, especially Graham Weddell, have greatly advanced our knowledge of the nerve-fibres and end-organs in the skin.

It is now widely considered that the receptors for pressure and touch depend upon mechanical deformation for their responses. It has been suggested that the hard capsules of the Meissner corpuscles situated in the dermal papillae protect them from being deformed except by pressure along their axes. They may thus act as levers to magnify the afferent impulses, and they may be important in the localization of tactile impressions. The discovery of certain areas of skin, for example in the lobe of the ear, in which there are no organized receptors but only free nerve-endings, has further complicated the position as all types of cutaneous sensation may be obtained from these areas. The further suggestion that all types of organized receptors are staining artifacts perhaps does little justice to the constancy and similarity of their appearance and to the technical ability of the older histologists. The work of Adrian on the impulses which determine cutaneous sensation is dealt with later (pp. 290 ff.).

(*h*) *Pathology and clinical neurology.* We shall confine ourselves to the mention of a few of the pathological conditions and of the clinical observations which were important in building up the very complex modern specialty, neurology.

One of the first observations on a nervous disease that had a scientific value was that of Johann Jakob Wepfer (1620–95) of Basle, who in 1658 published a work in which he showed that apoplexy is due to a haemorrhage from the cerebral vessels. He did much to elucidate the anatomy of these vessels. In 1686 Sydenham (p. 110) described the common form of chorea which bears his name.

In 1817 James Parkinson (1755–1824) of London published a small book entitled *An Essay on the Shaking Palsy*. This was the first description of cases of paralysis agitans. The pathological lesion in this distressing condition was not elucidated till 1921, when Charles Foix (1882–1927) of Paris showed that it was in the substantia nigra of the mid-brain.

In the early part of the nineteenth century two important infective diseases of the nervous system were definitively described. Polio-myelitis had been first described, briefly, by Michael Underwood (p. 226) in the second edition (1789) of his book on the diseases of children (p. 652) under the heading of 'debility of the lower extremities'. In 1840 Jacob von Heine (1799–1879) of Cannstadt, whose interests were orthopaedic, gave an excellent description of cases of the disease and of the resulting deformities. The site of the lesion in the anterior horn of the grey matter of the cord was not established until 1869 (Charcot and Joffroy), and it was not until 1890 that Oscar Medin (1847–1927) of Stockholm pointed out the fact that it was an infectious disease, following upon an epidemic outbreak in that city. The disease was long called the Heine-Medin disease. Cerebrospinal fever may have been described by Willis (p. 245) in his *Practice of Physick* (1684), but the first definitive account was given by Gaspard Vieusseux (1746–1814) of Geneva in 1805 following an epidemic of the disease in that city. The first book on this condition was that by Elisha North (1771–1843) of Goschen, Connecticut, published in 1811; by that time the disease was commonly referred to in many countries as spotted fever, or its equivalent.

Much attention soon came to be paid to lesions of individual nerves, mainly as a result of the writings of Sir Charles Bell (p. 154). In 1821, in a communication to the Royal Society, Bell described the long thoracic nerve, which now bears his name. In the same paper he showed that lesions of the seventh cranial nerve produce facial paralysis (Bell's palsy). In 1830 Bell summed up many of his ob-servations, and also described cases of pseudohypertrophic paralysis, in his excellent work, *The Nervous System of the Human Body*.

The first formal textbook on nervous diseases was written by Moritz Heinrich Romberg (1795–1873) of Berlin, who has claims to be considered as the founder of neurology as a specialty. Romberg was much influenced by Johann Peter Frank (p. 197), who in 1792 had made a plea for the study of diseases of the spinal cord. Two years after the publication of Bell's work of 1830 noted above, Romberg translated it into German. His own textbook, *Lehrbuch der Nervenkrankheiten des Menschen*, began to appear in parts in 1840, and it was completed in 1846. Seven years later it was translated into English, and it had a wide influence in Europe and in the United States. The diseases with which it deals are preponderantly those of the peripheral nerves, except for such conditions as apoplexy, epilepsy, and chorea which had long been known. One important exception to this statement was his description of tabes dorsalis (locomotor ataxia). In this is incorporated his description of Romberg's sign, the fact that a patient suffering from this disease sways and falls to the ground if he is asked to stand with his eyes closed. In 1846 Romberg also published a classical account of progressive facial hemiatrophy, a condition which was first described by Caleb Hillier Parry (p. 530) of Bath in a communication published posthumously.

Much of the important early writing on diseases of the spinal cord dealt with tabes dorsalis. Cruveilhier (p. 631) and others had described the condition. German physicians—such as Türck (1855)—had also written on it, but the account by Romberg was by far the best. There was, however, no recognition of the disease as a uniform group of symptoms. In Great Britain there had been lectures on it by Robert Bentley Todd (1809–60), physician and professor of anatomy at King's College Hospital, London, and founder and editor of the great *Cyclopaedia of Anatomy and Physiology* (1835–59). Todd stated that this disease was characterized not only by ataxia, but also by inco-ordination of movements, and he correctly predicted that the lesions would be found in the posterior columns of the cord; these lesions were found and published by Gull (p. 285) in 1856.

A masterly account of tabes was published in 1858 by Guillaume Benjamin Amand Duchenne (1806–75) who often signed his name 'Duchenne de Boulogne'. A son of seafaring people, Duchenne graduated at Paris, and then was a general practitioner at Boulogne. While there he became interested in the electrical stimulation of muscles (1830). Becoming dissatisfied with general practice for family reasons, Duchenne returned to Paris in 1842, and without any hospital appointments devoted himself particularly to electro-therapy and to neurology. He was dependent on friends such as Trousseau and Charcot, who gave him access to the patients in their wards. In Duchenne's first important paper he described progressive muscular atrophy of the Aran-Duchenne type. In 1855 appeared the first edition of his pioneer work, *De l'électrisation localisée* ('On the local application of electricity'), which dealt in masterly fashion with the use of electricity in physiology and in therapy. He employed two moistened electrodes applied to the skin. The third edition of this work (1872) contains his description of the Erb-Duchenne type of birth-palsy, affecting the brachial plexus. In 1860 Duchenne gave a classical description of progressive bulbar paralysis. He also wrote an important work on the analysis by electrical methods of the changes of facial expression under emotion (1862). Duchenne was a very individual worker, and he read little in the literature. He had therefore not read the accounts of the German physicians such as Romberg when he began to work on tabes. Nevertheless, the description of that disease which he published in 1858–9 is so complete that the condition was soon named 'Duchenne's disease'. He stated that the lesion was in the posterior columns of the spinal cord, and that it was syphilitic in origin.

Duchenne did no formal teaching and founded no school; but the same could not be said for his great contemporary Jean Martin Charcot (1825–93) of Paris. Charcot was early associated with the Salpêtrière, and he spent his life working and teaching in that hospital. He brought order into the classification of nervous diseases. He wrote enthusiastically of Duchenne's work on tabes, and himself described the joint conditions associated with that disease, now known as Charcot's joints (1868), and with Abel Bouchard (1833–99) the lightning pains in tabes (1866). In 1865 he gave the first description of amyotrophic lateral sclerosis, and with P. Marie the first description of the peroneal type of muscular atrophy (1886). In the same year this disease was independently described by Howard

Henry Tooth (1856–1925) in his Cambridge thesis. Some of Charcot's most important neurological work was done in connexion with the clinical aspects of cerebral localization; his three memoirs on this subject with J. A. Pitres (1848–1927) established the existence in man of cortical motor centres, previously worked out on the higher mammals (pp. 256 ff.), and Charcot's book, *Leçons sur les localisations dans les maladies du cerveau* ('Lectures on localization in cerebral diseases', 1876) dealt with the clinical aspects. With Alexis Joffroy (1844–1908) he showed that the lesion in poliomyelitis is in the anterior horn of the grey matter of the cord. One of his lesser-known activities was his courses of lectures on the diseases of old persons: in 1867 he published an important treatise on geriatrics, which deals mainly with gout and arthritic diseases. Charcot was outstanding as a teacher, and his *Leçons sur les maladies du système nerveux faites à la Salpêtrière* ('Lectures on nervous diseases delivered at the Salpêtrière', 1872–87) ranks as the second great textbook of neurology. He was equally well known for his work and teaching on psychopathological states, especially hysteria (p. 510).

Another important sign of tabes is the loss of accommodation of the pupil to light but not to near vision. This reaction was first described in 1869 by Douglas M. C. L. Argyll Robertson (1837–1909), after whom it is called the Argyll Robertson pupil. Mention has already been made of Westphal's discovery that in tabes the knee-jerk is lost.

The lesions of disseminated sclerosis were noticed quite early. They were illustrated by Cruveilhier in his great atlas (1829–42, p. 631) and also by Carswell (p. 632). The first clinical study of this disease was made by Friedrich Theodor von Frerichs (1819–85) in 1849. Frerichs held chairs in several German universities, and ended in Berlin where he had a great reputation as a clinical teacher. He discovered leucin and tyrosin in the liver in acute yellow atrophy, and his greatest work was his monograph on diseases of the liver (1858–61). He also did important work on the pathology of nephritis. The next important study of disseminated sclerosis is that by Charcot (1866), in which the classical picture of inco-ordination, intention tremor, and nystagmus is fully described. Other continental writers described cases of this disease, but it was nine years after the appearance of Charcot's study before the first case was published in Great Britain.

Frerichs is associated with another grave nervous condition. In his treatise on diseases of the liver he described a condition characterized by rigidity and contractures, together with cirrhosis of the liver. The most typical form of this disease was described by Samuel Alexander Kinnier Wilson (1878–1937), who named it progressive lenticular degeneration. It is now commonly referred to as Kinnier Wilson's disease, and variant types, all of which show cirrhosis of the liver, have been described by others.

The presence of abnormal cavities in the spinal cord was first mentioned by Estienne (p. 242) in his work on anatomy (1545), and following him many anatomists observed the condition. It was first associated with a peculiar form of spinal paralysis by the *baron* Antoine Portal (1742–1832), author of an early history of anatomy. The name syringomyelia was given to this disease in 1824, and thereafter many cases were described, including good accounts by Gull (p. 285) in 1862, and by Lockhart Clarke (p. 249) and Hughlings Jackson in 1867.

The disease now known as subacute combined degeneration, which consists of a progressive degeneration of the myelin sheaths of the axis cylinders, and then of the axis cylinders themselves, in the white matter of the spinal cord, was first described in 1884. It was then known that it was associated with a severe anaemia, and it was later recognized that this anaemia was pernicious in type. The definitive clinical and pathological description of the condition was given by James Samuel Risien Russell (1863–1939), Frederick Eustace Batten (1865–1918), and James Stansfield Collier (1870–1935) in 1900, and they also conferred on it the present name. It was long thought that the degeneration in the spinal cord was secondary to the pernicious anaemia, but it is now recognized that both conditions are due to a common factor.

Aphasia, a very difficult subject, has produced some distinguished memoirs. The area in the left temporal lobe of the cerebral cortex, which Broca (p. 256) designated in 1861 as the speech centre, subsequently became limited to the condition known as motor aphasia. Three years later Hughlings Jackson published the first of his many papers on aphasia; to explain the condition he introduced a dynamic conception. In 1869 H. C. Bastian (p. 257) described the type of impairment of speech known as sensory aphasia, and he localized auditory and visual word centres. Five years later this type was redescribed by Carl Wernicke (1848–1905), and it is now usually known by his name. Bastian stimulated interest in the study of various types of aphasia. The early ideas of Broca were upset by the critical work of Pierre Marie (1853–1940), who was probably Charcot's most brilliant pupil. Among the conditions which Marie first described was hereditary cerebellar ataxia (1893). The last important work on aphasia which will be mentioned is Head's *Aphasia and kindred Disorders of Speech* (1926). Head returned to the functional concepts of Hughlings Jackson and disregarded the approach to the problem through cortical localization; instead he regarded a speech defect as a disturbance of one of four defined types of symbolic formulation of ideas as related to the higher intellect.

Of the many works which have been written on injuries to the nervous system, mention should be made of the book on gun-shot wounds of nerves (1864) by Silas Weir Mitchell (p. 185). This work was written as a result of Mitchell's surgical experiences, working with William Williams Keen (1837–1932) in the American Civil War. Weir Mitchell is perhaps best known for the method of treating nervous diseases by rest called after him.

Three of Charcot's pupils reached the front rank as neurologists. Pierre Marie has already been mentioned. Joseph François Felix Babinski (1857–1932) is perhaps most widely known from his description of the cutaneous plantar reflex (1896) which bears his name. He wrote many papers on the clinical phenomena of affections of the nervous system, and he brought clinical diagnosis in neurology to a high degree of refinement. Georges Marinesco (1864–1938), a Rumanian, studied for years under Charcot and was afterwards appointed to a new chair of clinical neurology at Bucharest. He was the first to show experimentally that extirpation of the pituitary body is compatible with life, and he wrote successfully on several complex nervous disorders.

In this account of the rise of neurology we have concentrated on the main anatomical features of the nervous system and the diseases affecting them. But this merely constitutes the framework of neuro-logy. We have, for example, not written on the masses of association fibres which join the main tracts in the brain and cord. Any discussion of these and of the investigations which elucidated their role in certain diseases is impracticable in a brief account.

An illuminating survey of the progress made by neurology may readily be obtained by comparing the three great textbooks of the nineteenth century. That of Romberg (1846, p. 273) reads very differently from what we might expect. The emphasis throughout is on individual sensory and motor characters. Nearly half of the book is devoted to individual disorders of sensation, treated as isolated symptoms; and much of the rest of the book deals with various spasmodic conditions such as writer's cramp and torticollis. Individual symptoms had not at that period been grouped to form the patterns of the diseases, and practically the only nervous diseases mentioned are apoplexy, paralysis, epilepsy, chorea, and tabes dorsalis. To us, the presence of accounts of angina pectoris, ergotism, and tetanus in a work on neurology is strange. The great textbook of Charcot (1872–87, p. 275), on the other hand, contains descriptions of many more diseases, and symptoms and signs are integrated into the clinical picture. One feels that at that time clinicians were really coming to grips with nervous diseases as such. It should be appreciated that this five-volume work was the printed version of Charcot's lectures, and was not really designed as a textbook.

The modern outlook is expressed by the works of Bramwell and of Gowers. Sir Byrom Bramwell (1847–1931), the Edinburgh physician, did important work on intracranial tumours (1888), and in 1882 he published an excellent book on diseases of the spinal cord. Thirteen years later this work, which was arranged rationally by the sites of the lesions instead of by symptoms, had almost doubled its size and was in every way a modern work. The same characteristics are shown by the great *Manual of Diseases of the Nervous System* (1886–8) by Sir William Richard Gowers (1845–1915). Gowers was known for medical work apart from neurology, such as his invention of the haemoglobinometer (1875), and for his observation that the vessels of the retina show characteristic changes in Bright's disease. He localized the first tumour of the spinal cord to be removed in

Great Britain, the operation being performed by Horsley. Gowers's manual is on the same lines as the many textbooks on neurology which have succeeded it, and in the interval the general pattern of diseases and syndromes, apart from some additions, has not greatly changed. Of these later works on the various clinical manifestations of nervous disease perhaps the most comprehensive was the *Sémiologie des affections du système nerveux* ('Symptoms and signs of nervous diseases', 1914) by Joseph Jules Déjérine (1849–1917) of Paris. With his wife, Augusta Déjérine-Klumpke (1859–1927), Déjérine had already added greatly to our knowledge of the anatomical basis of these phenomena, especially in their joint work *Anatomie des centres nerveux* (1895–1901).

Of the recent generation of neurologists mention may be made of Walter Edward Dandy (1886–1946) of Baltimore who advanced knowledge of hydrocephalus and diseases of the ventricles. Dandy was responsible for the introduction of the methods of ventriculography and pneumoencephalography. Three men who had a life-long connexion with the National Hospital for Nervous Diseases, Queen Square, London, have made outstanding contributions. Sir Gordon Morgan Holmes has illuminated many subjects in neuroanatomy and clinical neurology, especially the origin of the pyramidal tracts, the analysis of the cerebellar syndrome, and the cortical localization of vision. He was associated with the first removal of a tumour of the adrenal cortex, the operation which established the relationship between adrenal tumours and sexual abnormalities. Sir Charles Putnam Symonds (1890–) was the first to describe the clinical features of spontaneous subarachnoid haemorrhage, and his work on hydrocephalus and cerebral abscess is also important. Finally, Sir Francis Martin Rouse Walshe (1885–) is internationally known as a clinician and as an acutely critical writer on neurological theories. Among his clinical studies are papers on decerebrate rigidity in man, on cerebellar ataxy, on the reflex phenomena of spastic paraplegia, and on the tremor-rigidity syndrome of extrapyramidal diseases. His critical writings include long reviews of the literature of special subjects, such as polyneuritis, cutaneous sensation, and cerebral localization. Not the least important aspect of his influence on neurology has been his constant attempts to correlate experimental results with the findings actually experienced in the wards.

SCHOOLS OF CLINICAL MEDICINE

Archibald Pitcairne (1652–1713), an original Fellow of the Royal College of Physicians of Edinburgh (founded in 1681), was asked to inaugurate medical lectures at the 'Town's College' in 1685. He is the effective founder of the Edinburgh School, which did not really progress until the time of Monro *primus*. In 1692 Pitcairne became professor of medicine at Leyden, where he taught Richard Mead and Boerhaave. For family reasons he resigned after a year.

In 1745 Gerard van Swieten (1700–72) was called from Leyden by the Empress Maria Theresa to reorganize medical studies at Vienna, where he established clinical teaching on a sound basis of observation. He was greatly influenced by Sydenham, and by Boerhaave, on whose *Aphorisms* he wrote a famous Commentary. Van Swieten founded the Old Vienna School. To it came Anton De Haen (1704–76) of The Hague, another disciple of Sydenham and Boerhaave. He introduced the use of the thermometer and the demonstration of autopsies. The School reached its greatest popularity with Maximilian Stoll (1742–87), who wrote on the epidemic constitutions of Hippocrates and Sydenham. Under Stoll the Allgemeines Krankenhaus was opened in 1784, and J. P. Frank (p. 197) later became its superintendent and a famous teacher. Auenbrugger is the greatest ornament of this School.

While the Vienna School was declining the Paris School was rising. It was in many ways a reaction against the systems of nosology which had been common in the eighteenth century. Supporters of these theories believed that diseases could be classified in the same way as plants, and that symptoms and signs must therefore follow pre-arranged patterns. These views took more tangible form with the publication of the *Systema naturae* (1735) by the great Swedish botanist Carl Linné [Linnaeus] (1707–78), and the system was especially applied to pathology and clinical medicine by François Boissier de la Croix de Sauvages [usually called Boissier de Sauvages] (1706–67). This in turn influenced Linnaeus who in 1763 published a medical work of this nature entitled *Genera morborum*. At a later date both Cullen (p. 148) and John Brown (p. 148) published noso-logical systems. One of the most detailed of such general systems was that of Pinel (p. 497), his *Nosographie philosophique* (1789). Pinel was essentially a scientist, intent on imparting scientific accuracy to his system of diagnosis and treatment. His system was therefore based on anatomical considerations, and in it he classified over 2,500 'diseases' into species, orders, and families. Such a classification is in no way possible, but it was even less so in Pinel's time, when there was little anatomical background on which to base it. It may be said that after Pinel the nosological system gradually declined except with a few enthusiasts. But in the sphere of dermatology it was remarkably persistent. Two great British pioneers of this specialty, Robert Willan (p. 204) and Thomas Bateman (p. 204), both wrote nosologies of skin diseases. But the best known of these works was the *Nosologie naturelle* (1817) of Jean Louis Alibert (1766–1837).

Pinel's great contemporary, Corvisart (p. 172), adopted a much more rational attitude to the problems of disease. His treatise on per-cussion laid the practical foundations of chest diagnosis, and made the principle known in a way that Auenbrugger's book had never done. His great work on diseases of the heart demarcated several dis-tinct lesions of that organ. He was a great teacher, and many of the leaders of the succeeding period were his pupils. All the men we have mentioned lived through the Revolution and the Napoleonic wars, and their careers were in part determined by their attitude to the events of the time. Corvisart became personal physician to Napoleon, and he disappeared from the stage with his master. Long before that Bichat (p. 320) had started the downfall of the humoral pathology and had placed the emphasis on the tissues.

Although Laennec (p. 172) is now recognized as one of the greatest of all physicians, his influence in France in his own day was not great. For one reason, he was a poor lecturer, and he was a royalist at a time when royalists were not popular. The greatest share in founding the Paris School therefore fell to François Joseph Victor Broussais (1772–1838), a colourful Breton who had a wide influence. He served in the Revolutionary wars and the campaigns of Napoleon, and he was later appointed an assistant professor at the Val-de-Grâce, the military medical school for the army. In 1808 Broussais published his *Histoire des phlegmasies ou inflammations chroniques*, which embodied much clinical material, and in which he set out his theory that many diseases are due to inflammation, especially of the gastro-intestinal tract. A brilliant but dogmatic lecturer, Broussais soon had a wide following in Paris. In 1816 he launched a full-scale attack on Pinel and the nosological school in a small work entitled *Examen de la doctrine médicale généralement adoptée* ('Examination of the accepted medical doctrine'). This was the opening salvo of a twenty-year campaign which petered out only with Broussais's death.

There are many points in Broussais's doctrine which seem paradoxical. He stimulated the study of morbid anatomy, and when the results seemed to show that some diseases at least presented clear-cut anatomical pictures, he denied that individual diseases existed and protested that different illnesses were merely the physiological expressions of varying degrees of over-stimulation, or less frequently under-stimulation, manifested by inflammation. Fever was a symptom of inflammation, and the 'essential fevers' of Pinel were cast aside. According to Broussais most diseases were due to gastroenteritis, and the main treatment of all diseases was anti-phlogistic—that is, a spare diet and blood-letting by leeches. Under his guidance the doctors of Paris leeched as they had never done before, and in hospitals they sometimes prescribed the number of leeches to be applied to newly admitted patients before they had even seen the patients. In the year 1833, when Broussais was at the height of his fame, over 41 million leeches were imported into France. The leaders of the opposing school—Laennec, Gaspard Laurent Bayle (1774–1816), the author of an important pathological work on tuberculosis, and other men—hit back as well as they could. Broussais's counter-attacks took the form of successive increases in the size of his *Examen*, which grew from 460 pages in the first edition to over 2,200 in the third; his system was now dignified by the name of 'physiological medicine'. As a result the anatomico-pathological school, led by Laennec, Cruveilhier (p. 631), Bretonneau (p. 204), P. C. A. Louis (p. 721), and Gabriel Andral (1797–1876), the author of an important work on anaemia, gradually won the day. The French School, in spite of—or perhaps because of—Broussais, was now fully established. One of the greatest ornaments of this school was the

Paris physician Armand Trousseau (1801–67), whose *Clinique médicale de l'Hôtel-Dieu de Paris* (1861) contains many important observations on diagnosis and treatment, especially of the acute infectious diseases. Diagnostic methods were possibly advanced by the influence of Pierre Adolphe Piorry (1794–1879), who for the practice of percussion invented the pleximeter, or small plate which was placed on the chest and was percussed with a rubber-tipped hammer (the plessor). Although Broussais's theories are now merely curiosities, his direct and indirect influence on the development of French medicine during the two decades following 1815 was very great. By the end of that period the emphasis had shifted from the symptoms of the nosologists to the organic lesions of the morbid anatomists, and diseases were by then regarded essentially as changes in function.

While these heated battles over medical theories were going on in France, less dramatic but equally important developments were taking place in the British Isles. The Irish School at Dublin had as its leaders two men who rank among the greatest physicians of their time. Robert James Graves (1796–1853) was a physician to the Meath Hospital and a founder of the Park Street School of Medicine. He had studied on the Continent, and he introduced in Dublin the methods of bedside teaching which were practised in the continental schools. Graves published in 1835 the best account to that date of exophthalmic goitre, and his name is frequently attached to that disease (pp. 530–2). His *Clinical Lectures* (1848) contain many important clinical observations, and he himself thought that perhaps his chief claim to fame was the fact that he reversed the current practice and 'fed fevers'. Graves's contemporary William Stokes (1804–78) was regius professor of medicine at Dublin and a physician to the Meath Hospital. When aged only twenty-one he published a useful guide to the use of the stethoscope, and his devotion to the teaching of Laennec was later more adequately confirmed by the appearance of his great works on diseases of the chest (1837) and on diseases of the heart and aorta (1854). He published definitive descriptions of Cheyne-Stokes respiration, and of the slow heart accompanied by signs of cerebral anaemia known as Stokes-Adams disease. Another sound Dublin physician of that period was Sir Dominic John Corrigan (1802–80), who is now chiefly remembered for his description of the water-hammer pulse of aortic regurgitation (1832, p. 245); he first described fibroid phthisis not occurring in miners. The great surgeon of the Dublin School was Abraham Colles (1773–1843), who is known for his daring ligations of the large arteries for aneurysm, for the fracture of the wrist named after him (1814), and for 'Colles' law', which states that a healthy mother may bear a syphilitic child without herself becoming infected.

In England the full flowering of the new art of clinical medicine was at first concentrated at Guy's Hospital in London. For teaching purposes it had for some time been joined with St. Thomas's Hospital as 'the United Hospitals', and on the combined teaching staff the greatest star was Sir Astley Paston Cooper (1768–1841), a surgeon of the first rank. His works on hernia and on fractures and dislocations are of permanent importance. In 1825 the two hospitals split, and Cooper's allegiance was thereafter to Guy's. A year earlier Richard Bright (1789–1858) had been elected a full physician on the staff of Guy's. Bright, a native of Bristol, had studied at Edinburgh and at Guy's, had travelled in Iceland and through Hungary, had become known for his botanical and zoological work, and had studied widely in France, Germany, Italy, and the Low Countries. He was a staunch supporter of the view that the physician must learn his art as much in the post-mortem room as in the wards, and all his clinical work was based on morbid anatomy. In 1827 Bright published his *Reports of Medical Cases* in which he drew attention to the fact that fatal cases of dropsy often showed disease of the kidneys. It had long been known that some cases of dropsy had albumen in the urine, and Morgagni had described a small contracted kidney; but until Bright published his work no one had associated dropsy with essential nephritis. The value of this work to medicine was immense; by it renal dropsy could easily be differentiated from cardiac dropsy. Bright gave the first accounts of several other conditions such as tuberculosis of the larynx, otitis following scarlatina, acute yellow atrophy of the liver; and his work on abdominal tumours is of great importance.

Thomas Addison (1798–1866) was also a physician to Guy's, and as an original observer he ranks almost equal to Bright. In 1849 he published a paper in which he described cases of pernicious anaemia (later known as Addisonian anaemia), and also three cases of a similar condition in which disease in the suprarenal capsules was found *post-mortem*; these latter were the first cases of Addison's disease. In 1855 he expanded this paper into his monograph *On the Constitutional and Local Effects of Disease of the Supra-renal Capsules*, one of the most important of all works on clinical medicine. With John Morgan (1797–1847) Addison wrote the first book in English on the action of poisons on the living body.

The third member of the Guy's triad, Thomas Hodgkin (1798–1866), was a lecturer in the medical school. Although a man of great distinction, he tended to be always in opposition, and perhaps for that reason he was never elected to the hospital staff. He was the first (1832) to give a clear description of lymphadenoma, which was later called Hodgkin's disease.

The names of three later Guy's physicians may be mentioned here. Sir William Withey Gull (1816–90) was one of the most distinguished and successful physicians of any period. His most important contribution to knowledge was his description of myxoedema (pp. 524 ff.); but his accounts of arteriocapillary fibrosis and of intermittent haemoglobinuria are also important. Sir Samuel Wilks (1824–1911) was in early life much engaged with morbid anatomy, and he published excellent lectures on that subject. He was one of the first to direct attention to the effects of syphilis on the viscera, and to show that one result was aortic aneurysm. He probably published the first accounts of bacterial endocarditis and of alcoholic paraplegia, and possibly also the first account of myasthenia gravis. Frederick William Pavy (p. 232) was for many years lecturer in physiology at Guy's. He had worked with Claude Bernard, and he devoted the remainder of his life to the study of diabetes and carbohydrate metabolism.

About the middle of the nineteenth century Vienna again became the European centre for medical teaching with the rise of the New Vienna School. Pre-eminent in this movement were the pathologist Rokitansky and the physician Skoda, but very soon the anatomist Hyrtl and the dermatologist Hebra began to attract pupils in great numbers. The medical specialties were also generally outstanding at Vienna from that date until the outbreak of the First World War.

Mention has already been made of Rokitansky's vast experience in morbid anatomy (p. 171). He was appointed extraordinary professor in the Pathological Institute of the Allgemeines Krankenhaus in 1834. He was much influenced by Andral, P. C. A. Louis, and other members of the French School. About the time of his appointment a new hospital regulation greatly increased the number of bodies available for autopsy, so that when Rokitansky finally retired he had personally done over 30,000 post-mortem examinations. His contemporary Josef Skoda (1805–81) was greatly interested in the work of Auenbrugger, Corvisart, and Laennec, but these new methods of diagnosis were not practised in Vienna, so that Skoda had to learn them himself, working from basic principles. In 1833 he was appointed assistant physician to the Allgemeines Krankenhaus, and he intensified his studies on the living patients and checked his results with Rokitansky in the post-mortem room. His *Abhandlung über Perkussion und Auskultation* ('Treatise on percussion and auscultation', 1839) sets out his detailed analysis of the sounds heard. He tried to obtain from these methods more than they would give; but some of his signs, such as Skodaic resonance, are still used. Skoda's whole interest was centred on diagnosis, and he cared nothing for treatment. The therapeutic nihilism of the Vienna School was largely due to him; it served its purpose in counteracting the polypharmacy which was so widely practised in his time.

Rokitansky and Skoda became the most popular teachers in Europe and students from other countries flocked to them. Many students also studied under Josef Hyrtl (1810–94), who from 1844 was professor of anatomy at Vienna and the most popular and successful teacher of that subject in Europe. His textbooks of general and of topographical anatomy were widely used, and he is the author of scholarly works on anatomical terminology and on Hebrew and Arabic elements in anatomy.

The fourth famous teacher in the New Vienna School was Ferdinand von Hebra (1816–80), the dermatologist. Hebra discounted the humoral theory which still lingered in dermatology, and by 1845 he was able to put forward a new classification of skin diseases founded on histological observations. Though not a simple classification, it left room for further advances, and by 1860 Hebra was able to publish the most comprehensive and stimulating textbook on skin diseases which had so far appeared.

We may turn back to consider those who have been the immediate progenitors of modern physiology. Among these, three men stand out beyond all others. In order of seniority, and perhaps of genius, they are Johannes Müller, Claude Bernard, and Karl Ludwig. The results of the movement that they represent, together with the knowledge of the cellular structure of the body (pp. 320 ff.) and of the life-histories of the disease-producing organisms (pp. 381 ff.), are the three main groups of ideas which separate the physician of our day from Laennec (p. 172).

(a) The Work of Johannes Müller

Johannes Müller (1801–58) was the greatest physiologist Germany has produced, and perhaps the greatest physiologist of all time. His genius was of the universal type and, despite his early death, he attained equal distinction in every department which he touched. Among these were comparative anatomy, embryology, physiological chemistry, psychology, and pathology. He was a careful scholar, well versed in the history of the subjects which he taught, and as great a teacher as he was an investigator. A very large number of the best-known men who have advanced medicine during the nineteenth century were his pupils while he was a professor at Berlin. His lovable character was pervaded by a mystical tendency.

Müller's textbook of physiology began to appear in 1834. It introduced into the subject the comparative and psychological points of view, which were not fully appreciated until the generation that followed. One of his interesting aphorisms says that 'No one can be a psychologist without being a physiologist'. The most remarkable generalization associated with his name—and one further developed by Ewald Hering (1834–1918)—is the Law of Specific Nerve Energies. According to this law each sensory nerve, however stimulated, gives rise to its own specific sensation and to no other. Conversely, the same stimulus applied to different organs of sense produces a different sensation in each organ—that sensation, in fact, that is its specific attribute. Thus electrical, mechanical, thermal stimulation produce only the sensation of light when applied to the optic nerve. On the other hand, any particular form of stimulation, for example electrical, produces sensations of light, smell, hearing, or taste if applied respectively to the optic, olfactory, auditory, or gustatory nerves.

A moment's reflection will enable the reader to realize the very great philosophical importance of these conclusions. They provide experimental evidence that the things of the external world are not in themselves discernible by us. Such external things we know only by the events to which they give rise acting on our senses, and yet from one and the same event utterly different sensations arise within us. To beings with senses different from ours the world also would be different. The Law of Specific Nerve Energies is thus fundamental for our view of the range of validity of the scientific method.

Among other important contributions of Johannes Müller to the physiology of the nervous system were his experimental confirmation of Bell's researches on the spinal roots (p. 154) and his experiments on the production of the voice. He launched important theories in explanation of colour vision, of the mechanism of hearing, and of the phenomena of fever. He was one of the first to use the microscope in pathology, and his great book on tumours, of which only the first volume was published, is based on the conception, introduced by his pupil Theodor Schwann (p. 322), of the cell as a functional unit. Müller foreshadowed the fundamental change in pathological outlook later to be more fully enunciated by Virchow (p. 325). Müller was also one of the founders of physiological chemistry.

Subsequent work on the electric phenomena of nerve. In the first edition of his textbook Müller stated that he could not detect electric currents in nerves. With reference to the speed of the nerve impulse he pointed out that different calculations or estimates from Haller onwards had varied from 150 feet to 57,000 million feet per second. Müller said frankly that we should probably never be able to measure it. Within twenty years the speed had been measured by one of Müller's most brilliant pupils, Hermann Ludwig Ferdinand von Helmholtz (1821–94). Primarily a physicist, Helmholtz made valuable contributions to medicine. With a special pendulum-myograph which he invented he measured the velocity of the nerve impulse in the frog (1852) and found it to be about 20 metres per second. (It was later shown that in human nerve the rate is 100 metres per second, but these rates vary with temperature and other conditions.) In 1847 Charles Babbage (1792–1871), who spent much of his life trying to perfect his 'calculating engine', invented an ophthalmoscope by means of which the retina of the eye could be studied. He asked a friend, a surgeon, to try it out; but the latter took it and did nothing, and a great opportunity was missed. In 1851 Helmholtz independently invented an ophthalmoscope, and in this case it was taken up by the medical profession. This simple invention has enabled ophthalmology to develop along scientific lines, and it has been of great value also to the general physician. The work of Helmholtz on colour vision and the sensation of tone is also important. His great physical doctrine of the indestructibility of energy arose out of physiological work on the heat generated in muscle.

Emil Du Bois Reymond (1818–96) took up the subject of animal electricity where it had been left by Galvani and Volta, and in 1845 he proved the existence of a resting current in nerve. He next studied the electromotive changes which are produced by excitation of the nerve. He invented a still well-known induction coil and other apparatus for use in his experiments. Du Bois Reymond was a pupil of Müller, and he succeeded his master in the Berlin chair on the latter's death.

During the early years of the twentieth century the most outstanding worker in this field was Francis Gotch (1853–1913) of Oxford. He was using the capillary electrometer for the detection of currents in nerve, and with it he showed that when two successive stimuli are given, the response to the second stimulus cannot be evoked if the charge produced by the first stimulus is still in progress. Gotch investigated this refractory period and also the effect of temperature on the nerve impulse. These problems were also dealt with by Keith Lucas (1879–1916) of Cambridge, who showed that in the contraction of muscle fibres the 'all-or-none' law prevails. He demonstrated the fact that the nerve-impulse leaves behind it a phase of diminished excitability. He was a man of great mechanical ingenuity, and by the outbreak of the First World War he was contemplating the method of valve amplification for the finer detection and study of currents in nerves. These methods were probably first actually used by Adrian in the United Kingdom, and also by Joseph Erlanger (1874–) and Herbert Spencer Gasser (1888–) in the United States. We shall discuss briefly Adrian's work as representative of activities now carried out in many research centres.

Most of the experiments of Gotch and Lucas dealt with motor and not sensory nerves, and the latter class has been the special field of study of Lucas's pupil, Edgar Douglas Adrian (Baron Adrian of Cambridge, 1889–). In one of his later works he says that the final objective of physiological work is to find out how the activity of the brain is related to that of the mind. Starting from work in a limited field, he has gradually widened its scope to include activity of the sensory nervous elements in the brain itself. Gotch, Keith Lucas, and other physiologists had worked mainly with isolated nerves, and the characteristic features of the action current had been demonstrated. It had also been shown that stimulation of a nerve-fibre by the usual form of stimulus which attained its greatest value almost instantaneously, produced an accumulation, or segregation, of ions in certain parts of the fibre which reached its maximum in 0·001 second or less. But a current of forty times this voltage will not act as a stimulus if it takes one second to reach this maximum—the assumption being that there is a leak of ions and that they never accumulate to the concentration necessary to produce a reaction.

Adrian now used the cathode-ray tube, or more commonly the capillary electrometer, for the more sensitive detection of the nervous impulses, and valve-amplification for their recording. Within a few years a 5,000-fold amplification was obtainable. These very sensitive methods were necessary because it had been found possible to set up a preparation consisting of one single end-organ in a frog's muscle, together with its related nerve-fibre. On stimulating the end-organ it was found that the nerve-fibre showed regular impulses at a frequency of 30 per second. By these methods records were obtained of the discharges in single nerve-fibres produced by tension on a muscle, pressure, touch, the movement of a hair, and the pricking with a needle. When Adrian published his first book in 1928 he had reached the following position: a stimulus of constant intensity applied to the skin causes immediate excitation of an end-organ. This excitation diminishes progressively as long as the stimulus continues. Concurrently, sensory impulses of a constant intensity pass along the nerve-fibre from the end-organ. At first they are very frequent, but the frequency gradually diminishes, and as this takes place the sensation experienced in the brain progressively falls away.

It is of interest to note the attitude adopted by Adrian and other workers in this field to Müller's law of specific nerve energy. It became clear that Müller's law had long been interpreted in a sense different from that for which he intended it. As taught by him it was a law of modality and not of quality. Modality may be explained by pointing out that we cannot say that a bitter taste is more like purple than red. But we can say that purple is more like blue than yellow— an example of quality. During nearly the last seventy years the law has been interpreted as referring to quality rather than modality. From his experimental work Adrian now pointed out that there is no specific activity in the sensory nerves. All the sensory nerve-fibres from the different types of receptors conduct impulses which are common to all and fundamentally alike, though there are quantitative differences in the impulses which are definite enough to appear amplified in the photographic record.

These conclusions were carried farther by Adrian in his *Physical Background of Perception* (1947). Gasser and Erlanger had shown that the sensory fibres in mixed nerve trunks can be arranged in decreasing orders of various physical properties, and that in general pain reactions are conducted by the smaller fibres. Adrian had shown that 'slow' impulses appeared whenever the skin was stimulated in a manner likely to cause damage or pain; but it was also found that the electrical signs of activity with pain fibres were almost negligible. He now argued that, since there is no radical differences in the messages sent from different kinds of sense organ, the mental results must differ because different parts of the brain receive them. It was found that the pain fibres probably do not ascend farther than the optic thalamus—a theory which had previously been advocated by Henry Head on clinical grounds. But in the case of all other sensory impulses their signals could be clearly distinguished in the sensory area of the cerebral cortex. Adrian also showed very clearly that the area of the cortex devoted to any particular type of end-organ is related to the animal's special needs. In man and the monkey a relatively large area of the sensory area of the cortex is devoted to the face and hand, and relatively little to the trunk. In the pony the nostril area is as large as that for the whole of the rest of the body; whereas in the pig, which uses its snout more than any other part of its body to explore its environment, practically the whole of the tactile sensory area in the cortex consists of fibres from the snout. Adrian's later work, on the interpretation of the waves of the encephalogram, first described by Hans Berger (1873–1941) of Jena in 1929, and on the olfactory sense, lies beyond our scope.

The mechanism of muscular contraction. It was known late in the nineteenth century that lactic acid is formed in muscle tissue when it contracts. The significance of its presence was not then understood; but in 1907 Gowland Hopkins (p. 611) and (Sir) Walter Morley Fletcher (1873–1933)—who later became the first Secretary of the Medical Research Council—showed that if a muscle is stimulated in an oxygen-free atmosphere, lactic acid accumulates rapidly until it reaches a certain concentration. The muscle then ceases to contract. If oxygen is now supplied, the lactic acid gradually disappears.

About 1911 the Cambridge physiologist and mathematician Archibald Vivian Hill (1886–) began to apply very sensitive physical methods to the difficult problems of muscular contraction. If the ends of a muscle are fixed so that it is unable to contract, when it is stimulated, the energy which would, had it been free or attached to a reasonable load, have produced a contraction, manifests itself by the production of heat. Hill showed that in a single twitch the temperature of the muscle rose only 0·003 degree Centigrade. He then made the significant observation that during a 'continued' (tetanic) contraction the heat production can be divided into two phases: (*a*) initial heat, and (*b*) delayed heat. He also showed that only the initial heat is produced during the actual contraction of the muscle; the temperature rises rapidly and then falls rapidly. The remainder— often more than half—of the heat evolved in the whole process of contraction and recovery is evolved slowly as delayed heat for some minutes after the muscle has ceased to contract.

Hill now demonstrated that, if the muscle were made to contract in an atmosphere of pure nitrogen, the initial heat was not affected, whereas the delayed heat was not produced at all. This showed that, while the recovery of the muscle depended on oxidative processes, the actual contraction of the muscle did not. It was also shown that a muscle can contract actively for a period in a complete absence of oxygen, and this confirmed the previous findings. Hence Hill's conception of the oxygen-debt; the muscle can up to a certain point continue to carry out work without receiving an adequate oxygen supply, but at the end of this brief period of exertion the required amount of oxygen must be provided in order to pay off the debt and to effect a recovery.

During this period Otto Fritz Meyerhof (1884–1951), then of Kiel, was studying the chemical changes associated with muscular activity. He confirmed the observations of Fletcher and Hopkins, and noticed further that as the lactic acid progressively accumulated in the muscle, glycogen, the muscle carbohydrate, progressively diminished. The inference was that glycogen disintegrated into lactic acid with the production of heat. If an extra supply of oxygen was provided during the contraction, the glycogen still disappeared, but there was no accumulation of lactic acid. Quantitative estimations of the oxygen consumed and of the carbon dioxide evolved now showed that the increased oxygen consumption was sufficient to explain the combustion of not more than a quarter of the lactic acid which had accumulated. The rest of the lactic acid must have been changed by some other process. Meyerhof now found that the glycogen content of a muscle contracting in oxygen was higher than that of one contracting in nitrogen, and he hence concluded that in the former case the extra glycogen was formed from the bulk of the lactic acid. In muscular contraction therefore glycogen is broken down into lactic acid during the phase of contraction, and during the recovery phase it is resynthesized from the greater part of the lactic acid present; the energy necessary for this reaction is derived from the complete combustion of the remaining part of the lactic acid. After certain adjustments had been made the physical factors associated with these chemical changes were found to agree with the production of initial and delayed heat obtained by Hill. For this work Hill and Meyerhof were jointly awarded a Nobel Prize in 1922.

At this time Gustav Embden (1874–1933) was working at Frank-fort-on-Main on the chemical changes during muscular contraction and recovery. From the juice expressed from muscles hexose-diphos-phate ('lactacidogen') was obtained, and it came to be accepted by Meyerhof and others that the transformation of glycogen to lactic acid was not a direct reaction, but involved the intermediate forma-tion of various compounds of phosphoric acid through the action of enzymes. It also came to be accepted that the actual contractile ele-ment in the muscle fibre is probably the muscle protein myosin. It is now known that the chemical changes involve a long sequence of reactions, many of which are reversible; in these adenosine triphos-phate and adenosine diphosphate play important parts. These com-plex reactions are still *sub judice* and are beyond our scope. But mention should be made of the work of Carl Ferdinand Cori (1896–) and Gerty Theresa Cori (1896–1957) of Washington, who isolated a new ester of hexose-phosphate ('the Cori ester') from muscle. This discovery led to new work and an altered concept, and the Coris were awarded part of a Nobel Prize in 1947 (see also p. 296).

(b) The Work of Claude Bernard

Claude Bernard (1813–78), the great French physiologist, was Müller's junior by twelve years and was in almost every respect a contrast to him. His mind was of that peculiarly French type to which anything mystical is abhorrent. He had few eminent pupils who owed much to him directly, but the influence of his ideas, through his writings, can hardly be exaggerated. Bernard was the founder of experimental medicine, that is, of the artificial production of disease by chemical and physical means. This is one of the most important scientific movements within our field.

Bernard's greatest investigation, which with its implications occu-pied him from 1843 until practically the close of his life, was the dis-covery of glycogen from liver tissue and a study of its formation and its fate in the liver and elsewhere in the body. The events in this investigation were briefly these. In the early decades of the nineteenth century it was held in France that only plants synthesized complex substances; fats, sugars, and proteins could be broken down but not built up in the animal body, but no one knew the changes through which these substances passed in the animal. Bernard decided that he would investigate the whole matter, and he started with sugar. He never went any farther, since the study of this food substance occupied him during the rest of his life.

Bernard showed that if an animal was fed on a diet containing sugar, glucose could be recovered from the portal vein which leads from the gut to the liver, and also from the hepatic veins which transmit the blood from the liver to the general circulation. The inference was that the sugar had passed through the liver. If he now fed an animal on a diet consisting entirely of meat and containing no sugar, he found that there was no sugar in the portal vein—the finding which would be expected. But to his surprise he discovered that the blood in the hepatic veins contained a high concentration of glucose. He even found that sugar could be extracted from the liver tissue itself. Bernard concluded in 1855 that the sugar was secreted by the liver. He called the process an 'internal secretion', and this is the first use of this term. While investigating this process later in the same year there occurred one of those accidents which sometimes lead a careful investigator to the correct solution. He was in the habit of carrying out his analyses in duplicate in order to compensate for experimental errors. He was investigating the extract from the liver of an animal and he was interrupted after his analysis of the first sample, made immediately after the animal's death. He left the second sample until the next day, and when he analysed it then he found that it contained much more sugar than the first sample. Repetition of this procedure on another animal gave the same result. He then removed the liver from yet another animal and flushed it with water for forty minutes. By the end of that time the washings contained no sugar, and neither did the liver tissue itself. Bernard now allowed the sugar-free liver to remain at a moderate temperature for twenty-four hours, and he then found abundant sugar both in the fluid from the liver and the liver tissue. He concluded that the sugar was not formed from materials in the blood but was a result of some sugar-forming substance in the liver having been changed into sugar. Two years later, in 1857, Bernard discovered this substance and called it glycogen. Since his demonstration that such a substance was present in the liver others had tried to isolate it, and in one case at least glycogen appears to have been isolated independently though not in a pure form.

In the course of these long researches Bernard had many critics. One of the most persistent of these was his former assistant F. W. Pavy (p. 232), who claimed that there is a standard amount of sugar in the arterial and venous blood and that even in a meat-fed animal there is sugar in the portal vein. Pavy believed that the liver absorbs sugar and stores it as glycogen. The final proof that Bernard was essentially right and that Pavy was wrong did not come until the twentieth century. But Bernard's views were really only the beginning of our knowledge of carbohydrate metabolism. Even at the end of his life he considered that sugar from the food was not converted directly into glycogen in the liver, but that it in some way acts as a stimulant to the secretion of glycogen. In recent years the use of radio-isotopes has demonstrated that a small proportion of the glucose in the diet is converted directly to liver glycogen and to muscle glycogen.

Some reference has already been made to the role of glycogen in muscle and to the work of the Coris in that field (p. 294). They showed that the lactic acid formed as a consequence of muscular activity is converted to glycogen in the liver, not in the muscles themselves. The Cori Cycle is the term given to the conception that the glycogen stored in the liver is converted to glucose in the blood, then to muscle glycogen, to lactic acid, and so back to liver glycogen. The Coris showed that the breakdown of glycogen is due to an enzyme which they named phosphorylase, and that the end-product is glucose-1-phosphate. They later demonstrated that several enzymes are concerned in the complete breakdown of glycogen to glucose, and in the subsequent reconversion of glucose to glycogen. The steps involved in the conversion of glucose to glycogen by enzyme action are still by no means clear, but it is possible that the main events may be represented as follows: glucose→glucose-6-phosphate→glucose-1-phosphate→glycogen. Bernard's discovery of glycogen has already given fruitful results both in biochemistry and in the practical treatment of diabetes mellitus and the glycogen-storage diseases.

Pancreatic juice. Bernard's earliest important research related to the function of the pancreatic juice. This was a subject which had not hitherto aroused much interest among physiologists, although the juice from a living animal had been first collected nearly 200 years earlier.

For this pioneer operation we are indebted to Regnier de Graaf (1641–73), a Dutch anatomist and physiologist. He studied under Franciscus Sylvius (p. 142) at Leyden, and while still a very young man he declined the offer of Sylvius' chair. Before his early death he discovered the follicles in the ovary which contain the ova, and to these Haller gave the name which they still bear—the Graafian follicles. While he was a student at Leyden de Graaf catheterized the pancreatic duct in several dogs. After opening the abdomen and the duodenum, he passed into the pancreatic duct the quill of a wild duck containing at its tip a plug which could be removed by a thread passed down the quill. The broad end of the quill was left outside the body when the abdomen was sewn up, and it was fixed in a flask suspended from the abdominal wall. When de Graaf pulled the plug out by means of the thread, pancreatic juice began to drop into the flask. In this way from one dog he collected an ounce of juice. It must be admitted that, having obtained the juice, de Graaf did not make very good use of it. He made no chemical examination, but on the supposed evidence of its taste he wrongly asserted that it was acid. He therefore argued that its function is to cause an effervescence when mixed with the alkaline bile; the effervescence attenuates the viscid mucus which is found in the intestine and also helps to separate the useful parts of the food from the useless. In these matters he was simply expressing the theories of digestion taught by his master Sylvius.

When Bernard began this work Magendie, Tiedemann and Gmelin, and others had obtained pancreatic juice from a living animal. Friedrich Tiedemann (1781–1861) and Leopold Gmelin (1788–1853) in their book, _Die Verdauung nach Versuchen_ ('Digestion studied experimentally', 1826–7), confirmed the work of Prout. Gmelin also did important work on bile (1826). But though the juice had been analysed chemically, nothing was known of its physiological functions. It was suspected that the pancreas was a salivary gland. Bernard was attracted to the problem by an accidental observation. While carrying out a post-mortem examination on a rabbit which he had induced to eat only meat, he noticed that the lacteals in the mesentery were filled with a white fluid, but only below a point at some distance from the pylorus, the outlet of the stomach. The white fluid indicated the digestion of the fat from the meat. But in a dog the lacteals would have contained white fluid almost up to the pylorus. Bernard knew that in the rabbit the pancreatic duct opens to the intestine much lower down than in the dog. He at once concluded that the different appearances of the mesenteries of the two animals after digestion of fat must be due to the fact that the neutral fat which passed from the stomach into the duodenum began to be acted upon at the point of entry of the pancreatic duct in each case, and that therefore the pancreatic juice plays a part in the absorption of neutral fats.

Bernard now showed that when he mixed crushed pancreatic tissue with neutral fat and kept the mixture at body temperature for a short time, the fat was split into a fatty acid and glycerol. He then carried out experiments similar to those of de Graaf, fixing a silver cannula in the pancreatic duct of a dog. He showed that there is no secretion of juice in a fasting dog; but that after food the passage of the acid chyme into the duodenum stimulates the flow of the juice. He attempted unsuccessfully to extirpate the pancreas in dogs; but he did succeed in blocking the duct, and he then found that fat in the food passed out of the body undigested. He also showed that the pancreatic juice transforms starch into sugar (maltose). He was doubtful whether the juice exerted any true chemical action on the proteins. His error is explained by the fact that the proteolytic enzyme (trypsin) in pure pancreatic juice is present in an inactive form (trypsinogen) which requires the presence of enterokinase from the succus entericus to activate it. Since his pancreatic juice came direct from the duct it had no contact with the secretion of the intestine, and the change to trypsin in his samples did not take place.

Vasomotor nerves. The action of the vasoconstrictor and vasodilator nerves, Bernard's third great contribution to physiology, is dealt with elsewhere (p. 261).

Bernard also did important work on certain poisons, notably carbon monoxide and curare. As a result of his work on carbon monoxide he correctly concluded that it is the red corpuscles of the blood which carry the oxygen from the lungs to the body tissues.

Curare is a South American arrow-poison. Bernard was one of the first to experiment with it. He showed that after the application of this drug to the muscle, the latter can no longer be stimulated through its nerve, though it can still react to a stimulus applied directly to the muscle tissue. Recent developments in the use of curare as an adjuvant to certain anaesthetics can therefore be traced back to him.

In 1857 Bernard introduced the very important conception of the internal environment, which implies that the proper regulation of the parts of the body in relation to each other, and even life itself, depends on the constancy of the composition of this 'internal environment'— the blood and lymph which bathe all the cells of the body.

(c) The Work of Karl Ludwig

Karl Friedrich Wilhelm Ludwig (1816–95) held chairs at Marburg, Zürich, Vienna, and Leipzig. He was, after Müller, the greatest of German physiological teachers, and he surpassed even Müller in the number of his pupils. As a physiologist he was chiefly remarkable for his ingenuity as an inventor, for his wide and deep knowledge of the physical sciences, and for his extreme generosity in handing over the results of his work to his pupils for publication.

Among the many lines of investigation of fundamental importance initiated by Ludwig, some of the most remarkable depended on the discovery of new methods. Just as the microscope had opened to the anatomist unexplored fields of research by bringing him into closer relation with objects which were hitherto beyond his scrutiny, so the rapid progress of physics and chemistry had placed more exact modes of observation and of measurement within reach of the physiologist. But the application of these methods was attended with great difficulty; there were no physiological laboratories, no instruments, no capable technicians to whom the physiologist could apply for assistance. Under such conditions, ingenuity and resource were indispensable to success; and in these qualities Ludwig was pre-eminent.

Accordingly we find that two of the most important of the early investigations of Ludwig were as much due to his ingenuity as an inventor as to his clear grasp of the physiological questions which his inventions were intended to elucidate. The most interesting of these inventions, or rather adaptations, is the mechanically rotating drum or kymograph. The word itself is derived from two Greek words which mean 'wave writer'. This instrument is now widely used, not only in physiology but in every department of science in which

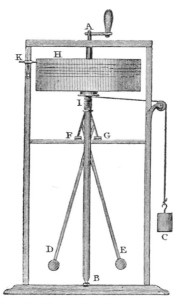

FIG. 86. Thomas Young's kymograph
(T. Young, *Course of Lectures*, vol. i, 1807, Pl. xv)

The cylinder *H*, rigidly fixed on the axis *AB*, is rotated by a handle at *A*. Manual rotation raises the weight *C*, and when the handle is then released the falling weight rotates the cylinder, a constant speed of rotation being obtained by the centrifugal governors, *FG*, *DE*. The writing point *K* produces a graphic record of its movements on the rotating cylinder.

permanent records of any continuous movement are desired. The most familiar instance is the self-recording barometer. The kymograph—the use of which had been suggested by Thomas Young (p. 642, and Fig. 86) in 1807—led to much wider applications of the method of automatic recording. Ludwig himself applied it to indicate the movements of respiration, as well as the variations in arterial pressure. Subsequently it became further adapted to the graphic method, and it serves not only for the investigation of animal movements of every conceivable kind, but even for the transient and delicate electrical changes which are associated with vital action.

An instrument invented by Ludwig is the mercurial blood-pump, the purpose of which is to separate from a known quantity of blood, derived directly from the circulation, the mixture of gases which it yields in a vacuum. This is an indispensable apparatus for the investigation of the physiology of respiration.

Ludwig devoted much attention to the physiology of secretion. Here his work has been of great importance in connexion with the time-honoured discussion between the vitalists and the mechanists. He succeeded in showing that the process of secretion can be so transformed experimentally as to do external mechanical work. This was a victory for the mechanistic theory. The idea has since been applied to many structures.

We can mention here only a few of Ludwig's important discoveries. In 1851 he found the secretory fibres for the submaxillary gland in the lingual branch of the fifth nerve, and five years later he discovered the secretory power of the sympathetic. He was the first to show that in the submaxillary gland the secretory pressure may be higher than the blood-pressure, and he demonstrated that during activity heat is produced in the gland. In 1848 Remak (p. 246) showed the presence of ganglia in the sinus venosus of the frog's heart, and this discovery was rapidly followed by Friedrich Heinrich Bidder's (p. 582) demonstration of the atrio-ventricular node, and Ludwig's of the ganglia in the interventricular septum. In certain mammals a fine nerve runs down the neck near the vagus. In 1866 Ludwig showed that when it is stimulated the heart beats more slowly and there occurs a marked fall in blood-pressure. He therefore named it the depressor nerve. He had already shown that there is a connexion between blood-pressure and respiration; a rise of pressure occurs during inspiration. He was the first to localize a vasomotor centre (in the medulla oblongata), and he did important work on intestinal movements.

Ludwig's fame will possibly rest most securely on his theory of the secretion of the urine. Bowman (p. 640) had advanced the theory (1842) that water and possibly salts passed out through the glomerulus into the tubules, and that it there dissolved the solid constituents, such as urea, which had been secreted by the tubules. Two years later Ludwig asserted that the blood-pressure causes a dilute solution of non-protein substances to escape through the glomerulus, which acts as a filter. In the tubules the solution is concentrated by osmosis. Bowman's theory was not tested experimentally until 1874, when Rudolph Peter Heinrich Heidenhain (1834–97), as a result of much experimental work, advanced a theory very similar to that of Bowman. In subsequent years many investigators, including Cushny (p. 685), studied this problem without conclusive results. But in 1924 Alfred Newton Richards (1876–) was able, by the methods of micro-experimentation, to collect and analyse the fluid from a single glomerulus. As a result of many experiments of this type Ludwig's theory, with certain modifications, has been upheld.

(d) Later Physiological Investigators

It is impossible even to attempt here any general summary of the conclusions reached by physiological research since Ludwig, but a brief attempt will be made to indicate the vast field opened up. The experiments of William Beaumont on the gastric juice (p. 157) were extended in brilliant fashion and far beyond any conception of their originator by Pavlov (p. 266). By an abdominal operation a portion of the stomach of a dog was fashioned to form a tubular pouch, opening to the external skin surface and separated from the main stomach only by mucous membrane. This miniature stomach reacted to stimuli in the same way as the main stomach, so that the composition of the gastric juice—which is the same in both the main stomach and the miniature stomach—could be ascertained at any time. In this way Pavlov was able to study the quantity and composition of the gastric juice under various physiological conditions, and to carry out the experiments on conditioned reflexes already described (pp. 267–8).

The work of the London University physiologists, Sir William Maddock Bayliss (p. 518) and Ernest Henry Starling (p. 518), first showed by their discovery of the substance that they called secretin that the secretions of some glands are regulated not only by nervous impulses, but also by chemical substances produced elsewhere and transported to the gland by the blood. This discovery

opened up the wide subject of chemical regulation of metabolism.
The work of the Harvard physiologist, Walter Bradford Cannon
(1871–1945), in which he used X-rays (p. 375) to study the passage
of opaque substances in the digestive tract, clarified the movements
of these organs, and was of great practical use in clinical medicine.
Cannon also did much work on the conception of homeostasis, the

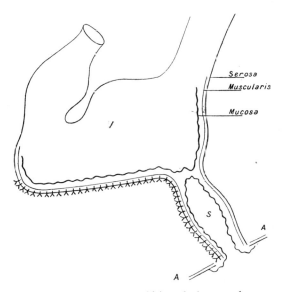

FIG. 87. 'Pavlov's pouch' in a dog's stomach
(I. P. Pavlov, *The Work of the Digestive Glands*, London, 1910)

condition of uniformity which results from the adjustment of the
internal relations of the cells of the body to its external relations.

Respiration. During this period the developments which occurred
constituted a revolution in this subject. In 1857 Lothar Meyer
(1830–95) showed that oxygen carried by the blood is not merely in
solution, but is temporarily bound to a constituent of the blood
by chemical combination. In 1851 Otto Funke (1828–79) had
isolated a red pigment from the blood. It was named haemoglobin,
and it was obtained in crystalline form in 1862 by Ernst Felix
Hoppe-Seyler (1825–95), one of the greatest of biochemists, who was
then assistant in Virchow's institute at Berlin but later held chairs at

Tübingen and Strasbourg. It was shown that the oxygen enters into a loose chemical combination with it to form oxyhaemoglobin. In the tissues the reaction is reversed; oxygen is liberated and carbon dioxide, the product of the life-process in the tissues, is taken up by the blood and liberated from it in the lungs. The processes of respiration are modified by many external factors. These were studied especially in this country by John Scott Haldane (1860–1936) of Oxford and Sir Joseph Barcroft (1872–1947) of Cambridge.

About the close of the nineteenth century there was much uncertainty concerning the mechanism of respiration and about the way in which the oxygen is carried to the tissues. In 1878 the French physiologist Paul Bert (1833–86), one of Claude Bernard's most distinguished assistants, had published his work *La pression barométrique*, in which he studied on himself and animals the physiological effects of abnormally high and low atmospheric pressures. Bert gave correctly the main facts and his deductions from them were inspired. His work was of great importance in connexion with balloon ascents and with work in caissons, and he advised Tissandier on his ill-fated balloon ascent. The advice was not taken. Bert's most important conclusion was that the physiological effects of oxygen and other gases in the blood are due not to their proportions but to their partial pressures. His work was not readily accepted, but in 1943, long after he was proved right, his book had the honour of being republished in an English translation.

About 1900 it was known that the rhythm of the respiratory centre is interrupted by mechanically stopping inspiration or expiration, and that this effect is absent if the vagi have been divided; it was supposed due to the phenomenon of vagus apnoea. The term 'apnoea' had been introduced in 1862 by Isidor Rosenthal (1836–1915) for the condition produced by excessive ventilation of the lungs as a result of artificial respiration, and from his subsequent work it was accepted that the respiratory centre is stimulated according to its oxygen content at the time. But it had been suggested by certain other investigators, on experimental evidence that at the time seemed to carry some weight, that the chemical regulation of breathing is due to the accumulation in the blood of either carbon dioxide or of some other acid substance produced in the muscles. Towards the close of

the century a new theory of vitiation of air breathed was introduced
by certain French physiologists: they stated that expired air contains
a poisonous organic substance. Haldane was attracted by this problem, and with James Lorrain Smith (1862–1931) he showed (1893)
that the symptoms resulting from the breathing of vitiated air were
due to an increase in the carbon dioxide content above 3 per cent. If
the accumulated carbon dioxide were absorbed, distress did not
begin until the oxygen content of the air fell below 14 per cent. As
fresh air contains 20·93 per cent. of oxygen and 0·03 per cent. of
carbon dioxide, such a large diminution of oxygen is very unusual.

Haldane now worked on the curve which expresses the percentage
saturation of blood when exposed to increasing percentages of a gas
important in industry, carbon monoxide (1895). He used birds as
tests for the presence of this gas, and he showed that if the air containing it has a high percentage of oxygen, the poisonous effects of
the carbon monoxide are less marked. In the following year he had
the opportunity of examining the bodies of a large number of men
killed in a colliery accident, and he showed that in most cases death
had been due to carbon monoxide poisoning. With Lorrain Smith he
carried out personal experiments on the degree to which the body
could be trained to tolerate this gas. At this time he also investigated
the air of wells in which men had lost their lives and he showed that,
contrary to the usual view that it contained an excess of carbon dioxide, it might consist of almost pure nitrogen. From the start of his
work Haldane combined academic researches with investigations of a
practical character connected with conditions in mines, submarines,
and caissons, and in this field he became the outstanding expert.

In his investigations on the carbon monoxide content of the blood
Haldane had to use the Töpler blood-gas pump. This instrument
was slow and difficult to use, and it required a considerable amount
of blood. About 1898 Haldane introduced his ferricyanide method
for the estimation of oxygen. It could be carried out rapidly on a
small amount of blood, and he showed that the results compared
favourably with those obtained using the blood pump. The method
was published in 1900.

Meanwhile Barcroft, a recent Cambridge graduate, had embarked
there on his first research under Foster—on the gaseous metabolism

of the submaxillary gland. He was certainly in touch with Haldane regarding an apparatus for the estimation of the gases in the blood passing to and from the gland. The result was a joint paper in 1902 in which they described their rapid method for estimating not only the oxygen but also the carbon dioxide. Haldane had meanwhile made important modifications in the Gowers haemoglobinometer.

During the period up to about 1904 Haldane was investigating phthisis and other diseases in the tin-miners of Cornwall, the results of which were published as a Parliamentary Paper. He then embarked on the long series of investigations on respiration carried out in collaboration with many junior colleagues, among whom may be mentioned Claude Gordon Douglas (1882–), Edward Palmer Poulton (1883–1939), and John Gillies Priestley (1880–1941). From 1903 he was engaged with Priestley on a fundamental piece of research (published in 1905) regarding the method by which the body automatically controls the breathing to meet the demands of the tissues for constantly varying concentrations of oxygen. The control was brought about by the action of the blood on the respiratory centre, and consequently investigation would have to be directed to that place where the blood was brought into contact with the inspired air, viz. the alveoli. Haldane devised an ingenious apparatus by which alveolar air could be easily obtained and rapidly analysed, and with it he and Priestley showed on themselves and other human subjects that during rest the percentages of oxygen and carbon dioxide in alveolar air are remarkably constant. They then varied the oxygen percentage in the inspired air over a very wide range, and they found that, while these variations were reflected in the alveolar air, the percentage of carbon dioxide in it remained very constant. When alveolar oxygen fell below 8 per cent., the carbon dioxide content rose and increased respirations righted the position. But when they increased the carbon dioxide percentage in inspired air, the carbon dioxide content of the alveolar air remained very constant. The regulating mechanism depended on the carbon dioxide content of the inspired air. A very small decrease—later determined as 0·2 per cent.—in the alveolar carbon dioxide percentage caused apnoea, and a correspondingly small increase in that gas caused hyperpnoea. The regulating mechanism is therefore very delicate. In the same paper the theory of vagus apnoea was demolished. By carrying out similar experiments under increased pressure in a steel chamber Haldane and Priestley brought out the important fact that it is not the actual percentage of carbon dioxide which is kept constant by the body, but the partial pressure of that gas in the alveolar air. Paul Bert's forgotten dictum was therefore confirmed. In the same paper Haldane included his early work on the respiratory movements and showed that the completion of expiration permits inspiration, but does not excite it.

The follow-up of these discoveries occupied Haldane and his associates for many years. It is sufficient to mention here that in 1908, with Poulton, he studied the effects of diminution of the oxygen in the inspired air, and of diminution of the oxygen reaching the blood (anoxaemia) whether as the result of pulmonary disease or other factors. This work led later to the improvement in the methods by which oxygen was administered in disease and in gas-casualties in war. They also further studied the effects of rebreathing the same air. Working under Haldane, Douglas invented (1911) the bag method of determining the respiratory exchange which bears his name; and in the following year he and Haldane used this method to investigate the effects of muscular work on the respiratory exchange.

From about 1908 onwards it became clear that the original conception that the tension of carbon dioxide in the respiratory centre influenced the respiration directly must be given up. It was gradually demonstrated by scientists in various countries that the carbon dioxide is carried in the blood in the form of phosphates and bicarbonates, and intensive studies were now made on the hydrogen-ion concentration of the blood. In 1912 the Danish biochemists Karl Albert Hasselbalch (1874–) and Christen Lundsgaard (1883–1930) discovered a formula by which it could be easily measured. Important work was also done in this direction by August Krogh (1874–1949) of Copenhagen, who later received a Nobel Prize for his work on the anatomy and physiology of the capillaries (1920). The result of these investigations was to show that in a resting man the regulation of breathing is due to incredibly minute changes in the tissue reactions.

The method by which the oxygen is carried to the tissues

presented equally complex problems. Contradictory experiments had been carried out from Paul Bert onwards on the amount of oxygen which was given off by the blood under varying partial-pressures of oxygen. In 1904 Christian Bohr (1855–1911) of Copenhagen showed that the oxygen-dissociation curve for a solution of haemoglobin differs from that for blood; and with Hasselbalch and Krogh he showed that the oxygen is released from the oxyhaemoglobin more readily in the presence of carbon dioxide. In the tissues, therefore, the higher the concentration of carbon dioxide, the more readily is oxygen given up to the tissues.

Barcroft had meanwhile been engaged on studies of the gaseous metabolism of different organs, and in 1909 he began to publish with various colleagues a series of studies on the oxygen-dissociation of haemoglobin. It had been demonstrated in 1912 by (Sir) Rudolph A. Peters (p. 619) that the association between the oxygen and the haemoglobin in the blood is almost certainly chemical combination and not absorption, one molecule of oxygen combining with each atom of iron present in the haemoglobin. Much consideration was now given to the form of the dissociation-curve. Experiments made in 1890 had suggested that the curve is a rectangular hyperbola; but Bohr made and plotted actual observations and showed that in the case of blood the resulting curve has a double contour and that its right limb crosses the hyperbola. It is therefore not a hyperbola at all. These experiments gained in interest and importance because of the subsequent attempt of A. V. Hill (p. 292) to obtain an equation expressing the dissociation of oxygen in blood. Barcroft and his co-workers now showed that the form of the dissociation-curve of oxy-haemoglobin depends on the presence of salts (electrolytes) in the solution, and also that, while carbon dioxide and other acids shift the curve to the right, alkalis shift it to the left. Barcroft also worked on the dissociation curve for carboxyhaemoglobin. He also showed that the form of the dissociation curve for oxygen varies in different individuals. These and similar investigations engaged him until 1914, when he published *The Respiratory Functions of the Blood*. A much enlarged edition of two of the three sections of this work appeared later (1925, 1928).

While these events were in progress great interest had been

awakened in the subject of anoxaemia, mountain sickness, and the results of living at high altitudes. Although Paul Bert had in general explained that the symptoms at high altitudes were due to a lowering of the oxygen tension, his observations passed unheeded, and for many years an erroneous theory had held the field which asserted that the results were due to 'acapnia', an excessive loss of carbon dioxide. In 1910 Barcroft and Douglas were invited to be members of a small expedition of German and Austrian scientists, led by the physiologist Nathan Zuntz (1847–1920) of Berlin, who were to make physiological observations on the Peak of Teneriffe (12,000 ft.). As a result of his observations on this expedition Barcroft showed that the oxygen-dissociation curve of an individual is not altered by altitude provided that the estimations are made at the carbon dioxide tension found in the individual's blood at that particular level. In the following year Barcroft was with the expedition to Monte Rosa (15,000 ft.), the primary purpose of which was to investigate the effect of exercise on the dissociation curve at high altitudes. He found that at these heights the blood shows an acidosis even while the individual is resting, and during exercise it is very much increased. Concurrently with this expedition Haldane was leading an Anglo-American Expedition to Pike's Peak, Colorado (14,000 ft.), the specific purpose of which was to study acclimatization to the oxygen deficiency experienced at high altitudes. Other members of this expedition were Douglas and the American physiologist Yandell Henderson (1873–1944). The results gave new information on the cyanosis of high altitudes and on the methods whereby acclimatization is established.

Over a period of many years there had been differences of opinion regarding the method by which the oxygen passes from the alveoli into the blood. Pflüger, as a result of tests with his aerotonometer, concluded that the process was one of simple diffusion through the wall of the alveolus, but before the end of the nineteenth century other scientists were arguing, on the analogy of what was known to happen in the swim-bladders of fishes, that a process of active secretion of oxygen takes place. In 1910 Krogh, using the micro-tonometer which he had invented, reinvestigated the position and concluded in favour of simple diffusion. Haldane did not agree, and as a result of his own early experiments he favoured the doctrine of secretion. From his work on Pike's Peak he concluded that at high altitudes, though diffusion does take place, when the individual is acclimatized to the altitude secretion of oxygen by the alveolar wall occurs while muscular work is being carried out.

On grounds which cannot be entered into here Barcroft favoured the theory of pure diffusion, and he undertook two enterprises in order to prove it. The first was his famous 'glass-chamber' experiment of 1920. In this specially constructed glass chamber Barcroft lived, did muscular work, and slept for six days, during which time he was, by the introduction of nitrogen into the chamber, subjected to a gradually decreasing partial pressure of oxygen until at the end of the experiment he was in an atmosphere equivalent to that at 18,000 ft. On the final day during a period of two hours he had samples of blood from his radial artery withdrawn for analysis. Despite certain relevant criticisms put forward by Haldane, Barcroft claimed that this rather heroic experiment gave no support to the secretion theory. To meet the criticism of lack of acclimatization in this experiment another Anglo-American expedition, with Barcroft as leader, was organized by the Royal Society for 1921-2. The destination was Cerro de Pasco (14,200 ft.) in the Andes of Peru, where copper mining was carried out on a commercial basis. They found that on acclimatization there is a rough agreement between the increase in the haemoglobin and in that of the red blood corpuscles. They made observations on cyanosis and mountain sickness; and they attributed acclimatization to an increased oxygen pressure in the alveoli (due to an increase of total ventilation), to the increase of red cells and haemoglobin, and to a change in the oxygen-dissociation curve which enables the blood to take up an increased amount of oxygen. No evidence whatever was found for the secretion theory. Some important information was also obtained on the effect of high altitudes on the mind.

This account has had to be selective, and little has been said of the many ancillary investigations made by British and American workers. Of the latter, Y. Henderson (p. 309) made an attempt to measure the circulation rate in man directly, and introduced an automatic sampling method which was important. Donald D. Van Slyke (p. 597) of the Rockefeller Institute introduced a modi-

fication of the ferricyanide process and made many important contributions on oxygen-dissociation, hydrogen-ion concentration of the
blood, and other aspects of the physical chemistry of that fluid. Van
Slyke was also known for his work on the chemistry of proteins and
protein derivatives and on enzyme action.

In 1908 Haldane began his important studies on the 'bends' produced in the muscles during decompression from high pressures,
and his further work over the years included practical discoveries on
war gases, the emphysema of miners, the control of underground
temperature, and the measures necessary to deal with various
'damps' and other accidents of mining. In 1923 Barcroft published
the first of his important studies on the spleen with which he was
engaged for ten years. He showed that that organ is a store-house for
blood corpuscles which are only forced into the general circulation
by the muscular contraction of the organ, under the influence of
emotional and other conditions. In 1933 he published his first paper
on the foetal respiration, a subject which was to engage his attention
during the remainder of his life.

Circulation. In his experiments on blood-pressure Stephen Hales
(p. 155) measured it by allowing the blood to rush up into a vertical
glass tube. For a horse a tube at least eleven feet long was required,
and the method was extremely inconvenient and required patience
on the part of the operator. In 1828 the French physiologist Jean
Léonard Marie Poiseuille (1799–1869) first used a mercury manometer for the same purpose. The weight of the mercury allowed a
short column of it to counterbalance the pressure of the blood, and
his apparatus was therefore more convenient. In 1847 Karl Ludwig
(p. 299) provided a float for one limb of the manometer, and he
arranged it so as to record the changes of blood-pressure on the
revolving drum of a kymograph (p. 300). This apparatus, together
with Poiseuille's very important studies on the velocity of the blood,
made possible more accurate experimental work on the circulation.
All these methods involved the placing of a tube in an artery, so that
the blood flowed directly from the artery into the apparatus. They
were therefore unsuitable for clinical use. The first sphygmomanometer which could be used to determine the blood pressure without puncturing the skin was that of Samuel Siegfried von Basch

(1837–1905), described by him in 1881. The instrument consisted of a small capsule the floor of which was formed by a rubber diaphragm. The cavity of the capsule was connected with a manometer by a rubber tube. In use the diaphragm was pressed upon the radial artery until the pulse disappeared beyond the point of application. The reading of the manometer at this point indicated the arterial

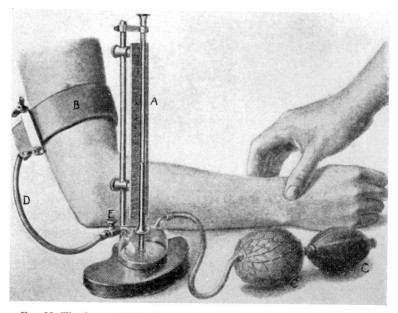

FIG. 88. The first model of the Riva-Rocci sphygmomanometer, for measuring the blood pressure
(S. Riva-Rossi, *Gaz. med. di Torino*, 1896)

pressure. The error with this instrument was very large, and it was not generally satisfactory. It was not until 1896 that an instrument was invented by Scipione Riva-Rocci (1863–1936) which enabled the blood pressure to be easily determined in the human subject. The illustration of the first model of this instrument is reproduced in Fig. 88. By compressing the bulb *C* air is forced into the mercury cistern and then through the tap *E* and the tube *D* into the rubber cuff *B* which surrounds the upper arm. After each compression of the bulb the mercury column in *A* registers the pressure in *B*.

Pumping is continued until the pulse at the wrist disappears. The tap E is closed and the pressure read. E is then opened slightly and the pressure is again read at the point where the pulse reappears. The mean of the two readings gives the systolic blood pressure.

In 1825 a very important work entitled *Wellenlehre* ('On wave motion') was published by the brothers Ernst Heinrich Weber (1795–1878) and Eduard Friedrich Wilhelm Weber (1806–71). In this work they discussed the hydrodynamics of liquids flowing in tubes, and they made the first measurement of the velocity of the pulse wave. These brothers, who were both professors at Leipzig, were responsible for other important discoveries. In 1867 Ludwig's invention of the 'Stromuhr' for measuring the velocity of the blood-flow in an artery was published by one of his pupils. Ten years earlier Étienne Jules Marey (1830–1904) had extended the work of the Webers to the flow of fluids in elastic tubes. The arterial system of the animal body is a very complex arrangement of muscular and elastic tubes, and the waves set up are only slightly distinguishable by the finger which feels the pulse. The instrument of Sanctorius (p. 115) was incapable of distinguishing the different waves. In 1855, however, Karl Vierordt (1818–84) of Tübingen first applied the graphic method to the investigation of these waves. Five years later Marey devised the first portable sphygmograph, with which a tracing of the pulse wave could be obtained on a strip of smoked paper. This instrument was important not only in physiology, but also in the clinical investigation of heart disease. In 1878 Marey's sphygmograph was modified by Robert Ellis Dudgeon (1820–1904) to its present form. The first serious study of the venous pulse was made by Mackenzie (p. 623) in 1902. He used a recording tambour applied over the jugular vein.

Much work had meanwhile been carried out on the heart itself. In 1837 Alfred Wilhelm Volkmann (p. 261) stimulated the vagus nerve and found that the heart's action was inhibited. Nothing was then known of the inhibitory action of nerves, and he therefore dismissed his observation as an accident; he thus missed an important opportunity. The chance was seized by the Weber brothers in 1845. They then demonstrated that Volkmann's observation had been correct and most physiologists then accepted the view that the result was a true inhibition. Some years later the vagus centre was localized in the medulla. Albert von Bezold (1836–68) demonstrated the accelerator nerve fibres of the heart in 1862, and he showed that they arose from the spinal cord. The discovery of the depressor nerve by Ludwig and Elie von Cyon (1842–1912) in 1866 has been mentioned (p. 301). In 1871 Ludwig and Schmiedeberg showed that the vagus also contains accelerator fibres. A classical paper on the innervation of the heart was published by Gaskell (p. 262) in 1882. He showed that the nerve ganglia in the sinus venosus play an important part. The regulatory effect of the carotid sinus was well worked out between 1923 and 1927 by Heinrich Ewald Hering (1866–1948).

Great interest had been shown in the cause of the heart-beat. The earlier physiologists, up to the time of Haller, had held that the heart-beat is caused by the direct action of the blood as it flowed through the cavities of the heart. It was then realized that a frog's heart would continue to beat for some time after it had been removed from the body. Haller and his early successors therefore adopted the myogenic theory, according to which the cardiac muscle possesses an inherent rhythmical power which acts automatically. In 1848 Remak (p. 246) showed that the sinus venosus of the frog's heart possesses groups of ganglion cells; and in the same year Ludwig discovered the ganglion cells in the interventricular septum. Four years later Friedrich Heinrich Bidder (p. 582) discovered at the junction of the atrium and the ventricle in the frog's heart the ganglion which bears his name. In the same year Hermann Stannius (1808–83) described the 'Stannius ligatures'. The assumption that the second ligature inhibits the action of the ganglia mentioned above was construed as a powerful argument in favour of the neurogenic theory of the heart-beat. In 1859 Michael Foster (p. 262) showed that any part of a snail's heart will continue to show rhythmical contractions when separated from the rest of the heart. Foster later demonstrated that in the frog's heart the ganglion-free apex is thrown into rhythmical activity if a constant current is passed through it; and in 1871 Henry Pickering Bowditch (1840–1911) working in Ludwig's laboratory showed that the same effect was produced by passing fluid under pressure into the apex. In the same paper Bowditch established the principle of 'all-or-nothing' in relation to cardiac muscle. (Bowditch later founded at Harvard the first physiological laboratory in the United States.) The whole question was then very thoroughly investigated by Gaskell (p. 262) using the hearts of frogs and of other animals. In the tortoise especially he demonstrated (1883) that if a section is made in the region of the auriculo-ventricular groove, the ventricle at first beats excitedly and then more and more slowly until it stops; but after a period it begins to beat again at a rhythm which is different from that of the atrium. Gaskell proceeded to give a very convincing proof that the heart-beat is of myogenic origin.

Most of the experimental work on the heart itself had up to 1880 been carried out on the hearts of the lower vertebrates, since mammals presented many difficulties. In order to study the effects of drugs and certain conditions on the work of the mammalian heart, the organ had to be 'isolated', that is, severed from all connexions with the nervous system. This meant removing it from the body. In the year 1880, however, this very important procedure was successfully carried out by Henry Newell Martin (1848–96), and he kept the heart alive by perfusion. (Newell Martin studied under Foster at Cambridge, and in 1876 he became professor of physiology at Johns Hopkins University. His early retirement and death was a great loss to science.) In the same year Sidney Ringer (1834–1910) did much work on solutions suitable for perfusion purposes, and he introduced that usually called after him. During the next few years Newell Martin investigated the effect of changes in arterial pressure and of temperature on the isolated mammalian heart. His method remained standard until well into the twentieth century, when attempts were made to isolate a heart-lung preparation. This was successfully accomplished by Starling (p. 518) in 1910, and was modified to its present form especially in 1912. In these years Starling studied with these preparations the manner in which the heart adjusts its output to the amount of blood which flows into it. He investigated the volume and pressure changes of the organ under varying degrees of venous filling and arterial resistance. By 1918 he was able to enunciate the Law of the Heart, that for cardiac muscle as for voluntary muscle, the energy of contraction is a function of the length of the muscle fibres. Briefly, if an excess of blood flows into the heart, or if it has to work against an increased arterial pressure, it is temporarily overfilled. The resulting increase in length of its fibres stimulates them to increase the force of their contraction, and the load or the obstruction is thus compensated. Later work on the conduction in the heart muscle is dealt with hereafter (pp. 624–5).

Sir Charles Arthur Lovatt Evans was associated with Starling in the early phases of these preparations, and from 1912 he worked for over twenty years on the metabolism of cardiac muscle. He devised a formula from which the work done by both ventricles can be calculated, and from which the mechanical efficiency is easily obtained. With his colleagues he measured the amount of oxygen consumed by the heart under various conditions. He also investigated the greatly increased consumption of oxygen under the action of adrenaline. In order to study the carbohydrate metabolism of the heart, using the heart-lung preparation, it is necessary to exclude the lungs. Evans devised a heart-oxygenator circuit and found that the glucose consumption of the heart muscle is much less than had been anticipated. With the ordinary preparation a great deal of the glucose taken up is consumed in the lungs. He also showed that in general lactates are burned by the heart muscle to replace energy, and that the sugar is changed to glycogen. The respiratory exchange of the heart was found to be directly proportional to the amount of work which it had to perform. Lovatt Evans has also worked on the physiology of plain muscle and on the hydrogen-ion concentration of the blood.

We have already mentioned the discovery of vasomotor nerves in 1852 (p. 261). A vasomotor centre was first discovered, in the medulla oblongata, by Ludwig and Carl Dittmar (1844–1920) in 1871, and in the same year Ludwig localized it very accurately. Gaskell observed the circulation in a frog muscle directly in 1877, and he measured the diameter of the vessels on stimulation of certain nerves. He showed that vasodilator fibres run in motor nerves. Ten years later Brown-Séquard (p. 261) showed that vasodilatation is produced by stimulation of the cerebral cortex. The control of the capillary circulation is more complex and is dealt with later (pp. 557 ff.).

The blood. John Hunter regarded the blood as a living tissue of the body. His work was carried on by one of his most distinguished pupils, William Hewson (1739–74), who published his *Experimental Inquiry into the Properties of the Blood* in 1771. Two further parts followed; the second of these also dealt with the blood (1777). He made important experiments on coagulation, and from the plasma he separated fibrinogen ('coagulable lymph'). Hewson gave many measurements of the 'red particles' (erythrocytes) in various animals, and he put forward the theory that the white corpuscles are derived from the thymus and the lymph glands; in the spleen they are transformed into red corpuscles. Lister discovered that coagulation of the blood in the vessels did not take place unless they were injured. In 1842 Alfred Donné (1801–78) announced his discovery of 'globules' (platelets) in the blood. During the next forty years several other descriptions of the platelets were published. Perhaps the best of these studies was that of (Sir) William Osler (1849–1919), published in 1874. This was probably the most scientific of the contributions to medicine made by this great physician. A Canadian by birth, Osler studied at Montreal, and later became professor of medicine at Philadelphia and then at the newly founded Johns Hopkins University at Baltimore. In 1905 he was called to the regius chair of medicine at Oxford. He was widely known in Europe and America, and by his very numerous occasional lectures and papers he exerted a great influence on the advancement of medicine. Of his more serious contributions to medical literature his studies on bacterial endocarditis (1885, 1908), on the cyanosis associated with increase in the number of blood-cells and enlargement of the spleen (1903) which had been first described by Louis Henri Vaquez (1860–1936), and his *Lectures on the Diagnosis of Abdominal Tumours* (1894) are the best remembered. His greatest work was his *Principles and Practice of Medicine*, first published in 1892, which saw many editions. This great book was for more than a generation the bible of medical students and practitioners in all parts of the English-speaking world. Osler was also one of the earliest and greatest of the modern collectors of medical literature, and his bibliographical and personal notes on his books formed the basis of the *Bibliotheca Osleriana*, the catalogue of his great library—left to McGill University, Montreal—which was published ten years after his death.

Accurate blood-platelet counts were first made by Georges Hayem (1841–1933) in 1878. Hayem, one of the founders of haematology, later published a valuable textbook on this subject. The platelets were given their present name by Giulio Bizzozero (1846–1901) in 1882, and he made the first study of their role in blood coagulation.

The first satisfactory attempt to determine the number of corpuscles in a cubic millimeter of blood was made by Vierordt in 1852. The method was not very convenient, and it was later superseded by that of the Gowers haemocytometer, which was a modification of an instrument devised in 1874 by Louis Charles Malassez (1842–1909). Gowers's haemoglobinometer has already been mentioned (p. 278). In 1910 Cecil Price-Jones (1863–1943) claimed that the sizes of the red cells were important in diagnosis, and he described a method for their measurement.

Early studies of the white corpuscles were those of Thomas Addison (p. 284), and the word leucocyte was first used in 1855. The first successful attempts to stain the white corpuscles were carried out by Ehrlich (p. 687) about 1875. He employed the newly discovered aniline dyes, and his tri-acid stain was long used. By these means he was able to revise the classification of these cells.

The later history of haematology is too complex for discussion here, but something may be said of the reticulo-endothelial system. In 1876 Karl Wilhelm von Kupffer (1829–1902), anatomist of Kiel and Königsberg, described in the walls of the liver capillaries star-shaped cells, now known to be phagocytic. In 1899 Louis Antoine Ranvier (1835–1922), the Paris histologist, best known for his nodes in the medullary sheaths of nerves, described branched cells in connective tissue generally. In 1901 Felix Marchand (1846–1928) of Leipzig showed their derivation from tissues and not from blood. In many other tissues similar cells were found, and although they showed wide morphological variations, those in the liver, the spleen pulp and sinuses, the lymph glands, the adrenal and pituitary glands, and the bone marrow were all characterized by their ability to ingest very actively certain dyes exhibited to them in weak concentrations. In the ten years from 1913 Aschoff (p. 638) worked on this problem, and having shown that these scattered cells form a homologous system, in 1922 he proposed for it the term reticulo-endothelial system. It has now been shown that the endothelial type of cells in this system contain very fine intracellular fibrils which emerge from the cells and form an intercellular network.

The reticulo-endothelial system is concerned with metabolism and the formation and destruction of blood cells. It is subject to its own type of tumour formation, and it is deranged in, and may be the cause of, a few rare metabolic diseases, such as that described by Philippe Charles Ernest Gaucher (1854–1918) in 1882.

Biochemistry. Under the stimulus of Liebig and Wöhler (p. 238) chemical methods began to be applied to the study of the body just before the middle of the nineteenth century. Qualitative tests for various body constituents were rapidly elaborated. Michel Eugène Chevreul (1786–1889) had already shown in a classical monograph that neutral fats can be split to fatty acids and glycerol. Nine years later he isolated creatine from animal tissue, and he was still carrying out important work even as a centenarian. Under the influence of Helmholtz (p. 288) physical methods were increasingly applied. Thus the chemist Robert Wilhelm Bunsen (1811–99) introduced spectrum analysis in 1859, and he improved the methods of gas analysis. The discovery of the spectra of oxyhaemoglobin and methaemoglobin (1862–4) by Hoppe-Seyler (p. 303) was followed by those of reduced haemoglobin and haemochromogen by Sir George Gabriel Stokes (1819–1903). Thomas Graham (1805–69) did important work on osmosis and introduced the analytical method of dialysis.

One of the earliest biochemists was Johann Ludwig Wilhelm Thudichum (1829–1901) who had studied under Liebig and Bunsen. For political reasons he migrated from Germany to London in 1853, and in his long tenure of the post of chemist to the Medical Department of the Privy Council he carried out a series of investigations which were far in advance of their time. Mention may be made of his work on the pigments of bile and urine. He discovered the carotenoid pigments, and also cephalins and myelins in brain tissue. He was the author of an early textbook of the subject, *A Manual of Chemical Physiology* (1872), and his last work, *Die chemische Konstitution des Gehirns des Menschen und der Thiere* ('The chemical constitution of the human and animal brain', 1901), is now recognized as a classic. In 1887 Gustav von Bunge (1844–1920) published his well-known textbook on physiological and pathological chemistry.

Since 1900 biochemistry has become a vast subject. The work of Gowland Hopkins, Pavy, and many other biochemists is dealt with later. Otto Knut Olaf Folin (1867–1934) of Harvard did important work on blood analysis, especially in relation to sugar. Johann Kjeldahl (1849–1900) introduced in 1883 his almost universally employed method for the determination of nitrogen in organic matter, and most important work was carried out on the amino-acids over many years by Emil Fischer (p. 595) of Berlin and Emil Abderhalden (p. 596) of Halle. Henry Drysdale Dakin (1880–1952) is known for his work on oxidations and reductions, though he is more popularly remembered for his part in the development of the Carrel-Dakin solution. The new conceptions of the internal environment raised by Rudolf Schoenheimer (1898–1941) in his important work on *The Dynamic State of Body Constituents* (1942) are briefly discussed in the section on Metabolism (p. 601).

It is safe to say that the more important conclusions of the three modern founders of the science of physiology, Müller, Bernard, and Ludwig, form the main scientific background of the clinical practice of our time.

THE CELL THEORY

We have seen (p. 132) how the wall of a plant cell was described and illustrated by Robert Hooke in 1665. Following him Nehemiah Grew (1641–1712) also illustrated plant cells. Less clearly, a similar structure was discerned in animals. No real understanding of the nature of cells was, however, reached. Little progress was made in the eighteenth century. But at its close Marie François Xavier Bichat (1771–1802), at the Hôtel Dieu, Paris, though he did not employ a microscope, encouraged the use of this instrument by his division of the materials of the body into twenty-one 'membranes' or 'tissues'. He compared the minute structure of the animal body to the substance of a web or woven fabric. The word Bichat used was the Old French term *tissu*. Hence arose the name histology (Greek *histos*, a web) for this new method of studying the structure of animals and plants.

During the early nineteenth century there were many developments. The cell nucleus had been first observed by Leeuwenhoek in 1700 in the red blood corpuscles of the salmon. Nuclei had been first clearly seen in cells, other than blood cells, by Felice Fontana

(1720–1805) in 1781. He may also have seen the nucleolus, but he named neither it nor the nucleus. The nucleus of a plant cell—in an orchid—was first seen and illustrated by Ferdinand Lucas Bauer (1760–1826) in 1802, but his drawings were not published until 1830–8. Robert Brown (1773–1858), the celebrated botanist, knew about Bauer's drawings, and in 1831 he coined the name nucleus, gave an excellent description of that organelle in plant cells, and recognized that it occurred very constantly in them. The nucleolus was now rediscovered by Rudolph Wagner (1805–64) in 1835. Meanwhile Purkinje (p. 246) had described in 1825 the germinal vesicle of eggs, but his paper was not published until 1830. In 1827 Karl Ernst von Baer (p. 237) discovered the mammalian ovum.

By about 1835 it was recognized that the nucleus occurred frequently in the tissues of plants, and that it was also found in unicellular organisms. Some emphasis had been placed on the cell wall or 'membrane', but there was a lack of curiosity about the material which lay between the nucleus and the cell wall. A substance which was obviously protoplasm had been mentioned by Abraham Trembley (1710–84) in 1744, but not in connexion with cells. About 1824 René Joachim Henri Dutrochet (1776–1847) clarified some of the biological problems, described the process of osmosis, and recognized that the viscous substance was important. Dujardin (p. 327) described many new species of protozoa. In order to explain some of the biological phenomena which they presented, he postulated a substance which he called 'sarcode' as constituting the bulk of these animals (1835). This was equivalent to what we know as protoplasm.

In the animal field pertinent observations of this nature were being made. Johannes Müller had shown that the notochord (chorda dorsalis) of fishes consists of separate cells with distinct walls. At this period some workers were inclined to use the word 'cell' literally, that is, as indicating a living wall surrounding a cavity. A definite advance was made by Friedrich Gustav Jakob Henle (1809–85), who had been a pupil of Müller at Bonn and later his assistant at Berlin. Henle early became professor of anatomy at Zürich and then at Heidelberg. In 1852 he was appointed to the corresponding chair at Göttingen, where he worked until his death. At first better known as a pathologist, he was the author of a well-known work on that subject. He was also the author of a famous and very popular work on gross descriptive anatomy. More important from our point of view, he wrote what might be called the first systematic work on general anatomy, in which the tissues were considered individually. Jakob Henle first described the microscopic structure of human epithelium (1837). He showed that the cells in the superficial layers of epithelium are larger, and what we would call more organized, than those in the deeper layers, indicating a gradual growth from the deeper layers to the more superficial. He also showed that the cilia which are found on the surface of certain types of epithelium stand up from the superficial layer of cylindrical cells. These cilia are in motion, and this circumstance is opposed to the view that epithelium is a lifeless substance. At this period there was no recognition of the fact that even in plants all tissues were made up of cells, each of which had a nucleus and protoplasm.

About this time Matthias Jacob Schleiden (1804–81) had been working on the microscopic structure of plants. In 1838 he was appointed assistant professor of botany at Jena, and in the same year he published his *Beiträge zur Phytogenesis* ('Contributions to phytogenesis'). In it he demonstrated for the first time the regular occurrence of nuclei in the young cells of the phanerogams, and he also saw the nucleolus. He thus directed attention to the nucleus as a characteristic part of a cell. Unfortunately Schleiden thought the nucleus was formed by crystallization in the structureless fluid which he called 'Schleim'; the nucleus later secreted the cell wall.

Schleiden made no mention of a Cell Theory. But before publishing anything he discussed his views with his friend Theodor Schwann (1810–82), who was also a friend of Henle and a pupil of and assistant to Müller at Berlin. Schwann later filled the chairs of anatomy at Louvain and at Liège. In 1839 he published his work entitled *Mikroskopische Untersuchungen über die Uebereinstimmung in der Struktur und dem Wachsthum der Thiere und Pflanzen* ('Microscopical researches into the accordance in the structure and growth of animals and plants'), which six years later was awarded the Copley Medal of the Royal Society. Schwann stated that the purpose of his work was to show that even complex animal tissues develop only from cells, and he referred particularly to Schleiden's work on plants. Although Schwann went much farther than Schleiden, he was certainly influenced and inspired by his conversations with the latter. Unfortunately he adopted Schleiden's idea of the development of cells, and neither Schleiden nor Schwann had any conception of the formation of new cells by division.

Schwann had already published the factual parts of his book in

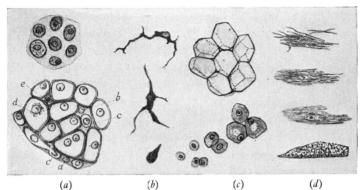

(a)   (b)   (c)   (d)

FIG. 89. Schwann's illustrations of the nature and origin of animal cells
(T. Schwann, *Microscopical Researches*, London, 1839)

three successive articles, the first of which appeared in January 1838 and the third in April of the same year. In these papers he confirmed that the notochord consists of cells with nuclei. 'Cartilage corpuscles' had already been seen by Purkinje. Schwann examined the branchial cartilage of the tadpole, and Fig. 89 (a), lower figure, shows what he saw. The surface of the cartilage is at the lower margin of the figure. As we pass inwards the cell walls become thicker and intercellular substance is seen. The upper figure shows more mature cartilage, from a foetal pig, with more intercellular material. Fig. 89 (b) shows pigment cells from the skin of a tadpole. In the primitive cell (lower figure) the nucleus is obscured by pigment, but in the more mature ramifying cells (above) the nuclei are seen. Fig. 89 (c) shows cells from the pith of the shaft of a feather. Schwann thought that the matrix contained many nuclei, each of which later formed a cell round it (left of lower figure). Fig. 89 (d) shows from below upwards the stages in the differentiation of the cells which form the shaft of the feather, from the nucleated cell below to the fibrillated cells above. Schwann examined the structure of other tissues in this manner. In fibrous tissue the fibres developed as prolongations of cells in opposite directions; areolar and adipose tissues were similarly modified from cellular tissue. He then formulated the Cell Theory, according to which animals are made up of cells modified in development in various ways for particular purposes, or of substances secreted by these cells.

Schwann concentrated his attention on the nucleus and the cell wall and made little reference to the cell protoplasm. In this he was following Schleiden, who regarded his 'Schleim' as not worthy of serious attention. At that time Schwann does not appear to have been very familiar with the current literature, since he seems to have been unaware of the contributions of several others. Dujardin's 'sarcode' was a pointer. In 1836 G. G. Valentin (p. 481) studied the substance lying between the nucleus and the cell wall and called it 'parenchyme'. In an address delivered on 16 January 1839 Purkinje made the first attempt to generalize about the living substance of cells. He used the word 'Protoplasma'. This term had previously been used in religious literature to mean 'the first created thing', but Purkinje was the first to use it in a scientific sense. His address was published in 1840. Four years later the Swiss botanist, Karl von Nägeli (1817–91), paid special attention to the gelatinous substance which lines the cell wall of certain algae. In the same year Hugo von Mohl (1805–72) of Tübingen gave a more detailed description of this viscous lining, which he called the 'Primordialschlauch' or 'utriculus primordialis'; he distinguished it from the watery sap that fills the interor of the cell. In 1846 he re-introduced the word 'Protoplasma'. He was obviously unaware of the fact that Purkinje had already used it seven years earlier.

By that time it was recognized that a plant cell contained a nucleus and a viscous substance which was now called protoplasm. The protoplasm was enclosed in a rigid cell wall. In the case of the lower animals it was recognized that nuclei were present, embedded in a contractile substance of sarcode. The next step was the realization that the protoplasm of plants was essentially the same as the sarcode of animals, and this was largely due to the botanist

Ferdinand Cohn (p. 336) in 1850. From that time it was increasingly appreciated that protoplasm is the essential living substance.

Scientists now turned their attention to the cell wall, which is so constantly present in plants and so often absent in animals. The first to suggest that in animals a cell need not have a cell wall was Franz von Leydig (1821–1908), professor of zoology at Tübingen. His statement of 1857 was followed by similar statements, based on observation, by the botanist Heinrich Anton de Bary (1831–88), then at Freiburg-im-Breisgau, in 1860, and by Maximilian ('Max') Johann Sigismund Schultze (1825–74), successor of von Helmholtz as professor of anatomy at Bonn. Both these men showed that in the Mycetozoa it was common to find a syncytium, consisting of a mass of protoplasm containing nuclei. Schultze's work in this field began in 1860, and in the following year he gave his famous definition of a cell as 'a small naked lump of protoplasm with a nucleus'.

By this time the Cell Theory was exerting much important influence in general biology. The work of John Goodsir (1814–67) was widely recognized in Germany. Goodsir was in 1846 called to succeed Monro *tertius* in the chair of anatomy at Edinburgh University, and he proved a worthy successor. He enriched science with many notable contributions in the fields of anatomy, comparative anatomy, and pathology. In a work published in 1845 he showed that in his microscopic observations he was far ahead of most others in the field. He had an advanced knowledge of the cell as a centre of nutrition and of the secretory functions of certain cells. Virchow was later to dedicate his work on Cellular Pathology to Goodsir with expressions of his indebtedness.

The British naturalist Thomas Henry Huxley (1825–95) opposed the Cell Theory in 1853 on very inadequate grounds. In an address delivered in 1868 he completely changed his view and described protoplasm as 'the bases of physical life'. By the following year this had been modified as the title of a popular article by him into the famous phrase 'the physical basis of life'. This was his sole contribution to the Cell Theory.

The reaction against a cell-covering was long in being overcome. Several botanists suggested that there must be some covering, even though a cell wall was not present. In 1895 Charles Ernest Overton

(1865–1933), then a Zürich botanist but later professor of pharmacology at Lund, as a result of a careful study of the osmotic properties of living cells, put forward the theory that the ground-cytoplasm was modified at the surface to form a cell-membrane. This theory was generally accepted and has been prolific in results.

Cell division seems to have been first observed by Barthélemy Charles Dumortier (1797–c. 1840), the Belgian botanist and politician, in 1832. Three years later it was seen and described by von Mohl. Both Valentin and Purkinje had recognized cell division by 1838.

It has long been the custom to refer to the Cell Theory of Schleiden and Schwann, but it is now coming to be recognized that the expression is incorrect. Several scientists had already laid the foundations before the works of these two men were published, especially Purkinje, Valentin, and Henle. Schleiden's part in the actual formulation of the theory is not great, and his many erroneous views also discount his importance. Schwann, on the other hand, despite his neglect of the work of others, made a careful study and deductions based on his own work. He formulated the Cell Theory. But it will be seen that it was many years before the theory could be justifiably applied to all plant and animal cells. Others before Schwann had played a part in the conception of the Cell Theory, and it was not due to the work of any one man. But if any single name is to be attached to it, Schwann has very strong claims.

The Cell Theory had important effects on the study of histology and embryology. Kölliker's textbooks on these subjects (p. 247) were remarkable expositions of the new views. It was inevitable that the theory should be applied to pathology and morbid histology, and this step was taken in 1858 with the publication of Virchow's famous book on *Cellularpathologie* (p. 635). This event was a landmark in the history, not only of medicine, but also of science in general. The study of diseased tissues still pays tribute to Virchow's genius.

ESTABLISHMENT OF THE DOCTRINE OF THE GERM ORIGIN OF DISEASE

As long as we can remember all of us have been familiar with the fact that certain diseases are caused by micro-organisms, and that in the case of some diseases the illness is caused by one particular micro-organism which is the specific cause of that disease. Yet even less than a hundred years ago virtually nothing was known of this vast field. The problem originally invaded the territory of several different subjects, and we shall review briefly some of the earlier history. It involved first the discovery of bacteria, as we shall usually call them; and, second, the proof that some bacteria cause diseases. Third, it necessitated a proof of the fact that the bacteria concerned arose from patients suffering from these diseases. Finally, this involved the overthrow of the doctrine of spontaneous generation.

(a) *Discovery and knowledge of bacteria.* We have already described how Leeuwenhoek definitely saw and described bacteria in 1683. No systematic description of different types of bacteria is found until the work of the Dane Otto Friderich Müller (1730–84). Several types of bacteria are clearly described and figured in some of his books, especially his posthumous *Animalcula infusoria fluviatilia et marina* ('River and marine animalcules', 1786). Of the early works on protozoology the most sumptuous is the main work of Christian Gottfried Ehrenberg (1795–1876). The title of this work, *Die Infusionsthierchen als vollkommene Organismen* ('The infusoria as complete organisms', 1838) indicates Ehrenberg's views. He fed the living infusoria with carmine and indigo, and the particles of the dyes appeared in their contractile vacuoles. Ehrenberg was therefore erroneously led to the view that they were all multicellular, with stomach, alimentary canal, and other organs, whence he included them in the group Polygastrica. This work contains a magnificent series of coloured plates, some illustrating forms which are definitely bacteria. Ehrenberg was soon shown to be wrong in this view; but his work had great influence and he continued to carry out further important researches during the rest of his life. Félix Dujardin (1801–60) published a simpler classification of protozoa in 1841. By the middle of the nineteenth century the existence of bacteria was widely accepted.

(b) *Specific pathogenic action of certain bacteria.* The discovery of bacteria and other minute organisms was one thing; the demonstration that some of them could cause specific diseases was quite another. The honour of having been the first to do so goes to the

Italian Agostino Bassi (1773–1856), who graduated in law and became a civil servant. He gave much of his early life to microscopy, and in later life he devoted himself to agriculture. He was especially concerned with the infectious disease called muscardine which is fatal to silk-worms; in an epidemic it can have devastating effects on the silk industry. Bassi spent twenty years in the investigation of this disease, and in his work published in 1835–6 he showed that it is due to a minute fungus, later named *Botrytis bassiana*; he also demonstrated the method of contagion. In 1839 Johann Lucas Schönlein (1793–1864), a distinguished Berlin physician and clinical teacher, discovered that another minute fungus, later called *Achorion schönleinii*, was the cause of the skin disease favus. In the following year Jakob Henle published his famous essay on miasma and contagion (p. 729), and the stage was set for numerous attempts to discover the causal organisms of many diseases. In the early stages most of these attempts were fruitless, but reference will be made later to the work of Pollender, Davaine, and other early bacteriologists.

(*c*) *Spontaneous generation.* The belief that even fair-sized animals can be generated spontaneously from decaying matter goes back at least to classical times. The first to dispute this theory was the scholarly physician Francesco Redi (1626–97) of Arezzo. He showed by a series of convincing experiments that maggots do not breed spontaneously in decaying flesh, but that they are the products of eggs laid in the meat by flies. Despite this bold advance Redi continued to believe that the grubs in oak galls are bred spontaneously. The discussion soon came to be centred round the animalcules which are developed in infusions of hay and other organic matter. The subject was then taken up by John Turberville Needham (1713–81), a Londoner who lived for years in Paris. As a result of many experiments on infusions he put forward the view that these animalcules are produced as a result of a 'vegetative force' in every microscopic particle of living matter. This doctrine was most effectively attacked in 1765 and 1776 by Spallanzani (p. 156), who showed that if an infusion was boiled, the air in contact with it heated, and external air completely excluded, no animalcules developed. He also demonstrated that the animalcules were of two types, a higher order which was easily destroyed by heat, and a lower order—probably including bacteria—which resisted boiling for half an hour. These experiments should have been conclusive; but the supporters of the theory of spontaneous generation now alleged that the heating of the air had destroyed its hypothetical ability to support life.

This point remained a subject of dispute for sixty years. Then in 1836 Franz Schulze (1815–73), a Berlin chemist, carried out an experiment in which unheated air was repeatedly aspirated through concentrated sulphuric acid and then through a previously heated infusion, which remained sterile. This experiment ought to have demonstrated conclusively that it was not the air in the flask which caused the growth of organisms, but something contained in the air. Unfortunately there were technical difficulties, and it was found possible by modifying the experiment to obtain a growth. The problem was now taken up by Theodor Schwann (p. 322), who devised several experiments. In his final experiment (1837) he showed that air which had been previously heated could be passed through a heated infusion for long periods without putrefaction taking place. His conclusion was that it was not the air *per se* which produced putrefaction, but something in the air that was destroyed by heat. Schwann's work was not universally accepted, because other experimenters who were technically less expert sometimes got putrefaction. A new principle was introduced in 1854 by Heinrich Georg Friedrich Schröder (1810–85) and Theodor von Dusch (1824–90). They aspirated air through a heated infusion; but instead of subjecting the entering air to treatment by heat, they filtered it through cotton-wool. The infusion remained sterile, and they thus showed that the agent which caused putrefaction is particulate and can be removed by filtration. Unfortunately, however, when they modified this experiment in various ways the results were not so conclusive. Four years later papers began to be presented to the French Academy of Sciences by Félix Archimède Pouchet (1800–72) by which he claimed that he had proved the existence of spontaneous generation in matter which had at one time been alive. He repeated all the previous important experiments in such a way as to prove his theory. In 1860 therefore the whole question was very confused.

(*d*) *Theories of fermentation.* Bound up with these difficult questions were opinions regarding the nature of fermentation. In modern times the first to express a relevant opinion on this subject was Adamo Fabbroni, who in 1787 published a book on the making of wine in which he expressed the view that the sugar in the grape is decomposed by a living substance in the grape itself. But until the fourth decade of the nineteenth century fermentation continued to be regarded as wholly in the province of the chemist. In 1836 and 1837, however, communications were published by three men who had for some time been working on the subject quite independently, the *baron* Charles Cagniard-Latour (1777–1859), Friedrich Traugott Kützing (1807–93), and Theodor Schwann (p. 322). All of these men gave clear descriptions of the yeast cell, and two of them described the process of budding. All of them disagreed with the current view that yeast is a lifeless chemical substance, and all were convinced that fermentation is a vital process consisting of the action of the yeast cells on chemical substances in the material which undergoes fermentation. Schwann's account is rather more detailed than that of the others and it is contained in the same paper in which he described his experiments to disprove the existence of spontaneous generation (p. 329). He really established many of the fundamental points, and he is regarded as the founder of the microbic theory of fermentation. This theory was not accepted by the scientific world of the time, which continued to believe that fermentation is a purely chemical process. This view was represented by the theories of two of the most famous chemists of the period, Berzelius and Liebig. In the middle of the nineteenth century the chemists were still stoutly holding the field.

(*e*) *The work of Pasteur.* Nearly all of these questions were virtually settled by the work of the brilliant French chemist Louis Pasteur (1822–95). While still a very young man Pasteur discovered that, though tartaric acid crystals were regarded as turning the plane of polarized light to the right (dextrorotatory), there is another chemically identical type of tartaric acid which is laevorotatory; he also discovered that racemic acid, which is optically neutral, is a mixture of equal parts of dextro-tartaric acid and laevo-tartaric acid. By further researches he founded the science of stereochemistry. He was later appointed to an academic post at Lille, in which city industries involving fermentation processes were of great importance. His work on amyl alcohol led him to embark on a long study of fermentation in all its aspects—the lactic acid fermentation of milk, the alcoholic fermentation of wines and beers, the butyric fermentation found in rancid butter, and finally the acetic acid fermentation of vinegar.

Liebig regarded a ferment as an unstable organic product, the character of which determined the type of decomposition of the medium in which it is placed. Pasteur, on the other hand, demonstrated that, as there is a specific alcoholic ferment, so there is a specific milk-souring ferment. Any nitrogenous matter present in a fluid containing it will serve as food for the development of a ferment, but will not of itself induce fermentation. Ferments have, he demonstrated, the power of reproduction. Pasteur rapidly seized on the idea of the specificity of ferments. An albuminous sugar solution can be converted into various products by the addition of various ferments. According as one sows, so will one reap. The milk-souring ferment, Pasteur concluded, is organized and living, and its action is correlated with its development and organization. No life, no ferment.

During the next years Pasteur applied himself to a study of ferments, notably of those which involve deterioration of wines and beers. This led him to perceive that there is a great multiplicity and variety of these organisms. Fig. 90 is an illustration taken from a much later book by Pasteur (1876), which makes clear the types of organisms which he had seen in his earlier work. Each of the seven compartments into which the figure is divided contains drawings of the organisms found by him in a particular type of souring of beer. (These organisms Pasteur called 'ferments', by which he meant the living cells which caused the fermentative or putrefactive action. We now know that the ferments are indeed chemical substances; but under natural conditions they are only produced by the metabolism of these organisms. At the time when Pasteur wrote such ferments could correctly be called living organisms, and his theory explained the facts in a way which Liebig's theory never did.) Each compartment contains a few yeast cells to indicate the relative sizes of the 'ferments'. It is now obvious to us that the organisms illustrated by Pasteur were various types of cocci and long slender bacilli. He conceived that they gained entrance to the wort or the beer by being borne on atmospheric dust.

It was an old and well-known view that fermentation, putrefaction, and the infection of disease had much in common. This being

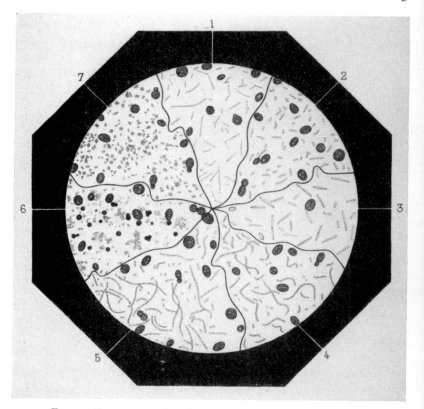

FIG. 90. Types of organisms found by Pasteur in the souring of beer
(L. Pasteur, *Études sur la bière*, Paris, 1876)

the case, it was perfectly natural, therefore, for Pasteur to regard the latter in the light of a vital process. A great difficulty was, however, the demand that any such doctrine made on the germ-bearing capacity of the air. Critics were not slow to avail themselves of this weakness, and pointed out that, according to Pasteur, the air must be one solid mass of germs. For the opponents of Pasteur the living organisms found in the process of fermentation or decomposition were the result, not the cause, of the process. These organisms were regarded by them as spontaneously generated in the fermentation process. Thus arose a discussion of the old theme of spontaneous generation.

By 1859—the year of publication of Darwin's *Origin of Species*— Pasteur was engaged in controversy as to the origin of life. The discussion specially turned round what were then regarded as the lowest forms of life, the bacteria. These are now classified roughly into spherical forms (cocci), rod-like forms (bacilli), and thread-like undulating forms (sphirochaetes or treponemata). The question was again asked whether such forms were, or were not, ever generated spontaneously. If a flask of broth, supposedly sterilized by boiling, went 'bad' and organisms appeared in it, was it certain that they came from without, or could they have been spontaneously gene- rated by the broth itself? Life must begin somewhere. Then why not here at its lowest stage? If this view is justifiable, Pasteur's doctrine of the nature of ferments must fall to the ground.

Pasteur had thus before him the task of proving a universal negative—a task impossible in formal logic, although the steps which he took to solve the problem were the most logical conceivable. His first task was to prove that living organisms actually existed in the air. He did this by aspirating air through a plug of gun-cotton or asbestos inserted in a glass tube which projected through a shutter to the air outside his laboratory. The gun-cotton was then dissolved and in the sediment were found microscopically organisms of the types present in fermenting liquids. Pasteur had thus demonstrated that the air contains organisms, but he had not proved that they are alive.

He then repeated Schwann's experiment many times, and modified it in such a way that he always had satisfactory results. He thus proved that it is possible to introduce air to a sterile infusion without the latter becoming infected, provided that the air has been previously heated. Into one of these sterile infusions he now introduced, with suitable precautions, one of his plugs of gun-cotton through which air had been aspirated. The infusion became infected within two days. If the gun-cotton was previously heated, no infection took place. He thus proved that the organisms naturally present in air are alive and can produce putrefaction; on heating they lose this power and are presumably killed. He next showed by an important experiment (Fig. 91) that an infusion can be sterilized and left open to the air indefinitely provided that the neck of the flask is drawn out into a tube which somewhere has a convexity pointing upwards. The air is able to pass up over this convexity but the organisms, being particulate, are prevented by gravity from doing so. If the neck has a double bend, the organisms are deposited in the concavity. Any

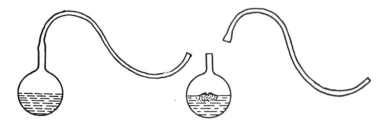

FIG. 91. Pasteur's demonstration that a putrescible infusion can be sterilized in a flask with an open neck
(L. Pasteur, *Mémoire sur les corpuscles organisés*, Paris, 1861)

suggestion that the boiling of the infusion or the effect of other factors may have made the infusion incapable of supporting life was disproved by simply breaking off the neck close to its entry to the flask, so that air together with organisms now had direct access; the infusion became infected within two days. Some of the flasks of putrescible fluids sterilized by Pasteur in this way are still in existence; although still open to the air, the fluid still remains sterile.

Finally Pasteur showed that these living organisms are not uniformly disseminated in the air. He took twenty sealed flasks containing a sterile infusion and broke and resealed the neck of each on a busy road. The number which became infected was noted. This experiment was repeated several times at different altitudes, and in general he found that in the still air of a high mountain very few of the flasks showed growth. These experiments were carried out over years and were the subject of several communications to the French Académie des Sciences. In 1861 Pasteur published a very important work detailing the whole of his researches on this subject. This was the *Mémoire sur les corpuscles organisés qui existent dans l'atmosphère* ('Memoir on the organized bodies which exist in the air'). It should be said that even these most convincing experiments did not completely silence the supporters of the theory of spontaneous generation. Further important work in support of the theory of Pasteur was carried out at the Royal Institution in London by the physicist John Tyndall (1820–93). By means of his optical culture chamber he showed that the ability of the air to develop organisms in an infusion and its power of scattering light are very closely related. Tyndall also showed that the organisms which are likely to be found in infusions of hay pass through two phases one of which is much more heat resistant than the other. Tyndall described his experiments fully in his important book, *Essays on the Floating-Matter of the Air in relation to Putrefaction and Infection* (1881). So far as bacterial life is concerned this virtually marked the passing of the doctrine of spontaneous generation.

The first disease which Pasteur was able to demonstrate as causatively related to a living organism was 'pébrine', which was devastating the silkworm industry of France. In 1866 he proved the contagiousness of the disease, showed that it was due to a living organism, and followed the organism through the life-history of moth, egg, caterpillar, and chrysalis.

In 1870 the Franco-Prussian war broke out. Pasteur now decided to make investigations into the diseases of beer, his object being to improve the French brews and to carry the war into the enemy's camp by making them equal to the German beers. He succeeded in isolating organisms, referred to above, which produced defects in beer (Fig. 90). This work naturally led to an enlargement of his views on the nature and action of micro-organisms.

About this time Pasteur was elected a member of the French Academy of Medicine, a very unusual honour for anyone who was not a medical man. Lister had already begun his teaching, based partly on the work of Pasteur, and his first important paper on antiseptic surgery was published in 1867. On entering the Academy Pasteur found himself faced by all kinds of ancient prejudices and misconceptions in connexion with his new doctrine, and especially with his denial of spontaneous generation. Among his supporters was the physiologist Claude Bernard (p. 294). His work proceeded to more and more triumphant issues.

The first disease affecting man on which Pasteur was able to throw light was anthrax, in relation to which his work interdigitates with that of Robert Koch and some other observers. Anthrax is a deadly and highly contagious condition which commonly affects cattle, but sometimes spreads to man. In 1849 Franz Aloys Pollender (1800–79) saw microscopic bacilli in the blood of cattle dead of anthrax. In 1868 Casimir Joseph Davaine (1812–82) showed that a bacillus is not simply the inseparable companion of the disease, but also is its cause and its only constantly acting cause. In fact he demonstrated that the disease can be communicated by the injection of one-millionth of a drop of anthrax blood. At this time the losses of cattle from anthrax in France were enormous. The character of the outbreaks had been studied and seemed wholly unexplained by what was known of the bacillus. Farmers found that they lost cattle in fields from which infected animals had been excluded for months or even years.

The explanation was first advanced in 1876 by the German scientist Robert Koch (1843–1910), whose work was now beginning. Koch had studied at Göttingen under Wöhler and Jakob Henle, and after graduating in 1866 he set up in general practice. He served as a surgeon in the Franco-Prussian War, and when the war finished he was appointed as district medical officer ('Kreisphysikus') in Wollstein, a small town in Posen. During the course of his work he had occasion to study anthrax in animals, and he proceeded to carry out experiments with the blood of animals dead of this disease. All this work he carried out in his own house. When he had completed an investigation which was later to be recognized as a classic, he wrote to Ferdinand Cohn (1828–98), the professor of botany at Breslau, asking that he might be permitted to demonstrate his discoveries to Cohn. Cohn was specially known for his work on the algae and fungi, and from about 1860 he had devoted himself intensively to the study of the bacteria. He was a staunch supporter of Pasteur against the doctrine of spontaneous generation. Cohn invited Koch to come to Breslau and for three days the latter demonstrated his experiments at Cohn's institute. Cohn was so much impressed by the work that he published Koch's paper immediately in the journal which he had founded (*Beiträge zur Biologie der Pflanzen*). Koch showed that the anthrax bacilli under certain conditions formed spores, that is, small encysted bodies, exceedingly resistant to heat and to other changes of external conditions (Fig. 92). This discovery opened up a new field which was cultivated by Koch and Pasteur and their followers.

While making his studies on ferments in 1863, Pasteur had

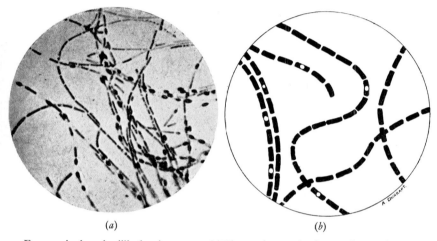

(a) (b)

FIG. 92. Anthrax bacilli, showing spores. (a) Photo-micrograph of smear from a three-days culture. × 1,000. The spores are the dark oval bodies. (b) Simplified drawing of similar preparation. The spores are shown as white, oval bodies

(a after Browning and Mackie, *Textbook of Bacteriology*, London, 1949)

witnessed the formation of spores in the organisms of butyric fermentation, but had failed to grasp their significance. In 1869 he had again found spores forming in the organisms of silk-worm disease, and had shown that they resisted prolonged drying. On the basis of their resistance he had explained the persistence and latency of the silk-worm disease. Other observers had had similar experiences. The investigations of none of them, however, approached in brilliance and completeness those of Koch.

Koch found that spores always form in the blood and tissues of animals dead of anthrax, provided that (1) the temperature is suitable, and (2) there is sufficient oxygen. These two conditions, temperature and oxygen, were found to be necessary. Below 18°

Centigrade spores are not formed; at 30° Centigrade they occur at the end of thirty hours; at 35° Centigrade in twenty hours. The rapidity with which spores are formed is, therefore, proportional to the amount of heat. Oxygen was also found to be indispensable. Anthrax blood, if deprived of oxygen, ceases to be virulent in twenty-four hours provided there is no putrefaction. When the blood is allowed to putrefy the virulence also disappears if putrefaction exhausts the oxygen quickly enough to prevent the spores from forming. If, however, the spores have already formed, putrefaction does not kill them, nor does it prevent them from developing later into bacilli if circumstances become favourable. The persistence of the disease and its return in an infected country was thus explained. It was the spore which was the agent of preservation, which persisted when the degree of temperature and of aeration had permitted it to form, and which always held itself in readiness to make new victims.

The matter was carried further by Pasteur in 1877. At that time he did not know of all the work of Koch. He succeeded in obtaining pure cultures of anthrax. The question then being debated in France was whether anthrax was caused by a 'virus', then used in the sense of a non-living poison, or by a microbe. Pasteur had long been a believer in the microbic theory, and it seemed to him probable that the blood of an animal infected with anthrax, if sown in a suitable medium, would stock it solely with anthrax bacilli which he could then keep pure for an indefinite time in successive cultures, as he had done with yeast and other ferments.

Experiment showed that the anthrax bacillus reproduced itself rapidly in neutral or slightly alkaline urine. The principle of the method employed by Pasteur was to inoculate 50 c.c. of this medium with one drop of anthrax blood. After an interval for growth of the organisms one drop of the culture fluid was used to inoculate 50 c.c. of sterile urine. This gave a dilution of about 1 in 1,000. Successive subcultures in this manner gave dilutions of 1 in a million, 1 in 1,000 million, and so on. After ten cultures it fell to such a figure that the original drop of blood had been drowned in an ocean. Everything that it carried with it, to which we might attribute the production of anthrax—red corpuscles, white corpuscles, granules of all sorts—was either destroyed by the change of medium or was widely disseminated in this ocean and lost. Only the organism could escape the dilution because it had multiplied in each of the cultures. A drop from the last culture killed a rabbit or guinea-pig as surely as a drop of anthrax blood. It was, therefore, to the organism that the virulence must be attributed. A conclusion of the first rank had been established.

In 1880 Pasteur discovered that by suitable cultural methods he could 'attenuate' the virulence of the bacillus of fowl cholera, and that inoculation of such attenuated organisms protected a chicken from the effects of the subsequent injection of a virulent culture. By similar methods he attenuated the anthrax bacillus and prevented it from developing spores. A much-publicized test of his method of inoculating sheep against anthrax, made near Melun in France in May 1881, demonstrated conclusively that inoculated sheep were completely protected against virulent anthrax bacilli subsequently injected.

Pasteur next turned to rabies. He found that by passing the virus from the saliva of a mad dog through the brains of rabbits, a virus of maximum virulence (the *virus fixe*) could be obtained. He then injected *virus fixe* into the spinal canal of rabbits and after death he suspended their spinal cords in sterile air. A cord thus dried for two weeks became almost non-virulent. He then treated dogs with emulsions of such dried cords, using first one which had been dried for a fortnight, and then cords dried for successively shorter periods. A stage was soon reached when the *virus fixe* could be injected into a treated dog without ill effect (1885).

By chance an Alsatian boy, Joseph Meister, who had been badly bitten by a rabid dog, was at this time brought to Pasteur. He treated the boy on these lines, and there was no sign of rabies even after the injection of *virus fixe* on 16 July 1885. In the same year Pasteur successfully treated his second case Jean Baptiste Jupille. Since then the success of Pasteur's method has been overwhelmingly demonstrated.

Pasteur was fortunate in having obtained a pure culture of the anthrax bacillus by the method described above. A similar method had been tried for various organisms by Edwin Klebs (p. 381) in

1873, without outstanding success. In general, with the fluid media employed about that time, success was usually only achieved with pathological material when it came from an animal suffering from a disease in which the organisms invaded the blood-stream. It was realized that solid media would be much more satisfactory, but several scientists had tried unsuccessfully to find a suitable method and medium. Koch declared the problem to be incapable of solution, but three years later he solved it. His search was for a solid medium on which most types of organisms would grow, which was transparent, and which could be sterilized. Being unsuccessful, he then tried solidifying well-known fluid media with gelatine. This 'nutrient gelatine' he melted and poured on glass slides. After solidifying, it was inoculated by the stroke method. During incubation the slides were covered by a bell-jar. Koch demonstrated this important new method at the International Medical Congress held in London in 1881. Two years later he introduced the poured-plate method: the material to be examined was mixed with the melted gelatine before it was poured on the slides. It was soon found that the gelatine does not remain solid at body temperature (that is, the usual temperature of incubation), and blood-serum and agar-agar were later substituted for it. Glass-covered glass dishes were substituted for the glass slides in 1887 by Julius Richard Petri (1852–1921), one of Koch's assistants. Today these are one of the most familiar of objects in a bacteriological laboratory, and they still bear the name 'Petri dishes'.

If Pasteur can be said to have laid the foundations of the knowledge of the nature of infection, it is to Koch that we owe the main basis of the technique by which such diseases are now studied. He it was who elevated bacteriology into the position of a separate science. Soon after his work on anthrax he published a remarkable research which placed our knowledge of wound infection on a firm footing. He is thus among those who helped to create modern surgical technique. Many other communications came from him. None was of more far-reaching importance than his demonstration in 1882 of the organism of tuberculosis, the tubercle bacillus. All subsequent work in connexion with phthisis and allied conditions has been rendered possible only by this discovery of Koch. Other investigations associated with his name are on cholera and on African sleeping sickness (trypanosomiasis, p. 481). Koch was unquestionably the greatest bacteriologist that the world has seen. His genius was limited as compared to that of Pasteur, but his exquisite technical skill and acumen have never been excelled.

Since the time of Pasteur and Koch, the study of infectious disease has developed along various special lines. The work of these two men, however, has determined their direction, and they themselves are the most typical, as well as the greatest, representatives of the most important of all movements in modern medicine.

ANAESTHESIA

The aspect of surgical practice was dramatically changed during the course of the nineteenth century by two discoveries, that of general anaesthesia and that of the antiseptic method. It will be convenient to deal first with anaesthesia. This discovery was in fact earlier than that of the antiseptic method. Further, the increase in the number of operations performed after the discovery of anaesthesia was directly responsible for the increase in the total number of unsuccessful cases, and these attracted attention to the defects in surgical technique.

From early times there had been crude attempts to diminish the pain of surgical operations. The *nepenthe* of Homer is thought to have been Indian hemp, which was probably then used as a soporific. The Arabian physicians appear to have used opium and hyoscyamus, among other drugs. Mandragora (mandrake) has a still longer history for this purpose. About the ninth century drugs for sedative purposes began to be applied by inhalation instead of by mouth. The 'soporific sponge', saturated with such drugs as opium, mandragora, and hyoscyamus, was held to the patient's nostrils. Alcohol had been used for centuries to stupefy the patient before operation. Nevertheless, these measures could have had little effect in preventing pain in cutting operations. Even in 1832 the great French surgeon, Alfred Armand Louis Marie Velpeau (1795–1867), thought that it was impossible to prevent pain during operations. Compression of the nerves to the site of the operation had often been tried, but there were difficulties. This severe method was tried by Benjamin Bell (1749–1806), a well-known Edinburgh surgeon. He published a *System of Surgery* (in six volumes, 1782–8) which ultimately reached a seventh edition. In this work Bell gives an illustration (Fig. 93) of a clamp proposed to be applied to the shoulder or groin in amputation of the arm or leg. It may be thought that this clamp was to compress the vessels, but that is not the case. Bell thought that compression of the nerves must be continued for at least an hour before the parts are rendered insensitive, and compression of the vessels during this period might be dangerous.

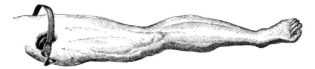

FIG. 93. Screw-clamp for the compression of the nerves to a limb
to produce anaesthesia during amputation
(Benjamin Bell, *System of Surgery*, vol. vi, 1788)

Mesmerism was tried for anaesthetic purposes in India by James Esdaile (1808–59). As a recently qualified doctor Esdaile accepted a medical appointment with the East India Company and was soon put in charge of a hospital. Inspired by Elliotson's (p. 509) declaration regarding the value of mesmerism, Esdaile tried it on a patient about to undergo a surgical operation. This was carried out without the patient awaking. Official support was given to his method, and when he left India he had carried out 261 painless operations under mesmerism. During his retirement in Scotland he again tried the method, but found that the natives of that country were much less susceptible to mesmerism than those of India had been.

Henry Hill Hickman (1800–30) occupies a place of his own in the history of surgical anaesthesia, since he recommended the inhalation of a gas, but the gas had no anaesthetic properties. While practising in Shropshire he induced 'suspended animation' in dogs, a mouse, and a rabbit by causing them to breathe carbon dioxide. While they were unconscious various parts of their bodies, such as ears or legs, were amputated painlessly. He also thought that other gases could be used but he did not name them. He never tried his method on a human subject. He was apparently unaware of Davy's previous suggestion.

The beginning of inhalation anaesthesia dates from 1799, when Sir Humphry Davy (1778–1829) himself breathed nitrous oxide (laughing gas), and suggested that it might be used during surgical operations. Its exhilarating properties soon came to be used for entertainment purposes; and in Britain and the United States it was not uncommon for parties of young people to spend an evening breathing the gas intermittently. It was contained in bladders which were not very convenient to handle. Then it was found that sulphuric ether—which is a liquid, and can therefore be carried in a small bottle—was equally satisfactory, and 'ether frolics' were for a time quite popular.

A chemistry student, William E. Clarke, of Rochester, U.S.A., had frequently attended such frolics, and he conceived the idea that ether could be used for another purpose. In January 1842 he administered it to a young lady, and under its influence she had a tooth extracted painlessly by a dentist. Clarke presumably considered his discovery of no importance, since he did not follow it up. Crawford Williamson Long (1815–78), a young practitioner of Jefferson, Georgia, had also had experience of 'ether frolics', and on 30 March 1842 he used ether as a general anaesthetic in a surgical operation. During the next four years Long gave ether four or five times. He has been hailed as the discoverer of anaesthesia, but it was not until 1849 that he made a statement in which he attempted to explain why he had not encouraged the use of ether by others.

The first real attempt to establish the practice of anaesthesia was made by a young dentist of Hartford, Connecticut. This was Horace Wells (1815–48). Influenced by a popular demonstration of the effects of nitrous oxide, Wells had one of his own teeth extracted under its influence, and he said afterwards that he did not feel 'so much as the prick of a pin'. After using the gas in about fifteen cases of tooth extraction, Wells went to Boston, and gave a demonstration at the Massachusetts General Hospital in that city in January 1845. Unfortunately, although the patient said afterwards that he had felt nothing, he groaned during the extraction of the tooth. The critical audience considered the attempt a failure. Although Wells was successful with his own dental patients, he did nothing to convince the world that general anaesthesia was a practical possibility.

This unsuccessful demonstration at Boston was witnessed by one of Wells's former pupils, William Thomas Green Morton (1819–68). He was advised to try ether, and on 30 September 1846 he used this substance to produce anaesthesia during tooth-extraction. He also requested a trial of his method at the Massachusetts General Hospital. The famous demonstration took place there on 16 October 1846. The operation was for the excision of a tumour of the neck, and Morton demonstrated successfully that ether produced satisfactory general anaesthesia. In the next few weeks Morton confirmed his claims during further operations at the hospital. Unfortunately, he attempted to patent his discovery, and he spent the rest of his life in trying to substantiate his claims. He played no further part in the development of his method. But the seed which he had sown bore abundant fruit, and for practical purposes he must be considered the discoverer of anaesthesia.

The first operation under a general anaesthetic in England was carried out by Robert Liston (1794–1847). Liston was at an early age appointed as a surgeon to the Edinburgh Royal Infirmary, but when the chair of clinical surgery in the University became vacant in 1833, he was beaten by James Syme (p. 351). In the following year, therefore, Liston accepted an invitation to become one of the surgeons to the newly founded University College Hospital, London, and in 1835 he became professor of clinical surgery in the University of London. His operations were carried out with incredible dexterity and rapidity. About 19 December 1846 Liston heard of the successful Boston operations, and on 21 December, in University College Hospital, he amputated a leg at the thigh and also evulsed a great toe-nail of another patient, ether being inhaled as the anaesthetic. During 1847 the use of ether spread rapidly throughout Europe and to many other parts of the world.

In January 1847 Sir James Young Simpson (1811–70) of Edinburgh first used ether in obstetrics. Many found ether unpleasant, and Simpson sought a substitute. Chloroform had been prepared independently in 1831 by Eugène Soubeiran (1793–1858) of Paris, by an American, Samuel Guthrie (1782–1848), and by Liebig, though pure chloroform was not prepared till 1834. By November 1847 Simpson was using it in obstetrics, and in the same month he used it as an anaesthetic in three surgical operations. Within a few weeks chloroform had almost displaced ether as a general anaesthetic.

The use of these anaesthetics spread very rapidly and almost as

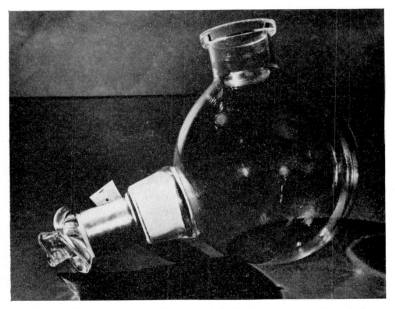

FIG. 94. Morton's ether inhaler, devised for his first demonstration, 1846
(Facsimile in The Wellcome Historical Medical Museum; original in the
Massachusetts General Hospital, Boston)

rapidly changed the character of surgical technique. Until the adoption of anaesthesia, speed had been of primary importance in surgical operations. Excessive speed now became a secondary matter, and neatness and thoroughness took its place as the hall-marks of good surgery. Moreover, operations of a more drastic character could be undertaken since the shock to the patient was now much reduced. Even then, the dreadful risk of sepsis still kept the abdomen as an unbreached citadel. But women in labour were found to stand chloroform very well, and its use in midwifery steadily spread despite some foolish and fanatical opposition on theological grounds.

Almost at once anaesthesia became a profession in England. The first professional anaesthetist was John Snow (1813–58), who practised in London. He made many memorable additions to our knowledge of the theory and practice of this subject. Snow was also a very distinguished epidemiologist (p. 730). The problem of the

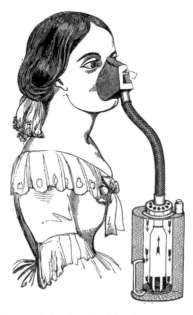

FIG. 95. John Snow's chloroform inhaler
(Snow, *On Chloroform and other Anaesthetics*, London, 1858)

best method of vaporizing the anaesthetic exercised the ingenuity of both anaesthetists and instrument-makers from the start. Morton invented for his first operation an inhaler consisting of a spherical glass flask with two necks, through one of which the external air entered; through the other the patient breathed this air after it had passed through the liquid anaesthetic contained in a soaked sponge (Fig. 94). The mouthpiece attached to the side neck had two leather valves. One of these allowed the ether vapour to pass from the globe into it only on inspiration; the other valve allowed the expired air to be expelled without passing through the globe, and prevented its outlet from opening during inspiration. Such rough methods did not permit the anaesthetist to vary the concentration of the anaesthetic. Before long other types of inhaler were devised for this purpose, among others by Snow and by his virtual successor, Joseph Thomas

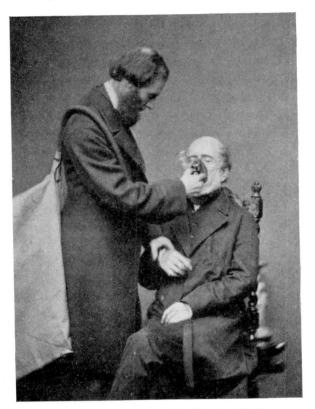

FIG. 96. J. T. Clover using his chloroform inhaler
(Photograph in the Nuffield Department of Anaesthetics,
University of Oxford)

Clover (1825–82). Snow's inhaler was designed to give a 4 per cent. mixture of chloroform vapour in air (Fig. 95). The inspired air passed, in the direction shown, through liquid chloroform in the inner chamber; the chloroform was distributed on a roll of blotting paper. In the case of Clover's inhaler (Fig. 96) the required concentration of chloroform vapour in air was prepared in advance and passed into an air-tight bag which was slung on the anaesthetist's back. The bag was filled with the mixture by using a special bellows, an evaporating box, and a syringe which held a definite amount of liquid chloroform. Clover's inhaler got over some difficulties and

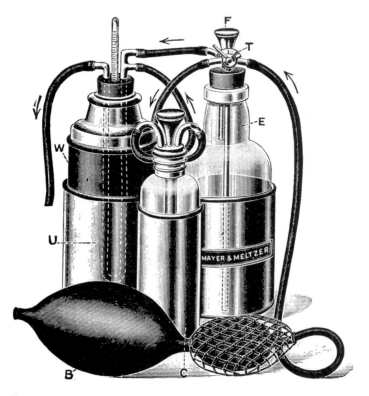

FIG. 97. Shipway's apparatus for inhalation of a warmed mixture of chloroform and ether
(Mayer and Phelps, *Catalogue of Surgical Instruments*, London, 1931)

he used it himself for many years, but it was found rather clumsy for general use. Various types of apparatus were invented, among others by Sir Francis Edward Shipway (1875–), which permitted the anaesthetist to use at the same time varying concentrations of chloroform and ether, and to combine these with oxygen (Fig. 97). Nowadays these types of apparatus have become even more complicated; the anaesthetist of fifty years ago would be unable to use such machines without tuition.

After the early successes of nitrous oxide for dental operations in the hands of Wells and his followers, this gas was almost entirely supplanted by ether and chloroform. In 1862 it was reintroduced for these operations in the United States, and by 1868 it was widely employed in America and Europe. It could only be used for very short periods since asphyxia was produced. To overcome this it was then combined with oxygen. Technical difficulties were, however, introduced by the great pressures produced by the gases. The next development was the introduction of liquid nitrous oxide, which greatly simplified the problem of the containers. Clover introduced rebreathing and the gas-ether sequence. From about 1885 onwards Sir Frederick William Hewitt (1857–1916) experimented with the various types of apparatus used. He found that the valves in the face-pieces were unsatisfactory, and that it was desirable to allow for some rebreathing. During the next few years he introduced various modifications, and his gas-and-oxygen apparatus, as described in his *Anaesthetics and their Administration* (1893), was the first really effective gas-and-oxygen apparatus to be produced.

Soon after the introduction of general anaesthetics efforts were made by various methods to secure a painless state of a part without the patient losing consciousness. From early times the natives of Peru knew about the anaesthetic qualities of the coca plant, and they used to chew the leaves and allow the saliva to run over the part of the body which had to be cut. About the middle of the nineteenth century certain German workers obtained from these leaves crystals of an alkaloid (p. 679) which they named cocaine. In 1872 a recently qualified Scot, Alexander Hughes Bennett (1848–1901), who later became a well-known London neurologist, showed in his Edinburgh M.D. thesis that cocaine has pronounced anaesthetic properties. It was not until 1884, however, that Carl Koller (1857–1944) in Vienna made further observations which led to the use of cocaine in the surgery of the eye, and later to that of the nose and other parts. At first cocaine was applied in solution to the part to be anaesthetized, but very soon it was injected under the skin for small superficial operations. Then it was found that good results could be obtained for larger operations by injecting it into the nerve trunks. The first to do this (1884) was the Baltimore surgeon William Stewart Halsted (1852–1922), and his method was extended in 1898 by Harvey Cushing. A number of derivatives of cocaine—such as novocaine and stovaine—have since been produced.

In 1885 James Leonard Corning (1855–1923) of New York made experiments which introduced another new anaesthetic method. He injected cocaine in the region of the spinal cord of a dog, and obtained weakness of the hind legs. In 1898 August Karl Gustav Bier (1861–1949) of Greifswald in Germany injected cocaine into the spinal canal and produced insensibility to pain (analgesia) in the legs. He then used the method for surgical operations, and its use has now become greatly extended.

In 1847 the Russian surgeon Nikolai Ivanovich Pirogoff (1810–81) attempted to produce anaesthesia by injecting ether into the lower bowel (rectal anaesthesia). It was soon found that the injected ether was very irritating, and no satisfactory attempt was made to produce anaesthesia by rectal injection until 1913, when James Taylor Gwathmey (1863–1944) combined the ether with carron oil. The introduction of the anaesthetic directly into the windpipe (trachea), without passing first through the mouth and nose, was first performed on an animal by John Snow. The tube through which the anaesthetic was introduced was passed into the trachea through an opening in the front of the neck made by the operation of tracheotomy. Friedrich Trendelenburg (1844–1924) first used the method on man in 1869. Eleven years later Sir William Macewen (p. 366) obtained the same result without the tracheotomy. His method led to the modern form of endotracheal anaesthesia, which is valuable in the case of operations on the mouth and jaws.

It was inevitable that attempts would be made to introduce anaesthetics into the body by way of the veins. Experiments were carried out by Pierre Cyprien Oré (1828–89), and in 1874 he reported his first success in a human patient. The substance which he injected was chloral hydrate, and he used the method frequently with success in surgical operations. Intravenous anaesthesia was much affected by the introduction in 1903 of the group of hypnotics known as the barbiturates. It would take us beyond our scope to deal with the more important barbiturates used for this purpose; but we may mention that evipan, first introduced in 1932, has been much used for certain types of operations.

The action of curare, the South American arrow-poison, in causing temporary paralysis of muscles came to be understood through the work of Claude Bernard (p. 298). It was found to be dangerous for surgical use. Recently, however, it has been purified, and even synthesized in a pure state, and it is found to be of great assistance to the anaesthetist, since it increases the muscular relaxation necessary in abdominal operations.

General anaesthesia was born in the United States, and much of the pioneer work has been done there. Even the word anaesthesia is an American invention. Five weeks after Morton's famous operation at Boston, Oliver Wendell Holmes (1809–94), the distinguished author of the 'Breakfast-Table' series, wrote to Morton to suggest that the loss of consciousness produced by ether should be called 'anaesthesia'. During its first fifty years relatively few substances were used to produce the state. The anaesthetist of today has a whole battery of drugs and methods at his command, and frequently several different methods are used on the same patient during a single operation.

THE REVOLUTION IN SURGERY

Although the surgical revolution was effected by Lister, there were signs that in allied directions surgery was awaking from the long stagnation into which it had fallen. Until the advent of general anaesthesia surgery consisted very largely in the amputation of limbs. But a few surgeons were endeavouring to introduce something of the scientific attitude into it, and to follow in the Hunterian tradition. In the United States Philip Syng Physick (1768–1837), who had studied under John Hunter and graduated at Edinburgh, was appointed to the chair of surgery at the University of Pennsylvania, for the first time divorced from the chair of anatomy. Physick was a worthy occupant. Besides inventing new operations he devised the forerunner of the modern guillotine for tonsillectomy. In 1816 he published an important paper on substances to be used for ligatures which would be gradually absorbed in the wound. At Edinburgh surgery was possibly the richer because of the rivalry between Liston (p. 344) and James Syme (1799–1870). When Syme was a young man he published a *Treatise on the Excision of Diseased Joints* (1831), in which he described some of the excision operations devised by himself. This work had a great influence in popularizing excision, thus enabling the limb to be saved with limitation of function, in preference to the final and more drastic method of amputation. Syme is also known for his method of amputation at the ankle, for his plastic operations, and for his work on aneurysms. He held the chair of clinical surgery at Edinburgh University for thirty-seven years, and he was an early adherent of general anaesthesia and of the antiseptic principle introduced by his son-in-law, Lister. Syme's caution in operating was also practised by his great contemporary Sir William Fergusson (1808–77), who after graduating at Edinburgh became at the age of twenty-eight a surgeon to the Edinburgh Royal Infirmary. In 1840 he was called to the chair of surgery at King's College, London, and during thirty years there he built up a great reputation as a speedy, dexterous, and cautious operator. To his methods he applied the term 'conservative surgery' to imply that his aim was always to save as much of the affected parts as possible. He had an unrivalled experience of the operations for cleft palate and for hare lip, and he is also remembered for his excisions of joints and his operations for vesical calculus.

Lord Lister. The fundamental revolution in surgery, the introduction of the antiseptic method, is inseparably linked with the name of Joseph Lister (1827–1912), later Baron Lister of Lyme Regis. Lister was born into a well-known Quaker family at Upton, then an Essex village east of London. The son of Joseph Jackson Lister (1786–1869) the distinguished microscopist, he inherited scientific ability. After graduating in arts at University College, London, Lister turned to medicine. While an arts student he had been present as a spectator at Liston's first operation under general anaesthesia. On qualifying he did histological work under William Sharpey (1802–80), who held the physiology chair at the College for nearly forty years and trained many British physiologists. The result was Lister's important paper on inflammation. He had decided to become a surgeon, and Sharpey advised him to study under Syme at Edinburgh. Lister did so, became assistant surgeon to the Edinburgh Royal Infirmary, married Syme's eldest daughter, and in 1860 was appointed to the regius chair of surgery at Glasgow University. It should be emphasized that it was while he held this post and that of surgeon to the Glasgow Royal Infirmary that Lister carried out the most important parts of his life's work. It was in the Glasgow Royal that antiseptic surgery was born. In 1869, after it had become widely accepted abroad, Lister returned to Edinburgh as professor of clinical surgery. There he remained till he was invited to accept the chair of surgery at King's College, London, in 1877. In some ways his acceptance may be regarded as a mistake. He held that chair for fifteen years, but during the early part of this period he was deprived of the enthusiastic support which he had had in Scotland, and was faced instead by the opposition of the London surgeons to his methods. In a few years the opposition was silenced, the antiseptic (later the aseptic) method was universally adopted in all civilized countries, and when Lister died, laden with honours, he was hailed as *medicorum facile princeps*. It was then said of him that by his work he had saved more lives than all the wars of history had thrown away.

When Lister arrived in Glasgow, surgery was cursed by the constant fear of sepsis. A vast amount of death and suffering was due to this cause, and surgeons were reluctant to perform many operations that we would now regard as trivial. Lister's first attempt to make any scientific analysis of the septic state is to be found in a paper by him 'On the early stages of inflammation' (1858). He showed that the effects of irritation on the tissues are twofold. Firstly, there is a dilatation of the arteries which is produced through the nervous system. Secondly, there is an alteration in the tissues on which the irritant acts directly. This alteration imparted, as Lister thought, an adhesiveness to both the red and the white corpuscles, making them prone to stick to one another and to the walls of the vessels, and so giving rise to stagnation of blood and ultimately to obstruction.

In 1847 Augustus V. Waller (p. 249), a pupil of Magendie, had shown that during the process of inflammation there is an active migration of white blood corpuscles through the walls of the capillary blood-vessels. Waller's observations attracted but little attention at the time. They were, however, amply confirmed in 1878 and the following years by the German pathologist Julius Cohnheim (1839–84), a pupil of Virchow. Cohnheim showed that this process of migration of white blood corpuscles is the essence of inflammation, and that when inflammation goes on to suppuration the pus that is formed consists largely of white blood corpuscles in a dead and disintegrating state.

Irritation, and the reaction of the body against it (the process known as inflammation), are encountered in all injuries in which the healing is not direct and healthy. It was those cases of injury in which the healing was indirect and unhealthy which then formed the surgeon's chief problem. Of these there are a variety, now rare, but then common and often fatal, such as blood poisoning, erysipelas, pyaemia, septicaemia, hospital gangrene, and simple suppuration of a wound, which was then so common as to be almost normal.

About 1861 Lister began to teach in Glasgow that the occurrence of suppuration in a wound is determined 'simply by the influence of decomposition'. Its nature was revealed to him about 1865 by the writings of Pasteur. From him he learned that putrefaction was, in fact, a fermentation, and that it was caused by the products of growth of microscopic organisms borne by the air. It was generally supposed that air was the cause of sepsis, and precautions were taken to exclude it from wounds. But Lister now saw that it was not the air but that which it carried which was responsible.

The general course of action was now clear to him. As a laboratory proposition the destruction of the organisms in the air was simple. The problem was to exclude them from wounds during and after operation. The solution of that problem developed as antiseptic surgery, which later became aseptic surgery. Antiseptic surgery means the destruction of germs in wounds by the use of chemical agents. Aseptic surgery means the procedure by which everything which touches the wound or the patient's skin before the wound is made is freed from germs by the methods now to be discussed. Lister's name is especially associated with antiseptic surgery; aseptic surgery came later. At first Lister paid most attention to air, as the source of infection. He recognized, however, that he must also deal with the germs present in the wound and on his hands. Of the methods available for destroying germs, viz. heat, filtration, and chemical action, he chose the last.

At that time carbolic acid was in use as a means of treating sewage. At first, therefore, Lister tried lint soaked in crude carbolic. This he found liable to cause superficial sloughing and death of the tissues. He next obtained a purer acid, using a solution of it in oil. A putty formed of common whitening and a solution of carbolic acid in linseed oil was used as a dressing.

Lister's carbolic acid sprays are well known, but there is much misconception regarding their functions and uses. Very frequently the spray, even at the time when it was used, was regarded as a basic principle of Lister's method—which it never was. The essential facts are these. On 12 December 1870 Lister operated on a young man who sometime previously had fractured his ulna near the elbow. The fragments had united with great displacement, and to render the arm functional it was necessary to break and reset the ulna. Lister failed to break the bone by forcible measures and he had to resort to a cutting operation, which meant transforming a simple into a compound fracture. In order to prevent infection from the air he used a Richardson's hand-spray—designed to produce local anaesthesia in a part by a spray of ether—to throw over the area of operation a fine spray of dilute carbolic acid. There was a perfect result, the wound healing without suppuration. The feasibility of operating through unbroken skin was hitherto established, even in regions, such as the joints, where suppuration was very likely to ensue. Lister then introduced a spray worked by foot, but found it rather unsatisfactory. Shortly afterwards he introduced the large hand-operated tripod model (Fig. 98), familiarly known as 'the donkey engine', which had to be carried from house to house in the surgeon's brougham as he proceeded to change his dressings. In 1875 Lister first described the small metal steam spray which gave an effective cloud of carbolic vapour. This apparatus is seen in action in Fig. 103.

No one liked the carbolic spray since the carbolic acid was deleterious to the surgeons, the nurses, and the patient. Lister himself said that it was 'a necessary evil, incurred to attain a greater good'. At the time of the introduction of his steam spray he said 'If we could dispense with the spray, no one would rejoice more than myself'. This action he was very disinclined to take. But in Germany especially it came to be realized that the likelihood of infection of a wound with *pathogenic* organisms from the air was not great, and surgeons gradually began to drop it. The current view was not openly voiced until the surgeon Victor von Bruns (1812–83) of

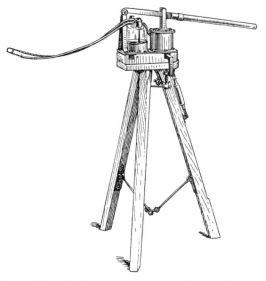

FIG. 98. Lister's hand-operated tripod model carbolic spray
('The donkey engine')
(Sir R. J. Godlee, *Lord Lister*, London, 1917)

Tübingen published in 1880 his paper entitled 'Fort mit dem Spray' ('Away with the spray'). At the International Congress of the following year Lister said he thought it likely that all ideas of atmospheric contamination of wounds during operations would be thrown to the winds, but he himself did not abandon the spray until 1887. By then his ideas were completely in accordance with current views, and in 1890 he stated that he was ashamed that he had ever recommended the spray for the purpose of destroying microbes in air. In truth, it was not an integral part of Lister's method.

When Lister began his work, amputation of a limb was often a fatal operation. Yet it had to be performed in most cases of severe fracture in which the bone was exposed because, without it, death from sepsis was almost certain. The improvement in Lister's own records of amputation, incident upon his adoption of the antiseptic method, is well brought out by his own figures:

Years	Total cases	Recovered	Died	Case mortality per cent.
1864–6	35	19	16	45·7 without antiseptics
1867–70	40	34	6	15·0 with antiseptics

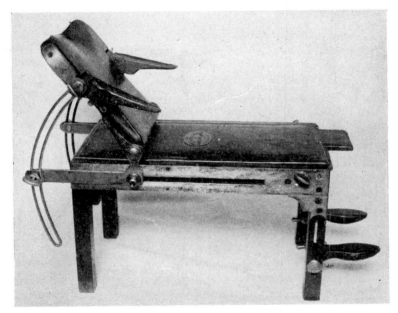

FIG. 99. Operating table used by Lord Lister
(In the Glasgow Royal Infirmary)

These results were considered extraordinarily good in their day. It is an index of the further advance since Lister's first attempts that results many times as good would now be regarded as unsatisfactory. Moreover, not only has the further development of Lister's method rendered amputation safer, but it has also enabled the surgeon to treat many cases without amputation, when before he would have been compelled to resort to that measure.

Lister first recorded his observations on the antiseptic system of surgery in 1867. Apart from the technical advances that he then set forth, he recorded also many new pathological facts that have since

proved of great practical importance. Thus he showed that an uninfected clot, if undisturbed, can become organized into a living
tissue, and that a piece of dead bone may be absorbed in an aseptic
wound. These are now matters of common knowledge, but then they
were instrumental in introducing a radically new outlook.

Lister gradually perfected his technique, chiefly in the direction

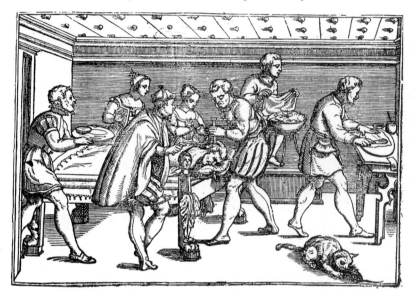

FIG. 100. Trephining the skull in the sixteenth century
(Andrea della Croce, *Chirurgia*, Venice, 1573)

of using milder antiseptics and adopting heat for the sterilization of
instruments and dressings. The antiseptic system was given its
military application in France during the war of 1870. It was soon
taken up also by German surgeons. The history of surgery since
Lister's day has been very often told. An important element in it is
the gradual supersession of antiseptic by aseptic methods (p. 367).

In addition to his discovery and development of the antiseptic
system, Lister made many other important contributions to surgical
methods. These were the result of long and patient research in his
laboratory. Thus, arteries were then usually tied with ligatures of
silk or hemp, which are not absorbed by the body tissues. Such

ligatures sometimes gave rise to an inflammatory reaction in the tissues and severe haemorrhage resulted. Lister devoted years of experiment to the search for a satisfactory ligature. He tested out each material in experimental animals and finally chose catgut, which is still in use. Even then the problem was not solved, since sterilization by most methods lessens the strength of catgut, but Lister at length evolved a satisfactory method.

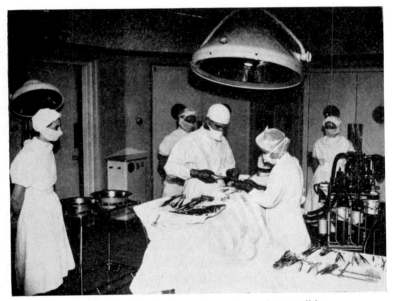

FIG. 101. An abdominal operation under modern conditions
(Whipps Cross Hospital, London. Photograph of 1946 by Pritchard)

The Listerian system, in rendering surgery safer, had also the effect of opening up many fields of operation that had previously been regarded as impracticable. Especially is this the case with abdominal surgery, which effectively dates from the introduction of the antiseptic system. Lister was often misunderstood and some of his contemporaries, and some even of those who opposed him, were really practising his system without knowing it.

There was no essential change in the conditions under which a surgical operation was carried out between the Middle Ages and the introduction of Listerian methods. Fig. 100 shows these conditions during this long period. A patient, lying semicomatose on an elaborate bed, is having his skull trephined. The surgeon rotates the trephine between his hands. He and all the others in the room are dressed in their ordinary clothes. A male assistant (right) is spreading a plaster. Behind are two women who may be either assistants or relatives. By the patient's head lounges an elegantly dressed young man who is probably a relative. In the foreground is a cat playing with a mouse. No photograph of a modern operating theatre, or even a casual visit to one, would indicate the enormous changes in equipment and methods which have taken place since the introduction of the aseptic system. It is a matter of technique and method as much as equipment, and these are not readily appreciated. However, an illustration of a modern operating theatre is given (Fig. 101). All persons present wear sterilized gowns, caps, masks, and rubber gloves. All instruments have been sterilized. Everything has been designed for ease of cleaning and to prevent the lodgement of dust. The surgeon operates under a light which casts no shadow.

Among the most important applications of the antiseptic method was its use in obstetrics. Here Lister had a predecessor, as he gladly and generously acknowledged. This was the unfortunate Hungarian genius, Ignaz Philipp Semmelweis (1818–65), who later became insane. In an obstetric unit of the great General Hospital at Vienna, in which he was an assistant, the death-rate in puerperal patients usually ranged between 10 and 30 per cent. of pregnant women admitted. The cause of this dreadful mortality was the condition known as puerperal fever. The women were attended by students or physicians who were visiting the post-mortem room. Semmelweis showed that the infective material that conveyed the fever was brought by the hands of the operator from the dead bodies, and he demonstrated also that puerperal fever was caused by decomposed animal matter. By insisting on the sterilization of the hands of the operators Semmelweis succeeded in 1846 in reducing the mortality at once to about 1 per cent. of pregnant women. This method of Semmelweis aroused great opposition, and he and his work were soon forgotten. But after the acceptance of Lister's antiseptic method in surgery which began a decade later, the procedures advocated by Semmelweis were universally introduced into midwifery practice.

XVII. LORD LISTER ON LIGATURING THE FEMORAL ARTERY

The letter and the objects enclosed therewith are in the Wellcome Historical Medical Museum

(*See p.* 358)

Semmelweiss was so disappointed that his method did not receive immediate recognition in Vienna that he very soon left that city and returned to Hungary. Shortly afterwards he became insane and he died in a lunatic asylum. It is perhaps because of his tragic story and the fact that his work was published such a short time before the surgical revolution that his investigations have so frequently been regarded as the first to elucidate the cause and prevention of puerperal fever. This, however, is not the case. Alexander Gordon (1752–99), a native and graduate of Aberdeen who practised and held teaching appointments in that city in the fifteenth-year interval between his two spells as a naval surgeon, was probably the first to demonstrate, on the evidence of the lying-in cases which he attended in his practice, that the infection was carried from an infected to an uninfected woman by the agency of the midwife or the doctor, that there was a definite connexion between puerperal fever and erysipelas, and that the application of putrid matter to the uterus would initiate puerperal fever. He did not recognize that the putrid matter was really the contagion. As preventive measures he stressed efficient cleansing of all parts of the operator's person which might have been in contact with the contagion. Gordon's book, *A Treatise on the Epidemic Puerperal Fever of Aberdeen.* was published in London in 1795. It was subsequently reprinted three times, and it seems to have exerted some influence on the obstetrical and medical practice of the next fifty years.

Previous to Gordon, Charles White (1728–1813) of Manchester published in 1773 *A Treatise on the Management of Pregnant and Lying-in Women.* White is often stated to have anticipated Semmelweis; but although he had much knowledge of the pathology and treatment of this disease, he held wrong views regarding the mode of spread. Hence in his preventive measures, although he emphasized general cleanliness of the room, clothing, and other articles which might be in contact with the patient, he overlooked the cleansing of the hands and persons of attendants. Many years after the publication of Gordon's book Oliver Wendell Holmes (p. 351), man of letters and professor of anatomy at Harvard, as a result of a discussion at a medical society, decided to examine the literature with reference to the possible transmission of puerperal fever from one patient to another by the midwife or doctor. In 1843 his paper was published: he quoted Gordon's book and many other instances of the transfer. Twelve years later his paper was reissued. Holmes had great influence, and it was due to him and other supporters of Semmelweis that the disinfection of the hands recommended by the Hungarian became common practice.

SOME MODERN SURGICAL ADVANCES

Ephraim McDowell (1771–1830) successfully removed an ovarian tumour in the patient's home in a Kentucky village in 1809, and he had two further successful cases. In 1852 James Marion Sims (1813–83) of New York introduced a sound operation for vesico-vaginal fistula. Nine years later he first reported his operation for amputation of the cervix uteri, and he was also well known for his work on the gall-bladder. Robert Lawson Tait (1845–99) of Birmingham was a pioneer gynaecologist who by 1883 had opened the abdomen in 1,000 cases. Lawson Tait was the first to popularize the operation of cholecystotomy.

Among the most capable surgeons of Lister's own day was Sir Thomas Spencer Wells (1818–97) of London. This great operator had been opening the abdomen successfully for ovarian conditions since 1858. In 1866 he performed the difficult operation of removal of the spleen. By 1867 his methods were approaching the Listerian. Under Lister's inspiration he further improved his technique and did more than any other man to raise the possibilities of abdominal surgery. Spencer Wells stands out for the extreme simplicity, directness, and effectiveness of his methods, and also for his exceptionally conscientious care as an operator. His name is commonly attached to an instrument of his invention for clamping the bleeding ends of cut blood-vessels. The illustration (Fig. 102) of the Spencer Wells forceps shows the catch near the finger-holes which locks the instrument as soon as the blades have closed on the bleeding-point. The forceps remain closed until deliberately opened by the operator. The familiar Spencer Wells forceps is at this day probably more frequently used than any other surgical instrument. An illustration (Fig. 103) showing Spencer Wells performing an abdominal operation gives an indication of the simplicity of his methods. Although published in 1882 the illustration depicts an operation of a few years earlier. It is really dated by the Lister steam carbolic spray on the left; as previously mentioned, this spray was first introduced in 1875. The anaesthetic is being given by means of a Junker inhaler, invented in 1867 and still used in Great Britain during the early decades of the twentieth century.

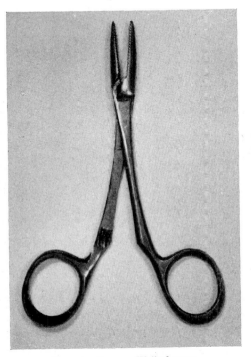

FIG. 102. Spencer Wells forceps

Cancer provides some of the most difficult problems which the surgeon has to deal with, and in the case of the surgery of the abdomen this malignant disease was the condition which gave rise to some of the earliest operations. It might be thought that other diseases would have provided nineteenth-century surgeons with better opportunities, but this was not the case. Any acute inflammation of the abdominal organs is liable to lead to generalized inflammation of the peritoneum, the thin membrane which invests all the abdominal organs. Without operation the localized inflammation has a chance to subside; with a badly performed operation the resultant general peritonitis often leads to a fatal result. It was long before the surgeon learned to attack the acute abdomen with confidence.

In 1833—long before the advent of Lister—the great French surgeon Jacques Lisfranc (1790–1847) had excised a cancer of the

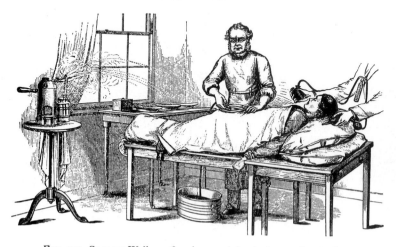

FIG. 103. Spencer Wells performing an abdominal operation *c.* 1875
(T. Spencer Wells, *On Ovarian and Uterine Tumours*, London, 1882)

lower bowel in nine cases, and in six of these death did not take place during the immediate post-operative period. But he used a method which avoided entering the abdominal cavity proper, and only the tumour itself was removed. In the case of malignant disease a much wider area of the tissues, or even the whole organ, must be removed. One of the first to perform successful operations for abdominal cancer was Christian Albert Theodor Billroth (1829–94). Billroth studied at universities in Germany, France, and Great Britain, and at the age of thirty-one became professor of surgery at Zürich. Seven years later he was called to Vienna, where his greatest work was performed. In 1872 he excised the gullet for cancer, and nine years later he was the first to remove the upper part of the stomach. Billroth frequently removed portions of the bowel, and by these pioneer operations he can be regarded as the founder of abdominal surgery. He was a keen follower of Lister's methods, and without Lister's work Billroth's advances would not have been possible.

In the meantime Richard von Volkmann (1830–89) of Halle had excised the lower bowel by the abdominal route for cancer (1878), and Ernst von Bergmann (1836–1907) of Berlin introduced steam sterilization for the destruction of organisms on instruments and dressings. He improved the design of operating theatres, and also performed a number of new operations. Excision of the kidney was first performed by Gustav Simon (1824–76) in 1869.

In surgical operations of this type the German schools at first outran their colleagues in other countries. One reason was that they at once adopted and practised vigorously the principles which Lister had so clearly put forward. In Britain, on the other hand, Lister's teachings were regarded with some disfavour by many surgeons; and in London, which ought to have been first to adopt the new methods, there was for years a positive hostility to Lister's work. When once this apathy had been overcome, British and American surgery entered new regions. In the realm of the acute abdomen some of their most important work was done.

Acute appendicitis is now a familiar condition, but at the middle of the nineteenth century it was unknown as such. Although Addison and Bright clearly recognized that the appendix can be the site of primary suppuration, inflammation in that region continued to be described as typhlitis or perityphlitis. Many cases of these conditions died of perforation of the appendix and general peritonitis. The first operation designed to treat peritonitis due to appendicitis (although it was not recognized as such) was carried out by Henry Hancock (1809–80), a surgeon to Charing Cross Hospital, in 1848. The patient had had a rupture of the appendix about twelve days previously, and the swelling caused by the suppuration could be seen in the right lower abdomen. Three days later Hancock opened this swelling and let out a large amount of offensive serum and pus. The patient had recovered five weeks later. The most influential voice in the new treatment of appendicitis in the Listerian period was that of Reginald Fitz (1843–1913) of Philadelphia. He pointed out the necessity for early diagnosis and operation. But this advice related to the abscess and not to the appendix. The first to remove the appendix itself was Rudolph Ulrich Krönlein (1847–1910); the organ had perforated (1886). In the following year Thomas George Morton (1835–1903) of Philadelphia performed the first operation in which a perforated appendix with an abscess was diagnosed and the appendix removed with a successful result. Charles McBurney (1845–1913) of New York emphasized the fact that in most cases of inflammation in the right lower abdomen the appendix was the affected organ. In 1889 he described the diagnostic point which bears his name. About this time Sir Frederick Treves (1853–1923) became interested in these conditions, and he decided that it was better not to operate during the acute stage of appendicitis, but to wait until the attack had subsided. In doing so he was taking the risk of perforation of the appendix, general peritonitis, and death. Against this risk he considered that the chances of a successful operation were greater during the quiescent stage. In 1887 he was the first to perform the operation on this principle. The result was successful, and Treves was the originator of the method which is now usually adopted.

Another acute condition of the abdomen fraught with the most serious consequences is the perforation of an ulcer of the stomach. The first successful operation to close a perforated gastric ulcer was performed in a private house by Ludwig Heusner (1846–1916) of Barmen in Germany in 1892. In the following year Hastings Gilford (1861–1941) of Reading did a similar operation. This case was not published until after that of Thomas Herbert Morse (1855–1921) of Norwich. Within two years it was almost a routine for surgeons to operate in such cases.

Macewen, asepsis, and the foundation of neurological surgery. Sir William Macewen (1848–1924), a native of Bute, studied medicine at Glasgow, and he remained there to adorn the University and the City during the rest of his life. As an undergraduate he studied under Lister, and at the early age of twenty-eight he became a full surgeon to the Glasgow Royal Infirmary (1876). Macewen at once made his personality felt, and soon large changes in equipment and staffing were in train. Between his appointment and 1890 he had established a severe aseptic routine, done important work on the transplantation of bone, introduced his operation for osteotomy and other bone operations, and founded neurological surgery. In 1889 he was invited to accept the chair of surgery at the newly founded Johns Hopkins University. Had he done so he would have been the colleague of Osler and probably the teacher of Harvey Cushing. But Macewen chose to remain in Glasgow, and in 1892 he succeeded Lister, at one remove, in the regius chair of surgery in Glasgow University, a post which he filled brilliantly for thirty-two years.

In the realm of asepsis Macewen early turned from the path beaten out so scientifically and so laboriously by his master. Even before he became a full surgeon to the Royal Infirmary his practice was essentially aseptic rather than antiseptic. By 1879 he had given up the carbolic spray—a year before von Bruns's pronouncement—and within about a year he was boiling the gauze used for dressings. He thus anticipated certain German surgeons. It has been mentioned that von Bergmann introduced steam sterilization for instruments and dressings. This was in 1886, but his full aseptic technique was not evolved till about 1891. Macewen had already been boiling everything used for some time, though he gladly acquired from Bergmann one of his specially designed sterilizers. Lister was the sole architect of the antiseptic system, but Macewen must be regarded as one of the principal architects of the aseptic system.

Macewen's greatest achievement is probably his foundation of neurological surgery. It will be appreciated that many surgeons through the centuries had trephined the skull, but they had all shrunk from opening the dura or from operating on the brain itself. These operations were skull surgery, not brain surgery. By brain surgery is meant the previous diagnosis of the site of the lesion by physiological and clinical methods, and then the performance of the operation at that site. Exact diagnosis and asepsis are essentials of the technique. By 1876 Macewen had both these essentials. In that year he diagnosed and localized a cerebral abscess. The operation which he advised was refused by the relatives, and death ensued. After death Macewen was allowed to perform the operation, and the abscess was found exactly as diagnosed. In 1879 he evacuated a sub-dural haematoma successfully. If there be any doubt about the previous case, this case most certainly initiated successful brain surgery. In the same year he successfully removed a fungus-like tumour of the dura (a meningioma). Between 1883 and 1886 Macewen reported five cases in which he had excised portions of the vertebrae and removed bodies—usually the products of inflammation—causing pressure on the spinal cord. In 1893 he published his great work *Pyogenic Infective Diseases of the Brain and Spinal Cord*. This book is an incredible record of ten years' achievement. He had operated on seventy-four patients with intracranial infections, and of these sixty-three were cured. Of these cases twenty-four suffered from cerebral abscess, and twenty-three of these were cured. Even today the specialist neurological surgeon finds it difficult to equal Macewen's results in the treatment of brain abscesses.

These results must be emphasized because there is a tendency to regard Sir Rickman John Godlee (1859–1925), Lister's nephew, and Sir Victor Horsley (1857–1916) as the founders of neurological surgery. It is the case that A. Hughes Bennett (p. 349) diagnosed a brain tumour in 1884 and Godlee removed it. This was a true neoplasm of the brain. But Macewen had already removed several tumours which, though not strictly neoplasms, were surgically equivalent. Horsley, a great physiologist and surgeon, removed a neoplasm from the spinal cord in 1887. This has been regarded as the first removal of a growth from the cord localized previously by the signs. But Macewen already had several successful cases of this nature to his credit, although none of the lesions removed happened to be true neoplasms. Macewen's book shows that by 1893 he was already the complete master in this field.

Macewen was by nature a biologist, a scientist who took his material and his examples from any part of the Realm of Nature. Throughout his career he was vitally interested in the process by which bone grows, and late in life he produced as a complement a work on the growth of the antlers of the deer. There are few branches of surgery which he did not adorn. His operation for hernia demonstrated that radical cure is possible and was the forerunner of many modifications. In 1895 he was asked to ease the last days of a man who had bilateral pulmonary tuberculosis, in whom a tuberculous empyema had developed on one side. Macewen diagnosed an abscess of the lung with advanced tuberculosis. He removed portions of ribs, evacuated the pus, and then proceeded to excise the whole of the lung on that side. The patient did well, and a month later the enormous cavity was partially closed by a thoracoplasty. The patient was still alive and well forty-five years later. This was the first total pneumonectomy.

Lister's first successes had been gained in the treatment of compound fractures, which were specially liable to become septic.

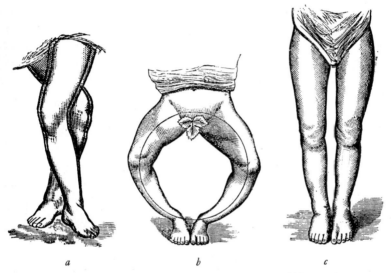

FIG. 104. Types of severe deformity following rickets, and result of Macewen's osteotomy
(a) and (b), two common types of deformity; (c) same case as (b), after operation
(W. Macewen, *Osteotomy*, London, 1880)

Rapid advances were made in bone surgery by applying his methods. As an example of the confidence which these methods bred in courageous surgeons, we may mention a problem with which Lister was himself quite familiar, that of rickets. This disease produces deformities of the bones in childhood, especially knock-knee or bow-leg. In the late nineteenth century such deformities were extremely common in Glasgow. Their correction then involved a major operation on both legs which few surgeons would risk. The results were often bad. In 1879 Macewen introduced a method whereby, working through a minute incision in the skin and soft tissues, he was able to cut the bone at the correct place and thus to straighten the leg. There were many technical difficulties which he overcame. The ordinary bone chisels were found to be unsuitable, and Macewen had not only to design his own osteotome, but even to determine the temper of its steel. His results with this pioneer operation were excellent. Orthopaedic surgery has since made many advances, and another landmark was the method of keeping broken fragments of bone in position by a metal plate screwed to the adjoining ends. This method was devised by Sir William Arbuthnot Lane (1856–1943).

Surgery in the twentieth century had the help of a method which was unknown to Lister and his immediate followers, radiology (p. 374). In the last two decades of the nineteenth century the practice of surgery was becoming surer. The technique of von Bergmann (p. 365) and other leaders in Germany was adopted and improved upon in other countries. In the pre-Listerian era the surgeon had operated in his ordinary clothes. In fact, it was common for each surgeon to keep handy an old frock-coat which he put on when about to operate. No special cleanliness was called for. About the eighties white gowns came into use. Efficient sterilization of the operator's hands remained a difficulty, but in 1890 W. S. Halsted (p. 349) introduced rubber gloves which are now universally used during operations. Operating technique has now developed to an elaborate and very rigid ritual.

Abdominal surgery continued to make notable advances. In the United States three of the leaders were John Benjamin Murphy (1857–1916) and the Mayo brothers, William (1861–1939) and Charles (1865–1939). The Mayos built up at Rochester, Minnesota, the great clinic which bears their name. They themselves advanced the art and practice of surgery, and under their leadership other men in their team developed the surgical specialties. In America and in this country an operation to short-circuit a portion of the stomach or bowel became common for the treatment of ulcers. In these developments a prominent part was played by Sir Arthur William Mayo Robson (1853–1933) of Leeds. More recently Berkeley George Andrew Moynihan (1865–1936), later Baron Moynihan of Leeds, was a pioneer in the surgery of the gall-bladder, and the doyen of surgery in Great Britain.

In neurological surgery the greatest advances of this century were made by Harvey Cushing (1869–1939) of Boston, a great and patient operator who performed long and detailed operations which would have been unthinkable before his time. Cushing made a careful study of the Gasserian ganglion as a preliminary to devising an operation for the cure of trigeminal neuralgia (1900). From about 1909 he worked on the hypophysis cerebri. This work culminated in his important monograph on *The Pituitary Body and its Disorders* (1912). He introduced an apparatus for cutting the tissues by electro-coagulation. Cushing had an unrivalled experience of brain tumours, and during his career he removed more than 2,000. He introduced the term meningioma in 1922, and in 1938 he published an important book on that subject. The work of Dandy has already been mentioned (p. 279).

With the acceptance of Listerian methods the treatment of compound fractures was gradually perfected, as has been mentioned, among others by Macewen and Arbuthnot Lane (p. 370). Simple fractures, which are far commoner, continued, however, to be treated with various types of splints in the traditional manner. Plaster of Paris bandages came into wide use in the seventies. They immobilized the fractured limb, but they had the disadvantage of also immobilizing the muscles. This led to subsequent pain and stiffness, and sometimes to wasting of the muscles. Moreover, with these plaster methods a faulty position of the fractured bone could often not be corrected. The increasing use of sandbags, laid on each side of the affected limb, instead of plaster splints, enabled the positions of the fragments of bone to be checked at intervals. This method also enabled massage to be applied to the muscles almost from the beginning.

Massage, employed for treatment in the ancient civilizations, was reintroduced into surgery by Ambroise Paré (pp. 95–97), but was little heard of in practice until the sixties of the nineteenth century, when it was strongly advocated by the Dutch surgeon, Johann Metzger (1839–1900). It was later strongly recommended by the French surgeon, Just Marie Marcellin Lucas-Championnière (1843–1913), whose principles were developed in the treatment of fractures and gun-shot wounds of the joints during the First World War. In this country James Beaver Mennell (1880–1957), who wrote an important work on this subject in 1917, was a pioneer of the new methods. Massage has since been broadened into the wider subject of physiotherapy, which plays such an important part in modern rehabilitation methods.

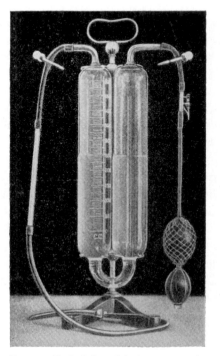

FIG. 105. Forlanini's original apparatus for
the induction of artificial pneumothorax
(C. Forlanini, *Die Therapie der Gegenwart*,
1908)

Thoracic surgery has shown dramatic advances in recent years. In 1888 Carlo Forlanini (1847–1918) of Pavia first carried out the minor operation for the induction of an artificial pneumothorax. The procedure had been suggested by James Carson (1772–1843) of Liverpool as far back as 1822, but no one had previously succeeded in the attempt. Forlanini injected an inert gas between the two layers of the pleura—that which covers the surface of the lung on the one hand, and on the other that which lines the inner surface of the chest wall. The result was a compression and collapse of the lung (Fig. 105). The enforced rest to the lung which resulted was of great value in the treatment of pulmonary tuberculosis. It was years before Forlanini's procedure became really popular with chest physicians. It was later learned that ordinary air could be effectively used to produce the collapse, and artificial pneumothorax was very widely used. Continued experience showed that in certain cases this minor procedure—it could hardly be called a surgical operation —did not give a sufficiently lasting collapse. The operation of thoracoplasty, in which after removal of portions of the ribs the chest wall falls in, was devised to effect this permanent collapse. At first this major operation was not very successful, but it was much improved by Ernst Ferdinand Sauerbruch (1875–1951) of Berlin. This operation was the forerunner of even more ambitious procedures, such as lobectomy or pneumonectomy. Pioneers of this work have been Hugh Morriston Davies (1879–), Arthur Tudor Edwards (1890–1946), and James Ernest Helme Roberts (1881–1948) in England, and Edward William Archibald (1872–1945) in Canada.

Related to the surgery of the lungs is that of the heart. Although a penetrating wound of the heart was repaired successfully as long ago as 1896, progress on these lines was at first very slow. Advances are, however, now being made, and in recent years deliberate operations have been successfully carried out on hearts which are the seat of certain congenital malformations. Diseases of the aorta and other large arteries have similarly been dealt with by direct operations on the arteries. Certain spasmodic diseases of the smaller arteries are now treated by operations on the sympathetic nerves which control their size.

Plastic surgery, which was initiated by Tagliacozzi (p. 98), was revived by Jacques Louis Reverdin (p. 524) in 1870; and by Karl Thiersch (1822–95), professor at Erlangen and later at Leipzig. Thiersch's work was based on his method of skin-grafting, which had an important influence on later work. Plastic surgery, which consists essentially in the grafting of tissue belonging to one part of the body to tissues of another part which have been mutilated, made rapid strides during the First World War, and since then it has made further rapid advances.

It is fitting to close this brief sketch of surgery since Lister with mention of a man whose outlook was basically that of Lister. Lister was essentially a scientist, and during much of his life he carried out experiments which had a direct bearing on the progress of surgery. Emil Theodor Kocher (1841–1917), who for nearly fifty years held the chair of surgery at Berne, was also a devoted scientist as well as a brilliant surgeon. In the practical field he enriched most departments of surgery. He is, however, best known for his pioneer operations for removal of the thyroid gland in certain types of goitre, for which work he received a Nobel Prize in 1909.

RADIOLOGY AND RADIUM THERAPY

The X-rays were discovered by Wilhelm Conrad Röntgen (1845–1923), professor of physics at Würzburg. In the autumn of 1895 he was experimenting with the new types of rays emitted from the recently devised vacuum-tubes of Crookes and of Lenard, and on 8 November he noted that when his tube was in action a screen of barium platino-cyanide which lay near by became brightly fluorescent. Within a few weeks Röntgen showed that this fluorescence was caused by a new type of rays. He was then ignorant of their nature, and he called them the 'X-rays'. During the next few weeks he worked intensively, and on 28 December 1895 he presented to the president of the Würzburg Physical-Medical Society a preliminary written communication in which he discussed all the more important physical features of the new rays. He showed that they passed easily through such materials as paper and wood, but that dense substances such as metals were more opaque to the X-rays. Röntgen also made X-ray photographs of objects (Fig. 106); and he had already taken an X-ray photograph of a human hand—his wife's (Fig. 107). In this photograph the bones stand out clearly, while a ring worn by his wife shows as a dense black shadow. Röntgen had thus pointed out from the start the importance of these new rays in medicine. His communication— *Eine neue Art von Strahlen* ('On a new kind of rays')—was printed and distributed to the members of the Society within a few days.

The contents of Röntgen's Preliminary Communication leaked out to the Vienna press almost at once. It was copied by some papers abroad, and on 6 January 1896 the London *Standard* sent a world

cable on the subject. This must be considered as the effective date
of the announcement of the discovery. The first X-ray photograph
for clinical purposes was made by Alan Archibald Campbell Swinton (1863–1930), a London electrical engineer who became a con-
sultant on X-ray plants, on 7 January 1896. At first the new method
of examination was used only to locate foreign bodies in the tissues,

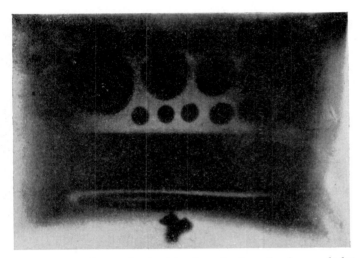

Fig. 106. X-ray photograph of weights in a closed wooden box, made by
Röntgen about December 1895
(O. Glasser, *Wilhelm Conrad Röntgen*, London, 1933)

and to diagnose fractures of bones. But efforts were soon made to
obtain relatively satisfactory X-ray photographs of the internal
organs. By 1897 W. B. Cannon (p. 303), then a student at Harvard,
had shown that if a bismuth compound was fed to an animal, it
appeared under the X-rays as an opaque mass in the stomach. The
progress of the bismuth-meal through the animal's alimentary tract
could be followed by means of the X-rays. This method was at once
put to practical uses, and a barium compound was soon substituted
for the bismuth in the test meal. These tests are of great importance
in the diagnosis of ulcers and other conditions of the stomach and
intestines. A similar method for the lungs was introduced by Jean
Athanase Sicard (1872–1929) and Jacques Forestier (1890–) in 1922.

This was the use of lipiodol—an oil containing a compound of iodine—which was injected into the bronchial tree in the lungs, and showed up abnormal pockets in the bronchial tubes. A similar method is also now used to delineate the cavities in the brain. Radiology of the heart and lungs was at first not very satisfactory, partly

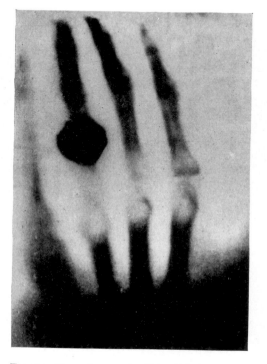

FIG. 107. X-ray photograph of his wife's hand, made
by Röntgen on 22 December 1895
(O. Glasser, *Wilhelm Conrad Röntgen*, London, 1933)

owing to the fact that the exposure to the rays had then to be of comparatively long duration, and hence movement of the organs was difficult to eliminate. As a result of co-operation between radiologists and manufacturers apparatus has been much improved, and for many years satisfactory radiographs of the lungs have been obtained. Rapid advances are now being made in the radiology of the heart.

Quite early in the history of radiology it was observed that those who worked extensively with the new rays tended to develop chronic ulcers and other skin conditions on exposed parts of their bodies. In some cases these ulcers developed into fatal cancers; and some workers died from a fatal type of anaemia. It was then discovered that such serious conditions could be prevented by stationing the operator behind a screen of lead or of lead-glass. More convenient methods for the insulation of the apparatus itself have since come into use. These accidents showed that X-rays have a harmful effect on living tissues, and attempts were soon made to use them for the treatment of certain skin conditions. They were also early used for the treatment of cancer and for some diseases of the blood-forming organs. They are still widely used in the treatment of certain forms of cancer.

Allied to treatment by X-rays is that by the radio-elements, especially radium. This element was discovered in 1898 by Marie Sklodowska Curie (1867–1934) and her husband Pierre Curie (1859–1906). Radium therapy began from an accidental burn sustained by the French scientist Henri Becquerel (1852–1908) through carrying radium in his pocket. In 1901 Pierre Curie confirmed this property by producing intentionally a burn on his own arm. In the same year radium was used in the treatment of lupus, and shortly afterwards in the treatment of malignant disease. The use of radium needles implanted in the tissues, and the bombardment of the tissues with rays from a 'radium bomb', have long been established methods for the treatment of certain forms of malignant disease.

Ultra-violet ray therapy. Although sunlight had long been thought to exert a beneficial influence on the human body, its scientific employment dates from very modern times. The ultra-violet rays in sunlight were discovered in 1801, and in the following year Sir Humphry Davy (p. 343) first produced the electric arc. This discovery later made light therapy possible, and Niels Ryberg Finsen (1861–1904) is regarded as its founder.

Finsen was born at Thorshavn in The Faroes. After graduating in medicine at the University of Copenhagen in 1890 he spent nearly three years as an assistant in the Anatomical Institute and thereafter devoted himself entirely to research. He engaged at

first on a physiological study of the effects of the various constituents of natural sunlight, and then of the light from an electric
arc. Finsen wished to treat lupus by means of ultra-violet light and
for this purpose local applications of the rays were necessary. He
therefore devised the 'Finsen Light', which consisted of a powerful
electric arc lamp, from which four brass collecting tubes, like large
telescopes, radiated downwards. The lower end of each tube could
be applied to a patient's lesion, so that four patients could be treated
simultaneously. Each collecting tube contained four convex quartz
lenses and it had a quartz window at its lower end. There was
distilled water in the compartments thus formed in the tube, and
cold water, to absorb the heat rays, circulated through an outer
jacket. Finsen treated lupus and certain forms of cutaneous tuberculosis very successfully by means of this apparatus. In 1896 he
opened at Copenhagen the first 'Medical Light Institute'. The
Princess of Wales, who as Consort of Edward VII was soon to become Queen Alexandra, was herself a Dane, and she was much
interested in Finsen's work. In 1900 she received from him a gift of
one of his lamps. She presented it to the London Hospital where it
gave excellent service for over thirty years. This historic Finsen
Light is now in the Wellcome Historical Medical Museum. Finsen
was awarded the Nobel Prize in 1903.

The Finsen Light is complicated, expensive, and non-portable.
In 1904 a portable water-cooled quartz mercury vapour lamp for
local treatment was designed by Ernst Kromayer (1862–1933), a
Berlin dermatologist. The Kromayer lamp is still used for certain
conditions, and its design has altered little. Four years later an air-
cooled quartz mercury vapour lamp was first used for general light
baths by Franz Nagelschmidt (1875–1952) of Berlin.

Two pioneers of natural heliotherapy, especially for tuberculosis
of the bones and joints, may be named. Auguste Henri Rollier
(1874–1954), a specialist in tuberculosis, established a famous
institution in the High Alps at Leysin before the First World War.
He achieved excellent results by the use of natural sunlight. In the
United Kingdom Sir Henry Gauvain (1878–1945) became medical
superintendent of the Lord Mayor Treloar's Cripples' Hospital at
Alton and Hayling Island, Hampshire, on its foundation in 1908.

He at once began to use heliotherapy for surgical tuberculosis, and, considering the differences of altitude and climate, his results compared favourably with those of Rollier.

BACTERIOLOGY BECOMES A SCIENCE

We have seen the microbic view of the origin of disease demonstrated as a reality by Pasteur (pp. 330–5) and extended to special disease conditions by him and by Koch (pp. 336–8). While the French observer stood above all men for the clearness and steadiness of his vision and for his persistence and resource in following what he had seen from afar, his German colleague had a genius for visualizing particulars and for adapting mechanical devices and scientific discoveries to particular ends. Koch thus vastly improved and elaborated the methods for detecting and examining minute organisms. The significance of his results was at once recognized, but the complexity of the technique involved, and the time and training necessary, demanded the elevation of the subject to the position of a special science.

With Koch's work on anthrax in 1876, on the bacteria that commonly infect wounds in 1878, and with his great discovery of the tubercle bacillus in 1882, the study of the infective diseases entered on a new stage. The enemy had been seen and was now known for what it was. The bacteriologist had succeeded in isolating disease-producing bacteria and had cultivated them in test-tubes. Moreover, the organisms had been compelled to exist alone without mixing with other species. In this way many of these organisms were obtained, and delicate methods of detecting and differentiating them were developed. With a pure culture of a particular disease-producing organism in his hands, the bacteriologist can determine the influences favourable or unfavourable to its growth, and he can investigate the conditions that exalt, destroy, or modify its activity (p. 340).

An important series of criteria established by Koch (1890) remain the tests by which the disease-producing character of organisms can be established. To prove that an organism is the inseparable cause of any disease we need to demonstrate:

1. The constant presence of the organism in every case of the disease.

2. The preparation of a pure culture, which must be maintained for repeated generations.

3. The reproduction of the disease in animals by means of a pure culture removed by several generations from the organisms first isolated.

These conditions—Koch's postulates, as they are called—have been fulfilled for many diseases. Evidently the third test can be applied only in conditions to which animals other than man are susceptible. Now in this matter the organisms that produce disease vary greatly. Some, for instance those of anthrax, are easily conveyed to a variety of species of animals; others, for instance those of syphilis, are with difficulty conveyed to a very few species of animals; yet others, for instance human malaria, cannot be conveyed to any animal save man.

Some light is thrown on the life-history of the second and third classes by recent discoveries. The science of comparative pathology, that is the knowledge of the relations of the diseases of different species of animals, is of quite recent growth. It has already demonstrated, however, the existence of organisms bearing some resemblance, for instance, to those of human syphilis and human malaria as the cause of disease in animals. By studying the life-history of these organisms in animals and by investigating their effect on animals, valuable side-lights have often been thrown on the allied diseases in man. Moreover, in exceptional cases and in some special diseases, it has been possible to convey a disease experimentally to man.

A second important factor has gradually come into prominence with the extension of bacteriological knowledge. It is evident that not all men are subject to all human diseases. Even in the most destructive epidemic there are some that escape. These lucky ones may be naturally immune. Many diseases, such as measles, seldom recur in individuals who have been infected, so our lucky ones may thus have an acquired immunity.

The general nature of immunity we shall presently discuss (p. 409), but we note here that it may be relative or absolute, and may, moreover, vary according to the circumstances of the individual. Thus, it has frequently been shown that pulmonary tuberculosis is, other factors being equal, relatively more common in the poor and ill-housed than in the rich, who live in much better conditions. During the Second World War there was a serious increase in the incidence of pulmonary tuberculosis in many belligerent countries, and defective nutrition probably played a part in causing this increase. The investigation of facts such as these on a large scale has demonstrated that the soil in which disease grows is of no less import than the seed from which it grows. The problem of disease causation is thus immensely complex. We are only just beginning to draw up general laws on the subject, and in approaching it we are beyond the frontiers of our positive knowledge. We shall now survey a part of the better-known territory, and we introduce the subject by considering a few specific bacteriological achievements under the headings of the diseases associated with them.

SOME IMPORTANT BACTERIOLOGICAL RESULTS

(a) *Diphtheria* is a disease for which physicians now habitually demand a bacteriological diagnosis. Bretonneau of Tours (p. 204), working on clinical and post-mortem material, and without the use of a microscope, was able to distinguish it as a specific disease (1826). In 1883 Theodor Albrecht Edwin Klebs (1834–1913) of Zürich, a pupil of Virchow, described the specific organism of the disease, the diphtheria bacillus (*Corynebacterium diphtheriae*). In 1884 F. Loeffler (p. 392), a Prussian and an assistant of Koch, succeeded in cultivating it. The organism has since been known as the Klebs-Loeffler bacillus (Fig. 108). Its study has thrown much light on the nature of bacterial action in general and has, moreover, led to important developments both in treatment and in prevention (p. 434).

(b) *Plague.* Of all diseases none is so dramatic as plague, the scourge of mankind throughout history. The plague bacillus (*Pasteurella pestis*, Fig. 109) was discovered independently by the Japanese, Shibasaburo Kitasato (p. 393), a pupil of Koch, and by the Frenchman, Alexandre Yersin (p. 394), a pupil of Pasteur, during an epidemic at Hong Kong in 1894. These two scientists cultivated the organism and reproduced the disease by inoculation of pure cultures in animals. It had long been observed that outbreaks of

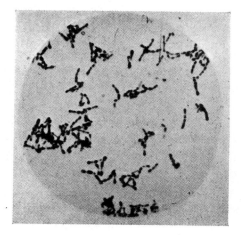

(a)

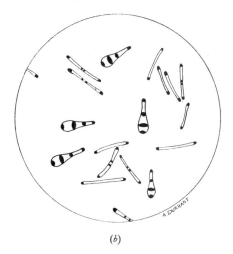

(b)

FIG. 108. Diphtheria bacilli

(a) Photomicrograph of smear from a 24-hour culture on Loeffler's serum, stained by Neisser's method. × 1000.

(b) Simplified drawing from an older culture, showing beaded appearance and swollen, involution forms.

((a) after Browning and Mackie, *Textbook of Bacteriology*, London, 1949)

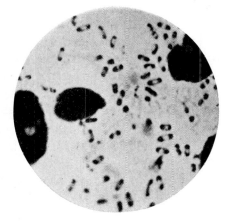

(a)

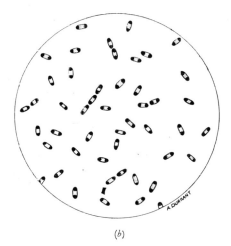

(b)

Fig. 109. Plague bacilli

(a) Photomicrograph of bacilli from a plague bubo showing bipolar staining. Leishman's stain. × 2000.

(b) Simplified drawing of similar preparation.

((a) after Browning and Mackie, *Textbook of Bacteriology*, London, 1949)

a deadly disease of rats and mice were liable to precede outbreaks of plague in human subjects. These epizootics which precede epidemics are now known to be due to the plague bacillus. A mass of evidence has been collected to show that the normal carrier of the plague infection is the rat flea. This knowledge has led to the formulation of effective measures for the control of plague. These measures are based on the wholesale extermination of the rat population which harbours the infective fleas. The study of the natural history of the plague bacillus has also led to prophylactic measures for the safety of individuals (see p. 439).

(c) *Undulant fever* (*Brucellosis*), formerly known as *Malta fever*, is a disease of much wider distribution than this last name implies. It was formerly thought to occur only in a relatively limited area of the earth's surface, and it was considered to have been conquered there by a simple procedure; but further investigation showed that the disease was literally world-wide in its distribution, and that it presented many difficulties. For centuries the peoples dwelling along the Mediterranean coasts had been afflicted with a low-grade fever, with pains in the muscles and joints. It had been called Malta fever, Mediterranean fever, Gibraltar fever, and similar names. In the Crimean War many of the British sick and wounded were sent to Malta to recover. There they contracted the disease, and it was shown that the fever was intermittent in type, lasted anything up to ninety days, and caused great loss of time in garrisons. It was investigated by medical officers of the British Army, and in 1886 Sir David Bruce (1855–1931) isolated the causative organism from a fatal case. Bruce thought the minute organism was of the spherical or coccus type, and he called it *Micrococcus melitensis* (from *Melita*, the Latin name for Malta). Measures to improve the hygiene and water-supplies of the troops and the drainage of camps were quite ineffective.

The British Government was much concerned about the problem, and in 1904 the Royal Society appointed a Commission, with Bruce as president, to investigate. By the following year the problem was virtually solved. Almost by chance it was found that the goat, which on bacteriological evidence had been thought to be resistant to the disease, was really very susceptible. The astonishing fact was soon elicited that about half the goats in Malta were infected, and a considerable proportion were excreting the organism in their milk. It was also found that large numbers of the native population were suffering from the fever in a very mild form, and many were excreting the organism in their excreta.

In the Malta garrison the drinking of goat's milk was at once forbidden. The resultant dramatic fall in the incidence of the disease in the armed forces is shown in the following table:

Year	Cases of undulant fever among		
	Navy	Army	Civilians
1905	270	643	663
1906	145	163	822
1907	12	9	714
1908	6	5	502
1909	10	1	456
1910	3	1	318

In Fig. 110 the monthly incidence of this disease in the British garrison at Malta is shown graphically for the years immediately preceding and immediately following the prohibition of the use of unboiled goats' milk. The size of the garrison remained practically constant throughout the period. There was a decrease in the maximum monthly incidence from 94 to 2 cases per 10,000. In other places where the use of goats' milk could be controlled there followed a similar sharp decline in the incidence of Malta fever.

There now followed investigations which showed how important an isolated finding can sometimes be in the control of a widespread disease. In 1897 the Norwegian, Bernhard Laurits Frederik Bang (1848–1932) had described a very small bacillus which he had found to be the cause of contagious abortion in cattle. It was soon discovered that this *Bacillus abortus* caused in man an obscure and intermittent type of fever which was very persistent. It was called undulant fever, and was shown to be present in southern European countries, in most of Africa, in many areas in America, and in Asia. In 1918 it was decided that the *Micrococcus melitensis* and the *Bacillus abortus* were really the same organism, a minute bacillus. The new name *Brucella abortus* was coined for this group of organisms in honour of Sir David Bruce, and the diseases caused by

C C

them were included under the term *Brucellosis*, or undulant fever. It is now known that these conditions are found over most of the inhabited world. They are not infrequently met with in the British Isles. Pasteurization of milk is the most important measure in their prevention, but in countries where this process is not carried out,

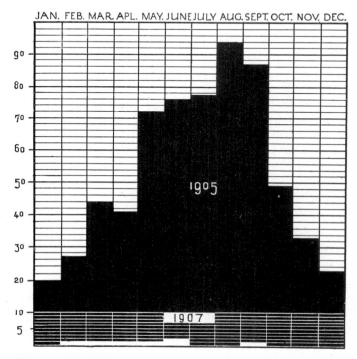

FIG. 110. Monthly incidence of Malta fever in the British garrison at Malta, 1905 (in black) and 1907 (in white). The ordinates represent case incidence per 10,000 garrison strength

their eradication will be difficult. The organism is found not only in cattle and in goats, but also in horses, pigs, and dogs, all of which may transmit the disease.

(*d*) *Tetanus.* This condition, also known as lock-jaw, is a very anciently described disease. There are unmistakable references to it in the Hippocratic Collection, notably in the *Aphorisms*. Two of these references we have already noted (p. 37). A general association of tetanus with wounds has long been recognized. In 1884 Nicolaier

(p. 392) produced tetanus in mice by inoculating them with garden earth. In such cases Nicolaier found constantly in the pus at the inoculation site a bacillus which was later shown to be the causative organism of tetanus. He was, however, unable to obtain the bacillus in pure culture. This was first accomplished in 1889 by Kitasato (p. 393), who then caused tetanus in animals by inoculating them with pure cultures of this organism (Fig. 111). He found the organism would grow only in the absence of oxygen. It is, in fact, a type of a large and now well-known group, the anaerobic bacteria. The natural habitat of the tetanus bacillus has been proved to be soil, and especially richly manured soil. The knowledge of the bacillus, of its habitat, and of its mode of growth has led to the development of a valuable protective measure.

(e) *Typhoid* (*enteric*) *fever*. On the basis of present knowledge we can trace this disease far back in history. Nevertheless, it was not till 1837 that the distinction between the two definite conditions known now as typhoid fever and typhus fever was first clearly made. This was the work of an American, William Wood Gerhard (1809–72) of Philadelphia. Gerhard's work was not well known in Britain and it was not until 1850 that Sir William Jenner (1815–98) confirmed his findings. The micro-organism of typhoid fever was first seen in 1880 by Eberth (p. 391), a pupil of Virchow. It was, however, not isolated in pure culture until 1884, when Georg Gaffky (1850–1918) obtained it from the spleen and investigated its cultural characteristics. Gaffky studied under Koch, became his chief assistant, and eventually succeeded him as the director of the Institute for Infectious Diseases in Berlin. The typhoid bacillus (*Bacillus typhosus* or *Salmonella typhi*, Fig. 112) is an inhabitant of the intestine, and its natural history was obscured by confusion with certain other very similar intestinal organisms such as the *Bacillus coli* (p. 399). These have now been well differentiated from each other, and in the course of this process the flora, both normal and pathological, of the intestinal canal has become well known. Moreover, it has been shown that typhoid organisms are not always of the same species, but that several closely allied forms produce several closely allied diseases. Lastly, certain of the effects wrought by the typhoid group of organisms on the body, which is their host, have

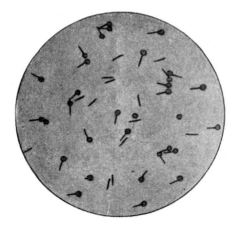

(a)

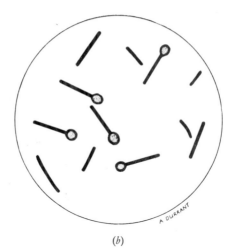

(b)

Fig. 111. Tetanus bacilli

(a) Photomicrograph of bacilli from an anaerobic culture, showing terminal spores. ×750.

(b) Simplified drawing of similar preparation.

((a) after L. E. H. Whitby, *Medical Bacteriology*, London, 1944)

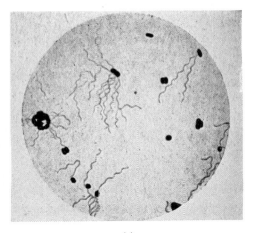

(*a*)

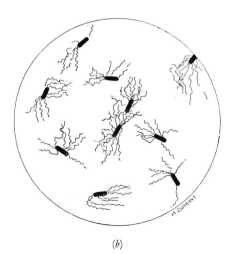

(*b*)

FIG. 112. Typhoid bacilli

(*a*) Photomicrograph of smear from a young
culture, stained to show flagella. × 1000.

(*b*) Simplified drawing of similar preparation.

((*a*) after Browning and Mackie, *Textbook of
Bacteriology*, London, 1949)

been exactly investigated. These investigations have led to improved methods of recognition of the disease, that is to say, diagnosis, and also of prevention of its incidence, that is to say, prophylaxis. These are referred to in a later section.

DISCOVERY OF THE MAIN PATHOGENIC BACTERIA

As an indication of the rapid development of bacteriology from about the time that Koch entered the field, reference may be made to the following table which gives brief particulars of the discovery of the specific organisms of certain diseases. It will be noted that in the twenty-one years between 1879 and 1900 inclusive the specific organisms of at least twenty-one diseases were discovered. It is true that later research showed that in a few instances the organism named in the table was not the specific cause of the disease associated with it; but this period does represent a record of success which could not be paralleled in any other medical field at the time. As a matter of interest a few brief notes are given on those discoverers named in the table who have not already been mentioned.

Gerhard Henrik Armauer Hansen (1841–1912), a Norwegian, was in charge of a leper hospital near Bergen, and he spent his life on the study of leprosy. Otto Hugo Franz Obermeier (1843–73) was an assistant in the Charité Hospital at Berlin, where he discovered the spirochaete which bears his name. He then went into practice in Berlin, and he died of cholera there. Otto von Bollinger (1843–1909) studied in several German universities, and from 1880 he was professor of pathological anatomy at Munich. He did much research on diseases of animals, such as anthrax, actinomycosis, and tuberculosis. James Israel (1848–1926) was a renal surgeon and director of the surgical division of a Berlin hospital. His important work on actinomycosis was done between 1878 and 1891.

With Albert Ludwig Siegmund Neisser (1855–1916) we reach the bacteriologists who are well remembered as such. Neisser was director of the Dermatological Institute at Breslau. He travelled much for the purpose of studying leprosy, and he confirmed Hansen's work. In addition to discovering the gonococcus he was an authority on syphilis, and he was associated with August von Wassermann (1866–1925), a famous assistant of Koch, in the discovery of the test for that disease.

Discoverers of the Main Micro-organisms

Year	Disease	Organism	Discoverer
1849	Anthrax	*Bacillus anthracis*	Pollender
1868	Leprosy	*Mycobacterium leprae*	Hansen
1873	Relapsing fever	*Treponema recurrentis*	Obermeier
1877 1878	Actinomycosis	*Actinomyces bovis*: (in ox) " " (in man)	Bollinger Israel
1878	" Suppuration	*Staphylococcus*	Koch Ogston (1881)
1879	Gonorrhoea	*Neisseria gonorrhoeae* (Gonococcus)	Albert Neisser
1880	Typhoid fever	*Salmonella typhi* (*Bacillus typhosus*)	Eberth
1881	Suppuration, &c.	*Streptococcus*	Ogston
1882	Glanders	*Pfeifferella mallei*	Loeffler
1882	Tuberculosis	*Mycobacterium tuberculosis*	Koch
1882	?Pneumonia	*Pneumobacillus*	Friedländer
1883	Erysipelas	'*Streptococcus erysipelatis*'	Fehleisen
1883	Cholera	*Vibrio cholerae*	Koch
1883–4	Diphtheria	*Corynebacterium diphtheriae*	Klebs (1883) Loeffler (1884)
1884	Tetanus	*Clostridium tetani*	Nicolaier
1885	..	*Bacterium coli commune*	Escherich
1886	Pneumonia	*Streptococcus pneumoniae* (Pneumococcus)	Albert Fraenkel
1887	Cerebrospinal meningitis	*Neisseria meningitidis* (Meningococcus)	Weichselbaum
1888	Food poisoning	*Salmonella enteritidis*	Gaertner
1889	Soft chancre	*Haemophilus ducreyi*	Ducrey
1892	?Influenza	*Haemophilus influenzae*	Richard Pfeiffer
1892	Gas-gangrene	*Clostridium welchii*	Welch
1894	Plague	*Pasteurella pestis*	Kitasato} independ- Yersin } ently
1895	Pseudo-tuberculosis of cattle	Johne's bacillus	Johne
1896	Botulism	*Clostridium botulismum*	van Ermengem
1898	Bacillary dysentery	*Shigella shigae* (*Bacillus dysenteriae*)	Shiga
1900	Paratyphoid fever	*Salmonella paratyphi*	Schottmüller
1905	Syphilis	*Treponema pallidum*	Schaudinn and Hoffmann
1906	Whooping-cough	*Haemophilus pertussis*	Bordet and Gengou
1915 1917	..	Bacteriophage phenomenon	Twort d'Herelle

Carl Joseph Eberth (1835–1926) was born at Würzburg and studied there under Virchow. He later held chairs at Zürich and Halle, and in addition to his discovery of the typhoid bacillus he did important work on the pseudo-tuberculosis of guinea-pigs.

Sir Alexander Ogston (1844–1929) was born in Aberdeen, and he studied there and at Vienna, Prague, and Berlin. In 1882 he became professor of surgery at Aberdeen. He was the first to identify the staphylococcus and to differentiate it from the streptococcus.

Friedrich August Johann Loeffler (1852–1915) was born at Frankfort-on-the-Oder and studied in Berlin. After serving in the Franco-Prussian War he became Koch's assistant. After a period as a professor at Greifswald he succeeded Gaffky, who had followed Koch as the director of the Institute for Infectious Diseases at Berlin. In addition to discovering the organisms of typhoid fever and diphtheria, he introduced many technical advances in bacteriology and recognized that the virus of foot-and-mouth disease is filterable.

Carl Friedländer (1847–87) studied at several German universities and eventually held a post in a Berlin hospital. A promising career was cut short by his long illness and death from pulmonary tuberculosis.

Friedrich Fehleisen (1854–1924) was a Würzburg surgeon who became assistant to von Bergmann in Berlin. His only important contribution to bacteriology was his discovery of the streptococcus found in cases of erysipelas.

Arthur Nicolaier (1862–?) was born in Silesia, and became a professor in the medical clinic at the University of Göttingen. He was later appointed to a chair in Berlin. In an article of 1884 he gave what is generally regarded as the first description of the tetanus bacillus, but he was unable to grow it in pure culture. This was not accomplished till 1889, when Kitasato grew it by anaerobic methods.

Heinrich Albert Johne (1839–1910) was born in Dresden, and he studied veterinary science, and also medicine under Cohnheim, and others. He became very well known as a specialist in veterinary pathology, and he made important contributions to the literature of actinomycosis, trichinosis and other conditions. His most important work was done on the pseudotuberculous disease of cattle now called after him.

Theodor Escherich (1857–1911), a native of Munich, became professor of paediatrics at Vienna. One of his main interests was the normal flora of the intestine, and he was the first to describe the commonest of the normal intestinal organisms, the *Bacillus coli communis*.

Albert Fraenkel (1848–1916), a native of Frankfort-on-the-Oder, became physician to a Berlin hospital and an authority on respiratory diseases.

Anton Weichselbaum (1845–1920), an Austrian, studied at Vienna and was at first a military surgeon. He later became professor of pathological anatomy at the University of Vienna. In addition to discovering the meningococcus he worked on the bacteriology of tuberculosis.

August Anton Hieronymus Gaertner (1848–1934), a native of Westphalia, was trained as a military surgeon, and later became a naval surgeon. He then studied under Koch, and became especially interested in the hygiene and bacteriology of food. At the age of thirty-eight he became professor of hygiene at Jena. One of the chief bacilli causing food poisoning, discovered by him, now bears his name.

Augusto Ducrey (1860–1940) was professor of dermatology in Pisa and Rome. The bacillus of soft chancre, which he discovered, was later called after him.

Shibasaburo Kitasato (1852–1931) studied at the Imperial University of Tokyo and graduated in 1883. Two years later he went to study under Koch at Berlin, and there he remained for six years. He then returned to Japan and founded a bacteriological institute. Of Kitasato's many noteworthy investigations the most important are his discovery of the bacilli of plague and tetanus, and his joint discovery of antitoxic immunity.

Richard Friedrich Johannes Pfeiffer (1858–1945), one of the greatest of German bacteriologists, was born in Posen and educated in Berlin as a military surgeon. He worked with Koch at the Institute for Hygiene at Berlin from 1887 to 1894, when he became professor of hygiene at Königsberg. In 1909 he was translated to the corresponding chair at Breslau. In addition to his discovery of the influenza bacillus he discovered in 1896 the *Micrococcus catarrhalis*, an organism found in the pharynx. His most important work was in connexion with the lysis of the organisms of cholera and typhoid (p. 414).

William Henry Welch (1850-1934), the most distinguished of American pathologists, studied at Yale and at several German universities. He held the chair of pathology at Johns Hopkins University, Baltimore, from its foundation in 1884 until 1918. He then became director of the School of Hygiene and Public Health at that University; he had been mainly instrumental in founding that School. He then founded, and became the first director of, the Institute of the History of Medicine at Johns Hopkins. In innumerable ways Welch advanced the sciences of pathology and bacteriology, and indeed the whole art of medicine.

Alexandre Émile Jean Yersin (1863-1943) was born at La Vaux (Lausanne), and became a surgeon in the French Colonial Army. He was later appointed director of the Pasteur Institute in Annam. For his discovery with Roux of diphtheria toxin, and for his independent discovery of the plague bacillus, see pp. 411 and 489.

Émile Pierre Marie van Ermengem (1851-1932) was born and graduated in medicine at Louvain. He also studied at Paris, London, Edinburgh, and Vienna, and he also worked with Koch at Berlin. From 1888 until 1919 he was professor of bacteriology in the University of Ghent, and he was then appointed perpetual secretary of the Académie royale de Médecine de Belgique. He made many important investigations in bacteriology.

Kiyoshi Shiga (1870-1957), a Japanese, studied at Tokyo and became assistant to Kitasato. After working for three years in Ehrlich's laboratory he held for sixteen years the post of director of a department in the Institute for Infectious Diseases in Tokyo. In addition to his bacteriological work he carried out important investigations in chemotherapy.

Hugo Schottmüller (1867-1936), a native of Brandenburg, became director of the Medical Polyclinic at Hamburg-Eppendorf. He discovered the disease paratyphoid fever and also its causative organism.

Fritz Richard Schaudinn (1871-1906), an East Prussian, studied the philology of the Germanic languages, but he soon turned to zoology, and after graduating in that subject he obtained a post in the University of Berlin. He became very well known for his researches in protozoology, and in 1904 he was appointed head of the laboratory of protozoology in the Kaiserliche Gesundheitsamt in Berlin. In the following year, with Hoffmann, he discovered the *Spirochaeta pallida* (*Treponema pallidum*), the causative organism of syphilis.

Paul Erich Hoffmann (1868–1959), a Pommeranian, studied in Berlin and was at first a military surgeon. He then turned to dermatology, in which he had a very distinguished career and he was for long professor of that subject in the University of Bonn. He was especially interested in the skin manifestations of syphilis, and in addition to his joint discovery with Schaudinn of the causative organism of that disease, he established its presence in the lymph glands in congenital and acquired syphilis.

The bacteriophage is dealt with on p. 406. Frederick William Twort (1877–1950), a Londoner, studied at St. Thomas's Hospital, and worked there and at the London Hospital. He then became superintendent of the Brown Institution and a professor of bacteriology in the University of London.

Félix Hubert d'Herelle (1873–1949) was born in Montreal, Canada. He studied at Lille and Leyden. He worked first in Guatemala and Mexico, and then from 1908 to 1921 he held important posts at the Institut Pasteur in Paris. In 1928 he became professor of protobiology at Yale University.

DEVELOPMENTS IN BACTERIOLOGY

Anaerobic methods. Leeuwenhoek was the first to show that some animalcules—almost certainly bacteria—could exist without oxygen (1680). Spallanzani (p. 156) also showed nearly a century later that some animalcules could survive for over a fortnight in a high vacuum. These observations were forgotten, and in 1861 Pasteur, while studying butyric fermentation, found that some bacteria were active where the concentration of oxygen was low, but that they became immobile and died when introduced to a normal oxygen concentration. The discovery of the gas gangrene bacillus and similar organisms led to a search for convenient methods of cultivation of such bacteria in an oxygen-free atmosphere. One of the most satisfactory of the early methods was the tube invented in 1888 by Hans

Buchner (1850–1902), who succeeded Pettenkofer in the chair of hygiene at Munich. The oxygen in this apparatus was absorbed by pyrogallol. A larger apparatus, depending on the absorptive power of potassium pyrogallote, was that of William Bulloch (1868–1941), of the Lister Institute and the University of London. With the London dermatologist James Harry Sequeira (1865–1948), Bulloch was the first to call attention to the relation between the suprarenal bodies and the sex organs (1905); and with Sir Paul Fildes (1882–), the London chemical bacteriologist, he was the author of an important work on haemophilia (1911). Bulloch also wrote the standard *History of Bacteriology* (1938). The anaerobic jar of James McIntosh (1883–1948) and Fildes, in which spongy palladium was used to absorb the oxygen, was also well known.

Investigation of types and varieties. A glance at the table on p. 391 will show that before the end of the nineteenth century the causative organisms of many of the commoner infectious diseases had been discovered. From about this period bacteriological research turned in the direction of the investigation of the differentiation of related organisms, and of the discovery of new variants. We select a few organisms for discussion, to show the manner in which these discoveries were stimulated.

The tubercle bacillus. The discovery of this organism by Koch in 1882 was a triumph for pure bacteriology, and, as Koch pointed out, it proved of great value in the diagnosis of the disease tuberculosis. But in his full account of his very numerous inoculation experiments, published in 1884, Koch missed a point which has since proved to be of the greatest importance in the prevention of the disease. His oversight is all the more inexplicable, since the point had been clearly made by his elder contemporary, Villemin.

Jean Antoine Villemin (1827–92) was a French military surgeon who became a professor at the military medical school, the Val-de-Grâce. During much of his early life Villemin's consuming interest was in tuberculosis. He had a theory that glanders, a disease of horses, was very similar to tuberculosis, and that since glanders was transmissible by inoculation, tuberculosis should also be transmissible in the same way. In 1865 Villemin inoculated tuberculous material, obtained from a lung cavity of a patient who had just died of pulmonary tuberculosis, into a healthy rabbit. Another rabbit from the same mother was used as a control, and both were kept in identical conditions and were killed after three and a half months. The uninoculated rabbit was free from tuberculosis, but in the inoculated rabbit the lungs were full of tuberculous lesions. This material was used to inoculate another rabbit, with the same result, and so on in six series. In an experiment with tuberculous material from a cow the inoculated rabbit became acutely ill after two months, and it was on the point of death when it was killed. Its organs showed an acute generalized tuberculosis. Villemin proved conclusively that, contrary to the opinion of many authorities at that time, tuberculosis could be transmitted to rabbits from a human patient or an animal suffering from the natural disease tuberculosis, and from these rabbits to other rabbits in series. He also made the specific point that tuberculous matter of bovine origin inoculated into a rabbit produced a more generalized and rapidly fatal disease than matter of human origin inoculated into a rabbit. Villemin's first statement of his very important experiments received a cool reception when he presented it at a meeting of the Académie de Médecine at Paris in 1867. In the following year he published his full account in his work *Études sur la tuberculose.*

Although Koch referred to Villemin's work in his definitive publication of 1884, he belittled its importance and suggested erroneously that a rather obscure German predecessor had already proved the transmissibility of tuberculosis. Koch specifically stated that, although there was no microscopical difference between tubercle bacilli obtained from different sources, such as tuberculosis of the lungs in human subjects, lupus, and tuberculosis in the cow, he thought they might well show cultural differences. But although he examined many cultures and devoted special attention to the question, he was unable to show that such differences existed. Koch therefore concluded that human and bovine tuberculosis were identical diseases. At first Koch also thought that tuberculosis in birds was also identical with that in man and in bovines, since the bacilli appeared identical microscopically. He had not been able to culture the avian bacillus. But this was done by Edmond Isidore Étienne Nocard (1850–1903) and Roux (p. 411) of the Pasteur

Institute at Paris. As soon as Koch received this culture from them he recognized that the avian bacillus was distinct from the mammalian organism, and he modified his view accordingly.

Koch's views were widely accepted, but Edward Emanuel Klein (1844–1925) disagreed. Klein was a German who studied in London and became a well-known London bacteriologist and the author of an outstanding early work on histology. He had inoculation experiments carried out under his direction, and he showed that in the rabbit tuberculous lesions are not caused by the injection of tuberculous material from a human source, but that generalized tuberculosis was caused by the injection of material from a tuberculous cow (1883). This was really a confirmation of Villemin's conclusion, since Villemin had killed his rabbits injected with human material at a period before a natural process of resolution of the tuberculous lesions would have taken place. Klein's work, like that of Villemin, received little attention. In 1896 Theobald Smith (p. 420) made a careful comparison of the morphology of two strains of tubercle bacilli, one from a bovine source and the other supposedly from a human source, and showed that there were differences; he also demonstrated that they showed marked differences in virulence for the ox and the rabbit. Two years later he investigated fifteen additional strains, and as a result he suggested that there are two distinct types of the mammalian tubercle bacillus, one human and the other bovine. Smith's work also received little attention.

This was the position when, at the British Congress on Tuberculosis which was held in London in 1901, Koch made an announcement of the greatest importance. He stated that as a result of his recent research he had concluded that human tuberculosis is different from bovine and cannot be transmitted to cattle, and also that bovine tuberculosis cannot be transmitted to man. Coming at a time when great efforts were being made in many countries to eradicate bovine tuberculosis in the interests of human welfare, this pronouncement was widely disbelieved, and it proved to be an enormous stimulus to further research. In Great Britain the outstanding result was the appointment of the Royal Commission on Tuberculosis which reported in 1911. Very extensive investigation of this and similar tuberculosis problems was carried out for this Commission and at later dates by Arthur Stanley Griffith (1875–1941) and Frederick Griffith (1879?–1941). It was conclusively proved that bovine tuberculosis is transmissible to man, and it was shown that the bovine bacillus causes lesions especially in the intestines and in the bones and joints. The report of the Royal Commission introduced the terms eugonic and dysgonic to indicate the types of growth obtained on suitable media in the case of human and bovine types of bacilli respectively. A very authoritative investigation of the extent and type of tuberculous lesions in Glasgow children was published by John William Stewart Blacklock in 1932. The material consisted of the bodies of 1,800 children upon which postmortem examinations had been carried out. Among many important findings it was shown that the bovine type of bacillus was four times more common than the human type in abdominal lesions.

The Coli-typhoid Group. It has already been mentioned that the typhoid bacillus was discovered by Eberth in 1880. It was first cultured by Gaffky in 1884. Up to that time this was the only recognizable organism which had been cultured from the bowel. In 1885 Escherich (p. 392) discovered the *Bacillus coli communis* as a normal inhabitant of the intestine of man. It is also found in many animals. In his original paper Escherich noted the existence of two types of the organism. One, *B. coli* proper, consisted of relatively long rod-shaped organisms, which were motile and clotted milk slowly. The other type, which he called *B. lactis aerogenes*, but which is now referred to as *B. aerogenes* or *Aerobacter aerogenes*, consisted of shorter and thicker rods which were non-motile and caused a more rapid clotting of milk. Similar organisms were soon described, and it was noted that they all resembled the typhoid bacillus in morphological appearance and that they could not be differentiated from it or from each other by the size or appearance of their colonies. Motility or non-motility was considered to be a characteristic of the individual strain and not of the species, so that this criterion was not of value in differentiating organisms. The fundamental test was introduced in 1887 by André Chantemesse (1851–1919), an associate of Pasteur who became professor of hygiene in the Faculty of Medicine at Paris, and Fernand Widal (p. 418). They showed that coliform organisms—that is, those of similar type to *B. coli*—readily fermented lactose, which the typhoid bacillus did not. This test was later shown to indicate a fundamental distinction between non-pathogenic lactose-fermenters of coliform type, found in the intestine, in the soil, or on various plants on the one hand; and on the other the non-lactose-fermenters which were generally pathogenic.

Tests for fermentation of various other substances, especially carbohydrates, were quickly introduced, and Durham (p. 418) introduced the use of a tiny test-tube, inverted in the culture tube, so that gas production could be easily seen. The organisms for which these tests were designed included not only coliform organisms, but also those of the typhoid and dysentery groups. In 1898 O. Voges and Bernhard Proskauer (1851–1915), chemist, hygienist, and associate of Koch, who held important posts in Berlin, introduced a simple test, now known as the Voges-Proskauer Reaction, which is carried out by adding a few drops of potassium hydrate to a culture of the organism grown in a dextrose medium. A positive reaction is constituted by the development of a red, fluorescent colour. It was shown by them, and later by other bacteriologists, that this reaction differentiated *B. coli* from *B. aerogenes*. It was demonstrated in 1909 by Alfred Theodore MacConkey (1861–1931), later of the Lister Institute, that this reaction was especially valuable in identifying strains which had been isolated from the faeces. Mac-Conkey also introduced a well-known medium—his bile-salt neutral red lactose agar—on which lactose-fermenters and non-lactose-fermenters gave rose-pink and colourless colonies respectively.

These investigations were especially important in the routine examination of the purity of water-supplies. Owing to the vast degree of dilution which results when a small infecting dose of typhoid bacilli are introduced to a storage-reservoir, it is often impossible to detect them, although consumption of the water may lead to cases of typhoid. In these circumstances it was decided that the presence of *B. coli* in water could be taken as indicating contamination by faecal matter of human origin, and therefore possibly by the typhoid bacillus. The interpretation of these tests is complicated. Many factors have to be taken into account, such as the fouling of the reservoir by sea-birds. One of the most successful bacteriologists in this field was Sir A. C. Houston (p. 232).

Other organisms. It was shown by Fred Neufeld (1861–1945) in 1900 that pneumococci can be differentiated from other types of streptococci by the fact that they are soluble in bile, and despite later criticisms it is now admitted that, if the test is performed with sodium deoxycholate instead of bile, it is essentially sound. Much work has been done on the separation of the pneumococci into various types by studying their antigenic relationships. This work was first undertaken in 1909 by Neufeld and Ludwig Händel (1869–1939), who studied the protective effect in mice of antipneumono-coccal sera made from different strains. During the First World War Alphonse Raymond Dochez (1882–), Oswald Theodore Avery (1877–1955), and their colleagues at the Rockefeller Institute typed strains of pneumococci from cases of acute lobar pneumonia in man. They recognized three well-defined types, which were labelled Types I, II, and III, and they recognized that the remaining strains constituted a large heterogeneous group. This work was confirmed in South Africa by Frederick Spencer Lister (1876–1939) in 1916. The heterogeneous group, labelled Group IV, has since been in-tensively studied, and it has been shown that at least seventy types of pneumococci exist, and that these cover most of the strains found in clinical pneumonia. The pneumococcus possesses a distinct capsule which can be demonstrated by appropriate methods of staining; and Avery, Michael Heidelberger (1888–), and their colleagues have shown that the type specificity of an individual strain of pneumo-cocci is due to certain substances in their capsules (1923). These they have isolated and shown to be complex polysaccharides.

The streptococci generally present a more difficult problem than that group referred to as the pneumococci. Alexander Marmorek (1865–1923), who worked in Vienna and later at the Institut Pasteur in Paris, noticed in 1895 that certain strains of streptococci were able to cause lysis of erythrocytes both *in vivo* and *in vitro*. Eight years later Schottmüller (p. 401) suggested that the ability of a streptococcus to cause lysis *in vitro* should be used as a differential test. Schottmüller found that in general the colonies of streptococci on a medium containing blood were surrounded by a ring which was either clear or of a greenish colour. He thus differentiated the *Streptococcus haemolyticus* and the *S. viridans* respectively. The ability to ferment various sugars was first extensively used to differentiate the various streptococci by Mervyn Henry Gordon (1872–1953), bacteriologist to St. Bartholomew's Hospital, London, in 1902 and the following years. These fermentation tests are still employed, but rather in an ancillary capacity. Although green-producing streptococci do not now constitute a very important type, the haemolytic streptococci differentiated by Schottmüller form one of the most important and difficult groups of organisms, causing as they do a heterogeneous array of diseases. Division of the haemolytic streptococci into main groups according to the serological reactions of their contained polysaccharides was extensively studied by Rebecca Craighill Lancefield (1895–) in 1928 and subsequent years. It was found that most strains isolated from pathological lesions in man contained the same polysaccharide and were placed in Group A. Similarly, strains from lesions in the cow and in lower animals contained different polysaccharides and were placed in Groups B and C respectively. Altogether at least twelve groups, distinguished by their individual polysaccharides, have been identified. In addition a vast amount of work has been done on the antigenic types of the streptococci within these various groups. This research is too complex for mention here, but it may be said that outstanding work in this field has been done by Lancefield and her colleagues; by Fred Griffith (p. 339), who differentiated thirty types in haemolytic streptococci isolated from human lesions; and by Edgar William Todd (1889–1950).

As a result of serious outbreaks of cerebrospinal fever much attention has been paid in past years to the various types of meningococci. In 1909 Charles Henri Alfred Dopter (1873–1950) found in the nasopharynx of certain persons organisms which resembled the meningococcus morphologically, but which did not behave like the meningococcus when treated with antimeningococcal serum. In the same year Sir Joseph Arthur Arkwright (1864–1944) tested forty-five strains serologically and found that they could be divided into two broad groups, and that this sharp division was rather more marked in epidemic than in sporadic strains. In 1915 he found that nearly 90 per cent. of strains could be classified in two types. In the same year, in epidemic cases occurring in troops, Mervyn

Gordon and Everitt George Dunne Murray (1890–) found that the strains obtained from the cerebrospinal fluid could be classified as Groups I, II, III, or IV. Much work since that date has not materially altered the position. In the years previous to the outbreak of the Second World War typing of the prevailing strain in an epidemic area was of great importance, because a serum made using one group of the organism was not usually effective against the disease caused by another. Since the demonstration of the great efficiency of the sulphonamides in the treatment of cerebrospinal fever the typing of the organism has become more an academic procedure than of practical utility.

In the case of *Corynebacterium diphtheriae*, the diphtheria bacillus, the differentiation of types was not made until 1931 as the result of an epidemic of diphtheria at Leeds in which the fatality rate was very high. In that year James Walter McLeod (1887–) and his colleagues used a blood tellurite culture medium and showed that two types of colonies, morphologically distinct, were produced. One type of colony was the result of the growth of organisms obtained from very severe cases of the disease, and the other type was produced by organisms obtained from mild cases. McLeod therefore named these types of organisms the *gravis* and *mitis* strains respectively. In 1933 he showed that some strains of the organism conformed to neither of these culture types but showed characteristics of both. To this type the term *intermedius* strain was applied, and biochemical differences were found between the three strains. These observations were rapidly confirmed in Manchester, and very soon the three strains were shown to be present in various parts of the world. So far as is known these strains are stable varieties of the diphtheria bacillus.

Bacterial mutation and variation. From the early days of the study of bacteria it had been noted that morphological variants of well-known organisms sometimes appeared spontaneously, and might even be produced intentionally. As far back as 1881 Pasteur showed that a change in the temperature at which the anthrax bacillus was cultured resulted in a great reduction in spore formation and a decrease in virulence, and it was later found possible by Bordet and others to produce a strain of the anthrax bacillus which did not form spores at all. These changes were permanent on repeated sub-culture. Early in the twentieth century many other variations were discovered, including pigment-producing organisms which gave non-pigmenting strains, and organisms which depended for their growth on the presence of a certain chemical substance in the culture medium suddenly developing the ability to utilize another substance when deprived of it. The basic conception of true mutation in bacteria is that the change is hereditable; once it has occurred it is passed on to succeeding generations. Temporary variations in morphology are common, but they are the results of transient reactions to changes in environment, and when the original environment is restored succeeding generations do not show the change in morphology. Familiar examples are the involution forms found in diphtheria and plague bacilli under certain conditions (Fig. 108).

An important aspect of variation in bacteria depends on principles dealt with in the next section, but will be discussed here. Much research has been done on the antigenic differences shown by bacterial variants. The fundamental observation was made in 1903 by Theobald Smith and Arthur Lincoln Reagh (1871–1949), who were working with the bacillus of hog cholera. The normal form of this bacillus has flagella and is therefore motile. They happened to isolate a variant which was without flagella, and they prepared agglutinating sera (p. 417) against both strains. As a result they concluded that the normal motile type of hog cholera bacillus has two types of antigens, one of which is contained in the flagella and the other in the cell body. Reagh and a colleague showed in the following year that a certain degree of heat destroyed the flagellar antigens while leaving the antigens contained in the body (the somatic antigens) unaffected. These observations were neglected by scientists generally until 1917, when Weil and Felix, who were then working on a test for typhus fever which involved the use of a certain strain (X.19) of the *Bacillus proteus*, found that there were marked differences in the type of growth produced by the normal flagellated form of this organism and that of a non-flagellated variant. The colonies of the normal form were connected by an 'exhalation' (*Hauch*), a thin spreading growth; while those of the variant were

DEVELOPMENTS IN BACTERIOLOGY

sharply isolated and not connected (*Ohne Hauch*). The type of colony was briefly expressed as 'H' or 'O' forms. As the type of colony was an indication of the antigenic activity of the strain, flagellar antigens and somatic antigens have long been referred to as H antigens and O antigens respectively.

In 1920 and subsequent years Arkwright, working with organisms of the coli-typhoid-dysentery group, described another type of variation which has become of great importance. These bacilli normally give smooth colonies on solid media and a diffuse growth in fluid media. The variant forms produced rough colonies on solid media and granular growths in fluids. The variants often showed a clumping-together (agglutination) of bacilli in groups when placed in normal saline, whereas this did not occur with the non-variant forms. The normal bacilli giving smooth colonies were referred to as the Smooth (*S*) form, and the variants giving rough colonies as the Rough (*R*) form. The change from the normal to the variant form —referred to as the *S→R* variation—often occurs spontaneously, and it may be induced artificially in various ways. It apparently occurs in a series of steps, and it is relatively irreversible, the *R→S* variation being very difficult to induce. The *S→R* variation is frequently accompanied by loss of virulence and changes in antigenic behaviour which are of great importance in medical bacteriology.

One further type of variation should be mentioned, more especially as it is of great practical importance. It is demonstrated by variations in agglutinating properties (see p. 418), and it is found especially in the typhoid bacillus and in certain other members of the *Salmonella* group. In 1934 Arthur Felix (1887–1956) and R. Margaret Pitt prepared an antiserum to a strain of the typhoid bacillus containing the O antigen. They then tested various other strains of typhoid bacilli for agglutination by this antiserum, and at the same time they tested the virulence of each of these strains by injecting them into mice. They found that the most virulent strains showed little or no agglutination, while avirulent strains were agglutinated very completely. In a later paper Felix and Pitt showed that the in-agglutinability of the virulent strains was due to the presence in them of a special antigen, named by Felix the Virulence or Vi antigen. It was further found that an O antiserum would protect mice from the toxic effects of large doses of killed typhoid bacilli, but that it gave no protection against living virulent bacilli. But mice which were injected with a Vi antiserum were fully protected against living typhoid bacilli.

Testing of the individual's serum for the Vi reaction is especially useful in the case of suspected chronic carriers of the typhoid bacillus (p. 408), since in them the bacilli are frequently temporarily absent from the stools, but a positive Vi reaction is given in over 90 per cent. of such cases.

The Spirochaetes. It had been shown in 1881 that if syphilitic material is inoculated into the eye of a rabbit, a syphilitic lesion in the eye results. Just after the discovery of the *Treponema pallidum* this experiment was repeated and the result confirmed. Further, the discovery of the specific spirochaete in the lesions proved that they were syphilitic. The rabbit may also be infected by inoculation at other sites. Syphilis was first consistently transmitted to the anthropoid apes by Metchnikoff and Roux in 1903–5, and in many of their inoculated animals secondary lesions developed. As most of the animals died from broncho-pneumonia after a few weeks, tertiary lesions did not have time to develop. The first pure culture *in vitro* of the *Treponema pallidum* was obtained in 1911 by Hideyo Noguchi (p. 475) using material from a syphilitic rabbit. In the following year he obtained a pure culture of the organism using material from a human subject. The difficulties associated with this work are very great, and some experienced workers assert that the organism has never been obtained in pure culture *in vitro* without losing its virulence for the rabbit. In both rabbits and mice the organism remains alive in the lymphatic glands without losing its virulence, and if a particular strain has to be maintained, a convenient method is to inoculate it into one of these animals.

The Bacteriophage. In 1915 Twort (p. 395) was investigating staphylococci derived from calf lymph, and he noticed that in some cultures the colonies tended to disintegrate and disappear. He took some of these disintegrating colonies, filtered them, and made a high dilution of the filtrate. A few drops of this filtrate, if allowed to flow over a healthy culture of the staphylococcus, produced a degenerative change in the colonies. In 1917 d'Herelle (p. 395) was working with mixed cultures of organisms obtained from the stools of dysentery patients. He filtered some of these mixed cultures and found that the diluted filtrate produced lysis of the organisms in a broth-culture of the dysentery bacillus. By filtering the lysed culture and adding the diluted filtrate to a new culture of the dysentery bacillus, and by continuing to repeat this process in series, he showed that the lytic change was transmissible indefinitely. These two reactions were essentially similar, and they were referred to as the Twort-d'Herelle phenomenon. These investigations were continued by d'Herelle until 1930, and he gave to the lytic agent a name which has been generally adopted—the *bacteriophage*, or simply the *phage*.

Twort and d'Herelle demonstrated that a lytic agent is most active against one bacterial species or related types. It has no action against unrelated types of organism. The lytic agents are most commonly found in the intestinal tract, and when a susceptible organism is exposed to phage action, variants appear which are resistant to it. D'Herelle maintained that the phage is a filterable virus which is parasitic on certain bacteria, and this view has not been substantially countered. But he erred in thinking that there is only one phage, since it is now known that their number is very large. Twort showed that his lytic agent could resist a temperature of 60° C. for one hour, and there is now evidence that different types of phage show different degrees of resistance to harmful physical and chemical agents, in the same way that bacteria do. D'Herelle thought that his phage was made up of minute living particles. When a particle obtained entry into a bacterium, it multiplied to such a degree that the bacterium was ultimately ruptured. The electron-microscope lends some support to this view.

Carriers. A few years after the discovery of the diphtheria bacillus it became known that that organism sometimes persisted in the throats of patients while they were convalescing from the disease. In 1900 Horton-Smith (later Sir Percival Horton-Smith Hartley, 1867–1952) in his Goulstonian Lectures on typhoid fever reported the case of an apparently healthy individual who was excreting the typhoid bacillus in his urine. Little attention was paid to these and similar reports. At the beginning of the twentieth century enteric fever was endemic in many parts of Europe, and it caused an especially serious problem in south-west Germany. In 1902 Koch gave a famous address on this problem in which he predicted that some persons who were convalescing from enteric fever still excreted the organism in their bowel discharges, and that these persons constituted the main source of continued infection in endemic areas.

As a result of Koch's influence an effort was made to reduce the incidence of enteric fever at Trier. Koch recommended the establishment there of an experimental typhoid station, and this was done in 1903. It was placed under the directorship of Paul Frosch (1860–1928), one of Koch's chief assistants. He quickly confirmed Koch's theory of the importance of mild or unrecognized cases of enteric fever in spreading the disease. The investigations of Frosch were not only bacteriological but also epidemiological. He found that there were still small outbreaks of the disease which he could not trace to patients who had suffered from it in some mild form. It was known that the typhoid bacillus could persist for a long time in the human body in association with gall stones or with abscesses in bones. Frosch therefore put forward the hypothesis that the organism might also persist for long periods in the human intestinal tract without producing any evidence of disease.

The success of the Trier station led rapidly to the establishment of others in south-west Germany. One of these was at Saarbrücken, and it was under the directorship of Karl Wilhelm von Drigalski (1871–1950). Drigalski was later associated with Heinrich Conradi (1876–), another bacteriologist at a German typhoid station, in the introduction of a well-known medium for the cultivation of the typhoid bacillus. In 1903, before his station at Saarbrücken had been in operation for a year, Drigalski had made the first discovery of an individual who gave no history of an attack of enteric fever but who was excreting the organism. Similar cases were soon reported by others, and to describe such individuals the word 'carrier' was introduced. In English the use of the word with this meaning dates from 1906.

It was soon realized that some carriers could excrete the organism for many years, if not for life, and several tragic examples were reported. In 1906 the case of the wife of a master-baker of Strasbourg was reported. She had had enteric fever ten years previously, and about the time of the report she had certainly infected two persons who had died of enteric fever, and she had also probably infected several others who had survived. The best-known example of the healthy carrier is the female cook—known as 'Typhoid Mary' —who in various places in the United States between 1900 and 1907 certainly infected twenty-six persons with enteric fever; one of the patients died.

The carrier state in relation to other organisms, such as the paratyphoid bacillus, the dysentery bacillus, the diphtheria bacillus, and the meningococcus was soon established. In 1912 Sir John Charles Grant Ledingham (1875–1944) and Sir Joseph Arkwright (p. 402) published their important work, *The Carrier Problem in Infectious Diseases*, which illuminated many aspects of the question and gave a great impetus to further research. In elucidating the incidence of carriers of the diphtheria bacillus and the virulence of the organisms which they carried one of the most active workers in this country was George Stuart Graham-Smith (1875–1950) of Cambridge. The meningococcus was found in the nasopharynx of healthy persons by Heinrich Albrecht (1866–1922) and Anton Ghon (p. 426) in 1901, and it was soon established that during an epidemic infection of the nasopharynx is common in persons who do not develop meningitis. In military camps during the First World War it was found by James Alison Glover (1876–) that there was a positive relation between the carrier-rate and the case-rate. By spacing out the beds to more than 3ft. apart Glover was able to reduce both the carrier-rate and the case-rate.

THE STUDY OF IMMUNITY

In the production of disease by living organisms two main factors are involved. There is, firstly, the multiplication of the organisms in the body, and there is, secondly, the production by the organisms of poisonous substances or toxins. The former phenomena constitute infection, the results of the latter come under the heading intoxication or toxic effects. The first toxins to be investigated were those isolated from putrefying substances and named ptomaines (1876, by false formation from Greek *ptoma*, 'a corpse'). These are, in fact, alkaloids (p. 679).

Theories of immunity. About this time, under the stimulus of the brilliant practical results achieved by Pasteur in his specific methods of preventing and treating certain diseases to which reference has already been made, intense interest was focused on the methods by which the body naturally protects itself against the inroads of organisms. The problem was soon seen to be very complex. It had been known from the early seventies that normal blood can destroy bacteria which may gain entrance to it, but little was known of the method by which this was accomplished. There was much experimentation and discussion on the question whether the bacteria were deposited by the blood in some part of the body where they could do no harm, or whether they were held in a clot in those experiments in which shed blood was used, or whether, on the other hand, their destruction was due to some substances in the blood serum. Many of the preliminary difficulties were cleared away by George Henry Falkiner Nuttall (1862–1937), the founder of the *Journal of Hygiene* and of the journal *Parasitology*, who in 1888 demonstrated quite clearly that, so far as certain organisms are concerned, the destructive (bactericidal) property resides in the serum, that it is lost naturally after a period, and that it does not survive heating beyond about 50 or 55 degrees Centigrade, the actual temperature depending on the species of animal from which the serum was obtained. In this way the humoral theory of immunity began to take form. The term indicates that the substances which kill bacteria in the blood, or which in some way prevent them from producing their pathogenic effects, are themselves of a fluid nature and are contained in the blood serum.

Meanwhile a contrary theory was being developed by Élie [Ilya Ilyich] Metchnikoff (1845–1916), the Russian zoologist and pathologist who was during that period working in Odessa and at Messina. In 1887 Metchnikoff was appointed sub-director of the Pasteur Institute in Paris. Thereafter he lived in that city, and his later writings were mostly in French. In 1908 he was awarded a Nobel Prize. Metchnikoff greatly extended certain observations which were already slightly known, namely, that certain body cells have the property of ingesting micro-organisms and minute particles of foreign matter. To these cells generally Metchnikoff gave the name phagocytes (from Greek *phagein*, to eat, and *kutos*, cell). The large mononuclear cells of the blood and tissues were called by him macrophages, and were especially concerned with the ingestion of foreign particles. To the polymorphonuclear leucocytes of the blood, which were active in the ingestion of micro-organisms, he gave the term microphages. This was the foundation of the cellular or phagocytic theory of immunity, which dates from about 1884. The theory became widely known owing to the publication in 1892 of Metchnikoff's *Leçons sur la pathologie comparée de l'inflammation* ('Lectures on the comparative pathology of inflammation').

Discovery of toxins and antitoxins. We return now to the humoral theory, in connexion with which discoveries of first-rate importance were meanwhile being made. Loeffler had suspected that the characteristic features of the disease diphtheria were caused by toxins elaborated in the bodies of the diphtheria bacilli, first grown in pure culture by him, and that these toxins were passed out from the bacilli into the blood-stream (exotoxins). He had, however, been unable to prove this point. In 1888 Pierre Paul Émile Roux (1853–1933), the greatest French bacteriologist after Pasteur, and Yersin (p. 394), working at the Institut Pasteur, filtered broth cultures of the diphtheria bacillus through bacteriological filters and showed that the filtrates—which contained no organisms—produced death with the characteristic lesions when injected into animals susceptible to the diphtheria bacillus. They concluded that the bacillus produced its effects by virtue of the exotoxins which were contained in the filtrate.

The next developments came rapidly from Koch's laboratory. His assistant Carl Fraenkel (1861–1915) had tried injecting cultures of diphtheria bacilli, killed by heat, into animals. He found that after a short time living diphtheria bacilli could be injected into these animals without any ill effects. The injection of killed cultures was not immediately employed practically to produce immunity because almost simultaneously an easier and more dramatic method had been evolved. While Fraenkel was carrying out these experiments in Koch's laboratory, two other assistants of Koch, Emil Adolf von Behring (1854–1917) and Shibasaburo Kitasato (p. 393), had repeatedly injected successively increasing non-lethal doses of tetanus toxin into rabbits and mice and had shown that the serum of these treated animals, even when freed from cells, had developed the property of neutralizing tetanus toxin. Mixtures of the serum from treated animals and tetanus toxin could be injected into susceptible animals without ill effects. Further, they found that anything up to 300 times the minimal lethal dose of tetanus toxin for a normal mouse could be injected into these treated mice without ill effects. The serum of the treated mice had developed the property of destroying tetanus toxin, and Behring and Kitasato called this property 'antitoxic'. This was the first use of the word in medical literature. As an indication of the speed with which Koch had envisaged the possibilities following the discovery of a toxin by Roux and Yersin, it only remains to be stated that Fraenkel's discovery was published on 3 December 1890, and that the paper by Behring and Kitasato appeared in another journal on the following day. One week later a paper by Behring alone announced that animals treated with repeated non-lethal doses of diphtheria toxin developed antitoxic properties in their serum. Behring and Kitasato were therefore the discoverers of antitoxic immunity.

Since the symptoms of diphtheria are due to the toxins circulating in the blood, it was at once apparent that antitoxic serum obtained from an animal previously treated with diphtheria toxin might be used effectively in the treatment of diphtheria in the human subject. The brilliant results obtained are dealt with later (p. 434). After his initial experiments on guinea-pigs, Behring used sheep and goats to provide the antitoxin. The horse was finally used, and this is the animal now universally employed in serum establishments. It is important to inject a correct dose of antitoxin, and various methods of standardization were used without much success. In 1897 Ehrlich (p. 687) published his paper entitled 'Die Werthbemessung des Diphtherieheilserums und deren theoretische Grundlagen' ('The estimation of the antitoxic power of antidiphtheritic serum and its theoretical basis'). Ehrlich adopted as his standard for toxin the minimal lethal dose, namely, the smallest amount of toxin which would cause death within four days in a guinea-pig weighing 250 gm. His immunity unit was the amount of the antitoxic serum under test which would neutralize 100 times the minimal lethal dose of toxin in a guinea-pig of 250 gm.; if these amounts of toxin and antitoxin were injected together, neutralization was assumed if the guinea-pig survived. This paper contains very important principles and methods, and it is one of the classics of immunological science. In point of fact, Ehrlich's use of toxin as his basic standard was soon abandoned, because toxin was shown to be a very unstable substance which is gradually transformed into harmless toxoid. In its place an arbitrarily chosen antitoxic serum, dried and preserved in a vacuum in the presence of phosphorus pentoxide, is now used as a standard. These standard sera are now prepared and distributed to manufacturers under the responsibility of the World Health Organization.

Among many consequences of this paper was controversy over the nature of the interaction between toxin and antitoxin. In the paper Ehrlich had given the first description of his side-chain theory. The essential basis of this was that the molecule of protoplasm consists of a central atom grouping with a number of side-chains or receptors which have a combining affinity for food molecules and for toxins. When a toxin molecule becomes anchored to one of these receptors, poisoning of the cell results. The group composed of the receptor with its anchored toxin is then shed into the blood, and the shed receptor is replaced by a new one. In certain circumstances the production of new receptors is greatly in excess of requirements, and the blood is flooded with free receptors which become anchored to toxin molecules before the latter can affect the cells. This is the basis of the famous theory, which was progressively modified by Ehrlich to meet criticisms as they were put forward. Ehrlich thus regarded the union of toxin and antitoxin as of a firm chemical nature. The theory that the combination is of a loose chemical nature according to the law of mass action, as in the combination between a weak acid and a weak base, was advanced in 1902 by the Swedish physical chemist Svante August Arrhenius (1859–1927) and the Danish immunologist Thorvald Johannes Marius Madsen (1870–1957), who became director of the newly founded Danish State Serum Institute at Copenhagen. According to a third theory put forward (1903) by Bordet (p. 414) the union is physical and not chemical, and is akin to the process of adsorption. The view currently held now is a combination and modification of all three theories.

Bacteriolysis. The demonstration of antitoxin in the blood of immunized animals soon led to the discovery of other important properties of immune sera. In 1894 Richard Pfeiffer (p. 393) discovered a test by which he could distinguish the cholera vibrio from other organisms closely resembling it. He found that if a guinea-pig is immunized against cholera, live cholera vibrios can be injected into its peritoneal cavity without ill effects. If he withdrew a loopful of peritoneal fluid a few minutes after the injection of the organisms and examined it microscopically, the vibrios were seen to become motionless, and they gradually swelled up and then disintegrated. They had been lysed by some substance in the peritoneal fluid. Other organisms which resembled the cholera vibrio were not thus affected. Pfeiffer also showed that the phenomenon occurred *in vitro*, but that the power of the peritoneal fluid to produce bacteriolysis is abolished if it is heated to 60° C. It was then shown by Metchnikoff that the heated immune peritoneal fluid could be reactivated by adding some normal peritoneal exudate. Pfeiffer's reaction was thus specific. This phenomenon had far-reaching immunological results. The phenomenon of bacteriolysis which it showed was studied by many different methods.

One of these was used (1898) by Jules Jean Baptiste Vincent Bordet (1870–), a Belgian who was then working at the Pasteur Institute in Paris. Bordet later enriched immunology by numerous valuable investigations. In 1901 he founded the Institut Pasteur in Brussels, and in 1919 he was awarded a Nobel Prize. Bordet repeated Pfeiffer's experiment *in vitro* using heated immune serum instead of the peritoneal exudate. No bacteriolysis took place, but on adding unheated normal serum the organisms were lysed. The normal serum lost its property of reactivating the heated immune serum if it was itself heated. Bordet concluded that two substances are necessary to enable the phenomenon of bacteriolysis to occur. One of these substances is present only in the immune serum and is resistant to heat. The other is present in both normal and immune serum and is destroyed by heat.

About 1898 it was shown that if the blood of a rabbit is injected into a guinea-pig, the serum of the guinea-pig becomes toxic for rabbits. It was suggested that the toxic property of the serum of the treated guinea-pig was due to certain substances liberated owing to the destruction of the rabbit blood-corpuscles previously injected into the guinea-pig. The same relationship was found when other animals were used, and in each case the phenomenon was specific. In 1898 Bordet began his active investigations into this property of haemolysis. He proved that the phenomenon was identical in type with bacteriolysis. He also showed that it could take place *in vitro*. To take the above example, the serum of the guinea-pig treated with rabbit blood is referred to as immune serum. If a small quantity of this serum is added to a suspension of rabbit blood corpuscles in salt solution, the corpuscles rapidly disintegrate and the haemoglobin passes into the fluid medium. Bordet then discovered that, if the immune serum is heated to 55° C., it loses its capacity to produce haemolysis, but that this capacity can be restored by adding a quantity of serum from a normal guinea-pig or a normal rabbit. As in the case of bacteriolysis, in the case of haemolysis Bordet postulated the presence in the immune serum of a thermostable substance which sensitized the foreign red corpuscles (or the bacteria), and also the presence in the normal serum of a thermolabile substance which caused the haemolysis of the sensitized corpuscles (or the lysis of the sensitized bacteria).

The whole subject was then taken up (1899) in its immunological implications by Ehrlich and Julius Morgenroth (1871–1924). They agreed in the main with Bordet, but they adopted a different terminology for the two substances actively concerned. The thermostable sensitizing substance in the immune serum they called the immune body or amboceptor; and the thermolabile dissolving substance in the normal serum they called complement. These terms were generally adopted, and they have long been basic elements in the vocabulary of immunological literature. Bordet believed that there is only one type of complement, which is active not only in bacteriolysis and haemolysis but also in similar kinds of immune reaction subsequently discovered. Ehrlich and Morgenroth, on the other hand, contended that each kind of these immune reactions involved a different type of complement. The question of the unity or diversity of complement was hotly debated by Bordet, Ehrlich, and many subsequent investigators, and it has possibly not yet been completely settled. There seems little doubt, however, but that the unitary theory will be finally adopted.

Complement-fixation. In 1901 Bordet and his assistant Octave Gengou (1875–1957) first observed and studied the phenomenon of complement-fixation which was to have wide implications. They were impressed by the similarity between bacteriolysis and haemolysis. In both phenomena the bacteria (or the red cells) were sensitized by a specific sensitizing substance (immune body); but the lysis of bacteria or of red cells did not occur until complement (in the form of normal serum) had been added. The complement used was identical in both reactions. In testing the possibilities they immunized an animal against plague. They mixed its serum with plague bacilli and added complement. To the resulting fluid they then added the serum of an animal which had been treated with red blood corpuscles, and also a quantity of washed corpuscles. There were therefore two separate systems, the bacteriolytic system and the subsequently added haemolytic system. The only difference between the systems was that the haemolytic system was not strictly complete, since no complement was included in the mixture of immune haemolytic serum and the red corpuscles. But theoretically this should not have mattered, since this haemolytic system was added to the bacteriolytic system which already contained complement. The addition of this complement to their partial haemolytic system, when the latter was added to the bacteriolytic system, should therefore have resulted in lysis of the red corpuscles. But in fact no haemolysis took place. Bordet and Gengou therefore concluded that the complement in the first system had been fixed by the sensitized plague bacilli, so that there was no free complement to cause lysis of the red corpuscles in the second system. They then made the important deduction that, if they had been given the plague immune serum without knowing that it had been obtained from an animal immunized against plague, they could have ascertained this fact by carrying out their complement-fixation test as described above. If no haemolysis occurred, the serum was from an animal or human subject who had been sensitized by experience of the plague bacillus. If on the other hand haemolysis did occur, the organism to which the animal or individual had been sensitized was not the plague bacillus. The importance of such a test in the diagnosis of infections was obvious, and Bordet and Gengou demonstrated its effectiveness in the case of the organisms of anthrax, typhoid fever, and other conditions.

The most brilliant and widely-used of all complement-fixation tests is the Wassermann reaction for the presence of syphilitic infection at some time in the individual's life. This was described by Wassermann (p. 390), Albert Neisser (p. 390), the discoverer of the gonococcus, and their associates in 1906. In this reaction the patient's serum provides the immune serum. At the time when the reaction was first introduced the *Treponema pallidum* (p. 689), the causative organism of syphilis, had been discovered in the previous year, but it had not yet been cultivated. In place therefore of the causative organism Wassermann used in his reaction a watery extract of the liver of a syphilitic foetus. This test gave a high proportion of positive results (absence of haemolysis in the haemolytic system) in syphilitics, and negative results (haemolysis) in normal controls. It was described as a complement-fixation test. But in 1907 Constantin Levaditi (1874–1953), a Romanian who held important posts at the Pasteur Institute in Paris, showed that extracts of normal liver gave identical results with those in which syphilitic liver had been used. It was later shown that better results could be obtained by using alcoholic instead of watery extracts. The addition of an alcoholic solution of cholesterol, an important modification, was introduced in 1924 by Carl Hamilton Browning (1881–), who had been assistant to Ehrlich and was then professor of bacteriology in the University of Glasgow, and his colleague the alienist Ivy Mackenzie (1877–1959). The Wassermann Reaction is therefore not a complement-fixation test in the true sense, and its real mechanism has not yet been explained.

Agglutinins and precipitins. From about 1890 Metchnikoff and other scientists had known that, in the case of certain organisms, if the organism was grown in the serum of an animal which had been immunized to it, the bacilli did not grow uniformly in the medium but tended to clump together into masses which sank to the bottom of the medium. This phenomenon was called agglutination. It was first systematically studied in 1896 by Herbert Edward Durham (1866–1945) and Max Gruber (1853–1927). Gruber then held a chair in Vienna, and Durham, later bacteriologist to Guy's Hospital, was working in his institute. Durham showed that if a uniform suspension of an organism was mixed with the serum of an animal which had been treated with that organism, clumping of the bacteria in the suspension rapidly took place. The bacteria were not killed by the agglutinating process, and their virulence was often not in any way affected. Within a few months of the publication of the reaction by Durham and Gruber it was used as a diagnostic test for typhoid by Georges Fernand Isidore Widal (1862–1929) and independently by A. S. Grünbaum (p. 259). The specific substances in the serum which produced the agglutination were called agglutinins. Since then these reactions have been widely studied.

Meanwhile Rudolf Kraus (1868–1932) had shown (1897) that, if the bacteria-free filtrates of cultures of the organisms of plague, cholera or typhoid were injected into an animal, its serum developed the property of causing a precipitate to form in the filtrate which had been injected. This process of precipitation is supposed to be effected by immune substances called precipitins formed by the treated animal. The reaction is specific. It has been much studied from the aspect of diagnosis. In 1899 Bordet showed that the phenomenon also occurred with non-bacterial substances such as milk. It has been used successfully to differentiate the various types of plant and animal proteins, and Nuttall and others have employed it to distinguish animal species.

In 1895 Joseph Denys (?–1932) and Joseph Leclef (? – ?), two Belgian biologists working in Louvain, made observations of some importance which were in conflict with the views of Metchnikoff. Metchnikoff held that the leucocytes from an animal immunized against a certain organism engulfed that organism more actively than did the leucocytes of a normal animal. Working with streptococci Denys and Leclef showed that, if the leucocytes from an animal treated with these organisms were placed in normal serum, they did not engulf streptococci more readily than did leucocytes from a normal animal. But if the same leucocytes from the immunized animal were then placed in immune serum the phagocytosis was very active. In 1902 (Sir) William Boog Leishman (1865–1926) independently showed the effect of serum in stimulating the phagocytic activity of leucocytes, but he did not investigate the mechanism of the phenomenon. Leishman was a professional military medical officer, and he ultimately became Director-General of the Army Medical Services of the British Army. He is better known for his work on the preparation of the anti-typhoid vaccine, for the stain for blood and organisms which bears his name, and especially for his discovery of *Leishmania donovani*, the protozoon parasite which is the cause of kala-azar.

The whole problem was now investigated by (Sir) Almroth Edward Wright (1861–1947), who had then left his chair of pathology at the Army Medical School at Netley to become the director of the Institute of Pathology at St. Mary's Hospital, Paddington. In co-operation with Stewart Ranken Douglas (1871–1936) he showed (1903, 1904) that the action of both normal and immune serum is due to the presence of certain thermolabile substances which act, not upon the leucocytes, but upon the organisms. In some way these substances change the organisms so that phagocytosis proceeds more easily. They were regarded as a kind of sauce which made the organisms more palatable for the leucocytes. They were hence called opsonins (Greek, *opsonein*, to prepare food for). Wright investigated this matter over many years, and his opsonic index was well known. His results were much criticized, and his methods have been discontinued. But in general no substitute to his main theory has been advanced. In practice Wright made use of these tests especially in connexion with his method of treatment by autogenous vaccines—that is, vaccines prepared from organisms cultured from the lesion of the individual patient. This method was very popular before the end of the first decade of the twentieth century, as is shown by Sir Ralph Bloomfield Bonington's injunction to 'Stimulate the phagocytes' in Shaw's *The Doctor's Dilemma* which was first produced in 1906, though in these exhortations 'B. B.' and Shaw mixed up humoral and cellular theories of immunity in a way that no bacteriologist of the period would have countenanced.

The reactions which have been described in this section have certain features in common. Thus, antitoxins, bacteriolysins, haemolysins, and agglutinins are all produced in the blood of an animal which has been treated in some way with an appropriate organism, the dose (or doses) of which must not have been sufficiently large to cause the death of the animal. Similar results can be obtained by injecting non-lethal doses of snake-venom, in which case antivenin is produced in the blood of the injected animal. In order to simplify the terminology adopted by investigators of particular reactions of this type, it became customary to refer to all substances, the injection of which produced such changes in the blood, as antigens. Antigens may therefore be bacteria, or their toxins, or poisons of various types, or indeed many other substances. Similarly, it became customary to use the term antibodies for all the different types of substances produced in the blood by such injections. Antibodies therefore include antitoxins, lysins, agglutinins, praecipitins, and opsonins.

Anaphylaxis and hypersensitiveness. The antigen-antibody reactions discussed in the preceding paragraphs all tend to protect the individual against the effects of the poisons produced by bacteria. They are in a sense 'prophylactic'. But even while the early investigations on these subjects were being carried out, it became evident that similar reactions could occur in the body which were destructive rather than preservative. About the beginning of the century Theobald Smith (1859–1934), then a professor at Harvard University and later of the Rockefeller Institute for Medical Research, noted that guinea-pigs used for the testing of diphtheria antitoxin became acutely ill if the test injections were separated by long intervals. No great attention was paid to these observations at the time. But in 1902 Charles Robert Richet (1850–1935), professor of physiology at Paris, and his colleagues discovered that certain animal poisons produced a type of hypersensitiveness when injected into dogs. Working with extracts made, first from the Portuguese man-of-war and later from the tentacles of certain sea anemones, they found the minimum dose which was actively toxic for dogs, causing death in two or three days. Smaller doses than this toxic dose produced only transient symptoms. But if a dog was reinjected with a similar small dose after an interval of several weeks, a violent reaction occurred and death ensued within a day. During the interval the first dose had sensitized the animal to the second dose, which was then able to exert very toxic effects. Richet somewhat erroneously regarded the reaction as one which produced the opposite of protection, and he hence called the phenomenon anaphylaxis. This term has persisted. In subsequent years Richet studied the phenomenon very thoroughly.

The Theobald Smith phenomenon was investigated (1905) by Richard Ernst Wilhelm Otto (1872–1952), who showed that it was not the toxin in the toxin-antitoxin mixture which produced the effect but the horse-serum in which it was contained. The reaction did not take place unless there had been an interval of about ten days between the successive injections, and large doses of the immune serum could be given at short intervals without producing any ill effects. In the following year the phenomenon was further studied by Rosenau (p. 234) and John F. Anderson (1873–1958). They showed that the reaction was specific; a guinea-pig which had been injected with horse-serum was not hypersensitive to the serum of other animals. Further, they demonstrated that an extremely minute amount of serum was sufficient to produce hypersensitivity.

With the increasing use of diphtheria antitoxin in treatment (p. 434) it was found that some patients suffered from a condition known as serum sickness. In its milder forms the patients exhibited drowsiness, excessive sweating, and urticarial rashes; in more severe cases pains in the joints were common. It was noted that these symptoms did not occur immediately after the injection of the serum; in the case of the generalized rash an interval of seven days was common. As further experience of antitoxin treatment was obtained in various countries it was found that the reaction after the injection of serum was occasionally accelerated and of considerable violence. Investigation demonstrated that the patients who showed this phenomenon had been injected with horse-serum at some time previously. The phenomenon after reinjection resembled true anaphylaxis.

In 1903 Nicolas Maurice Arthus (1862–1945) found that if rabbits were injected subcutaneously with horse-serum, with suitable intervals between the injections, local reactions appeared at the site of injection. After a few injections the tissues at the site became swollen and red. Such reactions were at first transient, but as the injections proceeded the site became indurated, and ultimately there was breaking down of the tissues, leading to an ulcer. This was an example of local anaphylaxis, and such a phenomenon was occasionally seen after serum injection in human subjects. Mild general serum reactions were quite common during the early days of serum-therapy; but as purified and concentrated antisera have become available in recent years they have become much less frequent. The incidence of serum sickness led, in cases where it was known or suspected that serum had previously been given, to the practice of desensitizing the patient by several very small doses before the therapeutic dose was administered.

It has already been mentioned that in 1882 Koch discovered the tubercle bacillus. He was obsessed by the ambition to discover a serum or some similar biological measure which would be effective in combating the dreadful mortality then caused by 'the Captain of the Men of Death'. In his investigations carried out during the next ten years he made certain significant observations which are not even now completely understood. In 1891 Koch showed that if a healthy guinea-pig is injected subcutaneously with live tubercle bacilli, only a slight local lesion is caused by the injection, and this heals in a few days. But about a fortnight later a nodule appears at the injection site, and this nodule soon breaks down and forms an ulcer which does not heal. The lymph glands which drain the area become swollen, and exhibit the typical cheesy change (caseation) found in the tuberculous process. The guinea-pig ultimately dies of tuberculosis with the ulcer still unhealed. If, however, this inoculated guinea-pig is injected again with live tubercle bacilli at another site about a month or more after the first injection, the response is quite different. The glands of the area show no change, but at the site of injection there appears a shallow ulcer which heals quickly. There is thus a marked difference between the response to a first injection with live tubercle bacilli and the response to a second injection. Years later it was shown that certain conditions had to be satisfied to enable these results to occur; among these was the condition that the first injection had to be sufficiently large to produce a chronic tuberculous process, but not large enough to cause acute tuberculosis.

This important result is known as Koch's phenomenon. In the same paper he reported his findings on the injection of dead tubercle bacilli. In the case of a normal *un*infected guinea-pig no constitutional effects of any kind were produced, though sometimes a sterile cold abscess, of no consequence, was produced at the site of injection. On the other hand, if dead tubercle bacilli were injected into a tuberculous guinea-pig—that is, a normal guinea-pig that had been injected with live bacilli at least four weeks previously—Koch's phenomenon resulted. Koch therefore deduced that the phenomenon must be due to some chemical substance which was present not only in living but also in dead tubercle bacilli. This led him to his search for a product of the tubercle bacillus which would be immunizing without being toxic.

Later in the same year (1891) Koch announced his discovery of this substance, which he had named tuberculin. He grew tubercle bacilli on a glycerine medium for six to eight weeks. The culture was then killed by heat, and reduced by evaporation to a tenth of its previous volume. The resulting fluid was then passed through a bacteriological filter so that the dead bacilli were removed. The resulting filtrate was a clear, brown, syrupy liquid. It contained substances produced in the medium by the growth of the bacilli, and also the products of disintegration of the bacilli themselves. Koch, and many other persons, subsequently prepared various modifications, so that Koch's original preparation is referred to as 'old tuberculin'.

Koch found that the injection of 2 ml. of old tuberculin into a normal guinea-pig produced practically no effect, whereas the injection of a very small amount (0·01 ml.) into a guinea-pig which had been injected with living tubercle bacilli about two months previously resulted in a highly significant threefold reaction. The guinea-pig died within a few hours. At post-mortem examination a local reaction, consisting of swelling and a dark-red colour at the injection site, was found. There was also a focal reaction, consisting of congestion of the related glands, and a constitutional reaction, which led to the death of the animal. This typical tuberculin reaction is also obtained in human subjects. An uninfected infant will stand the injection of 1 ml. of old tuberculin without reacting. An adult, who at some period of his life has been infected by the tubercle bacillus but who is not showing any clinical signs of the disease tuberculosis, will experience only malaise and slight pains in the limbs on the injection of o·oi ml. On the other hand, the injection of this amount into a patient suffering from clinical tuberculosis results in severe malaise, an exacerbation of his symptoms, and a transient increase of temperature. It should be said that in all the experiments mentioned in these paragraphs the injections were given subcutaneously.

These important observations of Koch set in train extensive investigations which are still being continued today. We cannot devote space to their discussion, but we give a very brief summary to show the influence which they had on the general problems of immunity. Koch originally put forward tuberculin as a cure for tuberculosis, though he later modified this claim. For many years there were supporters of this view, and until comparatively recently tuberculin was used by some physicians in a few special types of tuberculosis. From the other point of view, evidence accumulated to the effect that the subcutaneous tuberculin test gave fairly reliable proof that the individual tested had at one time been infected by the tubercle bacillus. It took many years to bring out the fact that, from the diagnostic aspect, what was wanted was not so much an answer to the question whether the individual had at one time been infected, as some visible reaction indicating whether the disease from which the patient was suffering was, or was not, clinical tuberculosis. Still, it was agreed that in many instances information of value could be supplied by the test. There was, however, a drawback in the fact that the reaction in an apparently normal individual was at times severe, and in a person suffering from clinical tuberculosis it was sometimes serious. In these circumstances other methods of testing which dispensed with the necessity of injecting the tuberculin subcutaneously were introduced. Two of these have had a very wide application. The von Pirquet test was introduced by Clemens Peter von Pirquet (1874–1929). Von Pirquet, an Austrian paediatrician, held the chair of paediatrics at Johns Hopkins University at Baltimore for two years before he returned to Europe in 1910 to fill the corresponding chairs at Breslau and at Vienna. His test, which consists in scarifying a small area of skin through a drop of Koch's old tuberculin, was first described by him in 1907. It is not followed by any focal or constitutional reaction, and the only local reaction in a positive case is the appearance of a red indurated area at the site of application. In 1908 another Austrian, Ernst Moro (1874–1951), who was then an assistant at the University of Munich, introduced a method of testing in which a piece of tuberculin ointment was rubbed into a small area of skin; a positive reaction is shown by the development of papules in the inuncted area within twenty-four hours.

Both of these tests have the disadvantage that the operator has very little control over the amount of tuberculin which is introduced into the skin of the individual tested. In 1910 Charles Mantoux (1877–1947), who was then a physician and specialist in tuberculosis near Cannes, introduced the intracutaneous test which bears his name. This test combines the advantages of Koch's subcutaneous reaction without its disadvantages. The test is performed by injecting a weak dilution of old tuberculin intracutaneously—that is, into the substance of the skin, and not under the skin as in the subcutaneous test. There are no constitutional or focal reactions, and the local reaction usually permits fairly accurate readings. If the reaction is negative the test is repeated on several occasions, using stronger and stronger dilutions of tuberculin. In recent years more rapid modifications of the von Pirquet test have been introduced, and much work has been done on the purification of Koch's tuberculin and in the search for its active principle. Growth of the tubercle bacillus on synthetic media has enabled a substance known as P.P.D. (purified protein derivative) to be isolated, and this substance is now used instead of Koch's old tuberculin in most of the tests.

From the time of their first introduction these percutaneous and intracutaneous tests were used to ascertain the degree of tuberculin sensitivity of urban and rural populations. Von Pirquet published in 1909 an extensive series of tuberculin tests in inhabitants of Vienna at different ages. Among these were over 1,100 children who showed no clinical evidence of tuberculosis. His results proved that about 70 per cent. of these children had been infected by the tubercle bacillus by the age of ten years, and probably over 90 per cent. by the age of fourteen years. In other large continental cities similar results were speedily obtained by Calmette, Mantoux, and others. It was admitted by these workers that the subjects upon whom they had carried out the tests came from the lowest social classes, in which overcrowding—and consequently opportunity to become infected by the tubercle bacillus—was common. About that time the tuberculin test began to take on a new significance, since in 1912 the Austrian, Anton Ghon (1866–1936), then professor of pathological anatomy at the German University in Prague, pointed out that in the bodies of most children a small pea-like body, really an arrested tuberculous focus, can be demonstrated. This he called the primary focus, and it is now often called Ghon's focus. Years later Karl Ernst Ranke (1870–1926) showed that the development of the focus is accompanied by a tuberculous process in the lymph gland which drains that part of the body in which the primary focus is situated. This important finding was published (1928) after Ranke's death. The combination of the primary focus and the diseased gland together constitute the primary complex, and the study of this phenomenon has provided an entirely new attitude to the development of pulmonary tuberculosis in the human subject. With improvements in X-ray plant in recent years the primary complex is more easily diagnosed during life, and its significance and its relationship to clinical tuberculosis has been increasingly studied. These discoveries stimulated interest in tuberculin tests, and the substance which Koch originally announced as a 'cure' has continued to give valuable information from the aspects of diagnosis and epidemiology.

Before leaving the subject of tuberculosis we may say that in the early years of the twentieth century various attempts were made to protect individuals against this disease by injecting them with tubercle bacilli, killed or treated in various ways. None was successful. But in 1906 Léon Charles Albert Calmette (1863–1933) of the Pasteur Institute and his collaborator Camille Guérin (1872–) introduced a new method, viz. the use of living bacilli so attenuated as to have lost their disease-producing properties, while retaining their power of stimulating a protective reaction when injected into an animal. They used a bovine strain of the tubercle bacillus—that type of the organism which has its natural habitat in cattle, but not infrequently causes disease in the human subject. They grew this

strain on a special medium for a period of several years. At the end
of this period they claimed, as a result of tests, that the strain had
become innocuous for all laboratory animals. The vaccine so produced was given the name 'B.C.G.' (Bacille-Calmette-Guérin), and
it was used for the inoculation of calves in France for many years.
In 1922 Calmette and Guérin first used it on human infants. It was
given in three doses by mouth during the first ten days of life.
Between 1922 and 1928 Calmette had treated over 50,000 French
children, and he claimed that he had by this method conferred immunity to the tubercle bacillus on a large proportion of these
children. Much work was done with B.C.G. on the Continent,
but in the United Kingdom, as a result of statistical and other criticisms, it was viewed with the greatest scepticism. It is now being
officially tested by the Medical Research Council; the original oral
method of administration has now been abandoned in favour of the
intradermal route, and the use of the vaccine at ten to thirteen years
of age is preferred to vaccination in infancy.

It will be appreciated that, when Koch introduced tuberculin as a
curative substance, he was certainly influenced by the brilliant
discovery of diphtheria antitoxin which had been carried out in his
institute. But while from the aspect of immunity diphtheria is one
of the easiest of diseases to understand, tuberculosis is certainly one
of the most difficult. A vast amount of work on the subject of
immunity in tuberculosis has been carried out during the last sixty
years, and it is still far from being understood. No antitoxin has
ever been discovered in the blood of patients recovering from this
disease, and it is now held that the skin reactions which indicate
sensitivity to tuberculin and immunity to the disease tuberculosis
do not necessarily go hand in hand.

Allergy and allergic diseases. During the early phases of this work
on tuberculosis investigations of a much less spectacular nature were
being carried out on certain diseases which were not dangerous
but which nevertheless caused great annoyance and inconvenience
to those addicted to them. The summer catarrh generally known as
hay fever had been known for over three centuries. It was first
described in 1565 by Leonardo Botallo (1530–?), who gave examples
of healthy men in whom it was caused by smelling the odour of

roses. The name summer catarrh was first given to the disease by John Bostock (1773–1846) in his description (1819) of his own personal sufferings in this disease. He and many others noted the tightness in the chest during an attack. John Elliotson (p. 509) gave a classical account of the condition (1831). One of Elliotson's patients suggested to him that the emanation from grass which presumably produced his attacks was pollen. Elliotson was much impressed. He argued in favour of the suggestion, and he described a similar condition due to the skin emanations from a rabbit.

Interest had also been shown in bronchial or spasmodic asthma, a disease which has an ancient history. It was described by Aretaeus of Cappadocia (p. 239), whose account of it is excellent. In the year 1552 the distinguished physician Jerome Cardan (1501–76) of Pavia was called especially from Italy to Edinburgh to advise treatment for John Hamilton, archbishop of St. Andrews, who had suffered from asthma for ten years. Cardan cured—or relieved—him by diet, regular exercise and sleep, and by prohibiting the use of feathers in his bed. In this last recommendation Cardan was centuries ahead of his time. The modern history of the disease begins with Thomas Willis (p. 245), who was the first to suggest tentatively that the disease consisted essentially in spasm of the bronchial muscles. The same theory was supported by Sir John Floyer (p. 171), and it was argued even more thoroughly from the clinical aspect by Laennec (p. 172). Physiological studies during the middle of the nineteenth century, especially by François Achille Longet (1811–71) in 1842 and by Alfred Wilhelm Volkmann (p. 261) in 1844. Volkmann demonstrated that stimulation of the vagus nerve produces constriction of the bronchi. But these experiments did not show what precipitated the attack. One of the most important of the early treatises was *On asthma; its pathology and treatment* (1860) by Henry Hyde Salter (1823–71). He described attacks of asthma due to hay, to ipecacuanha, and to the emanations of certain animals such as cats, dogs, cattle, horses, and rabbits. Salter recognized that asthma and hay fever were similar or even identical in nature.

The first fundamental experiments on these conditions were those described by Charles Harrison Blackley (1820–1900) in his book *Experimental Researches on the Causes and Nature of* Catarrhus aestivus (*Hay-fever*), published in London in 1873. These experiments were extended in what was in effect a later edition of this book, now published with the title *Hay Fever: Its Causes, Treatment and effective Prevention*, 1880. Blackley noted that if crude pollen is instilled into the eyes of hay-fever subjects, swelling of the membranes results. He also noted that pollen-grains rubbed into a scratch in the skin produced a local reaction. In certain quarters it was held that this reaction was due to the mechanical effect of the pollen grains, and it was not until 1903 that William Philipps Dunbar (1863–1922) showed that this was not the case, since the reaction could be produced by a saline or alcoholic extract of the pollen grains. Dunbar also claimed that he had found in hay-fever patients some of the phenomena associated with the production of toxins and antitoxins.

We now return to the subject of serum sickness. This condition had been first studied adequately by von Pirquet and his assistant Béla Schick (p. 434), then both working in Vienna. Their book, *Die Serumkrankheit*, published at Vienna in 1905, is important in that it had wider implications than its title suggests. In the following year von Pirquet discussed the reactions after serum in relation to what was known about conditions produced by substances such as pollen, and he adopted the view that such diseases and phenomena were due to antigen-antibody reactions. He coined the term allergy to indicate the state of hypersensitiveness in which man or animals react in an 'altered' or abnormal manner to contact with certain foreign substances. The abnormal reaction to a foreign serum is one example, and the classical case is the fatal general reaction to tuberculin in the guinea-pig, the most severe of allergic phenomena. This exemplifies a response to a non-living antigen. But examples of the response following sensitization with living bacteria are common, and Koch's phenomenon provides perhaps the most clear-cut example. In their investigations on serum disease von Pirquet and Schick had noted that reinjection of horse serum caused an intense oedema at the site of injection if more than seven to ten days had elapsed since the first injection. In 1907 von Pirquet introduced his tuberculin skin test, and he suggested that it was of a similar nature.

These observations led to the skin-testing of individuals for allergic reactions to various foreign proteins, and they made possible a new attitude to such conditions as hay fever and eczema. In 1911 Leonard Noon (1878–1913), working in what is now the Wright-Fleming Institute at St. Mary's Hospital, Paddington, introduced the method of testing individuals for pollen sensitivity by the instillation of a pollen extract into the conjunctival sac. As a pollen unit he fixed arbitrarily the amount of pollen toxin which could be extracted from a millionth of a gramme of the pollen of Timothy grass. The extract was prepared by alternate freezing and thawing, and then boiling. By using various dilutions it was possible to assess the subject's pollen resistance at any time. Noon then commenced immunizing the subjects by the subcutaneous injection of minute doses of pollen extract. He showed that if the doses were too large or too frequent the subject's resistance was diminished. Noon's work was carried on by John Freeman (1877–), who later made other contributions to this subject. It was shown in 1910 by John Auer (1875–1948) and Paul A. Lewis (1879–1929) that in true anaphylaxis in guinea-pigs death is due to asphyxia which is caused by a tetanic contraction of the bronchial muscles preventing any air from entering the lungs. In the same year Samuel James Meltzer (1851–1920) suggested that the mechanism of production of an attack of bronchial asthma was similar, and this condition was thus finally included among the allergic diseases.

During the last fifty years there has been much controversy over the nature of allergy. It is clear that anaphylactic phenomena are closely connected with the liberation of histamine (pp. 555 ff.) or histamine-like substances. Despite the fact that many allergic responses are not protective—as is the case in the immunity to specific antigens discussed in the following sections—it is probable that the basic mechanism which produces allergic responses is very similar to the antigen-antibody reactions which are the cause of specific immunity. To a more detailed consideration of this subject we now turn.

Types of immunity. The word immunity is from the Latin meaning exemption from military service. In medicine it means exemption, relative or absolute, from liability to become infected with a certain disease. Immunity in the medical sense is of various kinds. There is species immunity, some species not being liable to diseases to which others fall victims. There is relative and there is absolute immunity. There is natural (innate) and acquired immunity. Natural immunity refers to the fact that some animals (including man) are naturally very insusceptible to infection with certain diseases and more susceptible to infection with others. Acquired immunity may be of two kinds, active and passive. The distinction between active and passive immunity is not easy to define in a few words, but it is important to appreciate it.

Active immunity refers to the state which results in the body when the individual himself manufactures his own immunity as a result of some stimulus which he has received. The stimulus may be a natural happening. For example, the individual may be infected with measles. His cells are thereafter altered in such a way that they are at short notice able to produce substances which counteract any subsequent infection with measles. A second attack of this disease is therefore very uncommon; the disease gives a strong active immunity. The same state of readiness on the part of the body cells to produce adequate amounts of counteracting substances when required may be brought about more slowly. If an individual breathes in from time to time very small numbers of diphtheria bacilli, the cells are gradually sensitized, and a slowly acquired immunity to diphtheria is produced. This type of immunity is *active*, because the required protective substances are produced when needed by reason of the activity of the body cells. These examples are of *spontaneous active immunity*. They are caused by the individual taking into his body either large numbers of the infecting organism (with the consequent development of the disease itself), or very small numbers repeated over a long period (without the development of the disease, but with the acquirement by the body cells of the capacity to react rapidly and effectively should a large dose of the organisms be subsequently received).

In *passive acquired immunity*, on the other hand, the individual does not himself manufacture the specific protective substances, but has them manufactured for him. Most infants are immune to diphtheria. This is due to the fact that the infant before birth receives certain substances from the mother, and most adults have in their blood substances which protect against infection with the diphtheria bacillus. This is *congenital passive immunity*. On the other hand, if the blood serum of an individual or an animal which is known to contain these substances which protect against diphtheria is injected into a susceptible individual, the latter will be for a short time immune to diphtheria. This is *artificial passive immunity*.

Artificial active immunity is long-lasting. If small doses of the organism concerned are received into the body from time to time, the immunity may persist throughout life. Artificial passive immunity, on the other hand, lasts only a matter of weeks, and on it subsequent small doses of the organism have no 'boosting' effect.

For convenience we summarize here the different types of immunity:

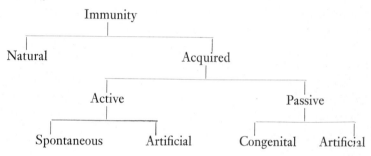

The early observers found that when organisms are cultivated outside the body they lose their virulence to a greater or less degree. Pasteur found this for chicken cholera (p. 339). He found, moreover, that such attenuated cultures, when inoculated, protect against the disease. By the use of attenuated cultures he succeeded in establishing a state of active immunity against chicken cholera. But there are many other ways of attenuating the virulence of an organism. Thus, in 1882, Pasteur showed that the virulence of anthrax bacilli could be reduced by growing them at a high temperature. These bacilli of reduced virulence could be injected into a sheep. If they produced any obvious effect, it was a febrile reaction and not characteristic of the disease, but the animals were protected against an attack of the disease itself.

It has been found, however, that the same kind of immunity which is produced by administering attenuated cultures is sometimes given even by dead cultures. Nearly all active immunization is therefore done by inoculating such killed cultures. Pasteur called these preparations 'vaccines' as a tribute to the work of Jenner. The most familiar and effective vaccine is that against typhoid fever. Moreover, it has been found that in certain cases the principle of the induction of active immunity may be applied directly in the treatment of disease. The conditions that respond best to this line of treatment are those which present some localized infection, such as a boil or carbuncle. In such cases we must suppose that, while the local capacity for resistance is lowered, yet reserves of resistance in other parts of the body can be brought into play. These reserves are called up by the signal that reaches them by the reaction of the body against the vaccine.

It has been shown that, for the production of active immunity, the actual bodies of the disease-producing organisms are not always necessary. In some cases, toxins obtained from these organisms are themselves sufficient to induce active immunity. The matter has long been of great medical importance and it has achieved brilliant results in the prevention of diphtheria (p. 436).

We turn to passive immunity. The production of passive immunity by the passive transfer of serum containing antibodies is most typically seen in the case of the new-born child, which is almost invariably immune to diphtheria. Most mothers are immune to this disease, and the immune substances are passed to the foetus in the mother's blood. After birth the immune substances in the infant's blood gradually disappear, so that in a few months it becomes susceptible to diphtheria. This is congenital passive immunity. In later life passive immunity is sometimes conferred artificially by injecting diphtheria antitoxin. The resulting immunity lasts only for a few weeks, but the method is sometimes useful where children in a ward have been exposed to infection from a diphtheria patient.

SOME PRACTICAL APPLICATIONS OF IMMUNITY

We may now consider a few special applications of our knowledge of the defences against bacterial action.

(*a*) *Diphtheria*. The use of diphtheria antitoxin in experimental animals has already been described. The first human subject treated with diphtheria antitoxin was a child in a clinic in Berlin; the injection was given on Christmas night, 1891. Antidiphtheritic serum was placed on the market in 1892. In a few years its administration had become a routine part of the treatment of the disease. Diphtheria antitoxin is one of the greatest additions to therapeutics. It came generally into use for treatment about 1895, and within ten years the case-mortality rate from all types of diphtheria had fallen to less than half what it had been in the pre-antitoxic era, and in later years it was to fall by half as much again. These figures are open to the objection that at about the time of the introduction of antitoxin many more cases of diphtheria, diagnosed as such, were established by bacteriological diagnosis. Consequently, mild cases which would previously have been called something else, were now included as diphtheria and automatically lowered the death-rate of the whole group. Nevertheless, when consideration is given only to some grave types of diphtheria, the diagnosis of which would never have been in doubt at any period, a very marked effect on the case-mortality is apparent after the introduction of antitoxin. For example, in the London fever hospitals the case-mortality of laryngeal diphtheria in 1894 was 62 per cent. After the introduction of antitoxin the mortality fell rapidly; in 1910 it was under 12 per cent. (Fig. 113).

An important aspect of the reaction of the body to the diphtheria toxin was revealed by Bela Schick (1877–) of Vienna in 1908. The technique of inducing it was perfected by him in 1913, and the test is known by his name. He showed that susceptibility to the disease could be detected by the skin reaction after injection of minute doses into it. It has thus been found that new-born infants are seldom susceptible and that the proportion of susceptibles increases up to one year of age, but after that it gradually diminishes. Many large series of results obtained by the Schick test at different ages have been published, and a general agreement in the results has been found. We may take the figures of Abraham Zingher (1885–1927) for New York (1923) as fairly typical. He found that by the age of 6 months about half the infants tested gave a positive result. The proportion of positives then increased rapidly until at the age of

I year over 90 per cent. were positive. Up to about 3 years of age this figure dropped very little. Then there was a rapid fall, succeeded by a more gradual decline. By the 7th year 50 per cent. were positive; at 12 years 25 per cent., and between 20 and 30 years, 12 per cent. Even in the age-group over 60 years about 5 per cent. of individuals were found to be positive.

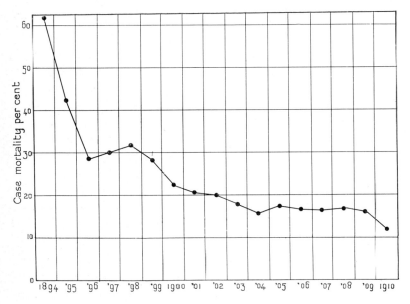

FIG. 113. Case mortality rate of laryngeal diphtheria, London fever hospitals, 1894–1910. Diphtheria antitoxin introduced in 1895, and used extensively from 1896 onwards

Actually, the figures for the older age-groups tend to be somewhat misleading. These older positive reactors are potentially more liable to react to a stimulus than are the younger positives, so that the disease in them is much less frequent than the figures might suggest. These data do bring out the reason why diphtheria is mainly a disease of childhood, and is relatively seldom encountered in adults. They also make it evident that steps for protecting individuals against contracting the disease—prophylactic measures, as they are called—need only be taken with a fraction of the population. The useful term prophylaxis is derived from a Greek word meaning a watchman or guard. It is used to describe preventive measures against disease in general, and the term 'specific prophylaxis' is applied to that form of protection which is achieved through the production of artificial immunity.

Such prophylactic measures have been available against diphtheria since 1913, when von Behring (p. 411) introduced toxin-antitoxin mixture. This consisted of a quantity of the toxin produced by the diphtheria bacillus, mixed with a quantity of antitoxin which was sufficient to destroy its toxic properties, but not enough to counter-act its immunizing effect. This method was used very widely in the United States and Canada, especially in New York City under the supervision of William Hallock Park (1863–1939) and Zingher. Many thousands of children were immunized in New York alone. It was, however, found that the temporary combination of the toxin and the antitoxin was not invariably stable. On a few occasions dissociation took place and serious occurrences were reported. Alexander Thomas Glenny (1882–) in Great Britain and Gaston Léon Ramon (1886–) in France showed that the toxin could be treated with formalin to produce formol-toxoid (F.T.), which is a very satisfactory prophy-lactic. Glenny later showed that the toxoid can be treated with alum (A.P.T.) to give a prophylactic which is more slowly absorbed, and thus produces a higher degree of immunity. The use of these prophylactics has spread very widely in this country, especially since the Second World War, and still more efficient prophylactics have been introduced. In the period just before the war the number of notifications of diphtheria in England and Wales yearly was over 55,000, and of these patients about 3,000 died every year. In 1956 there were only 51 cases of, and 8 deaths from, diphtheria in the whole of England and Wales. We can now look forward with some confidence to the day when the present type of diphtheria will be practically wiped out.

(b) *Scarlet fever.* This disease was not discussed in the section on bacteriology because, despite very extensive investigation over the last sixty years, no clear-cut results have ever been obtained. But from the immunological aspect certain investigations must be noted. In a later section (p. 735) it is explained that scarlet fever cannot be written-off as a disease of no consequence.

From the beginning of the present century streptococci were very frequently recovered from the throats of scarlet-fever patients, and when the haemolytic streptococci were differentiated from the non-haemolytic streptococci, if any organism was found it was the *Streptococcus pyogenes*. But the next step in proving that this organism is the cause of the disease was a complete failure. The streptococcus was found to be pathogenic for various laboratory animals, but on injection it hardly ever produced typical scarlet fever. But there were certain exceptions. For example, in 1911 Landsteiner (p. 700), Levaditi (p. 417) and Emil Prášek (1884–1934) of Vienna produced typical scarlet fever in monkeys by inoculating the throat with material from scarlet fever patients, and the *Str. pyogenes* was recovered from the throats of the monkeys. But these organisms did not produce the disease when transmitted to the throats of other monkeys.

In 1918 Werner Schultz (1878–1944) and Willy Charlton (1889–) of Berlin described a reaction produced by the intradermal injection of a small amount of serum obtained from an individual in the convalescent stage of scarlet fever, into an area covered by rash in a scarlet-fever patient at the height of the disease. In most cases an area of blanching appeared around the site of the injection. It was also found that the serum of many normal individuals would give the same extinction of the rash. At the time the phenomenon was explained by the assumption that normal serum contained some substance which was removed from it during an attack of scarlet fever. But in 1923 William Mair, a London bacteriologist, noted that of the normal sera which he had tested in this way, those obtained from young children failed to produce the blanching of the scarlatiniform rash much more frequently then did the sera of adults. Further, in the case of one child he had tested her serum and found that it failed to produce blanching. She then happened to have an attack of scarlet fever, and after her recovery Mair tested her serum again and found that it now produced blanching. He therefore suggested that the scarlet-fever rash is due to a circulating toxin. During the course of the disease an antitoxin is produced which neutralizes this toxin, and after recovery the antitoxin persists in the blood. If the serum of a person who has at some time had scarlet fever is used for the test, the small amount of antitoxin in his serum is sufficient to neutralize the toxin in the skin round the site of injection, and blanching of the rash results.

At the expense of anticipating the sequel it should be said that the Schultz–Charlton test is still used, but not in the manner described by its authors. If we assume that Mair's hypothesis was correct, and if we use as a test subject a patient suffering from an undoubted attack of scarlet fever, the test is for the presence of circulating antitoxin in the different sera injected. But a more rapid method was introduced to give this information. On the other hand, the physician sometimes needs to know whether a suspicious rash is or is not due to scarlet fever. He now uses a minute dose of scarlet-fever antitoxin and performs, as it were, the Schultz–Charlton test in reverse. Blanching indicates that the rash is due to scarlet fever.

Meanwhile George Frederick Dick (1881–) of the University of Chicago had in collaboration with his wife Gladys Rowena Henry Dick (1881–) embarked on this elusive question. In 1921 they inoculated the throats of a number of volunteers with organisms obtained from the throats of scarlet-fever patients. Some volunteers developed tonsillitis, but in no case was scarlet fever produced. Two years later they used a strain of the haemolytic streptococcus which they had isolated from the finger of a nurse who was suffering from surgical scarlet fever. The throats of ten volunteers were swabbed with this strain, and two of them developed typical scarlet fever.

It was known that some strains of haemolytic streptococci produced toxic filtrates, but in laboratory animals these filtrates gave rise to minimal effects. With the new interpretation of the Schultz–Charlton reaction in mind the Dicks now filtered broth cultures of strains of haemolytic streptococci obtained from scarlet-fever patients. They found that if a few drops of such a filtrate in a high dilution was injected intradermally into the skin of a person who had not had scarlet fever, an erythema developed round the site of injection, whereas in a person who had previously had scarlet fever no such erythema developed. If a larger amount of this toxic filtrate was injected into a specially susceptible individual, he sometimes developed a transient scarlatiniform rash with febrile symptoms.

The Dick test for susceptibility to scarlet fever is analogous to the Schick test for susceptibility to diphtheria, but it is much less reliable.

Scarlet-fever antitoxin is prepared in horses in much the same way as diphtheria antitoxin. The serum is certainly valuable against the rash and other toxic manifestations of the disease, and it sometimes has a beneficial effect on those symptoms and complications which are due to the invasive, in contradistinction to the erythrogenic, properties of the streptococcus. It is now used only for serious cases, and in some countries it has been entirely abandoned. No satisfactory toxoid has yet been produced from the erythrogenic toxin, so that active immunity can only be obtained by injecting successively increasing doses of the toxin itself. The resulting immunity against the toxin may prevent the occurrence of the rash should the individual be exposed to infection, but its inhibitory effect on the invasiveness of the organism is unfortunately much less.

(c) *Plague* differs from diphtheria in that the organisms, instead of remaining localized, multiply rapidly throughout the body of the victim. As in the case of most diseases of this type, the toxins of the plague bacillus are chiefly endotoxins, unlike those of the diphtheria bacillus, which are exotoxins (p. 411). Thus, the filtrate of a culture of plague bacilli is but little toxic and confers little or no immunity. The use of vaccines made from killed cultures of plague bacilli is especially associated with the name of the Russian, Waldemar Mordecai Wolff Haffkine (1860–1930), a pupil of Pasteur, who was for many years in the service of the British Government in India, the plague centre of the world. Figures which have been collected suggest that the use of Haffkine's vaccine confers a fourfold protection against an attack of plague, and a sixfold protection against death if the individual does become infected. In recent years, in Java, Madagascar, and other places, much use has been made of a vaccine made from living plague bacilli. The results appear to be satisfactory, and these vaccines can certainly be used with safety under proper conditions.

(d) *Tetanus.* In the same year (1889) in which Kitasato isolated the tetanus bacillus Knud Faber (1862–1956) obtained an exotoxin from a pure culture of the organism, and he showed that injection of this toxin into an experimental animal produced the symptoms of the disease. The discovery of tetanus antitoxin in the following year has already been described (p. 412). Kitasato also worked on the action of tetanus toxin, and he showed that after the injection of the toxin into an experimental animal there is a long period between the injection of the toxin and the appearance of symptoms, the period in general increasing with increase in size of the animal. Reference was made to this phenomenon in the *Aphorisms* of Hippocrates (p. 37). It was soon shown that after the injection of tetanus toxin into an animal, very little is found in the blood. The absorbing and difficult question of the fate of the toxin soon arose. Experiments on this problem were carried out as early as 1890 by Alessandro Bruschettini (1868–1932), who injected toxin into the sciatic nerve of a rabbit and produced tetanus; after death the lumbar region of the spinal cord contained toxin. In 1897 Auguste Charles Marie (1864–1935) showed that if a lethal dose of toxin was injected into the forepaw of a rabbit death took place; but if the nerve root of the peripheral nerves leading from the paw had previously been cut, tetanus did not develop. This strongly supported the view that the toxin was absorbed by the peripheral nerves and conveyed in them to the spinal cord. In 1902 A. C. Marie and Victor Morax (1866–1935), working at the Institut Pasteur, showed that a peripheral nerve can take up the toxin only if its nerve endings are intact. Their experiments suggested that the toxin passes only upwards towards the cord, and not centrifugally—that is, from the cord to the surface. The ultimate destination of the toxin is the cells in the anterior horn of the grey matter of the cord, where it becomes fixed. Symptoms of tetanus do not appear until this destination has been reached, and this fact explains the lag in their occurrence.

This is the classical theory of the action of tetanus toxin. It was essentially completed by the early years of the present century. From 1934 onwards it was severely criticized by J. J. Abel (p. 685) and his co-workers. According to their view the tetanus toxin exerts a local action on both the anterior horn cells and on the motor nerve endings; it reaches the anterior horn of the cord by way of the blood and lymph. Although we do not know the mechanism by which, according to the classical theory, the toxin passes up in the axis cylinders of the nerves, this theory is on the whole more favoured. The problem has, however, by no means been settled.

Soon after the isolation of the tetanus bacillus bacteriologists began to inquire about the function of the terminal spores. It was at this time that important experiments were carried out by Louis Vaillard (1850–1935), director of the French military medical school, the Val-de-Grâce, and his co-worker Jules Rouget (1864–1936). They found that if a tetanus culture was heated to destroy the bacillary forms and the toxin, the spores could be injected into an animal without the disease occurring. They showed microscopically that the spores were ingested by phagocytes. If, however, there was crushing of the wound with necrosis of tissue, or if there was secondary infection, the spores germinated and toxin was produced. Since then many research workers have investigated the problem, which has proved to be very complex. The problem became of great practical importance early in the First World War, when in the second month of the war nearly 1 in every 100 British wounded developed tetanus from the soil of the heavily cultivated fields of Flanders. As time passed many observers found tetanus bacilli and spores in the wounds of men who never developed tetanus. Further, it was reported that in some cases of tetanus the organism must have been introduced into the body years previously. Why did the organisms lie dormant during these long periods, and what caused their sudden activity? The first suggestion of an explanation arose from the work of William John Tulloch (1887–) of St. Andrews, who showed in 1919 that if tetanus spores which had been freed from toxin were injected into the tissues along with the toxins of certain other anaerobic organisms, such as the gas-gangrene bacillus, or with substances which generally lowered the resistance of the tissues, such as saponin or lactic acid, tetanus resulted. In the same year Bulloch (p. 396) and William Cramer (1878–1945), a notable writer on biochemistry and the cancer problem, showed that if ionizable calcium salts, such as calcium chloride, were injected along with toxin-free tetanus spores, tetanus resulted. In 1927 Fildes (p. 396) showed that the calcium salt produced necrosis, and that in necrosed tissue there was a lowering of the oxygen-reduction potential. This is probably the explanation, although many other factors have to be considered.

The discovery of tetanus antitoxin by Behring and Kitasato was an important advance in prophylaxis and therapeutics. The pure toxin is too powerful for the immunization of animals, and they used toxin modified by treatment with iodine tri-chloride. By 1892 Behring was by this method producing large quantities of antitoxin from horses. By 1921 Glenny (p. 436) and his co-workers were using toxin-antitoxin mixture for immunization. About 1926 the use of tetanus toxoid—that is, toxin modified by treatment with formalin— began to be used for the immunization of horses, and this method is still in use. The antitoxin has since 1950 been standardized on an international standard. For many years after its first production tetanus toxin was regarded as a prophylactic rather than a therapeutic measure. When injected in adequate doses soon after the infliction of the wound it was supposed to prevent the development of tetanus. Once spasms had developed, however, death was regarded as inevitable. The explanation is that the tissues of the nervous system have a strong affinity for tetanus toxin, but no such affinity for tetanus antitoxin. The antitoxin will neutralize toxin in the blood very effectively, but once the toxin becomes fixed to the nervous tissues its action is very problematical. When definite tetanus had developed the custom was to inject large doses into the arachnoid space in the lumbar region or in the bulbar region of the central nervous system. This technique was much influenced by experiments carried out by Sherrington (p. 263). Nowadays the intrathecal route has been largely abandoned, and the treatment of cases in which tetanus has actually developed has been much improved by appropriate surgical intervention, and by the employment of general anaesthesia, artificial respiration, and muscle relaxants.

Shortly after the introduction of tetanus toxoid it was used for the active immunization of human subjects, possibly first by Ramon (p. 436) and Christian Zoeller (1888–1934) of the Institut Pasteur in Paris (1927). The course, of two injections separated by an interval of six weeks, is followed by a marked rise in the antitoxin content of the blood, and a third injection about a year later completes the series. Booster injections are given every few years, and if a serious wound is suffered antitoxin may be injected or a further dose of toxoid may be given.

The test of any method designed to prevent the onset of tetanus is its efficacy in battle casualties, where wounds are often lacerated and contaminated with earth. The figures for British service cases during the First World War were published by Sir David Bruce and others. In 1914 few men received prophylactic antitoxin after wounding, and the highest monthly incidence was 9·0 cases of tetanus per 1,000 wounded. From 1915 until the end of the war practically every wounded man received antitoxin, and by 1918 the incidence of tetanus had been reduced to about 0·6 per 1,000 wounded. There was also a marked decrease of case mortality in wounded men who developed tetanus. During the whole war 2,385 wounded men developed tetanus.

The method of active immunization with toxoid introduced into the British Army previous to the outbreak of the Second World War was worked out by Sir John Smith Knox Boyd (1891–), who was later in a position to report on its efficacy in war conditions. In the conditions which supervened in the short period of active warfare prior to the completion of the Dunkirk evacuation a large proportion of the wounded did not receive any antitoxin upon wounding, yet no case of tetanus occurred in over 16,000 wounded men who had been actively immunized. In 1,800 wounded men who had not been actively immunized there were eight cases of tetanus. In the later stages of the war the figures were similar, although a few cases of tetanus did occur among the actively immunized.

(e) *Enteric fever.* Although the bodies of typhoid bacilli contain toxic substances, these do not pass to any degree into the surrounding medium, and there is no production of an exotoxin such as that obtained from the organisms of diphtheria and tetanus. The production of a true antitoxin in the case of the typhoid bacillus is therefore neither logical nor a practical possibility. Nevertheless, in 1907 Chantemesse (p. 399) immunized horses with dead cultures of the typhoid bacillus and used their sera in the treatment of enteric-fever patients. Between the wars others produced modifications of his sera, and in 1935 Felix prepared a serum by the immunization of horses with a typhoid antigen containing both the Vi and O principles (p. 405). None of these methods has been so clearly effective as were the diphtheria and tetanus antitoxins on their introduction.

Prophylactic immunization against typhoid fever is a more successful proposition. It was first introduced by Sir Almroth Wright (p. 419), and his preliminary note on the method appeared in 1896. His full description appeared in the following year, and from 1900 onwards he published several papers in which the results were discussed. Wright used cultures of a certain standard of virulence, killed them by heat, and then made up the vaccine to contain a pre-determined number of bacilli. It was given in two injections with a ten-day interval between them. Observations of results were made on British troops in South Africa during the Boer War and in India. The figures were collected and examined by an Antityphoid Committee, and a valuable statistical investigation was made by Greenwood (p. 736) and George Udny Yule (1871–1951) in 1915. During the siege of Ladysmith the incidence of typhoid fever in 1,705 inoculated soldiers was 2·0 per cent., whereas among 10,529 un-inoculated the incidence was 14·0 per cent. In the First World War the British Army was 90 per cent. inoculated against typhoid by the end of 1915. The overall figures for the incidence of this disease in British troops during the Boer War and the First World War respectively were 105 cases and 2·35 cases per 1,000 strength. These figures are impressive.

During the First World War, because of the incidence of para-typhoid fever on the Eastern Fronts, killed cultures of paratyphoid bacilli A and B were added to the vaccine, so that it became familiarly known as T.A.B. Between the wars the work of Felix on the Vi antigen emphasized the desirability of using virulent strains of the organisms, and the T.A.B. vaccine as used in the Second World War contained 1,000 million typhoid bacilli and 750 million each of paratyphoid bacilli A and B per ml. The results obtained were investigated by Boyd (p. 443), who showed that the British vaccine was very effective. When enteric fever broke out among Italian prisoners it was not controlled by Italian T.A.B., but was subsequently fully controlled by British T.A.B. On the other hand British prisoners of war in Italian hands, who had all been immunized before their capture, showed at one period no cases of enteric fever.

Despite the success of T.A.B. in preventing enteric fever among troops and in other circumstances where the vaccinated persons are under control, it is very doubtful if the use of the method on the general population would be successful in eliminating enteric fever. For the very great reduction in this condition in recent years we are indebted almost entirely to public health measures.

VIRUS DISEASES

We have been dealing so far with organisms which can be seen under a high power of the optical microscope, magnifying to about 2,000 diameters. Such organisms can be made more visible by appropriate stains and can be cultivated on suitable culture media containing protein and other substances. Despite the enormous urge to discover new organisms which marked the two closing decades of the nineteenth century, it was strange that a number of common diseases still eluded the efforts of the greatest bacteriologists. Measles, mumps, and poliomyelitis were cases in point.

In 1892 a new twist was given to the problem. All bacteriologists made use of special types of filters for the purpose of separating bacteria from any fluid which contained them. These filters, made of unglazed porcelain or a special type of natural earth, all had pores which were so small that no known organisms would pass through them. In 1892 the Russian botanist Dmitri Alexievitch Ivanowski was working with a disease of tobacco plants called tobacco mosaic. It was known that the sap of an affected plant would transmit the disease to a healthy plant. But Ivanowski demonstrated that the diseased sap will transmit the disease even after it has been passed through a bacteriological filter. Whatever it was that caused the disease was therefore so small that it would pass through these minute pores. Similar observations on tobacco mosaic were also carried out—more completely, and possibly independently—by Martinus Willem Beijerinck (1851–1931) in Holland in 1898. In this year also Loeffler (p. 392) and Frosch (p. 408) showed that foot-and-mouth disease in cattle was due to a virus which passed through a bacteriological filter. Hence diseases of this type could affect both plants and animals.

These infecting agents were therefore called filterable viruses, and filterability was regarded as a criterion of their nature. But it was found impossible to filter the virus of rabies and of vaccinia, and it soon became apparent that the possibility of these minute bodies passing through the pores of a bacteriological filter depended on other factors in addition to the relative size of organism and pore. The filtration could be affected by the electrical charges on the virus and on the filter respectively, by the temperature at which the filtration was carried out, the duration of the filtration, and other factors. Hence these agents came to be described more simply as viruses, using the word in a much more limited and specific sense than had been the case in previous centuries. Investigation soon showed that the agents of many other diseases were viruses, including smallpox, chicken-pox, cow-pox, herpes zoster, poliomyelitis, epidemic influenza, typhus, rabies, yellow fever, measles, mumps, and the common cold.

The vaccinia virus, and a very few of the other large viruses, can be stained and seen under the highest powers of the optical microscope as minute dots. All the others are too minute to be capable of optical resolution. Various methods have been used to make them visible. In 1925 Joseph Edwin Barnard (1869–1949) developed a reflecting microscope which utilized only the short ultra-violet rays, and with this he was able to obtain photographs of some of the larger viruses. Shortly afterwards the electron microscope was developed, and with its improvement excellent pictures of even the smallest viruses were gradually obtained. Theoretically this instrument will magnify up to about 200,000 diameters, but in virus work a practical limit of 50,000 diameters is convenient. The first pictures by this method were made in Berlin by Bodo J. H. H. A. von Borries (1905–56) and Ernst August Ruska (1906–) in 1938. It has been much improved recently by the technique of metal shadowing, in which the virus particles are thrown into relief by a coating of atoms of a suitable metal. The sizes of the individual viruses can be gauged in this manner. They can also be ascertained by filtration through specially prepared collodion membranes, each containing pores of a known size. These Gradacol membranes have proved very satisfactory. Of other methods in use that of the high-speed centrifuge, which throws down viruses of different sizes at different rates, may be mentioned. The unit of length for measuring viruses is the millimicron (one millionth of a millimetre), usually written 'mμ'.

On this basis the width of a staphylococcus—a globular organism, common in pus, which is easily visible with the conventional microscope—is 1,000 mμ, and the length of a rod-shaped bacillus, such as that of diphtheria, is about twice or thrice the width of a staphylococcus. The largest virus—that of psittacosis, a disease of parrots and of man—measures 275 mμ in diameter; it is about a quarter of the width of a staphylococcus. But there are many smaller viruses. That of influenza measures about 100 mμ, while the virus of infantile paralysis measures only 10 mμ.

The minute size of these bodies raised the question whether they really could be living individuals with something approaching organs in their structure. The doubt was increased when it was considered that the molecule of the globulin (a complex protein) which occurs in serum measures about 6 mμ, while that of egg albumin measures 4 mμ. Nevertheless, it was thought that these viruses were indeed living entities, even the smallest. Those who held these views received a more severe shock in 1935, when the virus of the mosaic disease of tobacco was obtained in what seemed to be crystalline form by Wendell Meredith Stanley (1904–), then of the Rockefeller Institute for Medical Research. Stanley, a biochemist, has been specially active in this field, and for his work on this subject and on influenza he shared the Nobel Prize in Chemistry in 1946. It was pointed out that the crystals were not true crystals; they had the appearance of crystals only in two dimensions. But three years later it was shown that the virus of a certain disease of tomatoes could be obtained as typical three-dimensional protein crystals. This observation, together with the results of subsequent researches, led to the supposition that viruses might after all not be living organisms in the generally accepted sense of the term. The whole question is of the greatest interest, not only to the bacteriologist but also to the biologist. It involves careful reconsideration of the fundamental characteristics of living matter. These difficult problems are beyond the scope of this book. It may, however, be said that the plant viruses are regarded as being rather different in nature from the viruses of animals and man. These latter viruses are considered to be minute organisms with the characteristic property that they grow only within living cells.

This property made cultivation of viruses difficult. In 1915 Noguchi (p. 475) obtained a pure culture of the vaccinia virus by growing it in the testes of living rabbits and bulls. Three years later he was able, by drying the virus, to keep it alive for over twelve months but with a decrease in its virulence. Methods such as these were not convenient for laboratory work. In 1925, however, Frederic Parker (1890–) and Robert Nason Nye (1892–1947) grew the viruses of herpes simplex and of vaccinia in tissue cultures prepared with material from rabbit's testis. This work was confirmed by Alexis Carrel (1873–1944) and Thomas Milton Rivers (1888–). The way was now open for many modifications of the method. If large-scale immunization against a virus disease is required, a large-scale method for growing the organism must be available. Such a method was discovered in 1931 by Woodruff (p. 697) and Ernest William Goodpasture (1886–1960), who inoculated the virus on the chorio-allantoic membrane of a developing chick embryo in the egg. It later became apparent that Ogston (p. 392) had tried this method in 1881 for the cultivation of bacteria. This technique is now used on a commercial scale for the cultivation of the influenza virus.

The practical application of work on virus diseases in man is generally of so recent application as to warrant only brief mention here. There is no evidence that any virus produces a toxin similar to that produced by the diphtheria bacillus, and, though the phenomena of immunity associated with the viruses are in general similar to those shown by the bacteria, practical methods for im-munizing are complicated by the fact that virus particles which are actually in the body cells cannot be influenced by circulating anti-bodies. In smallpox there has been no fundamental advance in the method of immunization since the time of Jenner, apart from the introduction of glycerinated calf lymph instead of the human lymph formerly obtained in arm-to-arm vaccination. Since 1931 two similar methods of producing the vaccine by using chick embryo tissue culture technique have been introduced by Rivers and by Good-pasture respectively. But there is no evidence that these vaccines are really better or more effective than calf lymph, which has generally been considered very satisfactory and which is manufactured by procedures that are now highly standardized.

Since the disastrous pandemic of 1918–19 influenza has demanded the earnest consideration of epidemiologists and immunologists. Research carried out after the discovery of the influenza bacillus in 1893 showed that it was frequently, though not always, present in patients suffering from epidemic influenza, and that, though it was probably not the actual cause of the disease, it was probably responsible for some of the complications. In 1918–19 no virus was discovered in influenza patients; but the technique for the isolation of viruses was then in its infancy. Within twelve years many technical advances were made. Late in 1932 Sir Patrick Playfair Laidlaw (1881–1940) and George William Dunkin (1886–1942) isolated the virus of distemper in dogs. In this work they found ferrets highly susceptible, and they perfected a technique to enable ferrets to be used experimentally without risk of adventitious infections. At the end of 1932 influenza broke out in London, and Laidlaw and his colleagues Christopher Howard Andrewes (1896–) and Wilson Smith (1897–), in search for an animal susceptible to the influenza virus, turned first to their ferrets which proved to be very susceptible. It was found that mice could be infected from them. In 1940 Sir Frank Macfarlane Burnet (1899–) showed that the virus would grow if it was inoculated into the amniotic cavity of a chick embryo. This 1933 London virus is now known as virus A. In 1940 also Thomas Francis (1900–), then of New York, isolated a virus which was not identical with the London virus, and is now named virus B. The influenza virus consists mainly of spherical bodies measuring 90 to 100 mμ in diameter, though elongated forms also occur. Much work has been done on the preparation of influenza vaccines, but although some success has been achieved, any immunity conferred is relatively short-lived.

The only other virus disease which we shall mention here is poliomyelitis. The history of this disease is dealt with elsewhere (p. 272). The virus is one of the smallest known, the globular elements measuring only 10 mμ in diameter. Electron micrograph pictures of these bodies have been made (Fig. 114). Landsteiner (p. 700) and Erwin Popper were the first to transmit the disease to monkeys (1909). This work was extended in the same year at the Rockefeller Institute for Medical Research by Simon Flexner (1863–

G g

1946) and Paul A. Lewis (p. 430), who showed that the disease could be transmitted to monkeys by using the nasopharyngeal washings from a patient. It is only quite recently that the virus has been cultivated in tissues other than nerve tissue, and monkey-kidney tissue is now extensively used. The very promising results obtained with vaccines made in this way are too recent for mention here.

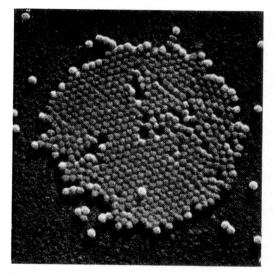

FIG. 114. Electron micrograph of poliomyelitis virus (MEFL). (×74,000) (after Schwardt *et al.*, *Proc. Soc. Exp. Biol. and Med.*, 1954, lxxxvi. 311)

RICKETTSIAL DISEASES

The pathogenic agents named the rickettsiae lie mid-way between the bacteria and the viruses. They are visible with high powers of the optical microscope and they are mostly held back by bacteriological filters. On the other hand, they resemble the viruses in that they tend to multiply intracellularly and are not culturable on the ordinary media used for bacteria. They cause several allied diseases of which the most important is typhus fever.

Two scientists who carried out extensive investigations on typhus fever early in the present century were Howard Taylor Ricketts (1871–1910) and Stanislaus Joseph Matthias von Prowazek (1875–

1915). They had similar careers, and both died of typhus fever during their investigations. Ricketts held a post at the University of Chicago, and in 1907 he transmitted Rocky Mountain spotted fever to guinea-pigs and monkeys. The organism was discovered in 1916 by Simeon Burt Wolbach (1880–1954), who called it *Dermacentroxenus rickettsi* after Ricketts. Prowazek, a Bohemian, was a protozoologist who worked with Ehrlich and then with Schaudinn. On the latter's early death Prowazek succeeded him.

The causative organism of typhus fever was described in 1916 by Henrique da Rocha-Lima (1879–1956), a Brazilian who held a chair at the University of Hamburg. He named the organism *Rickettsia prowazeki* in honour of his two deceased contemporaries. The generic name *Rickettsia* having been thus established, the name of the organism of Rocky Mountain spotted fever was gradually changed to *R. rickettsi*. More recently the rickettsiae of a few other diseases have been described, including *R. burneti*, the cause of the Australian Q fever.

Rickettsiae are generally about half the size of a coccus. They show various shapes and stain easily with the Giemsa blood stain.

An observation which had a very important bearing on the control of typhus fever was made in 1909 by Charles Jules Henri Nicolle (1866–1936) and his colleagues. Nicolle showed by experiments on man and monkeys that typhus fever is spread by lice. He was then director of the Institut Pasteur in Tunis, and he made many further contributions to infectious and tropical diseases, for which he received a Nobel Prize in 1928. It was later shown that most of the other rickettsial diseases are spread by either lice or mites.

Trench fever was first described by John Henry Porteus Graham in 1915 as 'a relapsing febrile illness of unknown origin' in troops on the British Front, and other cases were soon described by George Herbert Hunt (1884–1926) and Allan Coats Rankin (1877–1959), who called it 'trench fever'. By early 1916 it had been comprehensively studied by (Sir) John William McNee (1887–), Arnold Renshaw, and Edgar Harold Brunt (?–1922). In German troops it was described by H. Werner, and also by Wilhelm His, jun. (p. 623), son of the anatomist Wilhelm His, sen. (p. 247). His junior was then professor of clinical medicine at Berlin, and he had long been known for his important discovery of the bundle of His in the conducting mechanism of the heart. His encountered these cases of trench fever in Volhynia on the Russian front, and he hence called it Volhynian fever. Werner called it five-day fever. It was shown by McNee that the disease could be produced by inoculation with blood from a patient, and it was proved experimentally that lice could transmit the disease. Many points regarding the infectivity of the louse were cleared up by a War Office Committee, and the causative organism —named *Rickettsia quintana*—was described by Hans Willi Töpfer (1876–?) in 1916. There is little doubt that this rickettsia causes the disease, although absolute evidence has never been obtained.

THE CONQUEST OF THE TROPICS

Nowhere in medicine has the rational spirit been more triumphantly vindicated than in connexion with the diseases peculiar to hot countries. The increase in the habitability of the Tropics may be traced to two main causes. First is the application of the ordinary laws of hygiene. Second is the increasingly exact knowledge of the microbic origin of tropical diseases, leading to a more complete apprehension and a stricter application of these laws.

We have glanced at the great changes wrought in the social organization of temperate countries by the rise of modern hygiene (pp. 208–36), which commenced to be felt about the middle of the eighteenth century. The death-rate then began to fall, and has fallen steadily ever since. The mid-eighteenth century marks, for temperate countries, the end of the 'Middle Ages' of hygiene. But with the advent of the modern period the fall in the death-rate in temperate countries has not been the only change in the public health. Even more significant is a change in the causes of death.

Certain diseases have gradually receded from the more civilized and settled temperate countries, and are now almost unknown there. Thus, malaria, plague, typhus, leprosy, and dysentery, once of world-wide distribution, have come to be regarded almost entirely as tropical diseases. A time is approaching when we shall be able to place in the same category other diseases with which temperate countries are still afflicted, such as typhoid fever. The ultimate exclusion of typhoid fever as a disease of civilized communities is suggested by the death-rates for England and Wales.

Typhoid in England and Wales: Average annual death-rate per million living

1871–80	1881–90	1891–1900	1901–10	1911–20	1921–30	1931–40	1941–50
332	198	174	91	35	11	5	2

It should be said, however, that Malta fever, a disease until recently regarded as tropical, is now known to have a very wide distribution (pp. 385–6).

These diseases are rife in the Tropics because it is there that the general environmental conditions most favourable to their development are still found. If the environmental conditions of the Tropics could be raised to those of the civilized temperate countries—a task, it is true, of very great difficulty—these particular diseases might become as rare there as they are with us. Indeed, it is possible to foresee a world in which a number of these so-called tropical diseases will have disappeared altogether.

There are, however, other diseases that are tropical in another sense. Such diseases have seldom or never visited the shores of temperate countries, or at least have obtained no lasting foothold there, even when the conditions have been favourable to them. Among such diseases are yellow fever, African sleeping sickness (which must not be confused with encephalitis lethargica, a disease which was epidemic in Britain and some other countries about thirty years ago; it was often referred to as 'sleepy sickness'), dengue, kala-azar, and many less known conditions.

It must be said, to avoid misunderstanding, that 'the Tropics' in the medical sense is a region considerably wider and far less well-defined than the geographical Tropics. Moreover, despite the existence of diseases peculiar to the Tropics, 'tropical diseases' form no natural group based on any common organic causation. Organisms that give rise to the various 'tropical diseases' differ from one another just as much as those that give rise to the diseases of temperate countries.

Tropical diseases thus form a group, not from their nature but in the mode of their prevention. We therefore select five diseases, the history of which illustrates the processes by which the Tropics have been made safer both for Europeans and for native peoples. Malaria is an example of a disease which is gradually being eliminated from temperate climates. Yellow fever and trypanosomiasis are examples of truly tropical diseases which do not invade temperate climates. These three diseases are all spread by the bites of insects. Most cases of leishmaniasis are also spread by insects. Finally, we discuss briefly the problem of plague, which is now a tropical disease, spread by two intermediate hosts.

(a) Malaria

Malaria was, till recent times, a disease of temperate as well as of tropical countries. The old name for the disease is ague. The word 'malaria' is of no great antiquity in the English language. It came into use only in the eighteenth century. Like the word influenza, it is of Italian origin, and, like influenza, it carries with it a forgotten pathological theory. Malaria is simply *mal aria*, that is, bad air. So influenza is 'the influence', that is to say the influence of unpropitious planets or comets that were held to rain down poison. These diseases were thought to result from atmospheric conditions. In the Campagna the natives still believe that as the sun goes down the air becomes specially poisonous. In English the word malaria has been used for the disease itself only since about 1887.

While the *term* malaria is comparatively modern, recognizable accounts of the *condition* are perhaps more ancient than those of any other disease. Of all diseases that are produced by micro-organisms, malaria has perhaps changed its type least during the course of historic time. The disease is distinctly described in several places in the Hippocratic Collection.

The conception of diseases as separate entities is, of course, modern. In the case of most infectious diseases, therefore, we cannot hope to follow the history very far back. But the symptoms associated with a malarial attack are so definite that there is no difficulty in tracing the disease with certainty as far back as 1000 B.C. The real division into ancient and modern times comes, for this disease, with the use of cinchona, which is the plant from which quinine (p. 680) is derived. Very soon after the introduction of cinchona in the seventeenth century fevers came to be habitually divided into those which respond to cinchona and those which do not. Cinchona—and therefore its derivative, quinine—is one of the drugs that we owe to the

discovery of the New World. The bark of the cinchona tree was
taken as a remedy by the aborigines. In Europe, where it was introduced by Jesuit missionaries, it became known as 'Jesuits' bark'.
It was popularized by Sydenham (p. 110) and has ever since been
widely used in medicine.

Sydenham gave a good description of malaria. During the seventeenth and eighteenth centuries wave upon wave of 'ague' swept over

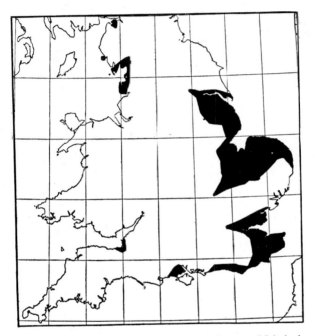

FIG. 115. Geographical Distribution of Indigenous Malaria in
England and Wales 1860

Europe. They spread from their endemic centres, the low-lying, ill-
drained, swampy districts, where the species of mosquito which
carries malaria could breed freely in the still water. Such places
in England were the Fens of Cambridgeshire, Lincolnshire, and the
surrounding counties, the marshes on either side of the estuary of
the Thames in Kent and Essex, the marshes of Romney and
Pevensey on the south coast, and those around Bridgwater near the
Bristol Channel (Fig. 115). There malaria was never absent, though

it differed greatly in prevalence and severity in different years. Ague remained prevalent in London as late as 1859. The proportion of ague cases to the total number of in- and out-patients at St. Thomas's Hospital in London from 1850 to 1860 varied from 12 per 1,000 at its lowest to over 60 per 1,000 at its highest. Thus, over one-twentieth of the patients in a large London hospital suffered from what we now regard as a tropical disease, within the lifetime of men who are only recently dead.

In London the rise in the value of land led to the erection of the Thames Embankment, which effectually reclaimed the land around the river. Extensive works of drainage were at the same time being undertaken in other infested districts. These soon had their now well-known effect. In 1864 malaria was found to be rapidly diminishing everywhere, and to have left many of its old haunts. The disease retreated rapidly. At the beginning of the twentieth century a systematic search was made for native (or indigenous) cases in England. After much labour a very few were at last found. It may safely be prophesied that malaria will never again be anything but a rare disease in any temperate country with an efficient sanitary service.

The malaria parasite. The presence in the tissues of malarial subjects of a grey-black pigment had been known since 1716, when it was first described by Lancisi (p. 196). With the birth of bacteriology attempts were made to incriminate one of the bacteria as the cause of malaria, and a bacillus described in 1879 had supporters for nearly twenty years. But in 1872 Francis Delafield (1841–1915) of New York had already stated that the pigment granules in malaria patients were embedded in small, transparent, finely granular bodies, which also existed without pigment. Though he did not know it, these were the malaria parasites.

The real discovery of the parasite was due to Charles Louis Alphonse Laveran (1845–1922), the son of a professor at, and later director of, the Val-de-Grâce (p. 281). Laveran followed in his father's footsteps, became a military surgeon, and later occupied his father's chair. While stationed in Algeria he saw that the pigment in malarious blood was contained in cyst-like bodies within the erythrocytes, but he had no indication that these bodies were alive. However, on 6 November 1880 he saw several long flagella being

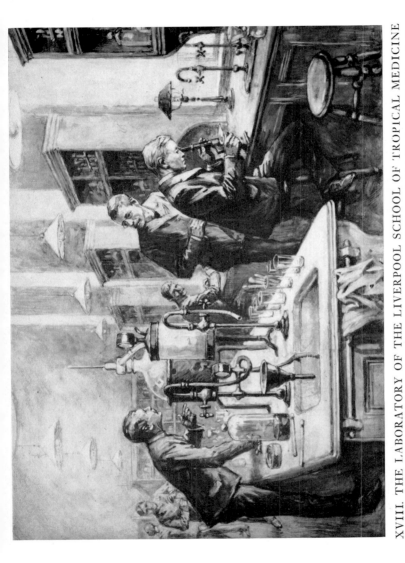

XVIII. THE LABORATORY OF THE LIVERPOOL SCHOOL OF TROPICAL MEDICINE

The School was founded in 1898. Rubert (later Sir Rubert) Boyce (1863–1911), Holt Professor of Pathology in the University of Liverpool, first Dean of the School, is seen examining a blood-film. On his left is C. S. (later Sir Charles) Sherrington, then Holt Professor of Physiology. In the left foreground is Surgeon Major (later Sir Ronald) Ross, first lecturer in tropical diseases in the School

(Drawing of June 1899 in body-colours by W. T. Maud, in the Wellcome Historical Medical Museum)

extruded from one of these hyaline bodies. They were obviously
alive, since they were actively motile. If we now refer to Fig. 116,
which shows in diagrammatic form our present knowledge of the
malaria parasite, it may be said that by 1882 Laveran had seen the
flagella shown in h^2 and had realized that they were alive. (We now
know that these gametes, which are normally formed from the male
gametocyte (g^2), appear in human blood only after it is removed
from the body.) He had also seen the gametocytes g^1 and g^2, and
some of the intra-corpuscular forms, certainly a and b, in the erythrocytes, together with c and d, though he had not interpreted these
latter properly; but he had no evidence that they were alive apart
from the fact that they appeared to grow in size. In 1882 Laveran's
observations were confirmed by Eugène Richard (1844–1926). In the
same year Laveran went to Rome and showed his preparations to
Italian malariologists, especially Ettore Marchiafava (1847–1935).
Marchiafava, like Laveran and practically all bacteriologists, was
then using high-power dry objectives. He was not convinced by
Laveran's supposition, made many preparations of malarious blood
himself, and finally decided that the pigmented bodies in the affected
red cells were melanin, produced by degenerative changes in the
haemoglobin. A little later he thought the pigment granules might
be cocci, but not unnaturally he failed to culture them. Then, in
1884, Marchiafava started to use an oil-immersion objective, which
greatly improved the magnification and the resolution of the image,
and he then saw amoeboid movement in the annular and other
bodies in the red cells. The bodies were therefore parasites, and
Laveran had been proved correct. But, while Laveran held that the
filamentous forms were the perfect forms of the parasites, Marchiafava and his co-workers were convinced that the annular forms—
which they thought were actually in the corpuscles, and not simply
adherent to them, as Laveran thought—were the essential parasites.
Laveran also thought that the parasite was itself pigmented, whereas
the Italians correctly held that the pigment was formed in the
erythrocytes after they had been invaded by the parasites.

During the next few years the Italians cleared up the asexual cycle
of the parasite in human red corpuscles. They showed that the ring
form (a) increases in size within the corpuscle and that eventually its

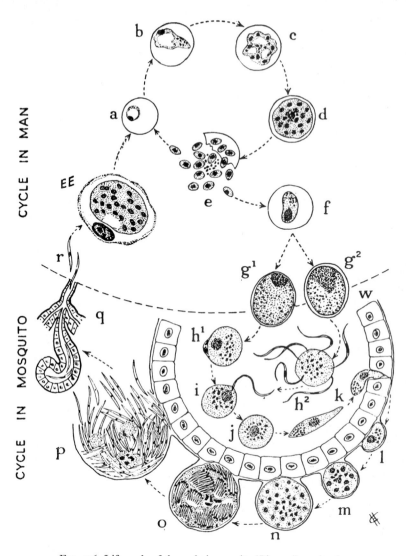

FIG. 116. Life-cycle of the malaria parasite (*Plasmodium vivax*)
(After C. A. Hoare, *Handbook of Medical Protozoology*, London, 1949)

Cycle in man. r, inoculated sporozoite. *EE*, exoerythrocytic stage (*schizogony*) in liver cells. *a–e*, asexual development (*schizogony*) in erythrocytes: *a*, ring form; *b*, trophozoite; *c*, *d*, development of schizonts; *e*, release of merozoites from red cell. *f*, *g*, sexual development: *f*, immature gametocyte; *g¹*, *g²*, female and male gametocytes.

Cycle in mosquito (sexual development). *g–k*, in interior of stomach: *h¹*, female gamete; *h²*, male gametes (*exflagellation*); *i*, fertilization; *j*, zygote; *k*, ookinetes (one penetrating stomach wall, *w*). *l–p*, oocysts undergoing *sporogony* on outer wall of stomach: *o*, formation of sporozoites; *p*, rupture of oocyst, with liberation of sporozoites which pass to salivary glands (*q*).

nucleus divides to form about twenty daughter nuclei. This is followed by the division of the cytoplasm to form the merozoites (*e*), each containing a little nucleus. Each merozoite then invades a healthy erythrocyte, and this asexual cycle, named schizogony, is repeated. In 1885 Golgi (p. 247) showed that the fever paroxysm in malaria coincides with the phase when the merozoites rupture the red cells and invade new cells. Golgi also noted the differences between the parasites of tertian and of quartan malaria. Then in 1889 Marchiafava and Angelo Celli (1857–1914) demonstrated that the parasite of malignant malaria is a separate species, in which the gametocytes are crescentic in shape. These crescent forms had been first described and figured by Laveran. He had called the parasite *Oscillaria*, and various other generic names were subsequently suggested. The genus was finally known as *Plasmodium*, and by 1890 the three species *P. vivax* (benign tertian), *P. malariae* (quartan malaria), and *P. falciparum* (malignant malaria) were known. In 1922 John William Watson Stephens (1865–1946) described a fourth species, *P. ovale*. Laveran was awarded a Nobel Prize in 1907 for his discovery, and Golgi received one in the previous year for his histological researches on the nervous system.

It was a fairly obvious step to produce malaria in human volunteers by inoculating them with human blood in which the parasites had been observed, and this was done by Marchiafava and Celli as early as 1885. But subsequent research showed that the problem was not as easy as it appeared to be, and it was suspected that part of the parasite's life-cycle was still unknown. In 1892 Richard Pfeiffer (p. 393), on the basis of the life-history of the coccidia, rather similar parasites which affect certain animals, predicted that in the case of malaria it would be shown that part of the parasite's life-history occurred outside the human body. In the following year Amico Bignami (1862–1929) and Giuseppe Bastianelli (1862–1959) made some very significant experiments. They inoculated human volunteers with blood known to contain malaria parasites. They found that a paroxysm of malaria supervened only when the blood contained the young forms, and not when the only parasites present were crescent forms.

The method of transmission of the parasites from one individual to another was now much discussed. For many centuries it had been suspected that a mosquito acts as a carrier, but all these beliefs were unscientific. The first proof that any insect spreads disease was given in 1877 by Sir Patrick Manson (1844–1922), one of the greatest of all research workers on tropical diseases. Manson showed that the embryos of the parasite *Filaria bancrofti*, which causes great swelling (elephantiasis) of soft tissues, are transmitted by a Culex mosquito, the parasite going through a necessary part of its life-cycle in the body of the insect. Among other noteworthy discoveries of Manson was his realization of the part played by the fluke *Paragonimus westermanii* in the causation of certain lung diseases. He was the founder of the London School of Tropical Medicine.

It need hardly be said that Manson had had great experience of the disease malaria, and that he was intensely interested in its problems. He saw the possibility that malaria was transmitted by a mosquito, but, like many other great authorities, he was at first inclined to the view that the disease was transmitted by the individual drinking water in which the bodies of malaria-infected mosquitoes had collected. The possibility of transmission by the bite of the mosquito was considered, but was not seriously held because it was known that mosquitoes were unable to transmit malaria for some short time after they had bitten a malaria patient. Manson had seen the flagellated bodies which had been observed by Laveran, and he knew that they were not formed until after the blood had left the vessels. He therefore concluded that the function of the flagellum lay outside the patient's body, and that it was the first stage in an extracorporeal phase of the parasite's life cycle. He was convinced that the flagellum was the key to the problem. By a bold deduction he formulated in 1894 his mosquito-malaria theory, according to which the flagellum, or some related form of the parasite, was sucked up by a blood-sucking insect, probably a mosquito, and that after a period of development it was in some way transmitted to another human host.

In the meantime a young officer in the Indian Medical Service, (later Sir) Ronald Ross (1857–1932), had become interested in malaria in 1889, but he had been unable to see Laveran's parasite.

It was not till five years later, when Manson showed him the parasite while Ross was on leave in London, that he became convinced. Inspired by Manson, Ross devoted himself to the problem after his return to India, and he spent two years in intensive research. He dissected over a thousand mosquitoes, which had been allowed to suck malarious blood, in order to find out what happened to the flagella and what species were able to transmit the parasite. The mosquitoes were bred from the larval stage, each in a separate bottle, so that they had had no previous contact with malarious blood. Ross was able to watch the process of exflagellation taking place in the mosquito's stomach after it had fed on blood containing crescents, but he saw no further development of the parasites. The mosquitoes in the district were entirely *Culex* and *Aëdes* mosquitoes, and Ross was unable to make them infect volunteers with malaria after they had fed on malarious blood.

In April 1897 Ross first saw an *Anopheles* mosquito in another district, and he thought that this 'dappled-winged' insect might transmit malaria. He intensified his researches, and on 20 August 1897 he saw pigmented cyst-like bodies projecting from the outer surface of the stomach wall of anophelines which had fed on malarious blood. He had no doubt that he had seen another stage in the life-cycle of the parasite. Within the next few days he had seen these oocysts in stages *l*, *m*, and *n* in the diagram (Fig. 116).

During the same summer an important intermediate stage was seen for the first time by William George MacCallum (p. 639), later a distinguished pathologist, but who in 1897 had just graduated at Johns Hopkins Medical School. In unstained fresh blood, within a minute or so after it had been drawn from a patient suffering from malaria, MacCallum saw the process of exflagellation—the male gametocyte (Fig. 116, g^2) throwing off flagella (male gametes) from its surface (h^2). Further, he was lucky enough to see one of these flagella penetrating a female gamete (Fig. 116, *i*) and thus fertilizing it. It was thus definitely proved that a sexual phase occurred in the life-cycle of the malaria parasite.

Just after his discovery of the oocyst Ross was ordered to another area where there was no malaria. But Manson and others then influenced the authorities to transfer him to Calcutta for further work on this disease. Unfortunately, owing to certain circumstances human volunteers were not there available at that time for malaria work. Ross therefore turned to the study of bird-malaria, which is caused by the parasite Proteosoma, closely allied to Plasmodium, the malaria parasite. Proteosoma is transmitted by the bite of *Culex*. He saw all the stages in the mosquito which he had already seen in the case of human malaria, together with exflagellation and fertilization in the lumen of the mosquito's stomach, the fertilized zygote (Fig. 116, *j*) and its passage through to the outside of the stomach wall (*k*). He then showed that the oocyst becomes mature by the development in it of large numbers of minute spindle-like bodies (sporozoites, *o*). He found also that shortly afterwards the oocyst bursts (*p*), and that the sporozoites are discharged into the insect's body cavity. In efforts to discover what ultimately happened to the sporozoites, Ross—as he wrote to Manson—went at mosquito after mosquito spending hours over each, until he was blind and half silly with fatigue. Then on 4 July 1898, in a structure which he had deduced was the salivary gland of the mosquito, he found some of the cells packed with sporozoites. By allowing culicine mosquitoes to feed on infected birds and then to feed on healthy birds he proved this method of transmission. The final stage, the demonstration that the sexual cycle of the human malaria parasites was the same as that of Proteosoma, was within Ross's grasp; but once again the authorities stepped in and he was ordered to Assam to investigate kala-azar. A few months later he retired from the Indian Medical Service.

Meanwhile the Italians had been active. Bignami, for example, believed in the mosquito theory, but he thought the insect obtained the parasite from the soil. Most of the Italians believed that the flagella were of no significance in the parasite's life-history. By the autumn of 1898, however, their attitude had been altered by Ross's discoveries. In November and December 1898 Bignami, Bastianelli, and Giovanni Battista Grassi (1854–1925) showed by various experiments that if some species of anopheline mosquitoes were fed on malarious blood, they could transmit the infection to healthy volunteers by their bite. By 1899 they had observed the complete sexual-cycles of *Plasmodium falciparum* and of *P. malariae* in the mosquito, and about the same time Bastianelli and Bignami demonstrated that of *P. vivax*. In 1900 Grassi published his important work *Studi di uno zoologo sulla malaria* ('Studies of a zoologist on malaria'), which contained the finest illustrations of the various stages of the parasite published up to that time. Ross had gone to Sierra Leone after his retirement from the Indian Medical Service, and there in 1899 he confirmed the work of the Italian investigators on human malaria. He received a Nobel Prize in 1902. Meanwhile, there had been criticism of the feeding experiments of the Italians, on the grounds that the volunteers resided in a malarial district and that the fever supervening after the mosquito had bitten might have been a natural attack of the disease. But in 1900 some infected anopheline mosquitoes were sent by Bastianelli from Rome to Manson in London, where there was no malaria. They were allowed to bite Manson's son, and fifteen days later he developed malaria. After he fell ill a laboratory assistant allowed some of the mosquitoes which had not been used to feed on his own arm. Fifteen days later he also developed malaria. This was a very convincing proof of the correctness of Manson's hypothesis.

If reference is made again to Fig. 116 it will be realized that by 1900 all the stages in the life-cycle of the malaria parasite had been seen and well described, except the stage marked *EE*. It was assumed that after the mosquito bit a human subject the sporozoites (r) immediately, as Ross wrote in 1898, began to develop into malaria parasites. This view, universally accepted, was apparently clinched by Schaudinn's (p. 394) report in 1902 that he had seen a sporozoite penetrating into an erythrocyte, and by his illustrations of the stages in that event. But it soon appeared strange that this observation was not confirmed, and despite much search it is still unconfirmed. From 1898 onwards various observers had noted that, in patients whose red cells had already been invaded by the parasite, similar but unpigmented forms of the parasite were sometimes found in endothelial and other tissue cells. These '*E-E* forms' constitute the exoerythrocytic stage. They may persist long after the blood-forms have disappeared, and they are probably responsible for relapses.

In 1940, however, forms of one of the bird-malaria parasites were found in the tissues, before the invasion of the erythrocytes had begun, by Henry Edward Shortt (1887–) and his colleagues in India, and independently by Lili Mudrow [-Reichenow] (1908–) in Germany. These were named pre-erythrocytic forms. Clinicians had long known that, after an individual had been presumably infected, there was an interval before the parasite appeared in the erythrocytes and before he developed a clinical attack of malaria. The crucial experiment was carried out on Australian volunteers during the later stages of the Second World War by Sir Neil Hamilton Fairley (1891–) and his colleagues. Fairley showed that after an infected mosquito bit a volunteer, the sporozoites could be found in the blood stream for about half an hour. They then disappeared altogether for a period—nine days in the case of tertian malaria and six days in the case of malignant malaria—during which the blood of the infected subject could be injected into other volunteers without transmitting malaria.

The final stages in the demonstration of the importance of pre-erythrocytic forms was shown by Shortt and Percy Cyril Claude Garnham (1901–), who found them in the liver cells of heavily infected monkeys in 1948. Then, in the same year, with their collaborators, they demonstrated these forms in the liver cells of infected human volunteers.

Malaria control. Since the demonstration of the life-cycles of the malarial parasites of man the chief attention of hygienists interested in malaria has been directed to the mosquito. It was early noticed that in countries where malaria is prevalent the incidence of that disease is low during the first half of the year. The number of cases increase sharply about midsummer, and reach their maximum by the ninth month. (These features are shown in the graph of the seasonal incidence of malaria in Italy, Fig. 117.) This seasonal incidence corresponds to the known facts of the life-history of the mosquito. It has been found that the best method of reducing the incidence of the disease is to control the breeding of the insect vector. Engineering and sanitary works in some places previously infested with malaria have had the effect of almost entirely eliminating the disease. The classical instance is the Panama zone, where the two mosquito-borne diseases, yellow fever and malaria, have disappeared

(p. 473). There are now many areas in the Tropics, previously infested, in which malaria is almost unknown.

Nevertheless, the early hopes that malaria would be eradicated from tropical regions by clearing trees from the neighbourhood of stagnant water, and by covering the water with a film of a thin oil, have on the whole proved disappointing. The measures are themselves costly, and the oil has to be renewed frequently. More

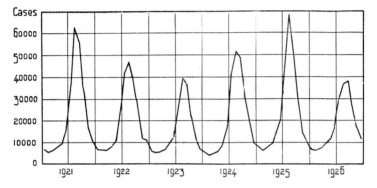

FIG. 117. Seasonal incidence of malaria in Italy, 1921–6. For each year the midsummer ordinate stands above the date

effective results have been obtained in many areas by concentrating on the particular species of mosquito which are known to transmit malaria in each particular area. Their habits are studied and selective measures are employed against them. This 'species control' is giving good results in many areas. The oil is now combined with powerful insecticides, such as DDT, and large areas can be treated by spraying the fluid from an aeroplane. Attention is now focused on the destruction of adult mosquitoes, especially by spraying habitations with pyrethrum. DDT is also widely used for this purpose, but there are signs that some strains of the mosquito are becoming drug-resistant. Especially is this the case in Greece and Java, where the local mosquitoes are so resistant to DDT as to make the use of this insecticide impracticable.

The use of the newer drugs against malaria is dealt with elsewhere (p. 691). In addition to their use in treatment they now play an important role in prophylaxis. In the South-West Pacific theatre of war in 1942–3 Fairley (p. 464) and his collaborators showed that soldiers would be kept fit by taking one mepacrine tablet a day. There were no deaths from malaria, and no soldiers thus treated were infective to mosquitoes.

Malaria still causes about 250 million cases and two and a half million deaths in the world every year. Though the last sixty years have seen enormous advances, much still remains to be accomplished.

(b) Yellow Fever

Outbreaks of yellow fever have struck the public imagination, have given rise to folk tales, and have inspired poets. The legend of the Flying Dutchman is that of a ship stricken with yellow fever. The spectre ship is supposed by sailors to haunt the seas around the Cape of Good Hope, and to bode ill for those who see it. A murder was committed in the ship, and following it yellow jack broke out. All ports were closed to the wretched crew, who finally all died of the disease. The story was made the subject of an opera by Wagner and a novel by Marryat. Coleridge's *Rime of the Ancient Mariner* is also a picture of a ship smitten by yellow jack.

An historic case may be quoted. In 1837 the barque *Huskisson* was at Sierra Leone. She was lading when yellow fever appeared among the crew. All but two or three died. Yellow fever broke out in the colony, but gradually died down. In the meantime the *Huskisson* remained in port without hands for three months. At last hands were obtained, tempted by very high pay. Again yellow fever broke out among them and again nearly all died.

Many cases, no less dramatic, are on record. The disease is among those which are peculiarly common and fatal among medical men. Thus, Senegal has twice been denuded of medical men by yellow fever. In 1830 six died out of twelve, and in 1878 twenty-two out of twenty-seven.

It is now known that an attack of yellow fever confers immunity. In children it is normally mild, and therefore, in countries where it is endemic, the population consists largely of the survivors of attacks. On this account terrible outbreaks of the Flying Dutchman or Ancient Mariner type are always either on immigrant ships or in places which have remained long unvisited by the disease. In other words such outbreaks occur under conditions in which immune persons are few or absent.

During the seventeenth and eighteenth centuries, and even during the nineteenth there were repeated outbreaks of yellow fever far beyond the region to which it is now confined. Along the eastern shores of North America it has at times extended as far north as Boston, and there have been destructive outbreaks in Baltimore, Philadelphia, and even New York. The disease has been found along most of the littoral of South America. In the Old World it has visited chiefly West Africa, where it was imported very early by the slave trade, but it has also penetrated as far as the Sudan. It has visited at times Spain, Portugal, and Italy with devastating epidemics, and has even occasionally made a call in France and once in England. The last considerable outbreak in Europe was at Madrid in 1878.

The United Kingdom has always had important interests in the West Indies. During the eighteenth and first half of the nineteenth centuries, moreover, she had there large military establishments which were regarded as very bad stations. In Thackeray's *Vanity Fair*, which refers to the period just after the Napoleonic wars, the disreputable and unfortunate Rawdon Crawley is sent as governor to 'Coventry Island' in the West Indies, and is not expected to last long. There are many historic occasions on which the British forces in the West Indies lost almost incredible numbers from yellow jack, garrisons being practically wiped out. In Jamaica the mean annual mortality in the garrison was for many years 185 per 1,000. In the Bermudas the mortality was about 80 per 1,000. One should remember that soldiers are picked men in the prime of life, and that these mortality rates were in places now regarded as health resorts. About a hundred and fifty years ago Jamaica had the highest death-rate in the Empire with the exception of West Africa, where the mean annual mortality of whites at Sierra Leone was 362 per 1,000.

Conditions in the West Indies began to improve definitely from about 1850 onwards. At the time there was no effective knowledge of the organic cause of yellow fever, nor, indeed, of any other tropical disease. Half a century later the basic reason for this early improvement gradually became obvious. From about 1850 onwards the domestic water in more settled parts of the West Indies, and notably in larger towns, came to be supplied by pipes. Now these towns were special haunts of the yellow-fever mosquito. The removal of open standing water, the enclosure of water supplies, and the introduction of ordinary modern sanitation in the clearing away of rubbish, did good work without involving any knowledge of the organic cause of the disease. The breeding haunts of the mosquitoes were destroyed.

Mode of infection. From the end of the eighteenth century some courageous physicians carried out experiments on themselves to show that yellow fever is not contagious. Until a century later it was commonly thought that the turning over of the soil in construction work was a likely method of spreading the disease, since it was held that it might be caused by a miasma emanating from the earth in conjunction with an atmosphere infected by the aggregation of the sick. Benjamin Rush (p. 190) did heroic work in treating the patients during the great outbreak at Philadelphia in 1793, and he later published an excellent clinical account. He thought that the disease arose from damaged coffee beans left lying on the wharves.

The first suggestion that a mosquito might be in any way connected with the transmission of the disease was made by Josiah Clark Nott (1804–73) of Alabama in 1848. This and other suggestions regarding the role of the mosquito did not implicate it as a carrier of the disease between individuals. The credit for having been the first to suggest that the mosquito carries yellow fever from man to man goes to Carlos Juan Finlay (1833–1915) of Havana, Cuba. (Finlay was baptized 'Juan Carlos', but he later called himself 'Carlos Juan' to avoid confusion with his son. In his writings both forms of his name will be found.) He was the son of a Scottish physician and a French mother. When Carlos was an infant his parents emigrated to Cuba, and from his eleventh year he was educated in Cuba, London, France, and Germany. He studied medicine in Philadelphia and took his degree there. He settled down in practice in Havana, and among his contributions to medicine was his successful practical work to reduce the incidence of tetanus neonatorum. He began to write on the cause of yellow fever when he was still a young man, and in 1881 he delivered his famous paper on the role of the mosquito in this disease at the meeting of the International Sanitary Commission which met in Washington in that year. Finlay did not incriminate mosquitoes generally. As a result of his studies of the conditions under which yellow fever was common, and also of those which suited certain species of mosquitoes, he was able to deduce logically that the mosquito now known as *Aëdes aegypti* must be the transmitter. This is all the more remarkable in that news of Manson's work on the transmission of filariasis by culicines had not then reached Cuba. In all he published over seventy papers on yellow fever. He did not rest content with theoretical deductions, but he also carried out many experiments with infected mosquitoes, and he showed that a mosquito which sucked the blood of a patient during the first few days of the illness was able to transmit the disease to others. Finlay also experimented on the production of immunity by allowing infected mosquitoes to bite healthy subjects. This experiment was carried out on ninety persons and in 18 per cent. a mild attack of yellow fever—with subsequent immunity—resulted. Finlay received many honours, and at the age of sixty-five he was appointed Chief Health Officer and President of the Board of Health of Cuba. Nevertheless, he very frequently does not receive the credit which is his due; and it is surprising to find that in many accounts of the history of yellow fever his work is passed over briefly or is entirely omitted.

During the many years when Finlay was doing his utmost to teach the scientific world the lesson which he had so carefully prepared thousands of victims were dying of yellow fever. In 1898 American soldiers suffered a high mortality from this disease in Cuba. The United States Government therefore appointed a Commission in 1900 to investigate the problem. The Commission was headed by Walter Reed (1851–1902) of the Medical Corps of the United States Army, who was then professor of bacteriology at the Army Medical School. He had already been chairman of a Commission which successfully investigated an epidemic of typhoid fever among troops. The other members of the Yellow Fever Commission were James Carroll (1854–1907), Jesse William Lazear (1866–1900), and a Cuban physician Aristide Agramonte [y Simoni] (1868–1931). Reed first disproved some of the alleged causes of yellow fever commonly held at that time, and he then concentrated on Finlay's theory of the mosquito as the transmitter. A great authority on yellow fever, Henry Rose Carter (1852–1925) had just drawn attention to the fact that the incubation period of yellow fever was five days, but a house to which a patient suffering from that disease was conveyed did not become infected until after fifteen to twenty days from his arrival. Having in mind Ross's work on the life-cycle of the malaria parasite, this fact suggested to Reed a development in the infecting organism within the mosquito. With volunteer soldiers and civilians as his material he then embarked on a prepared series of experiments. The first to be bitten experimentally by an infected mosquito was Dr. Carroll. He was bitten on 27 August 1900, by a mosquito which had fed on a yellow fever patient twelve days previously. By the 31st he was very ill, but he made a good recovery. Dr. Lazear was bitten experimentally a few days later, but did not develop the disease. But on 13 September, while Lazear was going round his wards an Aëdes mosquito settled on his hand. He left it undisturbed to bite, and five days later he had a very severe attack of yellow fever to which he succumbed. This was fortunately the only fatality in the series of experiments. In this way it was proved that yellow fever could be conveyed by infected mosquitoes.

Reed then tried to ascertain whether yellow fever could be conveyed from a patient in any other manner. He caused a small mosquito-proof hut to be constructed in which seven beds were made up with the unwashed sheets, blankets, and pillows on which yellow fever patients had lain. Then the hut was occupied by a doctor and six privates in the hospital corps. They remained in the hut for twenty days, and none of them was infected. Reed also had another hut prepared, in which the interior was divided into two 'rooms' by a wire screen. Into one room fifteen infected mosquitoes were admitted. Three non-immune American volunteers took up their quarters in the other room. One of the volunteers went into the room containing the mosquitoes. He was bitten freely. In four days he developed an attack of yellow fever, from which he recovered. The other two volunteers who had not been bitten remained healthy.

The conclusions of the Commission, which were first known early in 1901, drawn from many experiments such as those described, were that the yellow-fever (Aëdes) mosquito serves as an intermediate host, and that the disease is spread to persons who are not immune by the bite of a mosquito that had previously fed on infected blood. The Commission demonstrated that an interval of twelve days has to elapse after the mosquito bites a patient before it becomes infective, and that if it bites earlier the bite neither causes the disease nor confers any immunity. They showed that the disease is not conveyed by fomites, and that disinfection is therefore unnecessary. They also showed that an individual can be infected if he is injected with blood drawn from a patient during the first or second day of the disease. Tests were carried out also by injecting blood serum from a patient, filtered through a bacteriological filter. This experiment was tried on two volunteers, and both developed the disease. Though not fully appreciated at the time, this observation was of great importance later since it showed that the organism is a filterable virus. The Commission thought that the mosquito which transmitted yellow fever was *Culex fasciatus*. But in the discussion which followed the announcement of their conclusions, at a congress in Havana in February 1901, it was pointed out that this mosquito belonged to the genus *Stegomyia*, and it was named *S. fasciata*. Apart from names there was never any doubt in the minds of either Finlay or the members of the Commission regarding the identity of the mosquito. Its name was later changed to *Aëdes aegypti*.

The first practical application of the findings of the American Yellow Fever Commission was made in Havana. This city had long been a centre of yellow fever, and malaria, enteric fever, and other tropical diseases were also rife in it. In the last decades of the nineteenth century the sanitary conditions of Havana were extremely bad. The streets were narrow and badly paved, so that numerous puddles were in evidence. The sewage drained down the gutters and eventually found its way into the harbour. The cleansing of these Augean stables fell to the lot of Gorgas.

William Crawford Gorgas (1854–1920) was born in Alabama and was the son of a general in the United States Army. He graduated in medicine in New York in 1880, and was at once commissioned in the Medical Department of the Army. In 1898, when he was a major, Gorgas was sent to Havana as Chief Sanitary Officer. The Spanish-American War was by then virtually over—though peace was not signed until the following year—and most of the Spanish Army had just returned to Spain. It was these troops which formed the susceptible, non-immune population so far as yellow fever was concerned, since many of the natives of Havana were immune owing to mild attacks in early life. The incidence of yellow fever in Havana from 1885 to 1904 is shown in the following table:

Deaths in Havana from yellow fever

Year	Deaths	Year	Deaths	Year	Deaths
1885 .	. 165	1892 .	. 357	1899 .	. 103
1886 .	. 161	1893 .	. 496	1900 .	. 310
1887 .	. 532	1894 .	. 382	1901 .	. 18
1888 .	. 468	1895 .	. 553	1902 .	. 0
1889 .	. 303	1896 .	. 1,282	1903 .	. 0
1890 .	. 308	1897 .	. 858	1904 .	. 0
1891 .	. 356	1898 .	. 136		

It will be seen that the mortality had reached its peak in the two years previous to the advent of Gorgas to Havana. Owing to the lack of susceptibles in 1898 the mortality was low that year, but on the other hand deaths from malaria, typhoid fever, and dysentery were numerous.

Gorgas, like most other authorities, then held that yellow fever was a 'filth disease', and he at once initiated measures to improve the sanitary amenities of Havana. A proper system of drainage was instituted; stable floors were cemented; active disposal of refuse was carried out; and effective action for the cleansing of every type of public or private building was taken. Carlos Finlay watched these activities with interest and sympathy. The effect on malaria, typhoid fever, and dysentery was startling. The incidence of these diseases fell remarkably, and it was expected that yellow fever would be affected similarly. But in 1899 the end of the war led to the introduction of many thousands of non-immune immigrants from Spain, and in that year yellow fever deaths began to rise again. In 1900 they were back to the region of their pre-war level.

As has been previously mentioned (p. 470), the findings of the Reed Commission first became known in February 1901. Gorgas at once realized that he must direct a specific campaign against the yellow-fever mosquito, *Aëdes aegypti*. This species is known as the domestic mosquito because it seldom breeds more than 100 yards from houses, and it lays its eggs in domestic collections of water or in storage tanks. Gorgas argued that the cycle man–mosquito–man could be broken by nursing all yellow-fever patients in mosquito-proof rooms. This proved practical up to a point, but the method obviously failed in the case of mild or unrecognized attacks of the disease. Gorgas therefore also pinned his hopes on destruction of the mosquito. Very stringent measures were introduced which made it an offence punishable by fine for any property-owner to have mosquito larvae on his premises. The sanitary authority had powers to abate such nuisances, and a report had to be submitted by the sanitary staff every month on each house in the city. All yellow fever patients had to be screened. These measures were dramatically effective. During the remaining nine months of 1901 there were only five deaths from yellow fever (making eighteen for the whole year), and in the following three years no deaths at all from that disease occurred. Yellow fever in Havana had been wiped out.

Gorgas was also mainly responsible for the next great victory over yellow fever. The attempt to cut a canal through the Isthmus of Panama had been made by French engineers under de Lesseps, who had been successful in constructing the Suez Canal. This forty-mile tract was one of the foulest places on earth. It was described by a contemporary writer as 'a damp, tropical jungle, intensely hot, swarming with mosquitoes, snakes, alligators, scorpions and centipedes; the home, even as Nature made it, of yellow fever, typhus and dysentery'. The French began work in 1881, and from the start the workers suffered and died from many diseases, and each season thousands died from yellow fever. In the month of October 1884 there were 654 deaths from that condition alone. The French project was persisted in for nine years before it was abandoned.

The Americans launched their attempt in 1904, and Gorgas, the foremost living authority on yellow fever, was with a small staff placed in charge of the sanitary measures. At that time there were few cases of yellow fever, but in November there was the beginning of what proved to be a considerable epidemic which affected the workers, and also the towns and villages right across the isthmus. Gorgas then had a law passed which made it a punishable offence to harbour mosquito larvae on private premises. These measures drove the mosquito into vegetation near the houses, and this was attacked with fire. It was then found useful to set out numerous containers with clean water, in which the mosquitoes deposited their eggs. Before they were hatched they were destroyed by the sanitary staff, the containers were refilled, and the process of destruction began afresh. Nevertheless, the campaign was not an easy matter. Though the status and views of Gorgas were universally accepted by the medical profession, his methods were not acceptable to his civilian superiors. On several occasions he was nearly superseded, and he had to suffer several years of such obstructive conduct before the personal intervention of the President of the United States removed many of the petty restrictions which had hampered his great work. The canal was finished in 1914, and by that time the death-rate from all diseases at Panama was below that for any American city or State. The last fatal case of yellow fever in the Canal Zone occurred in September 1906. It was later estimated that, had the Americans suffered yellow-fever casualties at the same rate as the French had done, they would have constantly had about 13,000 in hospital, and the deaths from that disease would have been between 3,000 and 4,000 each year. Gorgas was later instrumental in reducing the incidence of pneumonia in the miners of the Rand. In 1920 he was asked to investigate possible outbreaks of yellow fever in Senegal, and while *en route* for that destination he was taken seriously ill in London. He was visited in hospital by King George V, who then bestowed on him the insignia of the K.C.M.G. Early in July Gorgas passed away. He must be one of the very few men— perhaps the only one—who received the equivalent of a state funeral both in London (at St. Paul's) and in Washington.

The causative organism. From 1888 onwards various bacilli were described as the organisms which caused yellow fever. When Reed's Commission started its work in Havana the favourite was the *Bacillus icteroides*, described by an Italian bacteriologist in 1897. It was an early part of the Commission's work to dethrone this bacillus. In 1912 minute bodies, supposed to be composed of cytoplasm and chromatin, were found in the red corpuscles of yellow-fever patients. These bodies (*Paraplasma flavigenum*) were supposed to be the cause of yellow fever, but they were later commonly found in the corpuscles of young London guinea-pigs.

Most important of the organisms alleged to be the cause was the spirochaete described by the Japanese, Hideyo Noguchi (1876–1928) in 1919. In 1886 Adolf Weil (1848–1916), then of Heidelberg and Dorpat, described a severe form of infectious jaundice with enlargement of the liver with haemorrhages into or from various organs, especially common in sewer workers. This not infrequently fatal disease was named spirochaetosis icterohaemorrhagica, but is commonly known as Weil's disease. In 1915 the Japanese bacteriologists Ryūkichi Inada (1874–1950), Yutaka Ido (1881–), and their colleagues described the causal organism, the spirochaete named *Leptospira icterohaemorrhagiae*. Noguchi was than a world-renowned experimenter at the Rockefeller Institute for Medical Research in New York, and he had to his credit very important studies on snake venoms, the cultivation of spirochaetes and the finding of *Treponema pallidum* in the brains of paralytics (p. 507), on scrub typhus, and on trachoma. Between 1918 and 1924 he went on four expeditions, organized by the Rockefeller Commission, to South America in an attempt to discover the cause of yellow fever. In 1919, while working in Guayaquil, Ecuador, he injected the blood of yellow-fever patients into guinea-pigs. The animals developed jaundice, haemorrhages from various organs, and coma. In their blood, and after death in their livers and kidneys, he discovered a spirochaete which resembled that described by Inada and Ido. He called it *Leptospira icteroides*, and in the succeeding years up to 1923 he obtained positive results with this organism in Pfeiffer's reaction (p. 414), differentiated it by immunity tests from *L. icterohaemorrhagiae*, and prepared from horses an immune serum which he used both prophylactically and therapeutically. It was then fairly widely recognized that *L. icteroides* was the cause of yellow fever in South America. But for some time papers had been appearing which failed to confirm Noguchi's findings. This was particularly the case in papers emanating from West Africa, and on no occasion was the leptospira recovered from yellow-fever patients in that region. He was a sick man, but his friends persuaded him with difficulty that he must himself find his leptospira in West Africa. He arrived there in

November 1927, and threw himself with enormous enthusiasm into the attempt to prove that West African yellow fever was also due to his leptospira. As the months passed the fact was borne in on him that his attempt had ended in failure. In May 1928, while still working on the problem, Noguchi himself developed an attack of yellow fever, from which he died. All his work on this disease had been planned and executed with his outstanding ability, and there is some evidence for believing that the blood which he first used in his early experiments in South America came from a case of Weil's disease.

Even at the time when Noguchi was considering whether, in his poor state of health, he would undertake his last journey to West Africa, another worker was laying down his life in the cause of yellow fever. This was Adrian Stokes (1887–1927), a member of the famous Stokes family of Dublin physicians. After a distinguished student career at Trinity College, Dublin, Stokes was for a time with the Rockefeller Foundation. During the war he found the recently described leptospira of Weil's disease in troops on active service who were suffering from infectious jaundice. For three years from 1919 Stokes was professor of bacteriology at Trinity College, Dublin, and in 1922 he was called to the chair of bacteriology at Guy's Hospital, London. In 1920 he had been a member of the Rockefeller Commission on Yellow Fever, and in 1927 he again returned to field work on this disease in West Africa. One of the great practical difficulties in yellow-fever research had always been the fact that no one had succeeded in transmitting the disease to an experimental animal. As early as 1881 Carlos Finlay had tried to get Aëdes mosquitoes to infect experimental animals, but he failed because he did not realize that an incubation period might occur during which the virus had to mature in the body of the insect. Walter Reed in 1900 had tried to infect a small monkey in this way without success. It was a local Havana monkey, and we now know that it was probably already immune. In 1927 Stokes and his collaborators succeeded in infecting *Macacus sinicus* with blood from yellow-fever patients. They then found that the more easily procurable *Macacus rhesus* could also be easily infected. In these monkeys the lesions were typically those of yellow fever in fatal human cases. Stokes and his colleagues transmitted the disease from monkey to monkey by inoculation of blood in series and by the bites of Aëdes mosquitoes, and they also conclusively showed that yellow fever is caused by a filterable virus. These discoveries were of the greatest importance, since they opened up enormous possibilities in immunological and epidemiological research. Stokes did not live to see his discovery bear fruit; in September 1927 he died at Lagos of yellow fever contracted in the course of his post-mortem work on infected monkeys.

The virus of yellow fever was shown by George William Marshall Findlay (1893–1952) and John Constable Broom (1902–60) to be one of the smallest known; in 1933 by the method of ultrafiltration they demonstrated that the minimum size of the virus particle is from 17 to 28 mμ. In 1928 Edward Hindle (1886–) showed that if infected mosquitoes are kept at from 10° to 15° C. the virus does not develop in them. By delicate manipulation he also showed that virus is not found in the legs of a mosquito, whereas other parts of its body contain the virus (1929). Reference has previously been made to the difficulties of preserving certain organisms and viruses which may have to be sent long distances. It was a great advance therefore when Andrew Watson Sellards (1884–1942) and Hindle showed in 1928 that the virus could be preserved in infected tissues and blood by freezing them. A monkey suffering from experimentally produced yellow fever at Dakar, West Africa, was killed, and its liver was removed entire and at once frozen. It was then kept at a low temperature during the twelve-day journey to London. On arrival an emulsion of the liver was prepared and on injection into a normal monkey it produced a fatal attack of yellow fever. Hindle also showed that the virus was preserved if the liver was dried *in vacuo*, and other methods were soon introduced.

A very important modification of the virus was effected by Max Theiler (1899–), a South African who, after qualifying in medicine in London and spending some years as an instructor in tropical medicine at Harvard, became the director of the laboratories at the Rockefeller Foundation. In 1951 he received a Nobel Prize for Physiology and Medicine. It was well known that white mice are not susceptible to the yellow-fever virus by the ordinary methods of inoculation. But in 1930 Theiler found that if the virus was injected into their brains, they developed fatal encephalomyelitis without any post-mortem evidence of liver involvement—an important result, as the disease in human subjects and monkeys always produces characteristic liver lesions. Theiler now found that by passing the virus through the brains of several mice, a completely neurotropic strain was produced. He injected this into the brain of a monkey, which died of encephalitis without liver lesions. If this virus was injected subcutaneously into another monkey, no disease resulted but the animal was immunized to the virus. Although such variant strains are generally very stable, Findlay showed that a neurotropic strain could be converted into the ordinary virus of yellow fever by injecting it into the liver of a monkey.

Immunization and recent epidemiology. It had been borne out by historical epidemics and by consideration of the endemic centres that yellow fever was a disease which was found mainly along the Atlantic seaboard of the tropics and always in urban communities. While measures against Aëdes mosquitoes in these areas were effective, the desire to produce a satisfactory method of immunizing was always present, if only to protect laboratory workers who had to handle infected animals. As we have seen (p. 469) Carlos Finlay attempted to immunize human subjects by allowing infected mosquitoes to bite them. Had Finlay's mosquitoes been at a different stage of infectivity he might well have had some fatal results—as had others who later tried this method. Noguchi's attempts at immunization were doomed to failure from the start.

With the recognition of the fact that the disease is caused by a virus a new era dawned for this work. The first to prepare a vaccine for prophylactic purposes was Hindle in 1928. He attenuated the virus by treating the liver and spleen of infected monkeys with glycerine and phenol, or with formaldehyde. He considered that the virus had lost its power of producing the disease in monkeys though not that of producing immunity. The experimental results varied. Shortly afterwards similar chemical methods of inactivation of the virus were applied to infectious serum by Wilbur Augustus Sawyer (1879–1951) of the Rockefeller Foundation and his collaborators, with only partial success. By 1936 it was admitted that such methods were unlikely to lead to an efficient vaccine which could be used on a large scale. Meanwhile, from 1931 another method had been tried by Sawyer and his co-workers. They used the active neurotropic virus produced by Theiler and injected it along with immune serum from subjects who had suffered from yellow fever. The method gave a high degree of immunity lasting for at least six months. But owing to the difficulty of obtaining human immune serum in large quantities, the method had to be confined to laboratory workers.

The virus of yellow fever was first grown in tissue culture by Eugen Haagen and Theiler jointly in 1932, and from that date efforts were made to develop a satisfactory vaccine by this method. Theiler and his co-workers passed the natural virus of yellow fever through more than 150 subcultures during twenty months, and by certain other procedures they produced a strain which showed considerable reduction in its capacity to affect the liver. When injected along with immune serum it gave satisfactory immunity, and it was used in the field in Brazil from 1935 onwards. The difficulty of obtaining sufficient quantities of immune serum limited this method also, and laboratory work was now directed to the production of a vaccine prepared by tissue culture which could be given without serum. The strain used was named 17D. It was derived from the Asibi strain, one of the most virulent yellow fever strains known. By repeatedly subculturing the 17D strain in embryonic tissues, in the last stages in chick embryos from which the brain and spinal cord had been removed, the American workers produced in 1937 a vaccine which had satisfactory immunizing properties, and which did not produce severe reactions, thus permitting its use without accompanying serum. Under the auspices of the Rockefeller Foundation this vaccine was extensively used in the field. In 1938 in Brazil alone more than a million persons were vaccinated, and by 1951 it was estimated that it had been given to more than a million people with good results.

Before 1930 a 'protection test' was used in the diagnosis of doubtful cases of yellow fever. A definite amount of the patient's serum was injected intraperitoneally into a monkey, and four hours later a definite quantity of yellow-fever virus was given by the same route. If the patient was suffering from yellow fever, and therefore had antibodies in his blood, the monkey survived, but if the disease was not yellow fever the monkey died. The test was expensive and rather time consuming. But in 1930 Theiler demonstrated the production of encephalitis on injecting the virus into the brain of a mouse (p. 478), and he showed that the nature of an unknown serum could be ascertained by injecting it along with virus into the brain of a mouse (the intracerebral mouse protection test). Two years later Sawyer and Wray Devere Marr Lloyd (1902–36) showed that after preliminary treatment of the brain of the mouse the test could then be carried out more easily by injecting the virus and unknown serum into the peritoneal cavity (the intraperitoneal mouse protection test).

There had already been disquieting reports of the existence of persons whose sera, as shown by monkey-protection tests, contained antibodies to the yellow-fever virus in districts where there had been no outbreak of the disease. The advent of the mouse protection test enabled a survey to be made of a large district relatively quickly, and to give information on the incidence of present or past infection with the yellow-fever virus. By the help of the Rockefeller Foundation very large areas in South America and in Africa were thus surveyed, and in addition special post-mortem examinations were made in the case of every person who died within ten days from the beginning of any disease. These investigations revealed that yellow fever was by no means eradicated. On the contrary, its distribution was very much wider than had been suspected. In the urban districts the disease is transmitted by the Aëdes mosquito which is relatively easily destroyed. But in many districts free from this species, such as the bush, infection with yellow fever is nevertheless widespread. This so-called 'jungle yellow fever' is transmitted by a different species of mosquito. It is known to affect certain wild animals, and these probably form a reservoir of infection. In the Tropics it is found in many areas in South America and in Africa.

It is now realized that, though the yellow fever which is spread by its well-recognized mosquito-host in urban districts can be wiped out, the jungle-type of the disease cannot be dealt with by anti-mosquito measures. The only practical solution is to immunize as many persons as possible. The preparation of yellow fever vaccine grown in chick embryos has been outlined above. When properly stored at slightly under 0° C. this vaccine keeps for a year. As stated, it has been used on many millions of individuals in South America and in parts of Africa; and in the French African territories millions have been protected by the use of a dried mouse-brain vaccine. Compared with the total population exposed to risk in tropical areas, these figures are still relatively small. Further, although the protection conferred by vaccination is very efficient, it lasts only for about six years, so that repeat vaccinations must be carried out. Though much has been done, much still remains to do, and it may be long before yellow fever is completely eradicated.

(c) Trypanosomiasis

This disease, popularly known as African sleeping-sickness, is a source of considerable anxiety in Africa. The infected person develops within a few weeks a persistent fever and considerable swelling of the lymphatic glands. Then the stage of lethargy develops, sometimes after a long interval. The patient appears as if drugged, and he finally passes into a coma which leads to death.

The trypanosomes constitute the genus *Trypanosoma* of the family Trypanosomidae and are flagellates which are parasitic in the blood and certain organs of animal hosts. Though considerable variations in shape occur in different species and in different hosts, a trypanosome is characterized morphologically by its curved, elongated shape, the presence of a nucleus and a kinetoplast, of an undulating membrane and a flagellum which is often free. Reproduction in the vertebrate host is by binary fission. These facts were known long before the association of trypanosomes with disease in the human subject was recognized. The first member of the genus to be seen was found in a salmon by Gabriel Gustav Valentin (1810–83) of Berne in 1841. During the next two years similar flagellates were found in the blood of frogs, and the generic name *Trypanosoma* was conferred on them by David Gruby (1810–98). The first description of a trypanosome in the blood of a mammal was published in 1878 by Timothy Lewis (p. 492); he found it in the blood of a rat, and it was called *Trypanosoma lewisi* after him. These protozoa were then only regarded as of zoological interest; but in 1880 Griffith Evans (1835–1935), an army veterinary surgeon in

India, described a trypanosome (*T. evansi*) in the blood of horses and camels suffering from the disease called surra. In the human subject the trypanosome is often described as the cause of 'sleeping sickness', but this name applies only to the African form of trypanosomiasis. We deal first with this form, and later with the Central American form in which lethargy is uncommon.

The first authentic account of trypanosomiasis was published in 1734 by John Atkins (1685–1757) in his book *The Navy Surgeon* under the heading 'the sleeping distemper'. A good account of the condition was given by Thomas Masterman Winterbottom (1765–1859), a medical man, in the second volume of his *Account of the Native Africans in the Neighbourhood of Sierra Leone* (1803). Winterbottom referred to the cervical gland enlargement, but thought it was accidental. He observed, however, that slave traders considered that these enlarged glands indicated a disposition to lethargy and would not buy slaves who showed them. A further description was given in 1840, and about 1875 British and French medical writers noted the fact that the cervical glands were frequently enlarged, that cases are most frequent near water, and that drainage of the land prevented the disease. During the last decades of the nineteenth century the disease was well recognized by missionaries in certain parts of Africa, where it frequently caused the mission stations to be abandoned.

Meanwhile the natives in certain districts of Africa had been much troubled for at least a century by a serious disease of cattle. It was well known that it was caused by the bite of a tsetse-fly, and that ten days or so after the bite the animal died. David Livingstone (1813–73) the explorer met with it on the banks of the Zambesi in 1847, and in his *Missionary Travels* (1857) he not only gave a good description of the disease but even illustrated the fly (*Glossina morsitans*). He says that he and his party lived for two months in the area without any ill effect. It seems certain that human trypanosomiasis was not then present in East Africa. In the last decade of the century the disease nagana was causing a high mortality among horses and cattle in Zululand, and David Bruce (p. 384), who was then on military duty in Natal, was sent to investigate. He quickly discovered trypanosomes in the blood of the affected animals

(1895). Bruce showed by animal experiments that a tsetse-fly (*Glossina palpalis*) transmitted the disease, and he also showed that —contrary to local belief at that time—nagana was the same as 'fly disease'. Bruce then turned to the question of the source of the trypanosomes, and, by inoculating blood from wild animals such as buffalo and antelope into susceptible domestic animals, he showed that the wild game acted as 'reservoir hosts' for the parasites and were themselves unaffected. The trypanosome which causes nagana was named *T. brucei* in honour of Bruce.

The first recognition of the existence of a trypanosome in human blood was due to Joseph Everett Dutton (1874–1905) of the Liverpool School of Tropical Medicine. The discovery was made in 1902, and the facts are illuminating. The patient, an Englishman, was the master of a Government steamer on the Gambia river, and in the previous year he had been admitted to the hospital at Bathurst suffering from a supposed attack of malaria. He was seen by Robert Michael Forde (1861–1948), who later became the principal medical officer of the West African Medical Staff. The clinical features were not typical of malaria, and in the patient's blood Forde found bodies 'of a worm-like character', but he failed to recognize their nature. The patient was sent to Liverpool for investigation, and he was seen in hospital by Dutton. The disease was still not correctly diagnosed, but the patient improved and returned to Gambia. On the voyage he again became ill, and he was sent straight back to hospital. Meanwhile Dutton had arrived in Gambia on an expedition from the Liverpool School. He saw the patient again, examined his blood, and discerned in it the parasite which he at once recognized as a trypanosome and named *Trypanosoma gambiense*. On this expedition Dutton and his colleague John Lancelot Todd (1876–1949) examined the blood of over 1,000 natives over a wide area, and in six cases only did they find trypanosomes. Nearly all these individuals said they were strong and well, and no significant physical signs were elicited. About this time the term 'trypanosome fever' began to be used for anomalous fevers in which trypanosomes had been found in the blood. There was still no suggestion that these organisms had any connexion with negro sleeping sickness. Both Forde and Dutton published papers concerning these findings, and three years later Dutton gave his life in the service of medicine while investigating African relapsing fever, the cause of which, *Spiro-chaeta duttoni*, he discovered. Fig. 118 is a black-and-white reproduction of the coloured illustration of the trypanosomes found by Dutton and Todd in one of their native cases.

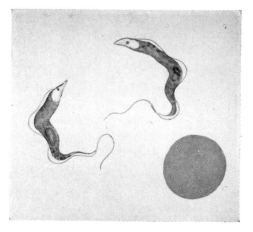

FIG. 118. *Trypanosoma gambiense* in the blood of a native of Gambia. × 2000

(From J. E. Dutton and J. L. Todd, *First Report of the Trypanosomiasis Expedition to Senegambia*, Liverpool, 1903. Original in colour)

During 1901 the British Government became concerned over a report which it had received of a very severe outbreak of sleeping sickness in Uganda; 20,000 were already dead or were beyond recovery. The Government therefore requested the Royal Society to appoint an investigating commission. This, the Royal Society's First Sleeping Sickness Commission, consisted of Cuthbert Christy (1863–1932), who had been an assistant to Haffkine in the Plague Laboratory at Bombay; George Carmichael Low (1872–1952); and Aldo Castellani (1877–). They arrived in Uganda in July 1902, and by November Castellani had seen trypanosomes in the cerebrospinal fluid, but he attached no importance to them. Early in 1903 the Royal Society appointed its Second Commission, which at first consisted of David Bruce and David Nunes Nabarro (1874–1958), a London pathologist. They arrived in March. Castellani mentioned his observations to Bruce, who stimulated him to find this organism in the fluids from other cases, before he left for London three weeks later. To Castellani is due the credit for having found trypanosomes in the cerebrospinal fluid of lethargic cases, and for having given a good description of those parasites. After his departure Bruce and Nabarro continued their routine search for trypanosomes in the fluid, and by the beginning of May they were finding them in every case of sleeping sickness, and in most cases also in the blood. They also found that the distribution of prevalence of sleeping sickness was the same as the distribution of the tsetse fly *Glossina palpalis*, and they showed that if these flies, caught in the area in which the disease was prevalent, were allowed to bite a healthy monkey, trypanosomes were later present in its blood. These results were published in a joint report, dated 29 May, by Bruce and Nabarro, who must be regarded jointly as the discoverers of the cause and mode of transmission of African trypanosomiasis.

Bruce and Nabarro continued to work steadily after the dispatch of their first report. On 25 May they were joined by Edward David Wilson Greig (1874–1950), who was then an officer in the Indian Medical Service. Before Bruce left for England on 28 August he had sent off a 'Further Report' written jointly with Nabarro and Greig, which cleared up many of the outstanding problems. At that time the type of case in which Dutton had originally discovered *Trypanosoma gambiense*—an anomalous fever, possibly with rashes, and in which trypanosomes were present in the blood—was described as suffering from 'trypanosome fever'. Bruce and his colleagues showed that it was probable that these cases were sleeping sickness in its early stages. They also showed that the trypanosomes found in lethargic cases were probably *T. gambiense*, and by extensive injection experiments in monkeys they demonstrated that typical sleeping sickness could be produced in these animals. They also investigated the susceptibility of various other animals. By experiments on healthy monkeys they showed that *Glossina palpalis* could by its bite transmit trypanosomes to them.

After the first reception of these important discoveries there was much discussion of the method by which the fly transmits the trypanosomes from infected to healthy individuals—whether it is a case of mechanical transmission, or whether there is a cyclical development of the trypanosome in the fly. In the light of later events it is now known that for several years experiments failed or were inconclusive owing to the fact that either wild flies which were already infected were used, or that the flies were also naturally infected with other species of trypanosomes. However, in 1909 Friedrich Karl Kleine (1869–1951), an associate of Koch and a leading member of the German Sleeping Sickness Commission, proved that, in the case of *T. brucei*, flies bred in the laboratory do not become infective until about twenty days after their infecting feed, and he demonstrated that in the fly changes in the trypanosomes occur, ending with the metacyclic infecting forms which are found in the salivary glands. These findings were confirmed by Bruce and his co-workers.

Until 1910 it was considered that the only species of trypanosome that effects man is *T. gambiense*. But in that year John William Watson Stephens (p. 459) and Harold Benjamin Fantham (1875–1937), both of the Liverpool School of Tropical Medicine, discovered a new species, *Trypanosoma rhodesiense*, which occurred in Nyasaland and Northern Rhodesia. In the following year it was shown by Allan Kinghorn (?–c. 1955) and Warrington Yorke (1883–1943), also of Liverpool, that the transmitting fly was *G. morsitans*.

Even with this knowledge the conquest of sleeping sickness has proved to be very difficult. A very desirable method is the destruction of the tsetse-flies, and it was thought that their breeding could be controlled by cutting down the trees near the streams where they bred. This often proved to be a costly process. In recent years a much more radical method has been employed in Nigeria. Where an area cannot be cleared of flies economically, a special tract of country in a more suitable region is made fly-free, and whole villages are removed to it. These heroic measures are meeting with considerable success.

Treatment of sleeping sickness has become fairly satisfactory with new drugs introduced in recent years. If the patient can be dealt with during the first phase, the results are good; but if the disease has entered the second stage, when the organisms are entering the nervous system, treatment can be very difficult. There is obviously no royal road to the conquest of this condition.

American trypanosomiasis is a very different condition from the African variety. In 1907 Carlos Chagas (1879–1934), of the Oswaldo Cruz Institute in Brazil, was sent to investigate an outbreak of malaria in the state of Minas Geraës. He heard that the inhabitants were much troubled by the bites of a Reduviid bug which they called the 'barbeiro'. He examined some of these bugs and found flagellates in their hind gut. He then found that most of the children in the region were affected at an early age by a disease marked by anaemia and weakness. Those that survived the acute attack were left as mental defects or paralytics. Chagas then found a new species of trypanosome in the blood of affected individuals. This was named *T. cruzi*. He was surprised that he found no signs of fission of the parasites in the blood. The mode of reproduction was cleared up in 1911 by Oliveira Gaspar de Vianna (1885–1914), who showed that the trypanosomes penetrate cells in many organs, for example the heart muscle, and there they multiply by a special process which produces leishmanial, crithidial, and finally trypanosome forms. A stage is reached when the cell bursts and the young flagellates attack other cells. Chagas showed that transmission to other individuals is affected by bugs such as *Triatoma megista*. He worked out the life-cycle in the insect host. Many papers on this parasite and its effects were written by Émile Brumpt (1877–1951), one of the greatest of the French protozoologists.

(d) Leishmaniasis

Reference has already been made (p. 419) to the discovery by Leishman of the parasite of kala-azar. The finding of the parasite occurred in 1900 in a case of 'dum-dum' fever (kala-azar), but Leishman did not publish until May 1903. In the following July Charles Donovan (1863–1951) described the same parasite in Madras, and it was named *Leishmania donovani*. In the same year the parasite of Delhi boil, which also goes under various other local names, was described by James Homer Wright (1870–1928) and was later called *Leishmania tropica*. This organism had in fact been described five years earlier by Petr Fokich Borovsky (1863–1932), but his article was in Russian and was not available in European medicine generally until forty years later.

Leishman–Donovan bodies were first cultivated in 1904 by Sir Leonard Rogers (1868–), who was associated with many other advances in tropical medicine. He showed that by using certain methods of culture the rounded parasite could be made to assume an elongated form resembling a trypanosome. He suggested that the organism was transmitted by the bed-bug. In 1911 Charles Morley Wenyon (1878–1948) suggested that the sandfly (*Phlebotomus*) was the transmitter of cutaneous leishmaniasis, and this inference was later shown to be correct. Wenyon was known for his work on kala-azar, on trypanosomiasis, on protozoa which inhabit the intestine of man, and as the author of the most comprehensive of all textbooks of protozoology.

(e) *Plague*

This grave disease has been mentioned several times in this book, and we must explain why it can now be regarded as a 'tropical' disease. It is of great antiquity. Some authorities think that this disease constituted the Plague of Athens (430 B.C.), so graphically described by Thucydides. In A.D. 542 there occurred the Plague of Justinian, which spread throughout the known world. It decimated the population, and although the heaviest mortality occurred during 542 and the years immediately following, the plague persisted until the close of the sixth century. The greatest pandemic in history, the Black Death, centred on the year 1348. It reached Europe in 1346, at the port of Caffa in the Crimea, and by 1347 Constantinople, Cyprus, Venice, and Sicily had been invaded. In the following year it had reached England, and practically the whole of western Europe was smitten by the dreadful mortality. Estimates of the deaths vary from a third to a half of the total population. The social and economic effects of the Black Death were widespread and long-lasting. The disease and the fear of it unloosed a flood of passion and violence. The mortality among men of learning was heavy, and the Church suffered grievously. The economic and agricultural structure of the land was radically altered, and plague became firmly re-established in Europe.

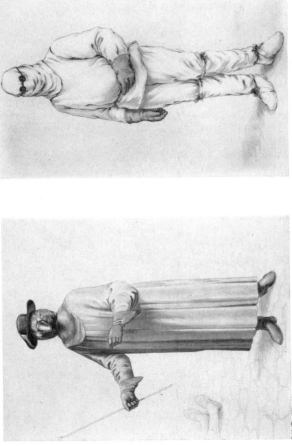

XIX. PLAGUE-FIGHTERS OF THE SEVENTEENTH AND
TWENTIETH CENTURIES

On the left, a modern drawing of a costume certainly employed in the early eighteenth, and probably also in the late seventeenth century. The mask is based on a photograph of a plague mask with a bronze beak; it was formerly in the Lazaretto at Venice, and was later transferred to a museum in Rome, but is now lost. Contemporary drawings of similar costumes are known.

On the right, a drawing of a costume successfully used during the Manchurian plague epidemic of 1909-10

(Drawings in the Wellcome Historical Medical Museum)

The next outbreak in the British Isles which has appealed to the popular imagination was the Great Plague of London in 1665. All the history books mention this outbreak, but few refer to the fact that plague was almost endemic in London from 1590 to 1665. Plague caused over 33,000 deaths in London in 1603, over 35,000 in 1625, over 10,000 in 1636, and over 9,000 in the four years 1644–47. In the great plague year, 1665, there were over 68,000 deaths from that disease. After this there were no further outbreaks of plague in Europe—apart from isolated incidents such as the violent epidemic at Marseilles in 1720. But plague continued to persist in remote parts of Asia, and there was a large epidemic in Egypt in 1834.

The plague bacillus (*Pasteurella pestis*) was discovered independently by Kitasato and Yersin in 1894 (p. 381), but this discovery of the microbic cause complicated rather than clarified the understanding of the method of spread. From early times until almost the last decades of the nineteenth century there were two opposing theories of the origin and spread of plague. The 'miasmatists' held that the disease was due to a 'miasma', a noxious influence which was found in the atmosphere or arose from the earth during plague periods. The 'contagionists', on the other hand, considered that a healthy person developed plague because he had been in contact with a plague-stricken individual or with something with which the latter had been in contact. For many centuries the battle continued between the opponents, and in practice preventive measures against plague assumed that both theories were right.

Plague prevails in great pandemic waves which persist for a very long time. The last great wave started in the year 1894, and it has not yet terminated. In that year it caused 100,000 deaths in Canton, and in that and the following year at least 1,300,000 persons died from it in India. It was expected that the discovery of the plague bacillus would solve the problem of the spread of plague, and consequently the problem of its prevention. But the event did not lead to the expected solution. Attempts were made to produce the disease by inoculating the bacilli, but these experiments had a very limited success. Some other mechanism was probably required, and research workers now turned their attention to an intermediate host.

In some ancient writings reference had been made to the association between rats and plague, and the same conditions were noted in China in 1792, in 1834, and again in 1894. In 1894 the plague bacillus was found on dead rats. But most plague authorities were still doubtful about the connexion, because cases of plague often occurred in places where no rats could be found. Further, it was noted that, while it was very dangerous to handle an infected rat which had just died, this could be done with safety a few hours later. This led Paul Louis Simond (1858–1947) to put forward in 1898 the theory that the rat-flea is the intermediary which transmits the bacillus from an infected rat to man. Even then the problem was by no means completely solved. It was not known whether the flea transmitted the bacillus from the rat mechanically or otherwise, and the actual method was not demonstrated until the experiments of Arthur William Bacot (1866–1922) and Sir Charles Martin (1866–1955) in 1914. What happens is that the rat-flea, in feeding on the blood of an infected rat, takes into its alimentary system large numbers of plague bacilli. These lodge in the fore-stomach of the flea, and as the process continues this organ eventually becomes blocked by a solid mass of bacilli. Thereafter, whenever the flea attempts to feed, the blood cannot pass to the true stomach, and it is regurgitated into the puncture made by the flea's mouth-parts. With the regurgitated blood go large numbers of bacilli, which are thus injected into the wound. If the flea is feeding on a healthy rat or a man, they are thus infected.

This new knowledge led to practical results. The importance of the rat in carrying plague in ships was recognized in 1906, and from that date rat-destruction in ships, together with inspection of passengers and crew where necessary, and quarantine, have kept the disease almost completely from the shores of the United Kingdom. In plague-ridden countries trapping and the use of various poisons are commonly employed. Opinion is now against the use of rat virus for this purpose. In ships the common method is fumigation by hydrocyanic acid, calcium cyanide, or other chemicals, which is very effective. Efficient rat-proofing of buildings, especially warehouses, is very important. These measures are not likely to give startling results unless they are combined with elimination of

rat-fleas. For this purpose all other insecticides have been superseded
by DDT, phenomenally successful since its introduction during
the Second World War. A third prophylactic measure is the use of
vaccines made either from live or heat-killed organisms. Such vaccines were first introduced by Waldemar Haffkine (p. 439), and their
employment has been the subject of much discussion.

In recent years three types of substances have been successfully
used in the treatment of plague—sera (p. 439), the sulphonamides
(p. 693), and antibiotics (p. 695). In 1896 Alexandre Yersin (p. 394)
first began to use for the treatment of plague patients a serum which
he had obtained by the immunization of horses with the plague
bacillus. Using different types of sera up to 65 per cent. of cures
have been obtained in plague cases. In 1940 the large-scale use of
sulphonamides in the treatment of plague was commenced. Sulpha-
pyridril and sulphathiazole were first used and gave good results;
but more recently sulphadiazine and similar synthetic drugs have
given up to 80 per cent. of cures in patients who had previously
been inoculated. In 1946 the antibiotic streptomycin was first used
for the treatment of plague, and it has proved eminently satisfactory;
from 90 to 100 per cent. of cures have been obtained in various series
of cases.

It might be thought that in this country at least all danger from
plague has passed, but this is not so. Of both the rat and the rat-
flea there are many species, some much more important than others.
The black rat (*Rattus rattus*) has been an inhabitant of the British
Isles from very early times, and it probably lived in harmony with
the brown (sewer) rat (*Rattus norvegicus*). It is possible that a great
influx of black rats entered England with returning Crusaders in the
twelfth century, and from then onwards the black rat was dominant.
In 1727 there occurred a westward migration of the brown rat from
the shores of the Caspian Sea, and it rapidly replaced the black rat
in western Europe and the British Isles. It so happens that the
rat-flea (*Xenopsylla cheopis*) which is particularly associated with the
black rat is the most effective of the flea-vectors of plague. The commonest flea (*Nosopsyllus fasciatus*) associated with the brown rat
carries the bacilli much less readily. This largely explains the disappearance of plague from Europe in the eighteenth and nineteenth

centuries. But in 1911 the black rat again appeared in London, and by 1937 it constituted over nine-tenths of all the rats found in the Metropolis. It is also common in other large ports. If at any time, therefore, the other factors necessary for a localized plague outbreak appear in the United Kingdom, the organism will have no difficulty in finding suitable animal hosts. But, considering the very efficient inspection carried out at our ports, such an event is not very likely.

There is another aspect of the plague problem which should be mentioned. The disease which we have been discussing is usually known as bubonic plague, because of the painful swellings (buboes) in the groin, armpits, and elsewhere which characterize most cases in a plague outbreak. There are, however, often a few in which the disease shows itself as a very fatal pneumonia. In some outbreaks these cases of pneumonic plague are relatively numerous. Since 1910 it has been known that the wild rodents, such as marmots, in certain parts of the world can also act as hosts of the plague bacillus. When the disease is transmitted to man from them the result is a comparatively few cases, but these are unfortunately nearly always of the pneumonic type and often fatal. This 'wild rodent' or 'campestral' type of plague is still causing many deaths in isolated regions of Asia, South Africa, California, and other areas, and its conquest may well mark the final stage in man's struggle with plague.

(f) Some other tropical diseases

The elucidation of the pathology and transmission of *filariasis* was effected in the last three decades of the nineteenth century. In 1863 Jean Nicholas Demarquay (1811–75) had found minute threadlike worms in the urine of a case of chylous hydrocoele in Havana. Not much attention was paid to this discovery, and it was made again independently by Timothy Richards Lewis (1841–86) in 1870 in a case of chyluria. In 1872 Lewis found these embryos in the blood, and they were called *Filaria sanguinis hominis*. After long search Lewis found the adult worms in the lymphatics in 1877. But they had already been found independently by Joseph Bancroft (1836–94) in 1876. The parasite was named *Filaria bancrofti*. There followed the classical investigations of Manson (p. 460) by which he showed that infestation with the worm was common, that the embryos appeared in the peripheral blood only at night, that this periodicity could be reversed by reversing the subject's hours of sleeping and waking; there followed also his proof that the embryos are transmitted from one individual to another by culicine mosquitoes which bite at night.

Hookworm disease (*ankylostomiasis*) has a history probably going back to Egyptian times. The worm itself was first seen by Angelo Dubini (1813–1902) in 1838. In 1878 it was shown by Grassi (p. 462), and by Ernesto (1849–1902) and Corrado Parona (1848–1922) that the presence of worms in the intestine could be deduced from the finding of their ova in the faeces. While the St. Gothard tunnel was under construction in 1880 there was a severe outbreak of anaemia among the miners. Against great opposition the Turin pathologist Edoardo Perroncito (1847–1936) demonstrated that the anaemia was due to hookworms. Until 1898 it was held that hookworm infestation arose through swallowing the ova. In that year Arthur Looss (1861–1923), professor of parasitology in Cairo, accidentally let a drop of a culture fluid containing hookworm larvae fall on his hand. He noticed only slight irritation, but he later suspected that the larvae might have passed through his skin. He therefore examined his faeces at intervals and eventually found hookworm ova. In his important monograph (1905–11) he traced the complicated path of the larvae by the blood or lymph channels to the lungs, and thence by the bronchi, larynx, pharynx, and oesophagus to the intestine where they develop into adult worms. These observations explained the 'ground itch' which is common in peasants who work barefoot in hookworm areas.

Amoebiasis has a long and complex history. The first account of an amoeba living in the intestine is probably that of Timothy Lewis (1870), who described this protozoon in cholera discharges. It was almost certainly the non-pathogenic *Entamoeba coli*. The *Entamoeba histolytica* was first described by Friedrich Lösch (? – ?) in 1875 in the stools of a Russian peasant from Archangel. Liver abscess was clearly described by William Budd (p. 731) in 1845. During the First World War much work was done on the amoebas by, among others, Wenyon (p. 483) and Clifford Dobell (1886–1949).

The use of emetine in treatment was proposed by Edward Bright Vedder (1878–1952), and a great improvement in its use, namely the subcutaneous injection of its soluble salts, was introduced by Leonard Rogers (p. 488).

THE CHANGED VIEW OF INSANITY

Insanity is as old as history. There are several references to madness in Homer. Ulysses simulated the condition, and Ajax had an attack of madness which led to his suicide. Orestes had hallucinations. Man's mental condition was conceived as being in the hands of the gods; those whom they wish to destroy they first drive mad. Mental derangement is mentioned many times in the Bible. Madness comes from the Lord. In Leviticus there is an injunction which was to have bloody consequences in later ages: 'a man also or a woman that hath a familiar spirit, or that is a wizard, shall surely be put to death.' Again: 'Thou shalt not suffer a witch to live.' References to possession in the Old Testament, which covers a thousand years, are very few. But in the New Testament, which covers only a few decades, examples of that condition are innumerable. In the Hippocratic Corpus there are also references to mental illnesses, and in the treatise on the Sacred Disease the first step is taken to remove these conditions from the sphere of theurgy.

This scientific basis was developed by later Greek writers, especially by Soranus, who not only made a real beginning in the classification of mental diseases, but also laid down principles of treatment which are based on sympathy, understanding, and a humanitarian attitude.

During the early centuries of the Christian era the practice of magic increased, and the Christian Fathers would not deny the existence of supernatural beings. The insane, for centuries regarded as being possessed by devils, were now subject to the wrath of the Church. The Codex Theodosianus of A.D. 429 officially prohibited magic, and legal sanction was given for the future prosecution of witches and those who were possessed. The physical evidence of possession was closely studied, and by the third century signs such as anaesthetic areas of the skin and mucous membranes—the *stigmata diaboli*—were accepted as being diagnostic of possession.

We now know that these signs occur in the hysterias. There are numerous paintings (cf. Fig. 119) of saints casting out devils.

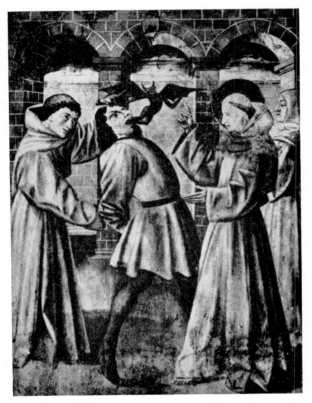

FIG. 119. St. Antony of Padua casting out a devil. Fresco by P. A. Mezzastri in the Church of St. Francis at Montefalco (From Laignel-Lavastine, *Histoire génerale de la médecine*, Paris, vol. iii)

Although the first official burning of a witch by the Church took place in 430, this was an isolated incident, and it was not until about the middle of the fifteenth century that the witch-fever really began to assume a definite place in the life of a community. Two Dominican monks, Jakob Sprenger and Heinrich Kraemer assumed for themselves the leadership in the campaign against witches, but they took care to arm themselves with a Papal Bull. They called themselves *Domini canes*, Hounds of the Lord, and their function was to bark against the rising flood of heresy. In 1489 they published a work called *Malleus maleficarum*, the Hammer against Witches. The second part of this work gives instructions for the recognition of a witch, and it is now known that many of the symptoms and signs described are those of true madness. It is evidence of the spirit of the times that this notorious book ran through ten editions before 1669, and nine further editions in the next century. For nearly 300 years it represented the spirit of the law against witches, and *ipso facto* the law which governed the 'treatment' of the insane, which was so frequently death by violence.

Asylums for the insane were in existence from about the thirteenth century, but they were far from being hospitals in which the patient's mental condition was treated. Bethlehem Hospital ('Bedlam') in London is one of the earliest, if not the earliest. It was founded in 1247, but it did not receive lunatics until 1377. An inventory of its equipment dating from twenty years later shows that it possessed four pairs of manacles, eleven chains of iron, six locks and keys, and two pairs of stocks. For centuries a visit to Bedlam to watch the antics of the poor suffering lunatics was one of the sights of London.

The first suggestion for the humane treatment of the mentally sick is to be found in the writings of Juan Luis Vives (1492–1540), a Spanish scholar and friend of Erasmus, well known in England and Flanders. Vives did significant work in pure psychology. More important from the aspect of practical results was the book entitled *De praestigiis daemonum* ('On the signs of possession') by the Rhineland physician Johann Wyer (1515–88). In this book, which was based on his own careful observations, Wyer showed that witches were persons afflicted by mental illness. He described optical hallucinations, and recognized that certain mental states affect masses of people simultaneously. Wyer was the first physician to devote himself to the study of the mentally afflicted, and he completed the divorce of medical psychology from theology. Wyer's work in this field was continued by Reginald Scot (1538?–1599) in his *Discoverie of Witchcraft* (1584), which produced a counterblast from no less a person than James I of England. Others who were equally interested in mental diseases were unable to follow Wyer's lead. For example,

Felix Plater (1536–1614), the professor of anatomy at Basle and an able clinician, went into the dungeons to study the insane. His general interest in nosology, the classification of diseases, led him to produce the first classification of mental diseases which has a modern character. But he was nevertheless unable to accept the fact that mental diseases might be due to natural causes, and he ascribed them mainly to diabolical agencies. Plater was a supporter of Vesalius, and he himself dissected 300 bodies and gave the first description of certain physiological conditions. He founded the botanical garden and the anatomical theatre at Basle. The new era in the actual treatment of insanity begins with the abolition of the old system of restraint. This was accomplished almost simultaneously by two noble-minded men, a Frenchman and an Englishman.

In 1793 Philippe Pinel (1745–1826), a Parisian physician and writer on medical subjects, was appointed physician to the notorious Bicêtre in Paris as a result of his essay on mania, written but not published in 1792. Shocked by what he saw, he decided at once to free from their chains the lunatics who were in his charge. One man had been incarcerated for forty years; another had been in chains for thirty-six years. The permission of the Commune for this scheme was reluctantly given, but the ultimate results of releasing the patients from their chains were wholly beneficial. As a result of the Revolution Pinel's essay was not published until 1801, when it appeared with the title *Traité médico-philosophique sur l'aliénation mentale ou la manie* ('Medico-philosophical treatise on mental alienation'). In it he developed his theories of the humaner treatment of the insane. Pinel was later appointed to the Salpêtrière, and from there he produced a second edition of his work. His book laid the foundation of the French School of psychiatry that remained important during the whole of the nineteenth century.

About the same time events in England took a slightly different form, but they led to a similar result. William Tuke (1732–1822) was a Quaker merchant of York who had devoted much of his spare time to philanthropical works. In 1791 a Quaker died in the York County Asylum in circumstances which suggested maltreatment. Tuke concluded that there was a need for an institution in which the mentally afflicted could be treated on humanitarian lines. In 1792 he

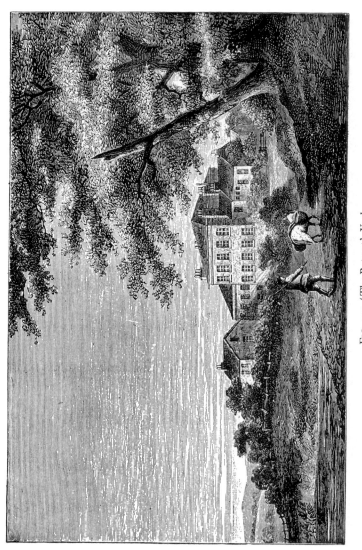

FIG. 120. 'The Retreat', York

(After Tuke, *Chapters in the History of the Insane in the British Isles*, 1882)

made this proposal to the Society of Friends in Yorkshire, and the scheme was enthusiastically adopted. It was resolved to erect a building to accommodate thirty patients, and in 1796 the first patients were admitted. Tuke's institution at York, The Retreat (Fig. 120), was run on his principles of reducing restraint to the minimum, of giving the patients as much personal freedom as possible, and of treating the mind by exercise of the body and by regular employment in industries. Tuke made these resolutions before Pinel had struck the fetters from the lunatics in the Bicêtre, and by the time he was putting them into practice in The Retreat news of Pinel's work had still not reached him.

Despite the interest which was shown in the work of Tuke and Pinel, there was for many years little improvement in mental hospitals. The York County Asylum again came to the public notice in 1814, as a result of the disappearances of several patients whose relatives had been forbidden to visit them. The outcry which resulted led to the appointment in 1815 of a select committee to study provisions for the better regulation of madhouses in England. The report revealed an appalling state of affairs. Filth and dirt were everywhere, and the keepers were ignorant and cruel. Chains and manacles were still being used extensively. In Bethlehem Hospital one man had been secured for twelve years by a series of iron rings round his neck and body; these were connected by very short chains to a vertical iron bar inserted into the wall (cf. Fig. 121). He could lie on his back on his bed, and he could stand upright; but practically all other positions were prevented by the apparatus. Pinel and Tuke were pioneers and their interests were mainly centred on their own institutions. What was now wanted was a man of courage and with the ability and personality to propagate the new doctrines. Such a man was John Conolly (1794–1866).

Conolly had practised medicine in two English provincial towns and at the age of thirty-three he came to London. In 1828 he was appointed professor of the practice of medicine at University College. He tried hard to induce the university to inaugurate a course of clinical instruction in insanity. Piqued at his failure in this matter, he left London and practised in Warwickshire until he was appointed in 1839 resident physician to the Middlesex Asylum at Hanwell, the largest mental hospital in England. William Tuke and his son, Henry Tuke (1755-1814), at York, and following them Edward Parker Charlesworth (1783-1853) and later Robert Gardiner Hill

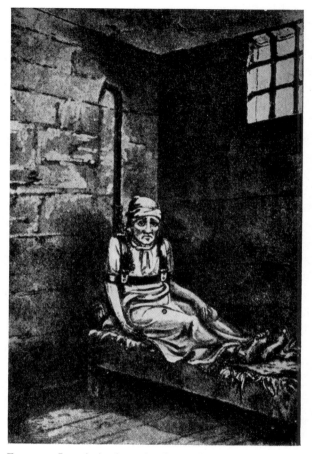

FIG. 121. Lunatic in the early nineteenth century, with body rings attached to a vertical iron bar (Drawing by G. Arnold, A.R.A.)

(1811-78) at Lincoln, had reduced restraint to the minimum compatible with the advantage and safety of the patient. On his appointment to Hanwell, however, Conolly at once abolished absolutely all forms of mechanical restraint. Within five years he wrote that 'there is no asylum in the world in which mechanical restraint may not be abolished not only with safety, but with incalculable advantage'. By his writings and his example Conolly disseminated the new doctrines.

The non-restraint movement spread slowly and with considerable opposition. In America it was first successfully practised by Thomas Kirkbride (1809–83) and Benjamin Rush (p. 190). In many asylums the abolition of the fetters led to the use of the padded cell, and it is only recently that this restrictive measure has been rendered unnecessary by appropriate management and the use of drugs. The most important single factor in all such cases is the necessity for the patient to be under constant observation both by day and night. In France the work of Pinel was continued by Jean Étienne Dominique Esquirol (1772–1840), who wrote a great textbook of psychiatry (*Des maladies mentales*, 1838), and Guillaume Ferrus (1784–1861). Ferrus did much to increase the number of asylums in France, and in them he first separated the lunatics from the criminals. He started a farm at the Bicêtre for occupational therapy, and became mainly responsible for initiating the law of 30 June 1838, which humanized the treatment of patients, improved the condition of mental institutions, and established new institutions in every department of France. In Germany progress was slower. Typical of the German attitude at this period were the methods adopted by Johann Christian Reil (1759–1813). Reil had the humane instinct, and he indeed reduced restraint in the treatment of patients. But he substituted for it, on psychological grounds, what he called 'non-injurious torture'. Patients were thrown into water, cannons were fired near them, and they were suddenly confronted with a tableau in which their physicians and keepers played the parts of judges, angels, and the dead newly risen from their graves. This primitive type of 'shock therapy' had a life-span out of all proportion to its merits, but it played its part in elucidating the psychology of mental diseases.

In England the next advances were most important in the field of local government and state control of the insane. 'Wynne's Act' for the better care and maintenance of pauper or criminal lunatics was passed in 1808, and four amending Acts were passed at intervals up to 1824. The first satisfactory law enforcing certification of patients before their admission into mental homes was passed in 1828, but it applied only to the Metropolis. The same Act appointed fifteen Commissioners in Lunacy for the Metropolis, and certifications were to be reported to them. About this time the great and good Lord Shaftesbury (p. 218) became interested in the subject, but it cost him many years of struggle against prejudice and apathy before he was able to see on the Statute Book his Bill regulating the conditions in private madhouses and establishing the Board of Commissioners in Lunacy for England and Wales (1844). It was a subject to which that great philanthropist devoted much thought. In 1845 the provision of asylums out of the local rates was made compulsory on the local Justices in England.

During this period the most potent force in the United States was certainly Dorothea Lynde Dix (1802-87). A school-teacher who had retired because of ill health, she became interested in institutions, and she made a personal investigation of the shocking conditions which she found in jails, almshouses, and asylums. She was responsible for the founding of about thirty-two new institutions for the insane, and for the improvement of many old ones. In 1848 she reported to Congress that she had seen more than nine thousand idiots, epileptics, and insane in the United States, destitute of appropriate care, bound with chains and fetters, scourged with rods, and abandoned to the most outrageous violations. She paid a visit to Scotland and in a few weeks she was responsible for the appointment of a Royal Commission to inquire into the condition of lunatic asylums in Scotland. Her cause was greatly assisted by the hearing which she obtained in the House of Commons.

The later decades of the nineteenth century saw further improvements in mental institutions. The period of non-restraint led to a system of seclusion, under which every patient had his own room, the door of which was frequently locked; padded rooms for violent patients were frequently in use. The gradual replacement of this system by more modern methods necessitated changes in the design of institutions. These more humane methods, based largely on efficient management of the patients, were made possible by an improvement in the number and training of attendants. Samuel Hitch (1801-81), founder of the Medico-Psychological Association, introduced female nursing of male patients into the Gloucester Asylum in 1841. In 1854 classes for the training of nurses were started at the Crichton Royal Institution, Dumfries. The revolution in nursing led by Florence Nightingale (pp. 704-9) was reflected in the quality of the nursing in mental hospitals. From 1880 onwards there was an increasing tendency to employ nurses who had received their full training in a general hospital.

Another Parliamentary investigation into the care of the insane in England and Wales took place in 1877, and in 1890 the duties of asylum administration were transferred from the Justices to the County Councils. This resulted in a great improvement in the extent of the accommodation and the quality of the treatment of the insane poor. At the same time the order of a magistrate became necessary for the consignment of a private patient to an asylum. In 1913 the Lunacy Commission was reorganized as the Board of Control, which also became responsible for the care and education of the mentally defective.

Mental conditions have given rise to some strange diseases, of which one may be mentioned here. This was tarantism, or the dancing mania, which was supposed to have been very common in Apulia for many centuries. Supposedly first-hand descriptions are found from the early seventeenth century. The most famous description appears in the dissertation on the disease by Giorgio Baglivi (1668–1707), who was adopted by a physician of Apulia and spent part of his early life there. Baglivi became one of the foremost physicians of his age. He was also an iatrophysicist, and he carried that theory to a degree that was almost ludicrous. In his mechanistic theory the body was made up of independent tools or machines, the teeth, for example, being scissors, the chest a bellows, and the heart and vessels a water-works. But as soon as he entered the sick-room he cast aside his mechanistic views and pinned his faith on astute observation and logical deduction. Baglivi gave a very interesting description of tarantism. The disease was said to be produced by the bite of the tarantula spider, and it occurred at the height of summer. Some saw the spider while others did not, but as soon as they were 'bitten' they ran to the market-place and began to dance. They were soon joined by others, who had also been 'bitten'. The poison remained in the system for years, and manifested itself only at the height of the summer. The population of a whole district might be 'affected' simultaneously. The dances were accompanied by riotous behaviour. The only cure was music, and especially the tarantella, which was written for that purpose. An outbreak of this behaviour might last several days till all were exhausted. This strange neurosis has never been satisfactorily explained.

Although this fanciful explanation of a neurosis was put forward as late as the time of Baglivi, there had been heard much earlier isolated voices calling for a more rational attitude to mental diseases. Among these was the voice of Paracelsus, who pointed out that the dancing mania was a disease, and was not due to possession. The teaching of Paracelsus was well known, although many of his books were not published until long after his death. About 1525 he wrote a small work entitled *Von den Krankheiten so die Vernunft berauben* ('On diseases which deprive the individual of his sanity', published in 1567) in which he distinguished between various forms of mental illness and included a class equivalent to the psychoneuroses. His division of mania into four major psychoses, and his insistence that these conditions are natural diseases of the individual and are not due to spirits, are far in advance of his time. He distinguished between the feeble-minded and those who are mentally ill, and he pointed out that while the former are so born, the latter are not. His therapy contains the germ of much that is modern, and some claim that his therapeutic use of the magnet foreshadowed the later development of mesmerism, suggestion, and psychoanalysis. Many of the observations of Paracelsus on mental conditions are found scattered in his general writings on medical subjects.

A contemporary of Baglivi was G. E. Stahl (p. 143), whose doctrine of Animism provided an effective counterblast to the Iatrophysicists, of whom Baglivi was himself an extreme example. Stahl's most important general work, his *Theoria medica vera* (1707), contains much relating to mental conditions; but in the following year he published a small book, *De animi morbis* ('On mental diseases', 1708), which helps to explain his attitude. Stahl was one of the first to emphasize that certain mental states are of physical origin, while others are functional. He was also one of the first to recognize the influence of the body on the mind, and vice versa. In his own day

Stahl's views on mental diseases had little influence in Germany. But in 1831 his *Theoria* was republished in a new German translation, and its significance was then recognized.

Although no great progress was made in the broad conception of mental diseases during the late seventeenth and early eighteenth centuries, this period was notable for several descriptions of individual diseases. Sydenham published in his *Dissertatio epistolaris* to Dr. Cole (1682) a classical account of hysteria, which he considered identical with hypochondria. His treatment of these conditions was logical, simple, and humane. Half a century later the physician George Cheyne (1671–1743) published a book entitled *The English Malady* (1733), by which he meant hypochondria. The significance of this book is that in it Cheyne described his own case, and ushered in a period when mental symptoms were much more fully discussed and described. Cheyne thought that a third of all his patients were neurotics. Trotter (p. 187), in his book *A View of the Nervous Temperament* (1807), put the proportion of his patients who were neurotics at two-thirds.

The eighteenth century closed with the publication of the three-volume work, *Della pazzia in genere e in specie* ('On mental diseases in general and in particular', 1793–4), by Vincenzo Chiarurgi (1739–1820) of Florence. He was the director of the Hospital of St. Boniface in that city, and in it he had improved the sanitation and abolished mechanical restraint. This comprehensive work is based on the case histories of a hundred cases which he records, and is notable for the numerous descriptions of the morbid anatomy of brains from mental cases. Despite the great amount of material in this book, Pinel criticized it as following stereotyped lines and as lacking in the spirit of research.

It was Pinel's *Traité* which ushered in the new outlook of the nineteenth century and laid the foundation of the great French School of psychiatry. Pinel's pupil Étienne Jean Georget (1795–1828) published his work *De la folie* (1820) at the age of twenty-five; it contains excellent clinical descriptions of his cases. Reference has already been made to Esquirol's famous book (p. 501). It epitomized over twenty years of clinical teaching and investigation. He introduced the term 'hallucinations' and the concept of depressions, and was one of the first to attempt an analysis of the psychological factors which may cause mental illnesses. Another French psychiatrist whose influence was felt in other countries was Benedict Augustin Morel (1809–73) who was interested especially in problems of degeneration. His large work on degenerations in general (1857), and his treatise on mental diseases (1860), gave prominence to conditions which were hereditary or supposedly due to toxins. In Great Britain, James Cowles Prichard (1786–1848) wrote a treatise on insanity (1835) in which he introduced the conception of moral insanity. A reaction to the prevailing trends was strongly shown by Wilhelm Griesinger (1817–68) in his book *Die Pathologie und Therapie der psychischen Krankheiten* ('The pathology and treatment of mental diseases', 1845). This work became a classic of psychiatry, although its author did not continue with his psychiatric work until over twenty years after its publication. Griesinger took little account of psychological causes and regarded mental conditions simply as evidence of brain lesions.

The natural history of mental diseases, that is, their causation, classification, and the consideration of the symptoms and signs which they produce in the patient, has long been the subject of the closest study and considerable controversy. It was at one time believed that an anatomical basis would be found for all mental diseases. Even at the present time this theory is far from being justified, and as the simplest type of classification we must therefore adopt a division into organic and functional disorders. A slightly more elaborate—but still by no means practical—classification divides the functional disorders into the neuroses and the psychoses. We may assume that there is an essential difference in kind between these two groups, though this assumption is not universally accepted. The neuroses are characterized by disorders of the emotions or of the intellect which are exaggerated examples of the symptoms found from time to time in all normal individuals. They are the normal reactions of the normal individual writ large. In the psychoses, on the other hand, the patient's reactions bear no relation to real life; they belong to a world of phantasy.

Consideration of the history of these subjects would lead us far into the vast ramifications of the human mind, but a brief discussion will indicate the steps by which the modern standpoint has been reached. Consider a disease long recognized as being due to an organic lesion of the brain, viz. general paralysis of the insane. It is characterized by a complete change in personality, impairment of memory, by increasing weakness, speech defects, various paralyses, and death in untreated cases. The disease is possibly to be identified with the conditions described in 1672 by Thomas Willis (p. 245) and in 1798 by John Haslam (1764–1844), apothecary at Bethlehem Hospital, though neither recognized its nature. The first undoubted cases of this disease to be clearly described were reported in 1822 by Antoine Laurent Jessé Bayle (1799–1858), who held that it was due to chronic meningitis. Four years later Louis Florentin Calmeil (1798–1895) showed that the chronic inflammation affected not only the meninges but also the substance of the brain itself. From then onwards it was increasingly suspected, on statistical and other evidence, that general paralysis was a late syphilitic manifestation, but the strongest evidence was not obtained until near the close of the century, when Richard von Krafft-Ebing (1840–1902) inoculated general paralytics with syphilitic matter without infecting them with syphilis. The conclusive proof was not obtained until 1913, when Hideyo Noguchi (p. 475) and Joseph Waldron Moore (1879–) announced that they had obtained the spirochaete which causes syphilis from 14 out of 70 brains of general paralytics which they had examined. General paralysis is therefore an organic disease of the brain. Of a generally similar type are the organic conditions produced by chronic intoxication with alcohol, morphine, and other substances. Other organic conditions may be caused by degenerative diseases of the brain substance, as in senile dementia, or by slowly increasing pressure on the brain, as in cerebral tumour and certain cases of injury to the brain.

In the case of the functional mental disorders the differentiation between the psychoses and the neuroses stems from a method of treatment which was practised by a man who is still considered something of a charlatan. Franz Anton Mesmer (1734–1815) studied medicine at Vienna, and his graduation thesis (1766) dealt with the influence of the planets on man. He believed that this influence could be exercised on patients by the use of a magnet. Next he

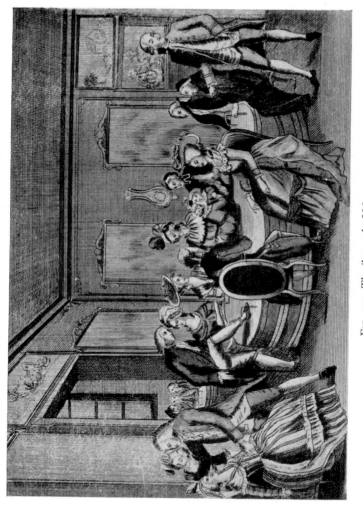

FIG. 122. The 'baquet' of Mesmer
(Woodcut after a contemporary engraving)

conceived the idea that the same power could be exercised by the human hand, and he ascribed the results to the influence of 'animal magnetism'. In consequence of his apparent cure of a young woman who was associated with the Austrian Court, and whose illness was probably due to a severe hysteria, Mesmer was asked to leave Vienna and in 1778 he arrived in Paris. He claimed that he could increase the flow of 'magnetic fluid' to or from a patient, even when he was acting at a distance. In Paris he at once began to practise his method on a large scale. He added to his method for group treatment much of the equipment of the charlatan, and he reaped a rich financial reward. He invented a sort of trough filled with mirrors and iron rods ('Mesmer's *baquet*') around which the patients were grouped with linked hands. Mesmer's practice caused much discussion in scientific circles, and in 1784 the French Academy of Sciences appointed a committee to report on the whole matter. The committee found that 'animal magnetism' did not exist, and that the violent effects produced by Mesmer in public treatments were due to the imagination. Mesmer was driven from France by the Revolution, but he returned several times in later years. Whatever his detractors might say about his magnetic theory, they overlooked two facts: Mesmer had a remarkable personal influence over the imagination of his patients, and during his cures somnambulism was a frequent phenomenon. He was in fact the first to produce the hypnotic state at will, and until recent times the verbs 'mesmerize' and 'hypnotize' have been practically synonymous. The transition of mesmerism into hypnotism occurred in 1820, when Alexandre Jacques François Bertrand (1795–1831) first observed the hypnotic state, and explained it on the basis of the laws of the imagination.

The first scientist of undoubted ability to adopt the new practice was John Elliotson (1791–1868), who attempted to introduce it in University College Hospital in London, but the reaction among the Hospital Governors was so violent that he had to resign his chair. Contemporaneously James Braid (1795–1860), a Scottish surgeon resident in Manchester, had been trying out the method, and he realized that the 'magnetic fluid' played no part in the conditions produced. In 1842 he published a paper on the subject, and in the following year there appeared his *Neurypnology, or the Rationale of*

Nervous Sleep, in which the terms 'hypnotism', 'hypnotize', and 'hypnotic' were first used. Twenty years later hypnotism began to be studied by Ambroise Auguste Liébeault (1823–1904) of Nancy, who was interested in it as a method of treating physical diseases. Associated with him later as pupil and colleague he had Hippolyte Marie Bernheim (1840–1919), who had studied under Charcot (p. 274) at

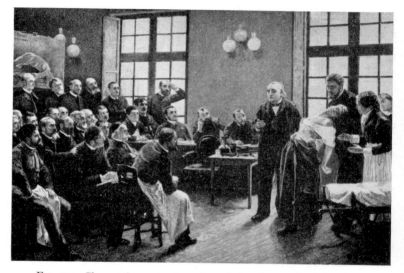

Fig. 123. Charcot demonstrating a hysterical patient at the Salpêtrière
(Etching by André Brouillet, 1887)

the Salpêtrière. Charcot had used hypnotism in his neurological work, and by its aid he had reduced the paralysis in patients suffering from hysteria.

Apart from their results in treating patients, the work of these last three men was important because of the insight which it gave into diseases of the mind. It was shown that, in addition to the graver psychoses—those diseases which popularly raise doubts about the patient's sanity—there exists a group of conditions which are now collectively known as neuroses, of which hysteria and anxiety-neurosis are important examples. The treatment of these conditions is now largely psychological.

A discussion of the psychoses—conditions associated with mania, extreme depression or melancholia—is too complicated for discussion here, but mention may be made of two men who have introduced far-reaching concepts. Emil Kraepelin (1856–1926), one of the greatest of systematizers in the history of mental diseases, described in 1898 the insanity which develops early in adult life, and which he named dementia praecox, although the term had been used earlier for a condition which was possibly not identical by Benedict Augustin Morel (p. 506) and others. Paul Eugen Bleuler (1857–1939) later modified some of Kraepelin's conceptions about this disease and renamed it schizophrenia (1911).

The beginning of the modern shock therapy for the treatment of certain types of insanity occurred in 1917, when Julius von Wagner-Jauregg (1857–1940) first succeeded with his work on general paralysis of the insane. Over twenty years previously he had used injections of tuberculin in order to produce fever. In 1917 he inoculated nine cases with malaria, and six of these were benefited as a result. This so-called 'shock treatment' by malaria is still being used, but more recently other methods of producing the shock—such as electrical methods—have been adopted. A dubious phase in the treatment of mental diseases is due to Manfred Joshua Sakel (1900–57), who described in 1937 the treatment of schizophrenia by the injection of insulin. The insulin produces a fall in the amount of sugar which normally circulates in the blood, and if sufficient is injected the patient passes through a stage of confusion into a deep sleep and a profound coma. The whole process has to be very carefully regulated and carried out under strict medical supervision. After about half an hour of coma the patient is aroused by giving him glucose. This method of treatment has not fulfilled its early promise, and it is now falling into disuse.

Another special method is the convulsive therapy for severe depressive and melancholic states, first introduced by Ladislas Jos Meduna (1896–) of Budapest in 1934. The aim is to produce a major epileptiform convulsion, and to repeat this up to twenty times over a period of several weeks. The convulsion is produced by the intravenous injection of the drug cardiazol (metrazol), and so far as the mental condition is concerned this method has given good results. In 1937 Ugo Cerletti (1877–) and Lucio Bini (1908–) of

Rome first used an electrical method to produce the convulsion, and this has advantages over the cardiazol method. In both these methods, however, special procedures have to be taken to prevent the patient under treatment from harming himself by the violence of the convulsion. Fractures of bones are common in both methods, and they also are being given up.

A further procedure may be mentioned. In 1935 Antonio Caetano de Egas Moniz (1874–1955), of Lisbon isolated the frontal lobes from the brain by injecting alcohol into the connecting white matter of the brain. This was done in patients suffering from extreme emotional tension of an apparently incurable nature. Later the bold step was taken of cutting through these connecting association fibres, which actually lie within the substance of the brain. This operation of prefrontal leucotomy is of a very delicate nature. In properly selected cases results have so far been promising, but the method has many disadvantages, and it is still the subject of much controversy.

The number of persons certified insane has been slowly increasing for many years. This increase is due partly to the increasing willingness of patients and their relatives to allow voluntary treatment to be tried, and partly to the fact that the insane now live longer than they used to do. There is no evidence at all of an actual increase in insanity. The great majority of persons treated for mental illness receive their treatment in mental institutions. In 1954 the number of patients treated in England and Wales was 152,144, and of these 140,487 were in mental hospitals. Although the quality of the treatment has improved vastly in recent years, the bed provision has not kept pace with the demands, and there is still a great shortage.

Amelioration of the lot of the mentally afflicted as a whole seems at present to depend more on official action than on further advances in medical treatment.

THE NEW MOVEMENT IN PSYCHOLOGY

The modern treatment of insanity is also closely bound up with methods which depend upon new ways of analysing the mind which have developed in the last hundred years. The study of the motives which direct man's thought and activity could not be properly studied except in relation to the actions of animals; and before a comparative and evolutionary psychology could be created, it had to be shown that man's mental development was continuous with that of the animal world. The evolutionary view of the origin of Man, both in his physical and mental aspects, was provided by Darwin in the *Origin of Species* (1859), and, so far as the mental aspect is concerned, more especially in the *Descent of Man* (1871) and the *Expression of the Emotions in Man and Animals* (1872). Much assistance has subsequently been provided in these studies by a consideration of the mind of primitive man, and it has been shown that there are constantly occurring in the mind conflicts between primitive emotions and the restraint imposed at higher evolutionary levels. These conflicts are normally quite unconscious. The study of the manner in which they are resolved has given rise to several Schools of Psychology.

From the medical aspect the founder of all such Schools was Sigmund Freud (1856–1939), who did most of his work in Vienna, but escaped to England a year before his death. Freud was at first a neuroanatomist and neuropathologist in Vienna, and in 1885 he was working with Charcot in Paris. He later studied hypnotism further under Liébeault and Bernheim at Nancy. Back in Vienna Freud associated himself with Josef Breuer (1842–1925), who a few years before had used hypnotism to enable the patient to express his inmost thoughts without any suggestion from the observer. The discharge of emotions in the hypnotic state led to great improvement in hysterical conditions, and to the discovery of the working of the unconscious mind. Freud and Breuer published their results in the treatment of hysteria in 1895. Briefly, it may be said that Freud divided the mind into three levels. In the conscious level emotions and the recollection of events were freely expressed. Below this was the pre-conscious level into which events which were inacceptable to the subject were consciously displaced; such events could be recalled under sufficient pressure. Lowest of all was the level of the unconscious or subconscious, from which the memory of events could not be recalled at all except by the methods which Freud was now adopting.

Freud now dispensed with the hypnotic state and allowed the patient to talk at random without suggestion. This was the method of free association. By its aid Freud divided the mind into the Ego, which is a subjective awareness of self, and the Id, which is the un-conscious reserve of primitive instincts. The libido, a particular division of the Id, was the source of the individual's emotional energy. In his works *The Interpretation of Dreams* (1900) and the *Psychopathology of Everyday Life* (1904) Freud entered the field of the psychology of the normal mind, and showed that the boundary between the normal and the abnormal was very indeterminate.

An important side-aspect of Freud's theories was his preoccupa-tion with sex. His conception of the Oedipus complex, which assumes that the young child's love for his mother leads to subconscious hatred of his father, is important. Freud conceived that this complex in the child's mind was repressed into his subconscious. Later in life these complexes may strive to pass from the subconscious into the conscious, and the result is a neurosis. Freud's methods of examination of such cases led to his practice of psychoanalysis under free association. The widespread use of this method has shown that painful or unwelcome experiences which have been repressed into the subconscious disturb the equilibrium of health. The psycho-analyst seeks to release the repressed experience into the conscious, since the patient often finds it easier to deal with the emotion or memory after it has been released than when it is in the sub-conscious.

Freud had several disciples who became famous, and some of these later broke with his Vienna School and founded schools of their own. For example, Alfred Adler (1870–1937) broke away in 1911 and founded his School of Individual Psychology. Instead of regarding sex as the driving force in personality, Adler substituted the need for superiority and power. He introduced the conception of the inferiority complex, and the method of compensation by which it is overcome. Carl Gustav Jung (1875–) broke away from Freud in 1913 and founded the School of Analytical Psychology. He thought that the libido was a fundamental force, which might on occasion be canalized in the direction of loving or hating or of achieving power, but which was essentially indefinable.

While these psychological methods of treating mental derange-ments have had great triumphs, the School of Freud and his asso-ciates has met with much opposition. A full analysis sometimes takes years to carry through and is therefore expensive. A celebrated American psychologist was analysed by Freud's leading disciple, and the analysis was discontinued after 168 sessions. At that stage it was doubtful whether the analysis had been a success.

SOME MODERN PHYSIOLOGICAL CONCEPTS OF CLINICAL IMPORT

The vast activity in the sciences of physiology and pathology during the last eighty years, and their repeated divisions into independent sciences, each prosecuted by its own specialists, have yielded many ideas which have been imported into the clinical practice of medicine. It is impossible to say which of these are of permanent value. All previous ages have had to discard part of the practice and a large proportion of the medical ideas that have been handed down to them, and there is no reason to suppose that the age that follows us will differ from those which have gone before us. Some ideas that have entered medicine from the physiological laboratory, pushed by interested parties or seized on in despair by physicians at a loss for a line of treatment, are already seen by men of experience and judgement to be no permanent addition to our store. Other lines of physiological thought are still under discussion by them.

There are, however, certain physiological conceptions which, apart from their general implications in the economy of the body, have received such wide application that their future, as an organic part of medical practice, seems assured.

(a) Ductless Glands and Internal Secretions

The nature and action of the various glands of the body has been a classical physiological field. Malpighi (pp. 124–6) was the first to investigate the structure of these organs, and he was followed by many others. It became evident that many glands, such as the liver, the salivary glands, and the tear glands, are provided with tube-like ducts, which carry off the characteristic secretion of the glands. The first of these special ducts to be discovered was the pancreatic duct. This discovery was made in 1642, and demonstrated on many bodies, by Johann Georg Wirsung (1600–43), a native of Augsburg who became prosector to the famous professor of anatomy and botany at Padua, Johann Vesling (1598–1649), whose textbook *Syntagma anatomicum* (in Latin, Padua, 1641) went through numerous editions, was translated into several modern languages, and had its last edition (in Italian) in 1804, over 160 years after the publication of the first edition. Wirsung's discovery, on the other hand, is recorded only on a single anatomical sheet of 1642, now very rare. In 1656 Thomas Wharton (1614–73) of London first described the submaxillary duct in his *Adenographia: sive glandularum totius corporis descriptio* ('Adenography or a description of the glands of the whole body', 1656). The parotid duct was first described in 1662 by Niels Stensen [Nicolaus Steno] (1638–86), of Copenhagen, in his *Observationes Anatomicae*. Stensen later wrote two important works on muscles (1664, 1667) in which he showed the action of individual fibrils is summed to produce the action of the muscle. Stensen was one of the founders of geology. He failed to obtain the chair of anatomy at Copenhagen, and he settled in Italy and became a bishop of the Church of Rome. De Graaf was the first to collect the secretion from a gland (p. 297).

Beginnings of the conception of ductless glands. One of the first to speculate that other organs might contribute secretions to the body's economy was Frederik Ruysch (1638–1731), a celebrated anatomist of Amsterdam who was the first to describe the valves in the lymphatics, and who brought anatomical injection to a very high pitch. About 1690 Ruysch suggested that organs such as the thyroid poured into the blood-stream substances which were of importance. Théophile de Bordeu (1722–76), a graduate of Montpellier who later practised in Paris, went much farther. In his *Recherches sur les maladies chroniques* ('Research on chronic diseases', 1775) he speculated on the possibility of many parts of the body giving off emanations which affected other parts; he argued from the results of castration, which had long been known. Although his views were based on speculation and not on experiment, there are grounds for considering de Bordeu as the founder of endocrinology.

The next events of importance occurred in 1849. In that year Arnold Adolph Berthold (1803–61) of Göttingen gave the first experimental proof of the existence of an internal secretion. It had long been known that castration of a cock leads to atrophy of its comb; but Berthold showed that if the testes are transplanted to another part of the bird's body, atrophy of the comb does not occur. This observation was completely neglected, and attention was not called to Berthold's paper until more than sixty years later.

The other event of 1849 was the publication by Thomas Addison (p. 284) of a paper which he had read in that year before a London medical society on the cause of idiopathic anaemia associated with disease of the suprarenal bodies. This paper also attracted little attention. But Addison was induced to expand it to a monograph, and in 1855 there appeared his *On the Constitutional and Local Effects of Disease of the Supra-Renal Capsules*. In this work he described eleven cases of a condition characterized by anaemia, increasing weakness, feebleness of the heart, gastric irritability, and a 'smoky' or bronzed pigmentation of the skin with a characteristic distribution. The cases were fatal, and at autopsy disease of the suprarenal bodies was found. In six of the eleven cases one or both suprarenals were tuberculous, and in four others they showed cancerous deposits. In the year following the publication of the monograph Trousseau named the condition Addison's disease. Addison had himself called it 'melasma suprarenale'. Although further work, including the observations of Addison's friend and staunchest supporter, Sir Samuel Wilks (p. 285), discredited a few of the eleven original cases, there was never any doubt of the fact that Addison had described a disease-entity in which the symptoms were characteristic, and in which frequently the only pathological lesion found *post mortem* was serious involvement of the suprarenals. Nearly three-quarters of these lesions were tuberculous, and the remainder were due to simple atrophy of the glands, or to fibrosis producing atrophy. (In recent years atrophy seems to have played the predominant role.) In the opening paragraph of this monograph Addison emphasized the fact that, though the suprarenals were very well supplied with blood, virtually nothing was known of their function.

In that same year, 1855, Claude Bernard (p. 294) introduced the term 'internal secretion' (*sécrétion interne*). He said that the external secretion of the liver forms the bile, whereas the internal secretion of that organ forms the blood sugar. This was a conception which was ultimately to bear rich fruit.

In 1856 the experimental study of the physiology of the endocrine glands was initiated by Brown-Séquard (p. 261). During the next two years he carried out excision of the suprarenal glands in animals, as a result of which he concluded that they are essential to life. It is now thought that many of his animals died as a result of post-operative shock or of sepsis, but his experiments paved the way for a vast amount of more detailed experimental work.

From this point investigation of several of the endocrine organs made steady progress. It is, however, convenient to deal with them separately, but before doing so we mention an important discovery which had a fundamental bearing on later research on the ductless glands. This discovery illuminated the process by which internal secretions produce their results. It is easy to say that the active substance is absorbed into the blood and passes in the circulation to the organs which it influences. But this statement overlooks the possibility of nervous and other factors. As was previously stated (p. 302) the solution of the problem was given in 1902 by (Sir) William Maddock Bayliss (1860–1924) and Ernest Henry Starling (1866–1927). They were investigating the flow of pancreatic juice from the duct which opens into the duodenum. It had long been known that the juice does not begin to flow until the pylorus opens and admits into the duodenum some of the acid gastric contents, but it was thought that the flow was regulated by a nervous mechanism. This is so, but only in part. Bayliss and Starling showed that there is a substance in the mucous membrane of the intestine which, when the acid gastric contents reach the pyloric valve separating the stomach from the first part of the intestine, is carried in the blood to the pancreas and stimulates it to activity. This substance they named secretin.

Bayliss was perhaps best known for his *Principles of General Physiology* (1915), a very individual work which included many biological observations not usually found in textbooks of physiology. He also wrote important monographs on *Enzyme Action* (1908) and *The Vaso-motor System* (1923), each of which embodies much personal research. A chair of general physiology was created for Bayliss at

University College, London, in 1912, and he was thus relieved of much teaching and administration. Starling was at that time the holder of the Jodrell chair of physiology in that College. Reference has already been made to his important work on the physiology of the circulation. His *Principles of Human Physiology*, the standard British textbook of its time, first appeared in 1912, and, under the subsequent editorship of Lovatt Evans (p. 316), is still a standard work.

Secretin was the first to be isolated of a whole group of substances called hormones (Greek *hormao*, I excite). The word was coined for Starling by a friend who was a classical scholar, and Starling first used it in his Croonian Lectures at the Royal College of Physicians in 1905. Hormones are active in very small amounts. They are secreted by one organ or tissue, pass into the blood and are carried by it to another secretory organ which they excite to activity. The action is very rapid, and is entirely independent of nervous activity. A very small amount of hormone only is necessary to produce a reaction, and the hormones are justly called chemical messengers.

This was the early conception of hormones. Since rapidity was part of the essence of their action, they had to be easily oxidizable so that they rapidly disappeared from the body. It should be said, however, that the modern tendency is to regard as hormones all internal secretions which are dispersed to other parts of the body in the blood-stream. Some of these act rapidly, but others—such as the internal secretion of the thyroid—are more stable and produce a more protracted effect.

(i) *The Thyroid*

This gland was known at least from the time of Galen, who thought it provided a fluid for the lubrication of the larynx, and the name 'thyroid' (Greek *thyreos*, a shield) was given to it by Wharton (p. 516), who considered that it was designed by Nature to give, especially in females, a rotundity and beauty to the neck. Microscopically it consists of vesicles lined with cubical cells. The vesicles contain a colloid material. About the middle of the nineteenth century it was held that the vesicles communicated with each other. But in his doctoral thesis of 1841 Heinrich Adolf Bardeleben

(1819–95), later a noted German surgeon and supporter of Lister's new methods, stated that the vesicles did not intercommunicate, a view which was not finally confirmed until about thirty years ago.

Sir Astley Cooper (p. 284) appears to have been convinced that the organ performed some definite function. He noted the large lymphatics which pass from it into the thoracic duct, and he suggested that they perhaps conveyed the secretion from the gland. About 1827 he carried out excision of the gland in puppies (thyroidectomy) and he found that they recovered and remained well. Cooper's results were published as an appendix to a paper of 1836 by his junior colleague Thomas Wilkinson King (1809–47) on the structure and function of the 'thyroid gland'. Already at that date the organ was confidently referred to as a gland, and King thought that it might form and store some material which on emergency was thrown into the circulation. King used a simple microscope and observed the thyroid follicles. He called them 'cells' and noted that each was filled with a gummy, translucent fluid. He was thus aware of the basic structure of the thyroid. Opinion was therefore turning from the view formerly held that the purpose of the rich vascular network in the thyroid was to protect the brain from the force of the circulation. By 1844 John Simon (p. 219), from comparative anatomical studies, was turning from this view to the idea that the thyroid was a secreting gland and that its product was thrown into the circulation. In 1856 and the following year Moritz Schiff (1823–96), who was then professor of comparative anatomy at Berne, but later held chairs of physiology at Florence and Geneva, did thyroidectomies on dogs and guinea-pigs with fatal results. His communication was buried in a work on another subject, and nothing further was heard of it for nearly thirty years.

Some consideration must now be given to diseases which affect the thyroid, especially in relation to the part which they played in clarifying its physiology.

(a) *Hypothyroidism.* From at least shortly before the beginning of the Christian era it was known that in certain districts the inhabitants had a tendency to develop a swelling in the region of the throat. Pliny refers to this condition, and Juvenal asks who would be surprised to see a swollen neck in the Alps. During the late Middle

Ages accounts of the prevalence of this condition in certain localities are found in the Lives of the Saints, and from this period dates the legend that the condition could be cured by the royal touch. The condition was known as goitre, and to distinguish it from a similar condition of different origin it is now known as *simple goitre*. In 1516 Paracelsus (p. 100) gave a good account of goitre in the Duchy of Salzburg, and he associated it with a condition now known as *cretinism*. It was shown that these two conditions were often endemic in certain mountainous districts. In the Alps, for example, they occurred in the deep valleys. In 1789 Michaele Vincenzo Giacinto Malacarne (1744–1816) published at Turin a treatise on these conditions as they existed in the valley of Aosta, and sixty years later it was shown that over a quarter of the inhabitants of that district were affected. From then onwards there were numerous studies of the geographical distribution of these conditions. In England goitre was especially common in the West Country (Somerset and Gloucestershire), and also in the Peak District, where it was referred to as 'Derbyshire neck'.

Simple goitre and endemic cretinism were superficially very dissimilar. In goitre the most prominent sign was the neck swelling, and the symptoms were directly attributed to it, such as dyspnoea, cyanosis of the head and neck, with cough and alteration of voice, due respectively to pressure on the trachea, the veins, and the nerves. On the other hand, cretins showed great retardation in development from infancy, with a characteristic facies—broad, depressed nose, enlarged tongue, wrinkled forehead, dry and scanty hair—spade-like hands, a protruding abdomen, and mental deficiency. There were pads of fat above the clavicles and the thyroid was usually enlarged. In many cases therefore cretinism could be regarded as simple goitre together with other prominent features arising in early infancy.

In 1850 Thomas Blizard Curling (1811–88) described two children who were mentally deficient and showed pads of fat above their clavicles, but neither of whom showed goitre. Both died, and in both cases post-mortem examination showed absence of the thyroid gland. Curling suggested that the presence of the abnormal fat might be due to 'the absence of those changes which result from the action of the thyroid'. These were cases of sporadic cretinism, which was distinguished from the endemic variety in 1871 by Charles Hilton Fagge (1838–83) of Guy's Hospital, who thought that cretinism might develop in adults. Fagge also pointed out that endemic cretins show goitres, but sporadic cretins show no signs of the presence of a thyroid. In the sporadic cretin the gland has undergone complete atrophy; whereas the endemic cretin has a thyroid which has been continually deprived of iodine before birth, and it is therefore born goitrous.

Although cretinism was still an obscure disease, certain definite views had long been held regarding the cause and treatment of goitre. Pliny considered that the water from some wells produces goitre, and this belief persisted. In fact, ever since then the view has nearly always been held that something in the water causes the disease, and at the middle of the nineteenth century the opinion favoured was that the cause was excess of magnesia. From the Middle Ages definite views had also been held regarding treatment. Roger of Palermo (*fl. c.* 1170–1200), an early surgical 'magister' of the School of Salerno, wrote about 1180 his *Practica chirurgiae*, in which he described the use of mercurial salves for chronic skin diseases, suture of the intestine, and the unfortunate doctrine of the healing of wounds by 'second intention', with the consequent production of 'laudable pus'. He also recommended the ash of burnt sponge and of seaweed in the treatment of goitre. About a century later this treatment was also strongly recommended by Arnold of Villanova (1235–1311), a master of the great and ancient medical school at Montpellier. Arnold wrote a commentary on the *Regimen Sanitatis Salerni*, and also on fevers and on the rational classification of diseases; he dabbled in alchemy, and is credited with having introduced tinctures into the pharmacopoeia. During the succeeding centuries burnt sponge and seaweed were given empirically in the treatment of goitre. In the eighteenth century they were widely used in a secret remedy by a family of doctors in Coventry, and this method was hence called the 'Coventry treatment'.

Iodine was discovered by Courtois in 1812, and four years later William Prout (p. 157) tested potassium iodide on himself to make sure that it was not toxic in small doses, and then used it as a remedy for goitre in one case. He made no secret of this experiment, and in 1818 it was also used by John Elliotson (p. 509). In 1820 Jean François Coindet (1774–1834) of Geneva gave the tincture of iodine to 150 goitrous patients without ill effect, and other physicians also used the tincture. In 1829 Jean Guillaume Auguste Lugol (1786–1851) of Paris introduced his well-known iodine solution for use in certain forms of tuberculosis. This consisted at first of a solution of iodine in water, and he later added potassium iodide. This solution was widely used in the treatment of goitre, and toxic effects from the iodine became common. A reaction set in about 1860, and soon iodine in treatment was abandoned.

Surgical treatment of goitre has an ancient, though rather uninteresting, early history. It was probably attempted by Albucasis, the great master of Arab surgery. The operation was probably revived towards the end of the eighteenth century by Pierre Joseph Desault (1744–95). Desault dissected an adherent thyroid from the trachea. During the next seventy years the operation of removal was seldom attempted, and then only partially and when death from suffocation was threatened. In 1869 Paul August Sick (1836–1900) performed the first total thyroidectomy. In passing, mention may be made of Timothy Holmes (1825–1907), who performed the heroic feat of removing from a patient aged sixty-five a pendulous suppurating goitre which hung down to below the waist and weighed 7 pounds. Surgeons were generally disinclined to attempt thyroidectomy because of the danger of severe or fatal haemorrhage from the very vascular thyroid. Really successful thyroidectomy was first made possible by Billroth (p. 364) while he was holding the chair of surgery at Vienna. By 1869 he had done twenty thyroidectomies with eight deaths. He was very cautious in his choice of suitable cases for operation, and in his lectures of 1877 he warned his students against attempting the operation merely for cosmetic purposes. Although much reduced, the death-rate during or following thyroidectomy was still considerable. The technique of the operation of thyroidectomy was progressively improved by Billroth's pupil, Theodor Kocher (p. 374) of Berne, who had at his disposal the great numbers of Swiss patients with goitres. From about 1878 other surgeons operated on the thyroid much more frequently. Kocher's own results were excellent. By 1895 he had done over a thousand thyroidectomies, and by about the beginning of the First World War he had performed this operation over 2,000 times with a mortality of only 4·5 per cent.

We now return to Hilton Fagge's work of 1871. In that year he prophesied that cretinism might develop in adults. Two years later his prophecy was fulfilled when Sir W. W. Gull (p. 285) described five cases of 'a cretinoid condition supervening in adult life in women'. This condition, now clearly recognized, is characterized by a dimming of the mental faculties, some loss of memory, a marked lowering of the basal metabolic rate so that the economy of the body is slowed down, a low temperature, and sensitivity to cold. The hair is dry and falls out; and the skin, especially of the face, the supra-clavicular region, and the extremities, present a puffy, oedematous appearance, but does not show pitting on pressure, the sign of true oedema.

This condition had previously been observed, but not published. In 1869 John Byrom Bramwell (1822–84) of North Shields demonstrated to his son, later Sir Byrom Bramwell (p. 278), all the important clinical features of this condition. But William Miller Ord (1834–1902), of St. Thomas's Hospital in London, first observed a case of this disease when he was twenty-seven, and in 1877 he published five cases. By then an analysis had been made of the swollen skin of the feet, which was reported to contain more than fifty times the normal amount of mucin. Ord therefore proposed *myxoedema* as the name for this 'cretinoid' condition of middle-aged women. A few years later it was shown by William Dobinson Halliburton (1860–1931) that the amount of mucin in the skin of these cases was very much less than had been stated, and that therefore the term myxoedema was a misnomer. Halliburton held the chair of physiology at King's College, London, for thirty-three years, and his works on the chemical composition of the blood, and muscle and nerve tissues were important in establishing chemical physiology as an independent discipline. Influenced by these criticisms, Osler in 1898 proposed the name Gull's disease, but by then the name myxoedema had become established.

Subsequent to Ord's publication there followed a very important period in the history of the thyroid. In 1882 Jacques Louis Reverdin

(1842–1929), a well-known teacher of surgery in Geneva, read a paper in which he described the occurrence after thyroidectomy of symptoms which resembled exactly those seen in cases of myxoedema. In the following year in a joint paper with his cousin Auguste Reverdin (1848–1908), also a distinguished Geneva surgeon, he further emphasized this relationship. In 1883 also Kocher reported that in 30 out of his first 100 thyroidectomies the operation had been followed by the development of a condition which he called cachexia strumipriva, and which he attributed to a chronic asphyxia. There then followed a controversy between Kocher and J. L. Reverdin regarding the nature of this post-operative condition. These discussions were reported in the German journals, but were unknown in Great Britain. They were read by (Sir) Felix Semon (1849–1921) who, born and educated in Germany, had come to London at the age of twenty-five and had by that year established himself as laryngologist at St. Thomas's Hospital. In November 1883 Semon stated at a meeting of the Clinical Society of London his view that cachexia strumipriva, myxoedema, and cretinism were all due to the same cause—loss of function of the thyroid gland. His opinion was ridiculed, but in the following month the Society appointed a committee to investigate the cause. (Sir) Victor Alexander Haden Horsley (1857–1916), then professor-superintendent of the Brown Institution, was a member, and he carried out experimental thyroidectomies on monkeys and other animals successfully. Moritz Schiff also repeated his previous experiments of 1856 on dogs (p. 520), and he also was successful. These results, with the other evidence collected by the Committee, proved that, as Semon had stated, cachexia strumipriva, myxoedema, and cretinism were all due to loss of function of the thyroid gland, and were all virtually the same disease. Horsley at first thought the function of the thyroid was to control the metabolism of mucus. Later it was considered that it neutralized or removed poisons, and thyroid deficiency hence led to toxaemia.

Both Horsley and Schiff had tried to treat the myxoedema arising after experimental operations by grafting the animal's thyroid into another part of its body. The results were only temporarily successful, since the transplanted thyroid was absorbed. In 1890 George

Redmayne Murray (1865–1939), who was then professor of comparative pathology in the University of Durham and later became professor
of medicine at Manchester, concluded that myxoedema ought to be
improved by the hypodermic injection of thyroid extract. Early in
the following year he published this suggestion, and in the autumn
he reported the progress of a woman of forty-six suffering from
myxoedema who had been treated during the previous six months by

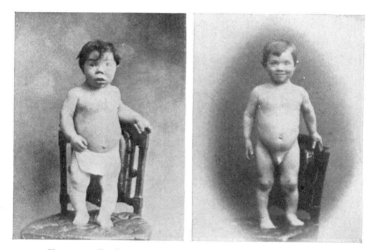

FIG. 124. Cretinous infant before and after thyroid treatment
(Photographs from the Collection of the Royal College of Surgeons of England)

the hypodermic injection of a glycerine extract of sheep's thyroid.
Under thyroid treatment this patient lived for a further twenty-eight
years. In 1892 cases in which thyroid extract had been given by
mouth instead of by injection were reported independently by
Hector Mackenzie (1856–1929) and Edward Lawrence Fox (1859–
1938), and the oral method was adopted and found to be satisfactory.
These results also confirmed that the function of the thyroid was to
control metabolism.

The nature of the metabolism controlled by the thyroid was
investigated late in the nineteenth century. In 1895 Eugen Baumann
(1846–96) investigated the thyroid chemically and found an organic
compound of iodine. On Christmas Day, 1914, Edward Calvin
Kendall (1886–) isolated the active principle, a tyrosine derivative,

which was named thyroxine. In 1927 Sir Charles Robert Harington (1897–) and George Barger (1878–1939) synthesized this substance.

Since these investigations were made there have been no significant additions to our knowledge of myxoedema or of cretinism, but simple goitre has been a different matter. The fundamental cause of the simple goitre is complete deprivation of iodine, as in these circumstances thyroxine is not produced. Complete deprivation of iodine is, however, rare. In goitrous districts of Switzerland and the United States goitre has been largely prevented by the provision of salt containing about 1 part of iodine in 200,000 parts of salt for table purposes. Deficiency of iodine in the diet leads to overgrowth of the cellular elements of the thyroid; the vesicles, which are normally full of colloid material, are compressed and contain little or none. Hence, although the gland as a whole is enlarged, its active elements are very deficient.

There were many cogent arguments against the theory that simple goitre is due solely to iodine deficiency, and of those who have illuminated the position in recent years a British and an American investigator must be specially mentioned. Sir Robert McCarrison (1878–1960) qualified in medicine in Ireland and then was commissioned in the Indian Medical Service, and in India he has spent the greater part of his active life. At Coonoor he started in 1918 a laboratory for research on nutrition, and it grew into a famous institute. In it he investigated scientifically the effects of various native diets, and he carried out many important investigations on deficiency diseases such as beri-beri. He began to study goitre in the foothills of the Himalayas in 1905 and continued this work intermittently for thirty years. In the area of Gilgit in this district there are nine villages. In eight of these goitre was endemic, while the ninth was free from goitre. The ninth village obtained its water from a very pure spring; the other eight villages were situated one below the other and had the same water supply, a snow-fed mountain stream. As the water descended to lower and lower villages it became more and more polluted from human and animal sources. A survey showed that the village which received the most polluted water had the highest incidence of goitre, nearly half of its population being affected. McCarrison tried treatment by intestinal disinfectants such as thymol, and found that a proportion of the cases were cured. He therefore thought that they acted by counteracting a goitrogen or goitre-producing agent in the food. This conception is important at the present time. In 1906 he carried out an interesting experiment on a group of non-goitrous young men who had just arrived in the district. They lived in a small goitre-free area in this goitrous district, and they drank only water from a spring which was known to be non-goitre producing. But each morning they consumed quantities of the suspended matter from the water-supply to the affected villages. An equivalent control group consumed the same suspended matter after it had been boiled. The experiment proceeded for 55 days. By the end of that time over a third of the test group had either progressively increasing or transient goitres, whereas the control group were quite free from goitre. McCarrison included himself in the test group and he developed a progressively increasing goitre. This is probably the only record of the artificial induction of an outbreak of goitre in human subjects. McCarrison concluded as a result of these experiments that goitre could be produced by the presence of some goitrogen in drinking water. This theory was the reverse of the theory that goitre is caused by the absence from the drinking water of some substance such as iodine.

Another important investigation was carried out by McCarrison in collaboration with the statistician Krishna Bindu Madhava (1895–). They weighed the thyroid gland and related it to the body-weight, age, and sex in rats, guinea-pigs, and other animals. They introduced the quantity r, which in any subject was obtained by dividing the weight of the gland by the body weight. For an associated universe of animals they plotted the values of r logarithmically and obtained a curve referred to as 'the life-line of the thyroid gland'. In this way they showed that there is normally a gradual relative increase in size of the thyroid up to puberty, when the demands on this organ are greatest. By application of these principles to the human subject they evolved logical methods for ascertaining whether a goitre was really present or whether the apparent increase in size of the gland was a physiological enlargement.

In the United States one of the most pertinaceous investigators of the physiology and pathology of the thyroid is David Marine (1880–). Goitre prophylaxis by the addition of iodine to the diet had been tried as early as 1860, but the method fell into disuse and was forgotten. In 1917 Marine and Oliver Paul Kimball (1889–) prevented goitre in schoolchildren in Akron, Ohio, by this method. It had long been known that the need of the body for the hormone of the thyroid may cause acute changes in thyroid structure. This theory was introduced by Halsted (p. 349) in 1896; he found that dogs which had had half of their thyroids removed developed hyperplasia (i.e. multiplication of its constituent cells) in the remaining half. Marine held that endemic goitre can be produced solely by iodine want. The normal functioning of the thyroid depends on the activity of the thyrotropic hormone of the anterior pituitary (p. 548). The colloid material containing iodine is stored in the thyroid follicles, and the thyroid hormone is passed into the bloodstream to maintain a minimum concentration. If the iodine supply is insufficient, this minimum concentration may not be maintained under increased need, as at puberty or during pregnancy. In 1924 Marine advanced the theory known as the Marine cycle. At such a time of increased demand the thyrotropic hormone stimulates the cells which line the thyroid follicles, and as a result the individual cells increase in size (hypertrophy). Further action of thyrotropic hormone causes the individual cells to multiply by cell division, so that the size and volume of individual follicles are increased. This constitutes hyperplasia. If an excess of iodine is now received, the enlarged follicles fill up with active colloid. This excessive secretion ceases after a time, but the follicles are permanently enlarged in their resting state (involution). A continuation of this state leads to degeneration of the gland substance, and the production of a simple colloid goitre. This is the typical sequence of the Marine cycle.

In 1928 the theory of the production of goitre by the presence of an active goitrogen—in contradistinction to the absence from the diet of some substance such as iodine—received a considerable stimulus as a result of the researches of Alan Mason Chesney (1888–) of Johns Hopkins University and his co-workers. While carrying out experimental work on syphilis they found that the rabbits in a colony which they were using were rapidly becoming goitrous. The rabbits had been fed mainly on cabbage, and Chesney later demonstrated that the cabbage was the cause of the goitre. This goitrogenic action of cabbage was confirmed by Marine and his co-workers, and also by McCarrison in India. Since then small outbreaks of goitre have been reported in human communities compelled by circumstances to exist mainly on cabbage. In 1941 Thomas Henry Kennedy and Herbert Dudley Purves, carrying out a similar series of experiments in New Zealand, found that rape seed would also induce goitre. This led to the discovery in 1943 by Edwin Bennett Astwood (1909–) of that type of goitrogens known as thyroid blocking agents, examples of which are thiourea and thiouracil which now have important uses in clinical medicine. Yet despite all the extensive research carried out on simple goitre during the last fifty years, its pathogenesis is far from being completely understood.

(b) *Hyperthyroidism.* During the first half of the nineteenth century accounts began to appear in the literature of another type of swelling of the thyroid associated with other definite symptoms, one of which was apparent protrusion of the eyeballs. The only earlier recorded association of these conditions appears to be an account by a twelfth-century Persian physician. The first modern writer to note it was Caleb Hillier Parry (1755–1822), the distinguished Bath physician who was a lifelong friend of Edward Jenner. In 1788 Parry read before a small country medical society a paper in which he attributed angina pectoris to disease of the coronary arteries. He did not publish this paper until 1799. In 1786 he observed a case of goitre associated with exophthalmos. During the remainder of his life he saw seven further cases in which goitre was associated with cardiac palpitation but not with exophthalmos. His account of these eight cases was published posthumously in 1825. Ten years later R. J. Graves of Dublin (p. 283) published three cases of cardiac palpitation with goitre, and in one of these he mentioned that exophthalmos was present. In 1840 Carl Adolph von Basedow (1799–1854) of Merseburg published four cases. In the following year Sir Henry Marsh (1790–1860) described two cases of enlarged thyroid and dilatation of the heart; he mentioned exophthalmos as being present. An excellent case showing typical exophthalmos was published in 1849 by

William White Cooper (1816–86), ophthalmic surgeon to St. Mary's Hospital, Paddington.

Possibly the best early account of this condition was that given by William Stokes in his book on diseases of the heart (1854, p. 283). Stokes regarded the disease as a cardiac neurosis, and he thought the cardiac condition was primary. This view was held for many years, but it was gradually superseded by the nervous theory of origin. Part of the nervous theory was bound up with the suggestion that the exophthalmos was due to excessive activity of the cervical sympathetic as a result of pressure exerted on it by the enlarged thyroid. On this theory it seems difficult to understand why exophthalmos does not occur also in simple goitre. Nevertheless, many of the great works of the last decade of the nineteenth century either stated that the disease was of nervous origin or associated it in some way with the nervous system.

It had meanwhile long been recognized that the two characteristic features of the disease previously mentioned—goitre and exophthalmos—were often accompanied by a third feature, viz. rapid action of the heart and nervous irritability or emotional disturbances. With the increase of knowledge of metabolism, it was thought that these and other features, including sweating and abnormal sensitivity to heat and cold, were an expression of an increase in basal metabolism. In 1880 Ludwig Rehn (1849–1930) of Frankfort-on-Main performed a thyroidectomy in such a case. The report of this case was not published till 1884, and in it Rehn suggested that the symptoms and signs were due to overactivity of the thyroid, and that thyroidectomy was thus a logical method of treatment. Despite the pertinence of this suggestion that the disease was due to overactivity of the thyroid it did not really receive much recognition until well into the twentieth century.

We are now in a position to consider briefly the various names which have been given to this strange and interesting disease. The first writers to describe the condition did not name it, but employed phrases descriptive of the main features. The name exophthalmic goitre was certainly in use before 1860, and about that period similar terms, none of which became at all popular, were employed. In 1860 Trousseau called it Graves's disease, and this name has been widely used. In Germany the term Basedow's disease is usually employed, and it also found a place in textbooks in English. The names of Stokes and Marsh have also been associated with it. In 1898 Osler, on the grounds of priority of observation, proposed that it should be called Parry's disease. The name hyperthyroidism was proposed by C. H. Mayo (p. 370) in 1907, and the name toxic adenoma has also been widely used although it does not adequately indicate the primary type of the disease. More expressive possibly is the name thyrotoxicosis, which is also widely used. On the whole the name Graves's disease is open to least objection; it has long been popularly known, and it is the term preferred by James Howard Means (1885–) of Johns Hopkins University, one of the great modern authorities on diseases of the thyroid. The difficulty in using for this disease any name which is not an eponym is that none of them covers the numerous cases in which one of the triad of signs is absent, and that nearly all of them suggest, if they do not actually indicate, that the cause of the disease is known.

Although Rehn's theory was adopted slowly, its progress was determined. In 1886 Paul Julius Möbius (1854–1907) of Leipzig suggested that in some way the abnormal activity of the thyroid poisoned the whole body. William Smith Greenfield (1846–1919), professor of general pathology at Edinburgh University, gave in his Bradshaw Lecture at the Royal College of Physicians of London in 1893 the results of his ten years' work on the histology of the thyroid in Graves's disease. He showed that there was increase in size and number of the cells lining the follicles, so that the volume of the follicles and of their contained colloid was reduced. Discussion then centred on the nature of the change in the thyroid secretion. Möbius had been inclined to consider that the changes in the gland produced an abnormal type of secretion. Henry Stanley Plummer (1874–1937) and Walter Meredith Boothby (1880–1953) of the Mayo Clinic advanced the view in 1924 that in Graves's disease the thyroid secretes an excess of normal thyroxine, and also an abnormal type of thyroxine deficient in iodine. Each of these two products was responsible for its own particular group of symptoms. Harington (p. 527) and others have, however, put forward cogent arguments against the theory of an abnormal secretion.

Twenty years ago it was held that true Graves's disease cannot occur without changes in the thyroid, but this view seems to have been abandoned. Though it is a fact that most cases show some thyroid abnormality, it is long since these changes were regarded as primary. Most authorities accept the fact that the disease is precipitated by some factor such as emotional strain, toxaemia, or the excessive action of some of the other endocrine glands. Discussion of these matters would, however, lead us beyond the scope of this book, but it must be stated that the fundamental cause of the disease is still unknown.

The prominence of the eyes (exophthalmos) seen in Graves's disease is different from that due to any other cause, and has long been a subject of research and discussion. The fact that the recognition of this particular type of exophthalmos as such may not be easy is indicated by the number of signs which have been described in connexion with it. The earliest of these was Dalrymple's sign, which consists of widening of the palpebral fissure due to retraction of the upper eyelids. It was used by John Dalrymple (1803–52), a London ophthalmic surgeon. He never published this sign, and it was left for his friend W. W. Cooper (p. 531) to do so (1849). The experimental study of exophthalmos began with the work (1858) of Heinrich Müller (1820–64), professor of comparative anatomy at Würzburg. Von Graefe (p. 647) described in 1864 the sign called after him, in which the upper eyelid lags behind the movement of the eyeball. In 1869 Carl Stellwag von Carion (1823–1904) noted that in Graves's disease the normal involuntary blinking movements of the eyelids are absent or much diminished (Stellwag's sign). Weakness of the power of convergence of the eyes on looking at a near object was described by Möbius (p. 532) in 1886; and in 1893 Alexis Joffroy (p. 275) of Paris described the sign known by his name—absence of wrinkling of the forehead when the patient looks upwards. At least eight other special signs have been described to differentiate this type of exophthalmos.

The cause of this condition is of some consequence, since in certain cases, especially after thyroidectomy, the exophthalmos may be extreme and may lead to corneal scarring and to inflammation of the eyeball sufficient to lead to the loss of the eye. William Stokes thought it was due to an increase in ocular humours, so that the size of the eyeball was increased. There is some evidence that weakness and degeneration of the external ocular muscles may play a part, as also may spasm of these muscles. The evidence is, however, on the whole in favour of an increase in the intraorbital contents, especially fat, pushing the eyeball forward. There is reason to believe that the condition can be produced by the anterior pituitary thyrotropic hormone without the agency of the thyroid hormone.

In the treatment of hyperthyroidism three methods deserve brief consideration from the historical aspect. On the analogy of simple goitre iodine was early used by Basedow, Stokes, and others. It subsequently fell into disuse, but in 1923 it was reintroduced as pre-operative medication by Plummer, and since then it has been almost universally employed. The earliest type of operative treatment con-sisted in the ligature of one or both superior thyroid arteries. About 1845 ligature of the inferior thyroid arteries in addition was described. Partial thyroidectomy was first performed for hyperthyroidism in 1872 by (Sir) Patrick Heron Watson (1832–1907) of Edinburgh. As an inventor of new surgical methods Watson stood very high. Before the introduction of Lister's antiseptic technique he had excised the whole larynx, removed the spleen, and excised joints with success. As already mentioned, sub-total thyroidectomy was first performed by Rehn in 1880, and this has become the operation of choice. Pioneers in these methods have been Kocher, Halsted, Cecil Augustus Joll (1885–1945), and Sir Thomas Peel Dunhill (1876–1957). The third method is the use of the so-called antithyroid drugs. The first attempt seems to have been the, only partially, successful use of potassium thiocyanate in Means's wards at the Massachusetts General Hospital in 1941. Shortly afterwards Astwood (p. 530) had much more promising results with thiourea and thiouracil (1943) in the United States, and thiourea was also effectively used (1943) by Sir Harold Percival Himsworth (1905–) at University College Hospital, London.

(ii) *The Parathyroids*

The extensive experience of thyroidectomy gained by the German and Swiss surgeons has already been mentioned. In their early days their results were not nearly so good as they were later, and some of their patients suffered from the condition named 'tetania thyreopriva' which was not infrequently fatal. This condition seems to have been first reported from Billroth's clinic in 1880, two years later by Reverdin, and in 1883 by Kocher. It also occurred about 1885 in the experimental thyroidectomies performed by Schiff and by Horsley. The cause of this condition was then unknown, but it was obviously closely allied to tetany of the idiopathic type. This condition may be acute or chronic, and is characterized by an abnormal irritability of the neuromuscular system, so that abnormal sensations are experienced in the extremities, and the muscles are subject to chronic spasms; when the laryngeal or bronchial muscles are affected death may result.

In children a condition known as tetany was first described in 1815 by John Clarke (1761–1815) of St. Bartholomew's Hospital. In 1816 George Kellie of Leith described a chronic contracture of the hands and feet in children, now known as carpo-pedal spasm and recognized as due to chronic tetany. Three years later John Cheyne (1777–1836), a Scots physician who migrated to Dublin, gave a good account of the condition. The name tetany was introduced in 1852 by Lucien Corvisart (1824–82), the nephew of the *baron* J. N. Corvisart (p. 172). Not much attention was paid to these observations, but gradually methods were introduced for the detection of minor degrees of the condition. Trousseau described in 1864 the sign which is known by his name—the production of a characteristic spasm of the hand on compressing the brachial artery. In 1878 Franz Chvostek (1835–84) of Vienna described a characteristic grimace which was produced in such cases by tapping over the facial nerve.

In another field the stage was meanwhile being set for the discovery of the true nature of tetany—atrophy or extirpation of parathyroid tissue. The parathyroid glands were first discovered by Sir Richard Owen (p. 237) during his dissection (1849–50) of an Indian rhinoceros which died in the London Zoo. His description was published in 1852, not—as is nearly always stated—in 1862. In man they were possibly described by Virchow in 1863, but the first systematic account in man was given by Ivar Victor Sandström (1852–89) of the University of Uppsala in 1880. Sandström described two parathyroids on each side in man, but subsequent workers—including Victor Horsley (p. 525)—found that the number appeared to vary in different species of animals. Until 1895 it was generally held that these glands consisted of thyroid tissue, but in that year Alfred Kohn (1867–1959) of Prague stated that the parathyroids were physiologically distinct from the thyroid.

The physiology of the parathyroids was extensively studied by Eugène Gley (1857–1930) of Paris. In 1891 he directed attention to Sandström's account; and as a result of surgical extirpation of the parathyroids then known in animals, he concluded that their function was the same as that of the thyroid. This conclusion was denied by Giulio Vassale (1862–1912) of Modena who, working with Francesco Generali about 1896, decided as a result of extirpation experiments that the thyroid provided an internal secretion, whereas the parathyroids exerted an antitoxic action, the loss of which gave rise to tetany. David Arthur Welsh (1865–1948), then at Edinburgh, Halsted and others then carried out further experiments about 1898 and showed that if the parathyroids were completely removed severe tetany resulted in death. For many years contradictory results were obtained by other experimenters, but it is now known that if a fatal result does not follow extirpation, the survival of the animal is due to the presence of parathyroid tissue outside the operation area.

In 1909 W. G. MacCallum (p. 639) and Carl Voegtlin (1879–), then of Johns Hopkins University, during their studies of the condition known as renal rickets, in which limitation of the function of the kidneys in early life leads to dwarfism, showed that the bone changes in that disease were accompanied by hypertrophy of the parathyroids. These changes consisted in the dissolution of the deposits of calcium salts in the bone, and they concluded that the parathyroids regulated calcium metabolism. They showed also that tetany following extirpation of the parathyroids could be prevented by the administration of calcium. Many attempts were made by others in later years to establish the manner in which this action is effected, and the steps are too complex for discussion here. It may be said, however, that in 1925 James Bertram Collip (1892–), then at the University of Alberta, Edmonton, but later at Montreal, isolated from the parathyroid an extract which he was able to standardize. This was named parathormone. Its administration leads to a depletion of the calcium in the bones and to a corresponding rise of the calcium content of the blood. Though it has important practical uses, especially in the treatment of tetany, its mode of action has not yet been completely elucidated.

A rare disease of bone, characterized by pains and weakness in the back and limbs, tenderness over the long bones, followed by deformity and bending of the bones of the limbs, had been known for about two centuries. The disease simulates certain other diseases of bone, especially osteomalacia, and an accurate differential diagnosis has been possible only in recent times by the chemical examination of the blood. The disease now in question is named generalized osteitis fibrosa cystica, but undoubted cases have in the past been described under other names. The symptoms are due to a gradual thinning of the bones, as a result of overactivity of the osteoclasts and a consequent mobilization of the bone calcium and an appearance of excess of calcium ions in the blood. This process often continues until cyst-like spaces are formed in the shafts of the long bones. Towards the end of the eighteenth century a nobleman suffering from this condition was graphically described as dying with liquefaction of his bones which 'melted like wax in the dog-days'.

The first hint of the true cause of this condition was given in 1904 by Max Askanazy (1865–1940), a well-known pathologist of Geneva. In a fatal case of generalized osteitis Askanazy found at autopsy a tumour of a parathyroid, but he did not associate the two conditions and it was long before this relationship was established. In 1906–7 Jakob Erdheim (1874–1937) reported several cases of osteitis in which there was parathyroid enlargement; but he regarded the bony changes as primary and the parathyroid enlargement as secondary to the supposed increased demand for calcium. By 1915 the suggestion was being made that parathyroidectomy was the correct treatment for generalized osteitis; but it was not until 1925 that Felix Mandl (1892–1957) removed a parathyroid tumour in such a case. The patient improved rapidly and remained well for six years. By 1931 thirty parathyroidectomies had been performed for the treatment of generalized osteitis, often with good results. In the same year, however, the effect of overactivity of the parathyroids in producing this condition was demonstrated experimentally in a human subject by the repeated injection of parathormone. This notable experiment was carried out by James McIntosh Johnson (1883–1953) and Russell Morse Wilder (1885–).

(iii) *The Adrenals*

Although physiological and clinical emphasis was not directed to the adrenals until the publication of Addison's monograph in 1855, they had been known long before that date. They were first mentioned by Eustachius (p. 243) who illustrated them, and they were called 'suprarenal capsules' in 1629 by Harvey's opponent Jean Riolan (1580–1657). Riolan thought that they were active in foetal life, a view which was accepted for many years. Even before that it had been considered that the adrenals did subserve some function, and in general the view of the famous Danish anatomist Caspar Bartholin (p. 627), to the effect that these organs excreted a humour named 'atrabilia' (black bile) in a cavity between the two constituent parts of the organ, the cortex and the medulla, was accepted. The first relatively satisfactory attempt to describe the microscopic appearance of the adrenal was made in 1840 by George Gulliver (1804–82). Reference has already been made to Brown-Séquard's extirpation experiments of 1856. More recent experiments of that nature show that in rats bilateral extirpation of the adrenals is fatal in at least three-quarters of the cases.

In 1894 there occurred an event of great importance not only in the history of the adrenals but also in that of the endocrine glands as a whole. In that year E. A. Schäfer (p. 258), then at University College, London, and George Oliver (1841–1915) proved that the adrenal medulla secreted a substance which had important physiological effects, notably the production of a rise in the blood-pressure due to vasoconstriction, mainly in the skin and splanchnic areas, and to relaxation of the bronchial muscles. J. J. Abel (p. 685) and Albert Cornelius Crawford (1869–1921) further investigated this pressor substance in 1897, and Abel called it epinephrine (the name still officially in use in the United States). In 1901 Jôkichi Takamine (1854–1922) and Thomas Bell Aldrich (1861–?) independently isolated it in a crystalline form. It was called by Takamine adrenaline (its official British name), and it was synthesized in 1904 by Friedrich Stolz (1860–1936). Adrenaline was the first hormone to be isolated and synthesized artificially. Since 1904 no fundamentally important new discoveries have been made in relation to the adrenal medulla, but much work has been done on adrenaline. In 1901 Langley (p. 262) showed that when this substance is injected into the circulation it produces those effects normally excited by stimulation of the sympathetic nervous system. In the first decade of the twentieth century a theory was advanced and widely supported that adrenaline is constantly being secreted into the blood-stream and that normal blood-pressure is thus maintained. This tonus hypothesis was attacked by W. B. Cannon (p. 303) in his *Bodily Changes in Pain, Hunger, Fear and Rage* (1919). Cannon deduced from his experiments that adrenaline is liberated when required in much larger amounts in response to emotional stimuli. This question has not yet been completely settled.

In the last thirty years much more research has been carried out on the adrenal cortex than on the medulla. In 1908 Schäfer and Percy Theodore Herring (1872–) concluded that the cortex did not produce any physiological effect. Brown-Séquard's extirpation experiments had been followed by the death of the animals in a few days; and the discovery of adrenaline had led to the assumption that the fatal result was due to deprivation of the medulla. But this conclusion was first shaken by experiments on lower vertebrates. Artur Biedl (1869–1933), then of Vienna but later of Prague, published in 1910 a book, *Innere Sekretion* ('Internal secretion'), which was probably the first comprehensive treatise on the ductless glands. In this he stated that in 1899 he had removed the inter-renal body in Elasmobranch fishes, but had left the medulla; the fishes died. In 1927 Julius Moses Rogoff (1884–) and George Neil Stewart (1860–1930), working at Cleveland, Ohio, also concluded that in dogs removal of the adrenal cortex was fatal, whereas removal of the medulla was not. They prepared an extract of the cortex, and later used it to treat adrenal insufficiency. In 1929 Wilbur Willis Swingle (1891–) and Joseph John Pfiffner (1903–) prepared an extract of the cortex which was named eschatin; it also was used with a similar effect.

These experiments ushered in a great advance in our knowledge of the cortex. In 1933 Jacques Loeb (1859–1924) showed that after adrenalectomy there is an increased loss of sodium salts from the body; and it was soon shown that the concentration of potassium salts in the blood is increased, as also are creatinine and the phosphates. These results pointed the way to the conclusion that the cortex regulates important elements in the blood, and that its removal results in a dehydration and marked reduction of the volume of the blood—a condition which is fatal. In 1934 Kendall (p. 526) and his colleagues isolated the hormone cortin in a crystalline form. Two years later they isolated nine steroids from the cortex, and the number has now been increased to over twenty. In the same year Tadeus Reichstein (1897–) independently discovered some of these important steroids. One of these was cortisone, which in 1949 was introduced by Kendall, Philip Showalter Hench (1896–), and their colleagues for the treatment of rheumatoid arthritis and rheumatic fever. In 1950 a Nobel Prize was awarded to Hench, Kendall, and Reichstein.

The treatment of Addison's disease was revolutionized by the use of some of these new products of the adrenal cortex, especially by the sterol desoxycorticosterone. The treatment was made still more effective by the synthesis of desoxycorticosterone acetate in 1937, and in 1939 George Widmer Thorn (1906–), then at Johns Hopkins, but now professor of medicine at Harvard, and his co-workers introduced the method of implanting pellets of desoxycorticosterone acetate in the abdominal wall. By this method without further hormone treatment absorption of the hormone goes on for many months, and the difficulties of daily injection are obviated. Although in Addison's original description no differentiation could be made between lesions of the cortex and of the medulla, it was shown experimentally, and confirmed by later pathological observation in human subjects, that it is the lesion of the cortex which produces the characteristic symptoms in this disease. Addison would be thrilled if he could know the wide implications opened up by the disease which he first described. Of the various other rare diseases due to lesions of the adrenal cortex one only will be mentioned here—the adreno-genital syndrome. This rare condition may affect males or females and begin at various ages. Onset in infancy or early childhood is, however, most usual. In both sexes the disease produces a masculinizing effect. There is precocious development, including that of the secondary sex characters. In boys the development may be of the 'infant Hercules' type, and there is a case on record of a boy of five years who was 4 feet 7 inches high; he could carry on his back a man weighing 14 stones.

The earliest case of this condition in which an autopsy was carried out was recorded in 1811. But there are much earlier reports of cases in which no autopsy was done. These possibly extend back to classical times. The lesion found post-mortem is usually a hyperplasia or an adenoma of the adrenal cortex, though malignant tumours are also known. The association between virilism and such adrenal lesions was first recognized in 1905 by Bulloch (p. 396) and James Harry Sequeira (p. 396), both of the London Hospital. The first treatment of the condition by removal of a cortical tumour was recorded in 1925 by Sir Gordon Holmes (p. 279); the operation in that case was performed by Sir Percy Sargent (1873–1933), surgeon to the National Hospital, Queen Square. Great surgical experience in such cases was obtained by Lennox Ross Broster (1889–) of Charing Cross Hospital, London. In 1933 Broster, in collaboration with the pathologist Howard William Copland Vines (1893–), published a classical work on the adrenal cortex.

(iv) *The Pituitary*

The pituitary body has been known since very early times, but until the last two decades of the nineteenth century its function was unknown. The fact that it consists of several divisions, recognized anatomically by the distinction between the anterior lobe and the posterior lobe, and the fact also that its embryological origin is from two very divergent primitive tissues, was disregarded in all physiological and clinical work on this gland until almost the close of the century. The history of our knowledge of the pituitary can be conveniently divided into three periods. In the first period (extending up to 1900) most of the diseases which are caused by dysfunction of the pituitary had been described, though without convincing evidence that this gland was responsible. In the second period (1901–20) the fundamental physiological work on the posterior lobe, which had been commenced towards the close of the first period, was completed. In the third period (1921–35) knowledge of the anterior lobe was much extended clinically, and its physiological functions were worked out in great detail.

(a) *Diseases produced by pituitary dysfunction.* The time-honoured view that the function of the gland was to secrete the mucus ('pituita') which escaped by the nose dates back at least to Galen. It was demolished in 1655 by Conrad Viktor Schneider (1614–80) of Wittenberg. In that year he described the membrane in the nose named after him, and also the cribiform plate of the ethmoid. Five years later he confirmed his views, and showed that the olfactory processes were cranial nerves. Théophile Bonet (p. 168), J. J. Wepfer (p. 271), and others towards the close of the seventeenth century or the beginning of the eighteenth described pituitary bodies which were much enlarged, but they did not associate the enlargement with any pathological condition.

Acromegaly. In 1886 Pierre Marie (p. 277) described two cases of a disease characterized by overgrowth of certain parts of the skeleton, especially the jaws and the bones of the face, the bones of the hands and feet, with a bending of the spine. The tongue was enlarged and the hair coarse and greasy. The disease has been aptly described as a reversion to the gorilla type. Marie also reviewed the literature and discovered five cases which he considered would accord with the features of his own two cases. The earliest of these five cases was that described by Nicolas Saucerotte (1741–1814) in 1772. This case was not actually published until 1801. The famous anatomist Broca (p. 256) had the opportunity to examine the skeletons of Marie's two cases, and he discovered that in each case the sella turcica (the saddle-shaped depression in the sphenoid bone which lodges the pituitary body) was enlarged. The inference was that in life the pituitary had also been enlarged in each case. Meanwhile Oscar Minkowski (1858–1931), then of Königsberg, had already noted that in fatal cases of acromegaly the pituitary body was indeed enlarged (1887). In 1893 Brown-Séquard recommended, without any experimental or logical foundation, the administration of extracts of the thyroid, spleen, and bone marrow in the treatment of acromegaly. It was realized fairly early that the abnormality of the pituitary in acromegaly was an adenoma or an overgrowth, and the next step was the recognition of the fact that it affected the anterior lobe. The histology of the gland was meanwhile being worked out. It was shown that the anterior lobe contains cells which by the aid of certain stains can be differentiated into two types, those which take the stain easily (chromophil) and those which do not (chromophobe). In 1900 Carl Benda (1857–1933) of Berlin found that in acromegaly the tumour consists of chromophil cells. Later research showed that it was the eosinophil, in contradistinction to the basophil, cells which were affected.

Gigantism. Some excessively tall individuals are regarded as healthy, while in others the tallness is pathological. The dividing line between the two conditions is sometimes narrow. Some giants show pathological changes in the bones other than those changes indicative merely of increase in length. In 1895 Édouard Brissaud (1852–1909) and Henri Meige (1866–1940) stated that gigantism is acromegaly during the period of growth, whereas acromegaly is gigantism of the adult. In the same year the American, Woods Hutchinson (1862–1930) argued that gigantism is acromegaly beginning in early or foetal life, and he suggested that the pituitary is a growth centre for the whole body. There was much discussion of this view, and Marie was against it. Within ten years, however, it was accepted that excessive action of the pituitary causes gigantism before, and acromegaly after, the epiphyses have united. About this time Harvey Cushing (p. 371) had begun his surgical and experimental work on the pituitary, and interest had also centred on some of the famous giants of the past. One of these was O'Brien, the Irish giant, whose body had been obtained after his death by John Hunter at considerable cost and no small personal risk. His skeleton, measuring 7 ft. 7 in. tall, is now in the Hunterian Museum of the Royal College of Surgeons of England. In 1911 Sir Arthur Keith (p. 623) opened O'Brien's skull and found the sella turcica much enlarged.

Infantilism. A deficient rate of growth, having regard to the age of the child, and deficient development of the sexual characteristics have been described in relation to lesions of various organs. The term 'infantilism' was first used by Paul Joseph Lorain (1827–75) in

1871 in describing a type of this condition of unknown origin. In 1908 Ettore Levi of Florence ascribed this condition to diminution of function of the pituitary beginning in childhood. The affected tissues are probably the eosinophil cells of the anterior pituitary.

Dwarfism. In 1886 Sir Jonathan Hutchinson (1828–1913) of the London Hospital described a case of congenital absence of hair and mammae with atrophy of the skin. In 1897 Hastings Gilford (p. 366) described a similar case—a boy of seventeen years who had died of senile decay. Gilford named the condition *progeria* in 1904. This condition is considered to be due to hypofunction of the anterior lobe of the pituitary.

Fröhlich's syndrome. In 1900 Babinski (p. 277) described a case of adiposity in a girl of seventeen years, associated with arrest of the sex characteristics. The patient had small ovaries and a tumour associated with the pituitary gland. In 1901 Alfred Fröhlich (1871–1953) of Vienna described the case of a boy of fourteen years with adiposity and deficient development of the sex organs. In a search of the literature he discovered other cases, the earliest being that described by Bernhard Mohr of Würzburg in 1840. Fröhlich failed to notice Babinski's case. In France and Germany the names of Babinski and Fröhlich are jointly used in the eponymous name of this syndrome. At a later date it was agreed that optic atrophy often develops in this condition as a result of the pituitary tumour. In 1908 the condition was named *dystrophia adiposo-genitalis* (or adiposo-genital dystrophy).

Simmonds's disease. In 1914 Morris Simmonds (1855–1925) of Hamburg described a case of weakness and wasting, with a failure of the sexual functions. There was a fatal termination, and at autopsy atrophy and fibrosis of the anterior pituitary was found. The patient had been suffering from puerperal fever, and the pituitary lesion was attributed to an embolus in the main artery supplying the anterior lobe. Since that date further cases were described by Simmonds and other writers. The destruction of the anterior lobe of the pituitary can be caused by other types of lesions, such as tuberculosis and syphilis.

Diabetes insipidus. In all the conditions described above it is now known that the lesion is in the anterior pituitary lobe. In 1794

J. P. Frank (p. 197) described a condition now known to be due to a lesion of the posterior pituitary or associated areas of the brain. This was diabetes insipidus, a disease in which very large quantities of urine free from sugar are passed. Children suffering from this disease may pass in twenty-four hours a weight of urine in excess of their own weight. Thomas Willis had noted the sweet taste of urine passed by patients suffering from diabetes mellitus (p. 245), but Frank distinguished this condition from diabetes insipidus, in which the urine does not contain sugar. Knowledge of the cause and treatment of diabetes insipidus is bound up with the physiology of the pituitary, dealt with later.

Cushing's syndrome. In 1932 Harvey Cushing (p. 371) described a syndrome in which the most characteristic features were excessive adiposity of the face and abdomen, sometimes of a painful nature; hypertension; rarefaction of the bones, with resulting deformities; virilism in the female and feminization in the male. Cushing found that in such cases there was an adenoma of the basophil cells of the anterior pituitary. It has since been shown that other types of the syndrome exist, and that in many cases the primary lesion is apparently a hyperplasia or an adenoma of the adrenal cortex. The whole question is still too much *sub judice* for treatment from the historical aspect.

(*b*) *The physiology of the posterior lobe.* The first physiological experiment on the pituitary was probably made by Horsley (p. 525), who excised the whole gland in two dogs; they were still well several months later. In 1895 Oliver and Schäfer (p. 538) showed that intravenous injection of an emulsion of the whole gland produced a striking rise of blood-pressure, mainly due to constriction of the peripheral vessels, together with slowing and increased force of the heart. This discovery followed very soon after their demonstration of the similar effects of adrenaline (p. 538). Three years later William Henry Howell (1860–1945), who had succeeded Newell Martin in the chair of physiology at Johns Hopkins, Baltimore, demonstrated that the pressor effect was confined to extracts of the posterior pituitary.

In 1906 H. H. Dale (p. 555) discovered that the stimulant action of adrenaline and the sympathetic on smooth muscle in the early-pregnant uterus of the cat is reversed by ergot preparations previously injected. He then found that the same uterus still contracted actively when the animal was injected with a dried extract of oxpituitary. The important conclusion was drawn that the pressor principle of the posterior pituitary acts on some constituent of the plain muscle fibre other than that which is excited by adrenaline and by impulses reaching sympathetic axon-endings. As a result pituitary extract (pituitrin) was soon extensively used to stimulate the contraction of the uterus in certain obstetric conditions, and this effect of the extract was referred to as its oxytocic action. In 1920 Dale's colleague Harold Ward Dudley (1887–1935) separated the pressor and oxytocic constituents of a pituitary extract into separate solutions, and in the following year they further established the existence of oxytocin, the active principle which causes powerful contractions of plain muscle.

The great importance of Dale's papers focused attention on the posterior lobe; but between then and the outbreak of the First World War a few experiments were carried out which suggested that the pituitary had other important functions. Cushing produced dystrophia adiposo-genitalis by excision of the pituitary (1908). In the same year, however, Schäfer and Herring said that the anterior lobe had no physiological action. As early as 1849 Claude Bernard had found that an injury to a certain point on the floor of the fourth ventricle produced polyuria. At later dates some clinical cases suggested that this effect might be produced by lesions of the pituitary. In 1913 Jean Camus (1872–1924), Gustave Roussy (p. 262), and their co-workers published the first of their researches which showed that the polyuria was due to injury to the floor of the third ventricle. The lesions may be in various parts in or surrounding the pituitary, but it seems that the hypothalamus must be involved. Meanwhile Schäfer and Herring had shown in 1908 that the posterior pituitary also contained a diuretic principle. It has since been shown that this action occurs only in certain conditions. The normal action of pituitrin after the injection of a large quantity of fluid is to delay diuresis for several hours by its effect on the renal tubules.

(c) *The physiological action of the anterior lobe.* It will thus be seen that by the end of the First World War, although all the disease resulting from pituitary dysfunction—except Cushing's syndrome—were known, in no case had there been any physiological demonstration of the cause. This was no doubt due to the concentration of experiment on the posterior pituitary. Since then very great advances have been made in our knowledge of the functions of the anterior pituitary.

In 1921 Herbert McLean Evans (1882–) and Joseph Abraham Long (1879–?) of Berkeley, California, showed that repeated injection of an extract of the anterior pituitary into rats produced gigantism. Oral administration produced no effect, as the growth hormone is destroyed in the stomach. It has since then been shown that this growth hormone of the anterior pituitary regulates especially the growth of the skeleton by action on the epiphyseal cartilages.

The next function of the anterior pituitary to receive attention was that associated with the female reproductive system—the gonadotrophic hormone. In 1898 the Swiss Louis Comte (1870–) had noticed that the pituitary was increased in size during pregnancy. Bernard Aschner (1883–1960) carried out a number of hypophysectomies on dogs in 1912, and he found that they developed hypoplasia of the genitals. H. M. Evans injected extracts of ox anterior pituitary into rats and thus inhibited the oestrous cycle and produced luteinization of the Graafian follicles (1924). Bernhard Zondek (1891–) and Selmar Aschheim (1878–?) found that the subcutaneous implantation of fresh anterior pituitary gland substance into young animals led to precocious sexual development (1927). The gonads matured early and produced other hormones which affected the secondary sex characters. In the same year Philip Edward Smith (1884–) and Earl Theron Engle (1896–1957) independently obtained similar results. Zondek and Aschheim described two gonadotrophic principles which they named prolan A and prolan B, and from their experiments arose the pregnancy test associated with their names. On the whole the existence of two separate prolans has not met with acceptance.

The influence of the anterior pituitary on metabolism was then investigated. In 1926 Goodwin LeBaron Foster (1891–) and P. E. Smith gave a convincing and important demonstration that experimental removal of the pituitary is followed by a fall in the metabolic rate. It was soon shown that in thyroidectomized animals injection of extract of anterior pituitary does not produce a rise in the metabolic rate, and it was therefore concluded that the pituitary acts indirectly through the thyroid.

In 1926 P. E. Smith showed that experimental hypophysectomy caused atrophy of the adrenal cortex. It was soon established that changes in the anterior pituitary are correlated with changes in the adrenal cortex. The adrenocorticotropic hormone (A.C.T.H.) was separated by Collip and his co-workers, and has since been considerably purified. Its use with cortisone in rheumatoid arthritis and certain skin lesions is still in the experimental stage.

Several other hormones have been found in the anterior pituitary. For example, it was thought to be associated with the increase in size of the mammary gland during pregnancy and with the secretion of milk, but hormones produced by the sex glands were also considered to be responsible. That the true cause lay in the anterior pituitary was shown in 1930 by George Washington Corner (1889–), then of Rochester, U.S.A., who is also known as a historian of anatomy, and especially as an embryologist of great distinction; much of his work therefore falls outside the scope of this book. The hormone which Corner had shown to exist was isolated a few years later and was named prolactin. A connexion between the anterior pituitary and the thyroid was shown in 1928 by Eduard Carl Adolph Uhlenhuth (1885–) and Saul Schwarzbach (1902–), and the hormone (thyrotropin) has been investigated by Collip and others. Lastly, the effect of the anterior pituitary on the pancreas may be mentioned. It had long been known that up to a third of patients suffering from acromegaly were also victims of diabetes mellitus In 1924 Bernardo Alberto Houssay (1887–) of Buenos Aires found that if the pituitary gland of an animal was removed no marked effects were produced under ordinary conditions. But if, by fasting or otherwise, the glycogen stores of the animal's body were lowered, the blood-sugar fell to a low level and the animal became much more sensitive to insulin. Even small doses of insulin considerably reduced the sugar content of the blood. Houssay was able to prevent this extreme action of insulin by injecting extracts of the anterior pituitary. In 1930–1 he and his co-workers demonstrated that in a dog from which the pancreas had been removed, the resulting diabetes could be checked by removing the pituitary. Such 'Houssay dogs' show an apparently normal, but really unstable, carbohydrate metabolism, so that in a condition of fasting the blood-sugar is easily tipped in the direction of the hypoglycaemic state. In 1937 Frank George Young (1908–) found that by repeatedly injecting extracts of the anterior pituitary into a dog a permanent diabetes could be produced. This was due to the action of the diabetogenic hormone, and there is evidence that the pituitary extract causes destruction of the islets of Langerhans in the pancreas. For his work in connexion with the pituitary and with carbohydrate metabolism Houssay shared a Nobel Prize in 1947.

From what has been written it will be clear that the anterior pituitary constantly exercises some effect on many of the other ductless glands. In fact, it is the leader of the endocrine orchestra—as was first said by Sir Walter Langdon Langdon–Brown (1870–1946), the regius professor of physic at Cambridge.

(v) *The Gonads*

(a) *The male gonads.* Mesuë the Elder (777?–857) advised the use of testicular extracts for impotence. In 1775 Théophile de Bordeu (p. 516) suggested that a specific substance was formed by the testis and was passed into the circulation. The experiments of Berthold at Göttingen have already been mentioned (p. 516); they were completely overlooked until attention was called to them by Biedl (p. 549) in the first edition of his book (1910). In 1869 Brown-Séquard (p. 261) suggested that the injection of semen into the blood of old men would stimulate their mental and physical powers, but he did not put this suggestion into practice. Six years later he carried out testicular grafts in guinea-pigs, and in 1889 he attempted self-rejuvenation by injecting into himself testicular juice and blood from the spermatic vein. Eugen Steinach (1861–1944) of Vienna introduced the operation of ligature of the vas deferens for rejuvenation (1920). Steinach had been working on this and similar physiological problems for over twenty years. He had castrated male guinea-pigs and then grafted ovaries into them; the animals developed some female characteristics. He then succeeded in grafting both testicles and ovaries on the same animals after castration, with the result that they developed both male and female characteristics. His rejuvenation experiments were excessively publicized, though for that he was probably not responsible. From 1919 onwards Serge Voronoff (1866–1951), of the Collège de France at Paris, carried out testicular transplants, derived from monkeys, into human subjects. At the time the medical profession was opposed to these operations, and the process has since been shown to be unsatisfactory.

The result of Berthold's experiment was confirmed in 1911 by Albert Pézard (?–1927), and he showed that the growth of the capon's comb after injection of testicular material could be used as a test for the presence of a hormone. The hormone androsterone was isolated in crystalline form by the chemist Adolf Friedrich Johann Butenandt (1903–) of Berlin in 1931. Three years later androsterone was synthesized from cholesterol derivatives by Leopold Ruzicka (1887–), the Zurich chemist. In 1935 Fritz Oscar Laquer (1888–1954) isolated another hormone—testosterone—from the testis. It was found to be about three times more potent than androsterone, and both Butenandt and Ruzicka independently obtained it from androsterone. For this and similar work Butenandt and Ruzicka shared a Nobel Prize in chemistry in 1939.

(b) The female gonads. The female sex hormones are more complex than those of the male, since two distinct sources are known, the ovary proper and the corpus luteum.

One of the first experimental demonstrations of the existence of a hormone in the ovary was given by the gynaecologist Emil Knauer (1867–1935), then of Vienna and later of Graz, who in 1896 transplanted ovaries into immature and castrated animals and found that the sex characters developed. In 1900 Josef von Halban (1870–1937), another gynaecologist of Vienna, carried out similar experiments. No further work of importance was done in this field until 1917, when Charles Rupert Stockard (1879–1939) of Cornell Medical College, New York, and George Nicholas Papanicolaou (1883–) demonstrated that the vaginal epithelium of certain mammals undergoes characteristic changes during each phase of the oestrous cycle. From this they derived their vaginal smear test which has been of great value in later work. In 1923 Edgar Allen (1892–1943) and Edward Adelbert Doisy (1893–) of St. Louis, Missouri, used this bioassay method in oophorectomized rats to show that there is present in the liquor folliculi an oestrus-producing substance. Such oestrogens were soon shown to be present in the solid ovarian tissue and in the placenta. That larger quantities are present in the urine of pregnant females was shown by Aschheim and Zondek (p. 547) in 1927. This led to the isolation of one of these substances in a crystalline form independently by Doisy and by Butenandt in 1929–30; it is now called oestrone. In 1930 also another hormone, oestriol, was obtained from urine by Guy Frederic Marrian (1904–), then of London. The most powerful hormone found in the ovarian substance is oestradiol, which was produced in 1933 from oestrone by Erwin Schwenk (1887–) and Fritz Hildebrandt (1887–) of Giessen.

Interest in the functions of the corpus luteum began to increase about the beginning of the twentieth century. Its important functions in relation to the oestrus cycle and to pregnancy were shown in 1929 by G. W. Corner (p. 548) and Willard Myron Allen (1904–) to be due to a hormone called corporin, but since then named successively progestin and progesterol. This hormone is excreted in the urine as pregnanediol.

An important development was the production of synthetic oestrogens by Sir Edward Charles Dodds (1899–) and his co-workers of the Middlesex Hospital, London. The first of these, stilboestrol, was produced in 1938, and the same year saw the production of dienoestrol and hexoestrol. Apart from the employment of these substances in menstrual disorders, they have other uses. The best example is stilboestrol, which is easily manufactured and is of great value in certain cases of carcinoma of the prostate.

(vi) *The Pancreas*

In ancient times various hypothetical functions were attributed to this organ, such as that it acted as packing for the stomach and neighbouring organs, or that it was the gall-bladder of the spleen. Recognition of its true function as a digestive gland dates from de Graaf's establishment of a pancreatic fistula and the collection of the pancreatic juice (p. 297). Excision of most of the pancreas in dogs was performed in 1673 by Johann Conrad Brunner (1653–1727) of Schaffhausen. He denied that this organ was an important digestive gland, but he noted that some of his dogs showed excessive thirst and polyuria after operation. All these observations were first published in Brunner's *Experimenta nova circa pancreas* ('New experiments on the pancreas', 1682). Five years later Brunner described the glands in the duodenum which are called after him. Purkinje (p. 246) showed that pancreatic extracts have proteolytic powers, and Lucien Corvisart (p. 535) proved in a series of experiments (1857–63) that this action of the juice is effected without the assistance of the bile. The fundamental work regarding this action of the pancreas was done in 1876 when Willy Kühne (p. 270) isolated the ferment trypsin.

Diabetes mellitus and the islets of Langerhans. A disease characterized by weakness, thirst, and polyuria was known from ancient times, and Aretaeus first applied to it the Greek word for a siphon (*diabetes*). It is possible that the sweet taste of the urine in this disease had been noticed by the physicians of ancient India, but in modern times this fact was rediscovered by Willis (p. 245). It may be mentioned that twenty-four years before Willis's observation there is a reference to the sweet taste of some urines in Molière's play *Le Médecin volant* (1650). Reference has already been made to the differentiation between the urine of diabetes mellitus and that of diabetes insipidus (p. 545). The proof that the sweet taste of the urine in true diabetes is due to sugar was given in 1776 by Matthew Dobson (1745?–1784) of Liverpool, who demonstrated that the residue after evaporation of such urine underwent vinous and acetic fermentation. Dobson made the further important observation that the blood serum in true diabetes also has a sweet taste, and he was thus the discoverer of hyperglycaemia. That the sugar in diabetic urine is glucose was first shown in 1815 by Michel Eugène Chevreul (p. 319). Chevreul, one of the greatest of French chemists and a pioneer in the chemistry of the animal fats and vegetable dyes, was still as a centenarian carrying out important research; he was also director of the famous Gobelin tapestry works.

Recognition of the association between the pancreas and true

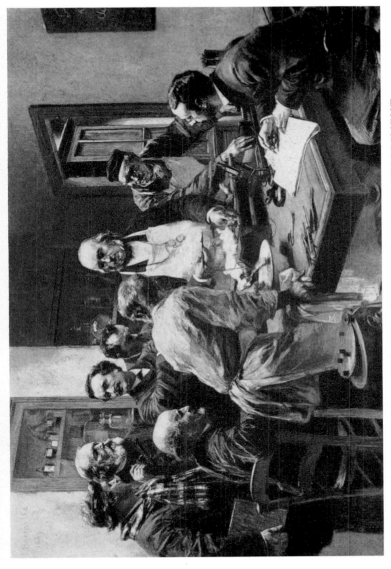

XX. CLAUDE BERNARD CARRYING OUT AN EXPERIMENT

From left to right standing: Nestor Gréhent; Amédée Dumontpallier, Trousseau's chief assistant and later physician to the Pitié; Paul Bert; and J. A. d'Arsonval (1851–1940), later director of a laboratory at the Collège de France. On left, seated, L. C. Malassez, assistant director of the haematological laboratory at the Collège de France. On right, seated and taking notes, J. A. F. Dastre, assistant to Bernard, and later professor of physiology at the Sorbonne

(Photogravure of the painting of 1889 by L. Lhermitte in the Sorbonne)

diabetes came comparatively late. In 1778 Thomas Cawley, about whom practically nothing is known, reported a case of diabetes in which there were numerous calculi in the pancreas. Richard Bright reported morbid changes in the pancreas in such cases in 1831, von Recklinghausen (p. 636) described the presence of calculi in 1864, and Frerichs (p. 275) stated in 1884 that 20 per cent. of his cases of diabetes showed gross changes in the pancreas. Meanwhile Claude Bernard had been carrying out his important experiments on glycosuria (p. 294).

In an inaugural dissertation published at Berlin in 1869 Paul Langerhans (1847–88) first described the islets of tissue scattered through the pancreas which were histologically distinct from, and had no direct connexion with, the glandular tissue proper. The name of Langerhans was attached to these islets by Gustave Édouard Laguesse (1861–1927) of Lille in 1893, and by this name they have since then been known. Meanwhile, the crucial experiment showing that true diabetes is due to a lesion in the pancreas was made by Joseph von Mering (1849–1908) and Oscar Minkowski (p. 542), then both at Strasbourg. In 1889 they excised the pancreas in animals and thus produced a rapidly fatal diabetes. They also showed that the production of this condition was not due to the loss of the flow of pancreatic juice to the bowel. The conclusion was that the pancreas not only secreted the pancreatic juice, but that some part of it was also closely associated with general metabolism. These experiments were confirmed by Laguesse, who in 1893 suggested that the islets of Langerhans produced an internal secretion. In 1900–1 Eugene Lindsay Opie (p. 639), then at Johns Hopkins, but later at St. Louis and the Henry Phipps Institute at Philadelphia, showed that in many cases of diabetes the islets have undergone hyaline degeneration. Other pathological changes in the islets have since been recorded, and a clear statement of the relation between lesions in this tissue and glycosuria was made by W. G. MacCallum (p. 639) in 1909.

Many attempts were now made to isolate the active principle of the islets, but the difficulties were very great, since the trypsin destroyed the internal secretion. It may be said retrospectively that there is no doubt that partial success was achieved in 1908 by Georg

Ludwig Zuelzer (1870–1949) of Berlin. Zuelzer succeeded in obtaining a pancreatic extract which was given to eight diabetics with good results. Unfortunately, symptoms later developed which were regarded at the time as toxic, and this important work was abandoned. Eighteen years later, when more was known about the action of the hormone, it was suggested that the supposed 'toxic' symptoms had really been due to hypoglycaemia, resulting from too large or too prolonged doses of a remedy which was successful.

The discovery and isolation of insulin, the active principle of the islets, was made in the summer of 1921 by (Sir) Frederick Grant Banting (1891–1941) and Charles Herbert Best (1899–) of Toronto. A method of preventing the destruction of the hormone by trypsin in the pancreas had been found by Leonid Vassilyevitch Soboleff (1876–1919) in 1902. Soboleff showed that ligature of the pancreatic duct led to atrophy of the glandular acini, whereas the islet tissue was unaffected. There were many technical difficulties associated with the further application of this principle. The laboratory of John James Rickard Macleod (1876–1935), who held the chair of physiology at Toronto, was peculiarly well equipped for work on carbohydrate metabolism, and it was for this reason that Banting asked Macleod's permission in 1921 to use his laboratory for the purpose of the investigation which he had in mind. Macleod gave this permission, and as it was expected that certain specialized work would have to be carried out, Macleod requested Best, who had had the necessary training in that laboratory, to work with Banting. Banting and Best carried out the whole investigation themselves. During most of the period concerned, and certainly at the time of the actual discovery of insulin, Macleod was absent from Toronto. In the late autumn a detailed communication on the technique and on the discovery was written by Banting and Best for the *Journal of Laboratory and Clinical Medicine*, in which journal publication could not be expected until some time during 1922. Meanwhile it was desirable that a preliminary announcement of the discovery should be made. Macleod arranged for a brief communication to be presented to a meeting of the American Physiological Society in December 1921. It was a rule of the Society that at least one member of any team which presented a communication should be a member of the Society. Neither Banting nor Best were then members, so Macleod attached his name also to the communication, which was published early in 1922 under the names of Banting, Best, and Macleod. In 1923 the Nobel Prize Committee awarded a Prize for Medicine to Banting and Macleod 'for their discovery of insulin'. Banting expressed his dissatisfaction with the award by sharing one-half of his prize with Best, and Macleod thereupon gave a half of his prize to Collip, who had with Macleod worked on the standardization of insulin after its discovery. The Committe was criticized for not having included Best in the award, but the statement has been made that it was not technically possible to do so, since he had not been nominated by anybody. Insulin was synthesized in crystalline form by Abel (p. 685) in 1926.

(b) Histamine

In this and the following section we refer repeatedly to the researches of Dale and his colleagues. Sir Henry Hallett Dale (1875–) studied physiology under Michael Foster, Gaskell, and Langley at Cambridge, and then did research there and at University College, London, in the department of Starling and Bayliss. In 1904 he was offered by (Sir) Henry Solomon Wellcome (1853–1936), and accepted, the post of pharmacologist to the Wellcome Physiological Research Laboratories which had been established ten years earlier. Almost from the start of his career there Dale was engaged on the ergot researches which are dealt with elsewhere (p. 682). These researches led him by a long series of steps not only to the discovery of successive increasingly active constituents in ergot, but also to the still not completely solved problems of histamine, and to the demonstration of the chemical transmission of the nerve impulse. After ten years in the Wellcome Laboratories, as pharmacologist and later as director, Dale was appointed pharmacologist to the newly established National Institute for Medical Research, of which he later became the first director. His tenure of the presidential chair of the Royal Society and his reception of innumerable honorary degrees from British and foreign universities mark, with the highest honours conferred on him by his Sovereign, his position as the doyen of British medical research.

In the following few pages we attempt to sketch briefly Dale's work in these fields, especially in its relation to the work of his colleagues and others. He has never written a book dealing with particular phases of his work. Many scientists have been honoured by having their scientific papers—or a selection of them—republished in volume form; in recent years perhaps the most notable of such collections were those of Hughlings Jackson and of Sherrington. But ten years after he relinquished active work in the laboratory Sir Henry Dale had the opportunity of producing his *Adventures in Physiology* (1953). This work, which is in many ways unique, consists of a generous selection of his most important scientific papers dealing with ergot, pituitrin, histamine, and chemical transmission written over a period of thirty-two years. The unique feature is the inclusion, at the end of each paper, of a commentary written especially for the book, in which the author criticizes and expands his earlier work in the light of subsequent research by himself and others. The advanced student who devotes a month to the serious study of this work will learn more than any textbook can tell him of research, its methods, its pitfalls and disappointments, and its final triumphs.

The histamine story begins in the year 1880, when Adolf Schmidt-Mülheim, a veterinary physiologist, found experimentally that the injection of a peptic digest of blood fibrin—a substance then much used in physiology under the name of Witte's peptone—into an anaesthetized dog was followed by a marked fall of blood-pressure. The phenomenon was most clearly and regularly produced in dogs kept overnight without food. This fact suggested that the liver was in some way responsible. If the abdomen was opened the liver was found to be intensely engorged with blood and was swollen to the limits of expansion of its capsule. The blood-vessels were markedly dilated, the blood had lost its power to form a clot, and the leucocytes and platelets had almost disappeared from it. At a later date E. H. Starling (p. 518) showed that the effects were due mainly to the action of the peptone on lymph formation and on the blood-vessels of the liver.

There was a long interval before the injection of other substances was found to produce a marked fall of blood-pressure. In 1895 Oliver and Schäfer (p. 538) observed that such a condition followed the

injection of extracts of the thyroid gland, and four years later Mott
(p. 260) and Halliburton (p. 524) also found that the same condition
followed the injection of extracts of nerve tissue. Within a few years
it was shown that extracts of many tissues would produce this pronounced depressor action. Leon Popielski of Lemberg put forward
the hypothesis that these extracts all contained a substance which he
called 'vasodilatin', but which up to that time had not been isolated
chemically.

Meanwhile, the chemists Adolf Windaus (1876–1959) and Karl
Vogt (1880–) had synthesized the substance which was later to be
called histamine (1907). It was not known to occur naturally. But in
1910 Barger (p. 527) and Dale had discovered this substance, which
for technical reasons they then referred to as β-iminazolylethylamine,
in an ergot extract. Almost simultaneously it had been obtained by
Friedrich Kutscher (1866–1942) from ergot, but Otto Heinrich
Rudolf E. D. Ackermann (1878–) and Kutscher had considered that
it was a slightly different substance. In the same year Biedl (p. 539)
and Rudolf Kraus (p. 418) had tried the experiment of the injection
of peptone, using not a dog but an anaphylactic guinea-pig. They
found that the anaphylactic shock manifested itself by an intense
constriction of the bronchioles.

When Barger and Dale isolated histamine from ergot they discovered that in the cat it produced powerful unco-ordinated contractions of the plain muscle of the uterus. This was the first indication
that histamine had any physiological activity, and its physiological
action was thoroughly investigated in the same year (1910) by Dale
and Laidlaw (p. 449). They found that the action varied with the
species of test animal; but in general the most characteristic action
was the direct stimulant effect on plain muscle, most marked in the
case of the uterus, but also very evident in the muscles of the bronchioles. One of the most interesting features was the fact that in carnivores, although histamine constricted the arterioles, there was also
what they called 'an antagonistic peripheral action' which led to a
general fall of blood-pressure. It is now known that this is largely due
to a wide-spread dilatation of the capillary network, which occurs even
after section of the nerves. Dale and Laidlaw noted that histamine
produced nearly all the effects of the shock following the injection of

Witte's peptone, except the abolition of the coagulability of the blood, and its action was thus closely parallel to that of Popielski's 'vasodilatin'. They also noted that the injection of histamine reproduces many of the immediate symptoms of anaphylactic shock following the injection of a protein into an animal previously sensitized to that protein.

Up to that time histamine had never been isolated from the living body; it was known only as a synthetic substance and as a constituent of ergot and certain other members of the vegetable kingdom. Dale recalled that when Bayliss and Starling discovered secretin (p. 518), they found that the intestinal extracts from which they obtained this hormone also contained another substance which had a profound depressant action. It now seemed that this substance might be histamine. In 1911, therefore, Barger and Dale directed their attention to the intestinal mucosa, and from it they recovered a substance which, apart from action on the coagulability of the blood, in its physiological action was indistinguishable from synthetic histamine. These experiments were later seen to be the first isolation of histamine from animal tissues. Their significance was, however, not at once appreciated. One reason was that there was no proof that the histamine was a product of the living cells of the mucosa. There was also more than a suspicion that, despite the precautions which had been taken to eliminate the possibility that the histamine had been produced from histidine by putrefactive processes in the intestine, this might actually have been the case. The suspicion received much support from the fact that in 1910 Ackermann had prepared histamine by the action of putrefactive organisms on histidine. As Dale notes, it would have been easy for them, even at that time, to have tried to isolate histamine from some other tissue which would have been free from such suspicions, but neither he and his co-workers nor anyone else attempted to do so. In point of fact histamine was not shown to be produced by animal tissues until sixteen years later.

Dale returned to these aspects of the action of histamine in the later years of the First World War. At that time the conditions then known as 'secondary' surgical and traumatic shock were of great interest and importance, and various suggestions based on experimental work had been made to explain them. In their paper in 1911

Dale and Laidlaw had been concerned mainly with the results of the injection of small doses of histamine, although they knew that large doses could kill the animal. The paradox that histamine, a potent stimulator of plain muscle, produced in the cat a fall of blood-pressure by vasodilatation was still unexplained. Edward Mellanby (p. 614) encouraged further work on this subject by his observations in 1916 that a large dose of histamine absorbed from the bowel produced a condition similar to surgical shock. In the following year Dale and Laidlaw returned to the study of the physiological results of the injection of histamine. A. N. Richards (p. 302) came over from the United States to work with Dale, and in 1918 they published a classic paper on the effect of histamine on the circulation—the experiments being carried out mainly in the cat. They concluded that small doses of histamine caused constriction of the arteries and also a general dilatation of the capillaries, this latter action being independent of any system of nerves.

Meanwhile Dale and Laidlaw had been investigating the results of the injection of large doses of histamine. They showed in 1919 that these consisted largely of a general vasodilatation, accompanied by a transudation of plasma from the capillaries due to an abnormal permeability of their endothelial lining. There was a consequent rise in the relative numbers of the blood-cells and a loss of blood-volume. To these effects were added a fall in the body temperature, drowsiness, and a depression of the respiratory centre. These features were virtually the symptoms and signs of 'surgical' shock. Certain characteristics of this condition were still not satisfactorily explained, so Dale then proceeded to test these by animal experiments. In his paper of 1920 he showed that the dose of histamine necessary to produce a condition of profound shock was very much smaller if the animal was under a general anaesthetic, or if there had been considerable haemorrhage, or if the suprarenal glands had been removed. These conditions were later shown to have important applications, but we do not follow these up here.

The striking analogy between histamine shock and 'surgical' shock could only be of direct practical importance if it was assumed that at least under conditions of injury histamine was produced by the body cells. At that time there was still no evidence that this was the case. About 1919 Sir Thomas Lewis (p. 623) was beginning his work on the response to injury—chemical, thermal, electrical, or mechanical—of the blood-vessels in the human skin, in the course of which he described his 'triple response'. Dale suggested to him that this response might be produced by pricking histamine into the skin, and Lewis found that this was indeed the case. While he agreed that the response was probably caused by a substance analogous to histamine, he was unable to feel sure that the response was normally caused by histamine itself. He chose noncommitally to indict an agent which he designated the 'H-substance'.

In 1919 Abel (p. 685) and Bennosuke Kubota (1885–) examined several tissues for the presence of histamine, but they obtained chemical evidence of its presence in only two, viz. in an extract of the gastro-intestinal mucous membrane, and in another extract of a dried preparation of pituitary gland. The original depressor activity of both these tissues had been considerable, and in both cases in relation to this activity the amount of histamine recovered was very small. Their results were therefore not considered to be completely convincing. In 1927, however, Best (p. 554), Dale, Dudley (p. 546), and William Veale Thorpe (1902–) made the crucial demonstration that histamine normally occurs in certain organs in quantities sufficient to account for the depressant action of extracts of these organs. They published their results in the case of extracts of liver and of lung. In both cases histamine was isolated from these extracts in quantities sufficient to account for their physiological effects. These investigators also found that the amount of histamine recovered from equal weights of extracts was many times greater in the case of the lung than in that of the liver. They were also able to ascertain whether the histamine was actually present in the cells of the organ during life, or whether it had been formed after death. Their evidence was strongly in favour of the view that it was either present during life or was formed actually at the moment of cellular death. As Dale has recently written, from the time of the publication of this paper onwards, the occurrence of a histamine-like activity in an extract from a fresh animal tissue was at least strong presumptive evidence that histamine itself was present in the living cells of that tissue.

From very early in these studies on histamine another aspect of its activity had been studied. This was its relation to anaphylactic shock. Reference has already been made (p. 420) to the observation of Theobald Smith that guinea-pigs are unusually sensitive to repeated injections of toxin-antitoxin mixtures provided that the successive injections are separated by suitably long intervals. The injection of substances such as Witte's peptone gave in the dog the characteristic picture already described; and it was soon found that the symptoms which followed such injections depended on the species of animal injected and not on the nature of the injection. The results in the guinea-pig were especially constant and dramatic. It was noted that if a sensitized guinea-pig subsequently received an intravenous injection of the specific antigen, the animal rubbed its face with its paws as if to clear an obstruction from mouth or nose and showed signs of acute respiratory distress. Within a few minutes it was dead. The post-mortem appearances of this condition were first described by Frederick Parker Gay (1874–1939) and Elmer Ernest Southard (1876–1920) in 1908, but a much fuller description was given in 1910 by John Auer (p. 430) and Paul A. Lewis (p. 430) of the Rockefeller Foundation. These authors showed that the acute distension of the lungs which resulted was not due to a simple emphysema, since the lungs remained acutely distended after removal from the body, and even a portion cut off from a lung still retained its air. They demonstrated that death was due to suffocation as a result of acute spasm of the muscles of the bronchioles. The endothelium of the bronchioles in the guinea-pig is normally thick and has a tendency to be thrown into folds. Hence the muscular spasm was sufficient to bring opposing folds together and so to produce complete blockage of the air-ways.

Interest now centred on the mechanism by which this sudden and dramatic fatal reaction was produced, and two conflicting theories were advanced almost simultaneously. Alexandre Besredka (1870–1940) of the Institut Pasteur at Paris, who later dealt comprehensively with his views in his book *Anaphylaxie et antanaphylaxie* (1917), propounded in 1908 his theory that the anaphylactic shock was due to a reaction between the antigen and a substance of the nature of a precipitin occurring on the tissue cells or actually in the cell protoplasm. In 1907 Victor Clarence Vaughan (1851–1929) suggested as a result of his work on the products of the cleavage of proteins that the first stage in the anaphylactic phenomenon was the formation in the blood of a non-specific poison, termed anaphylatoxin, produced by the action of a specific ferment which appeared in the blood following the sensitizing injection. This came to be called the humoral theory, in contradistinction to the cellular theory of Besredka. The humoral theory was modified by Ulrich Friedemann (1877–1949), who regarded the first stage of the reaction as the union of the antigen with a specific non-proteolytic antibody, the resulting substance being then subjected to proteolysis by a ferment in the blood plasma. These views received considerable support from the work of Ernst Friedberger (1875–1932) who became the chief protagonist of the theory and coined the term 'anaphylatoxin' for the toxic substance produced in the blood. In 1910 this humoral theory was generally accepted. But in that year William Henry Schultz (1873–?), of the Hygienic Laboratory at Washington, realized that the question might be further elucidated by utilizing portions of guinea-pig plain muscle, which is very sensitive to the anaphylactic phenomenon, and freeing them completely from blood and body fluids. He used isolated portions of small intestine from guinea-pigs sensitized to various proteins. His results gave support to the cellular theory, but for various reasons they were not completely convincing.

Dale had already embarked on work of this nature, but when he saw a preliminary account of Schultz's experiments he discontinued his own work. When some time later the full account of the Schultz experiments was published, Dale returned to his investigation and completed a classic study (1913). He took advantage of the fact— apparently not appreciated by Schultz—that the plain muscle of the sensitized virgin guinea-pig is exquisitely sensitive to the antigen in extremely minute doses and is very specific. By this method Dale demonstrated *in vitro* all the essential features of anaphylaxis. It had been pointed out by Harry Gideon Wells (p. 637) in 1908 that it was very improbable that the minute amount of the sensitizing protein which was necessary to produce an almost immediate shock in a sensitized guinea-pig could in that time undergo proteolysis with the production of toxic products. This was an argument against the humoral theory. Dale also used this argument, and his experiments were strongly in favour of anaphylactic shock being due to cellular disturbances initiated by the antigen-antibody reaction occurring on the cell surface or in the cell protoplasm. These results were confirmed by Richard Weil (1876–1917) of New York by independent experiments on rather different lines, using live guinea-pigs (1913).

In 1922 Dale returned again to this subject, working with Charles Halliley Kellaway (1889–1952), who subsequently did very important work on snake venoms, a subject not dealt with in this book. In a very extensive investigation they showed that, while in the guinea-pig histamine produces symptoms and post-mortem findings which closely resemble those found in true anaphylactic shock, in the case of the so-called 'anaphylatoxins' the resemblances are not nearly so close. They obtained further evidence in support of the view that the anaphylactic phenomenon is actually due to the location of the antibody, probably a precipitin, in the cell substance. They also showed that when the antibody circulates in the body fluids immunity results, whereas when it is located in the cells anaphylaxis is the result. Although they suspected that histamine might play a prominent role in these phenomena, this could only be a supposition, since the crucial demonstration of the presence of this substance in the animal body had not then been made (p. 560). In 1922 also Kellaway and Stuart Jasper Cowell (1891–) demonstrated the presence in normal serum of a shock-inhibiting substance which, if injected a few minutes before the injection of a shocking dose of antigen into a sensitized animal, prevented the onset of shock.

The final demonstration that histamine is released by the injured cells in the anaphylactic phenomenon was given almost simultaneously in 1932 by Wilhelm Siegmund Feldberg (1900–), then in Berlin, and his co-workers, and by Carl Albert Dragstedt (1895–) and his co-workers at the North-western University, Illinois. Feldberg used the lung of the anaphylactic guinea-pig, and Dragstedt the dog's liver. Since then other substances have been shown to be released by cells as a result of injury, and it has been increasingly realized that these were probably actively concerned in determining attacks of the allergic diseases. Previous to the outbreak of the Second World War it was discovered that certain substances protected animals from the effects of histamine. After the war much research was expended on the synthetic production of antihistaminic drugs of this type.

(c) The Chemical Transmission of the Nerve Impulse

When Henry Hallett Dale began his studies at Cambridge in 1894 his professor, Michael Foster, had just published the first volume of the sixth edition of his famous *Text Book of Physiology*, the first edition of which had appeared in 1876. In this volume Foster wrote: 'Putting aside certain cases which we cannot discuss here we may say that the series of shocks sent in at the far end of the nerve start a series of impulses; these travel down the nerve and reach the muscle as a series of distinct impulses; and the first changes in the muscle, the molecular changes which, sweeping along the fibre, initiate the change of form, and which we may perhaps speak of as constituting a muscle impulse, also probably form a series the members of which are distinct.' As if to emphasize the scantiness of the knowledge available to the inquiring student, Foster summarized the matter on the following page thus: 'Passing down the nerve fibres to the muscle, flowing along the branching and narrowing tracts, the wave [of the nervous impulse] at last breaks on the end-plates of the fibres of the muscle. Here it is transmuted into what we have called a muscle impulse, which with a greatly diminished velocity (about 3 m. per sec.), travels from each end-plate in both directions to the end of the fibre, where it appears to be lost, at all events we do not know what becomes of it.' Still later in the book Foster touched on the possibility that the transmission of the impulse from nerve to muscle was electrical: 'The curious disposition of the end-plates', he wrote, 'and their remarkable analogy with the electric organs which are found in certain animals, has suggested the view that the passage of a nervous impulse from the nerve fibre into the muscular substance is of the nature of an electric discharge. But these matters are too difficult and too abstruse to be discussed here.'

There was not much encouragement here for work on the nature of the neuro-muscular transmission. But in point of fact, despite Foster's disinclination to indicate that the question had been considered, both the chemical and the electrical theories had already been suggested. In 1877 Du Bois Reymond (p. 289) stated that either of two known physical processes could be responsible for the transmission—namely, an electrical process or a chemical process, possibly due to lactic acid. Although Du Bois Reymond favoured the chemical process, his views had little influence because they were not based on any experimental evidence, and also because in 1888 Willy Kühne (p. 270) put forward evidence in favour of the view that the endplate in voluntary muscle is stimulated electrically. Kühne's theory held the field for many years.

When Dale was at Cambridge he had as a fellow-student Thomas Renton Elliott (1877–), with whom he was to be much associated in later life. Both of them listened to the lectures, and worked under the supervision, of Langley and Gaskell. They were therefore spectators of the birth of modern knowledge of the autonomic nervous system. Langley coined the term 'autonomic' in 1898, and some seven years later he crystallized the conception of the two divisions of the system, the thoracic and lumbar enlargements forming the sympathetic (or orthosympathetic) system, and the cranial and sacral enlargements forming together the parasympathetic system. At this time physiologists were much concerned with the action of adrenaline, which had been discovered in 1894 (p. 538). Langley's work had been dependent largely on the action of various drugs, and in 1901 he pointed out that stimulation of nerves belonging to the sympathetic division of the autonomic system gave results which were closely parallel to the action of adrenaline. Two other drugs were then much used in experimental physiology. One of these was muscarine, the active principle of the fungus *Amanita muscaria* which for centuries had been known to be poisonous. The active principle, the alkaloid muscarine, had been extracted in 1869 by Oswald Schmiedeberg (p. 684) and Richard Koppe, who thought that it was closely related to choline. When used experimentally it simulates very faithfully the type of peripheral autonomic effect which is produced by stimulation of parasympathetic nerves. It was considered early in the present century to be produced by stimulation of these nerves; and although it is now known that muscarine is not found in the animal body, the term 'muscarine action' for this type of effect persisted. This term refers especially to a peripheral action on the effector organs. The other drug was nicotine, the chief alkaloid of tobacco, which has a complex action on different parts of the nervous system. In physiology it came to be used especially for its action on autonomic ganglia, which in small doses it first stimulates and then depresses.

In 1904 Elliott, in a short preliminary paper, made the suggestion that the true sympathetic fibres might act indirectly on the effector cells of plain muscle and glands innervated by them by the liberation of adrenaline. In the following year he showed in his main paper that there were analogies between the organization of the autonomic system and that of the central nervous system. He also showed that the adrenal medulla is a homologue of the sympathetic ganglia. He did not repeat in this paper the suggestion made by him in his paper of the previous year—which was in effect the first suggestion, based on experimental work, of the chemical transmission of a nerve impulse. Elliott's suggestion went unheeded, apart from the work of Walter Ernest Dixon (1870–1931) of Cambridge, who argued that the parasympathetic nerves must also release a chemical transmitter (1906). He removed the heart of a dog while it was still inhibited by stimulation of the vagus. He then made an extract from the heart, purified it as far as was then possible, and applied the purified extract to the beating heart of a frog, which was in its turn inhibited. Dixon was unable to isolate the substance responsible for the inhibition, and he suggested that it might be muscarine, which was not known to be present in the body.

Although muscarine was much used about the beginning of the twentieth century for physiological and pharmacological tests, actually the substance which was almost universally employed was not true muscarine, but the synthetic muscarine—or 'pseudo-muscarine' —of Schmiedeberg and Harnack, who supposed that it was an aldehyde. As early as 1885 it had been recognized that this substance differed slightly in its action from that of true muscarine. In 1914 Dale found in an ergot extract certain activities which were not explained by any of the known active constituents of ergot. These activities resembled rather those of muscarine, and it was expected that muscarine would be found. The active principle in the extract was isolated chemically by Dale's co-worker Arthur James Ewins

(1882–1957) and proved to be acetylcholine (1914). At the same time the opportunity was taken of investigating 'pseudo-muscarine', which was found to be the nitrous acid ester of choline; it showed to some extent a nicotine effect which is not found in true muscarine.

This discovery did not cause any particular enthusiasm, partly because the substance isolated was evidently not a normal constituent of ergot extracts, and partly because its physiological activity as then known was not remarkable. It was the acetyl ester of the substance choline, which is a constituent of lecithin and is widely found in the vegetable and animal kingdoms. Physiologically choline is a depressor, slowing the heart and increasing intestinal movements and the secretions of the lacrymal and salivary glands. Choline is chemically related to muscarine, and in some ways their action is similar. It was now recalled by Dale that in 1906 Reid Hunt (1870–1948) of Washington, a former pupil of Abel, and his co-worker René de M. Taveau had prepared several different esters of choline and had compared their activity with that of the parent substance. They found that the acetyl ester, acetylcholine, produced the same depressor symptoms as choline in less that a thousandth part of the dose. (It is now known that the comparative efficiency of acetylcholine is much greater than that.) Acetylcholine was indeed not a new substance. It was supposed to have been first synthesized by the German chemist Adolf von Baeyer (1835–1917) in 1867, and it was certainly synthesized by Günther Nothnagel of the University of Marburg in 1894.

This 1914 paper by Dale on 'The action of certain esters and ethers of choline' is of great importance as it foreshadowed the demonstration of the chemical transmission of the nerve impulse by acetylcholine. In it he described his physiological investigations of the actions of the choline-esters of acetic, nitrous and nitric acid, and also of the ethyl-ether of choline. He showed that when very small doses of the esters are injected they produce vasodilatation and slowing of the heart. This action is abolished by atropine, but if then a large dose of the ester is given, the result is a great increase in blood-pressure similar to that produced by an injection of nicotine. It was noted that, especially with acetylcholine, the depressor effect was very transient, but could be quickly reproduced by giving a further dose of the substance. Dale suggested that in the body this evanescent effect is due to the rapid hydrolysis of acetylcholine into choline and acetic acid, and with Ewins he showed that *in vitro* this hydrolyis of acetylcholine in aqueous solution occurs rapidly provided that the solution is rendered alkaline. Dale demonstrated that the action of acetylcholine on organs containing plain muscle, and on glands—apart from the sweat glands of the cat—reproduced closely the results produced by stimulation of the post-ganglionic fibres of the parasympathetic. Dale also showed that acetylcholine reproduces those effects of autonomic nerves which are absent from the action of adrenaline, and vice versa. They are therefore both complementary and antagonistic. It should be said that out of the very numerous samples of ergot extracts examined by Dale over a period of ten years acetylcholine was found only on a few occasions. It is not a natural constituent of such extracts, and its presence in these few samples was probably due to bacterial action. These observations on the physiological action of acetylcholine would have been very suggestive had this substance been known to be present in the animal body, but of this there was no evidence.

The next step in the demonstration of the chemical transmission of a nerve impulse was not made until 1921, by Otto Loewi (1873–), then professor of pharmacology at Graz. Loewi has himself told how in the night of Easter Sunday, 1921, he awoke and made a note for an experiment. Next morning he realized that he had written something important, but he was unable to decipher his note. During the next night he awoke at the same time—3 a.m.—and remembered what he had written. Instead of making another note, Loewi arose, dressed, went to his laboratory, and performed the experiment. By 5 a.m. one form of chemical transmission of the nerve impulse was conclusively proved. Loewi's experiment was briefly as follows. It had been shown in 1845 by E. H. and E. F. W. Weber (p. 313) that stimuli passing down the vagus nerve to the heart inhibit that organ. If the vagi are severed these tonic impulses are cut off and the heart beats more rapidly. Loewi isolated the hearts of two frogs. A quantity of Ringer's solution was introduced into the cavity of the first heart, and the vagus supply to that heart was stimulated. The heartbeat was inhibited. The Ringer solution was then transferred to the second heart and inhibition of its beat also occurred. As the nerve supply to the second heart had not been stimulated, the stimulus must have been due to a chemical substance. Since then Loewi and others have modified the experiment; a perfusion fluid is continuously passed from the first heart into the second, so that inhibition of the second heart follows quickly after the stimulation of the vagus to the first. This experiment was much more clear-cut and informative than that of Dixon. This latter experiment showed that an inhibiting substance was present in the heart tissues very soon after the heart had been inhibited by the vagus, but it did not show that this substance was not present when vagus inhibition was not acting. Neither did it show that each stimulation of the vagus produced this substance, the action of which was of short duration. Loewi's experiment demonstrated that each stimulation of the vagus produced a quantity of this substance in the cavity of the heart.

It should be noted that, though Loewi's experiment was crucial, it applied only to the heart and the vagus nerve. It might be thought that by analogy it could have been concluded that a similar mechanism was in action in the case of plain muscle, or even striated muscle. But analogy is a dangerous tool in such matters. Even up to 1933 Loewi did not believe in chemical transmission in the case of striated muscle. Loewi knew that a chemical substance was involved in his experiment, and he referred to it as the 'vagus substance'. Although he did not isolate this substance, he had a good idea that it was acetylcholine. He found that even the minute amounts of the vagus substance which he was able to collect gave all the physiological tests for acetylcholine. He also found that the substance was rapidly destroyed by an esterase in the heart muscle, and it could be restored by acetylating the residue. He discovered that eserine, the alkaloid known also as physostigmine, inhibited the action of the esterase. In the laboratories of both Loewi and Dale this fact was extended to supply a test for the presence of small quantities of acetylcholine. It was not until 1933 that Feldberg and John Henry Gaddum (1900–) gave the final proof that the 'vagus substance' is acetylcholine.

This, however, is anticipating. In 1921 acetylcholine was not known to be normally present in the animal body. It was probable that large quantities of animal tissue would have to be examined if its presence were to be demonstrated. During the course of their work on histamine which has already been mentioned, Dale and Dudley (1929) examined the spleens of freshly killed horses and oxen, and in addition to the histamine action they found a powerful action of the choline type. If it had been due to choline it would have meant—compared with the known histamine content—the presence of an incongruously high concentration of choline in the tissue. The substance was eventually isolated by Dale and Dudley and identified chemically as acetylcholine. This was the first proof that acetylcholine occurs naturally in the animal body. In 1930 Dale and Gaddum published a paper which lent considerable support to the view that the effects produced by the stimulation of the post-ganglionic fibres of parasympathetic nerves, and the contractures in denervated muscles accompanying this stimulation, are due to the liberation of acetylcholine at the end-organs.

The fact that acetylcholine occurs in very small amounts in the animal body, and the possibility also that it is rapidly hydrolysed, made its estimation in physiological experiments an extremely difficult proceeding. It is understandable therefore that no marked progress was made in the study of its effects for some years after its discovery in the animal body by Dale and Dudley in 1929. This is therefore a convenient point to mention the progress made in the study of the action of adrenaline and similar substances.

We have seen that Elliott's suggestion that stimulation of nerves of the orthosympathetic system might produce their effects by the liberation of adrenaline at their terminations continued to exert an influence on some workers in this field. The action of substances closely allied chemically to adrenaline had been examined by Loewi and his co-workers in 1905, and by Dakin (p. 320) in the same year. In 1910 Barger and Dale carried out a very extensive investigation of the amines, with special reference to the degree of similarity between their physiological results and that following stimulation of the sympathetic. They coined the word 'sympathomimetic' to indicate the relation of the physiological effects produced by intravenous injection of the substance to the effects produced by sympathetic stimulation, without any indication of the precise mechanism of the action. Many observers had noted that small doses of adrenaline sometimes give a depressor rather than a pressor effect, and this phenomenon was studied by W. B. Cannon (p. 303) in 1913. Cannon found that the vasodilatation only occurred after the administration of adrenaline when the blood-pressure was above a certain critical level. This result appeared to be bound up with the fact that ergotoxine reverses the normal action of adrenaline. Many years later Cannon and his co-workers advanced a theory to explain some of the anomalies between the action of adrenaline and the results of stimulation of different sympathetic nerves. The theory as originally advanced by Cannon and Zénon M. Bacq (1903–), now of Liège, in 1931 assumed that a hypothetical substance named sympathin was produced in the body when sympathetic nerves were stimulated. But stimulation of different sympathetic nerves may produce different effects on the same organ. Two years later, therefore, Cannon and Arturo Stearns Rosenblueth (1900–) postulated that there are two forms of sympathin. Sympathin E is formed when the action is of an excitatory nature, and sympathin I when the result is an inhibition. Different organs produce different proportions of E and I. The existence of another substance, a mediator (M), was also postulated, and the local action of the sympathins was supposed to be due to the combination of M with E or with I, or with both. Cannon and Rosenblueth gave a definitive statement of their theory in their joint work, *Autonomic Neuro-Effector Systems* (1937).

It should be noted that the substance sympathin has never been isolated. In 1934 Bacq suggested that sympathin E was 'arterenol', a substance which had been synthesized as long ago as 1904, but which was not then known to occur normally in the animal body. In Great Britain it is more familiarly known as *nor*-adrenaline, which is recognized as differing materially from adrenaline in many respects. For example, both adrenaline and *nor*-adrenaline raise the blood-pressure. But whereas adrenaline does so by increasing the cardiac output, it dilates the capillaries. On the other hand, *nor*-adrenaline causes vasoconstriction and has no effect on the cardiac output.

The suggestion that acetylcholine was responsible for the transmission of the impulses in post-ganglionic fibres of the parasympathetic system was not universally accepted. One of the fundamental difficulties was that while the vasodilatation produced by stimulation of the chorda-tympani nerve is practically unaffected by atropine, this alkaloid easily obliterates the vasodilator effects of acetylcholine. In 1930 Dale and Gaddum investigated this matter, and also the fact that, if voluntary muscle is denervated, contractures can be produced either by stimulation of the parasympathetic nerve to the muscle which causes vasodilatation or by injecting acetylcholine intravascularly, but that adrenaline diminishes or obliterates the latter action but not the former. From the very careful discussion of their experimental results they concluded that there was a strong case for acetylcholine being regarded as the chemical transmitter of parasympathetic impulses. They admitted that in the case of the sympathetic system the evidence was less clear, and that the only hint of the nature of the transmitter was its physiological similarity to the action of adrenaline. In the following year Ulf Svante von Euler (1905–) and Gaddum gave the first clear evidence of the existence of post-ganglionic fibres derived from the sympathetic system which gave effects similar to acetylcholine and not, as would be expected, to adrenaline. Such anomalous actions were to cause considerable difficulties in interpretation thereafter.

In 1933 Feldberg migrated to London from Berlin, and in 1934 he and Dale investigated the substance produced in the wall of the stomach on stimulation of the vagi. They found that if eserine was administered, sufficient of the substance collected in the perfusion fluid to make its identification possible. But on stimulation of the vagi this substance was increased fourfold. Although the substance could not be identified chemically, the physiological tests left no doubt that it was acetylcholine. The vagal fibres which were thus stimulated belonged to the parasympathetic system. In the same year Dale and Feldberg investigated one of the anomalous cases referred to above. This was the sweat glands of the cat which are innervated by post-ganglionic sympathetic fibres. As such they should produce an adrenaline-like substance on stimulation. On the contrary, Dale and Feldberg showed that the substance produced gave all the tests for acetylcholine. It was in order to avoid confusion in such cases that in 1934 Dale proposed to set aside the anatomical origin of post-ganglionic autonomic fibres, and to classify them as 'adrenergic' or 'cholinergic', according to the nature of the substance which was produced on stimulation. Post-ganglionic parasympathetic fibres are therefore predominantly, and perhaps entirely, cholinergic; while post-ganglionic sympathetic fibres are predominantly, though not entirely, adrenergic; and some, and probably all, the pre-ganglionic fibres of the whole autonomic system are cholinergic. This terminology was at once accepted. In the tests for acetylcholine in these experiments much use was made of the fact that the muscle of the leech is extraordinarily sensitive to acetylcholine, and this test was to play an increasingly prominent role.

In the investigations which followed increasing use was also made of the two actions of acetylcholine to which reference has been made —the muscarine action, paralysed by atropine, and the nicotine action, which is paralysed by curare (p. 565).

Meanwhile Feldberg and Gaddum had turned their attention to the transmission of a nerve impulse in a ganglion of the autonomic system (1933). They perfused the superior cervical ganglion with an inert solution, and found no result when the pre-ganglionic nerve was stimulated. But when eserine was added to the perfusion fluid, acetylcholine—as shown by the usual tests—appeared in it whenever the pre-ganglionic nerve was stimulated. Contraction of the nictitating membrane was taken as an indication of the activity of the ganglion cells. In the following year (Sir) George Lindor Brown (1903–), and independently (Sir) John Carew Eccles (1903–), showed that a single impulse in a pre-ganglionic fibre produces a corresponding impulse in a post-ganglionic fibre, and that the delay at the synapse is very short, probably a few milliseconds. The indication is that each impulse in the pre-ganglionic fibre causes the release in immediate proximity to the ganglion cells of a minute quantity of acetylcholine. This acts as a trigger to fire an impulse from the ganglion cell, and having done so it is itself at once destroyed by a specific esterase. Since the number of nerve-cells in a ganglion is very great, the perfusion fluid, after stimulation of the pre-ganglionic fibre in the presence of eserine, contains a high concentration of acetylcholine, and if this effluent is injected into the arterial side of the perfusion, an outburst of impulses from the nerve-cells in the ganglion is produced.

In 1934 also Feldberg and Armas Vihtori Vartiainen (1901–) proved that in such experiments the acetylcholine was liberated actually at the synapses. They were also able to calculate that the arrival of an impulse at a pre-ganglionic ending on one nerve-cell in a ganglion liberated about 10^{-15} gramme of acetylcholine, whether or not the cell was paralysed by nicotine. Brown and Feldberg (1936) showed that on repeated stimulation of pre-ganglionic fibres the amount of acetylcholine recovered in the effluent sank to a much lower level, but the ganglion continued to transmit its impulses. Their work suggested that normally there is a depot of acetylcholine at the end of the pre-ganglionic fibre, and that when this is threatened with exhaustion a synthesis of acetylcholine takes place.

Attempts had been made during the previous fifteen years to show that chemical transmission also occurs in the case of voluntary striated muscle. For example, Otto Loewi and Ernest Geiger (1896-) had made such an attempt in 1922. None of these experiments was satisfactory. The mixed nerve to the muscle was usually stimulated, and it was therefore impossible to decide whether, when a substance of the nature of acetylcholine was liberated, the result was due to stimulation of motor, sensory, or autonomic fibres. Neither had the substance liberated been satisfactorily identified.

This problem could be tackled by two complementary methods, with each of which certain considerable difficulties were associated. In the first method the motor nerve-fibres to a perfused muscle could be stimulated and an attempt made to identify some active substance in the effluent, as had been done in the experiments mentioned in the previous paragraph. This method had worked well in the case of the autonomic ganglia, in which each ganglion is crowded with nerve-cells so that the synapses are very numerous and the concentration of acetylcholine liberated in the effluent is relatively great. In the case of a voluntary muscle, however, since it contracts as a whole its whole bulk must be perfused. But the number of motor end-plates in the muscle is relatively small, and hence it is to be expected that the concentration of any active substance in the effluent will be low, and the difficulty of its identification correspondingly great. Assuming that a certain active substance has been identified or is suspected, the second method may be employed. This consists in the application of the substance to the end-plates of the muscle in order to ascertain whether a contraction results. There are obviously two ways in which this can be attempted. One is to immerse the muscle in a solution of the active substance and allow it to reach the end-plates by slow diffusion. In 1921 Otto Ludwig Maximilian Riesser (1882–1949) and Simon Marcel Neuschlosz (1893–) immersed frog's muscles in a bath containing a relatively weak solution of acetylcholine. The muscles contracted. But the contraction was really a prolonged contracture of low tension, and such a contracture was also produced in certain muscles of the tortoise by Hermann Sommerkamp in 1928. The other method is to inject the active substance into the muscle, or into its circulation. This had been tried using acetylcholine by various investigators, but as we show later the result in the case of the muscles of birds was found by Dale and Gasser (p. 290) to be a slow contracture, as also was the result in the case of denervated mammalian muscles. Feldberg had injected acetylcholine into normal mammalian muscles and, when large doses were used, had obtained contractions which were inconstant.

The whole problem was therefore surrounded by pitfalls when Dale and his co-workers embarked on it. In their first assault they endeavoured to stimulate the motor nerves to a muscle and to identify the substance produced. This paper by Dale, Feldberg, and Marthe Louise Vogt (1903–) was published in 1936. In the case of the gastrocnemius muscle of the cat or dog, the stimulation of the motor nerve-fibre was obtained by stimulating the ventral nerve-roots, the sympathetic chain on that side having been previously removed. In the case of other muscles also a suitable technique was adopted to ensure that only motor fibres were stimulated. The muscles were perfused with Locke's solution containing eserine, to prevent the destruction of any acetylcholine which might be produced. They found that stimulation of the motor nerve-fibres constantly caused the appearance of a substance, identified as acetylcholine by the usual tests, in the effluent; its production ceased when stimulation was stopped. When the nerve was made to degenerate, stimulation of the muscle caused contraction but no production of acetylcholine. If the end-plates were paralysed by adding curarine to the perfusion fluid, stimulation of the nerve produced acetylcholine but no contraction, showing that the production of acetylcholine was associated with the transmission of the impulse and was not produced by the contraction of the muscle. Very significant was the fact that the authors were able to calculate the amount of acetylcholine liberated when a single nerve-impulse in one motor fibre reached the end-plate of that fibre. They found that it was of the order of 10^{-15} gramme. This was virtually the same as the amount liberated by a single impulse at a synapse in a ganglion.

In view of the contractures or inconstant and inefficient contractions which had been found to be produced in various types of muscles by the application of acetylcholine, it was now necessary to show that when this substance was satisfactorily applied to the end-plates of mammalian muscle it would produce an efficient contraction of the type produced by the usual kinds of stimulation. This problem was attacked by Brown, Dale, and Feldberg (1936). They argued that stimulation of the nerve to a muscle produces—as had previously been shown—a low concentration of acetylcholine in the venous effluent, but that in reality the effective concentration of this substance at the places where it is required—the end-plates—must be high. Further, a volley of impulses caused by stimulation of the nerve must produce this concentration in all the end-plates in the muscle simultaneously. Because of the small volume of the end-plates in relation to the very large volume of the muscle, the blood and tissue-fluids would cause the resulting concentration of acetylcholine in the venous perfusion effluent to be very low, even in the presence of eserine, although at the effective points—the end-plates—it would be high. The failure of the application of acetylcholine by methods involving slow diffusion to the end-plates were therefore explained. Dale and Gasser (1926) had already tried injecting acetylcholine into the lower end of the aorta without interrupting the circulation, and André Simonart (1903–) had again used this method; but the results were inconstant since the acetylcholine reached the muscle under investigation at rates which were both variable and unknown.

Brown, Dale, and Feldberg therefore introduced a new technique whereby the muscle under investigation was temporarily drained of its blood, and then a small dose of acetylcholine was at once injected into the vessels. The result was that the acetylcholine reached all the end-plates as nearly as possible at the same time, and the condition approximated to that produced by a nerve volley. This small dose caused contraction of the muscle at not less than half the speed of a maximal motor twitch, and with a similar tension. The rapid, propagated contraction produced was abolished by curarine. These investigators also established the importance of a cholinesterase in regulating the action of the chemical transmitter in the case of voluntary muscle. They found that if an intravenous dose of eserine was also given, the contraction produced by the acetylcholine changed from a simple twitch to a series of twitches having the nature of an evanescent tetanus. The eserine antagonizes the esterase and thus allows the acetylcholine to remain in contact with the end-plates and to produce a series of rapid contractions. In the following year G. L. Brown cleared up some of the anomalies presented by frog's muscle. By employing the method of direct injection into the artery supplying the muscle he showed that acetylcholine could produce a propagated contraction, which, however, pertained rather to the response of denervated mammalian muscle.

For their work on the chemical transmission of the nerve-impulse Dale and Loewi shared a Nobel Prize in 1936. Since then their coworkers and others have further developed the theory, but the discussion of this later work falls outside the scope of this book. Suffice it is to say that the presence of cholinesterase in many tissues had been demonstrated, in work extending over twenty years, by David Nachmansohn (1899–). He and others found that acetylcholine was present not only at the nerve terminations, but also along the whole length of the fibres. Nachmansohn has therefore postulated a role for acetylcholine in the transmission of the impulse along the nerve fibre. Working with A. L. Machado he showed in a paper published in 1943 that the enzyme which synthesizes acetylcholine could be obtained in solution. They showed that it acts by the acetylation of choline in the presence of certain other substances, and they named it cholinacetylase. In 1935 Dale first suggested that acetylcholine might also act as a transmitter in the central nervous system. Since then Feldberg and his co-workers have obtained evidence of the presence of cholinacetylates in various parts of the central nervous system but not in others. Although the evidence for central transmission by acetylcholine is strong, it has not yet been accepted in all its implications.

(d) *Nutrition and Metabolism*

The experiments of Sanctorius on his steel-yard (p. 116) went largely unheeded for over two centuries. Physiologists were interested in the digestion of the foodstuffs from the time of Spallanzani and Beaumont onwards, but no outstanding worker was interested in the fate of the digested matter after it had been absorbed. In 1783 and the few years following Lavoisier made a great advance by showing that the extent of oxidation in the body—that is, the amount of oxygen absorbed—is increased after taking food, during muscular work, and when the temperature of the subject's environment is lowered. Early in the nineteenth century interest became focused on the three classes of foodstuffs which we now know as the proximate principles, the proteins, fats, and carbohydrates. The proteins had not long been recognized when François Magendie (p. 154), who later became much better known for his work in other fields, performed in 1816 a very important experiment. He fed dogs on sugar and distilled water alone and found that they died in about a month. The same result followed when others were fed on butter and water, or olive oil and water. Magendie rightly concluded that the proteins were necessary for life. He now tried adding gelatine, a protein, to his artificial diet and found that it did not save the animal. Meat protein, however, kept the animal alive. Evidently the necessary protein must be of a certain chemical constitution.

Shortly after this there followed a period when chemists were isolating various organic substances from the body, and about 1839 the conception of metabolism was first introduced. In that year the word 'Stoffwechsel' was used by Schwann for the changes produced in foodstuffs during their breaking-down and destruction in the body, and four years later it was found not infrequently in the German literature. This word was translated into English as 'metabolism', and in that form was soon widely used. This fundamental conception regards the body as being constantly in a state of change. The dead material derived from the foodstuffs is constantly being built up into living tissue (anabolism), and at the same time there is a process of breaking down of living tissue (katabolism). Lavoisier had indicated that the utilization of fats and carbohydrates depended on three main factors, and interest was now centred on the result of digestion of the proteins and on the relative amounts of each of the three proximate principles which were utilized for growth and repair of the body, for the maintenance of the body temperature, and for the performance of work. A balance-sheet of the food intake and the products of their combustion in the body was required, and this was first produced by Jean Baptiste Boussingault (1801–87) in 1839. He analysed the fodder of a cow, given sufficient food to maintain its weight under the conditions of the experiment, and determined the content of the food in terms of carbon, hydrogen, oxygen, and nitrogen. During the period of the experiment he also determined the amounts of the same elements lost in the urine, faeces, and milk of the cow. By subtracting, in the case of each element, the amount excreted from the amount ingested, the quantity of the element lost in the process of metabolism was obtained. Assuming that these quantities had been lost in each case by combination with oxygen derived from the air in respiration, Boussingault calculated the amount of oxygen necessary to effect this oxidation. He concluded that a cow would deprive 19 cubic metres of air of its oxygen content in twenty-four hours. He later repeated these experiments on a horse and on a dove.

Meanwhile the role of oxygen in these processes, first suggested by Lavoisier, was being further considered. Liebig (p. 237) was then at the height of his powers and was establishing the fundamental facts of organic chemistry. The theory then current was that the oxidation took place, not as Lavoisier had believed in the lungs, but in the blood. In 1837 Heinrich Gustav Magnus (1802–70) of Berlin showed that the blood contains large quantities of oxygen and carbon dioxide, and thus gave support to the theory. Liebig held, shortly after this date, the view that fats and carbohydrates were broken down by oxidation, but that proteins were disintegrated by muscle work. In 1840 Liebig presented to the meeting of the British Association in Glasgow the first part of a report in which he developed the doctrines of organic chemistry in their bearing on agriculture and physiology. At the meeting of the Association in 1842 he presented the second part of his report. This, a substantial book, was published with the title *Die organische Chemie in ihrer Anwendung auf Physiologie und Pathologie* (1842); in the same year a translation was

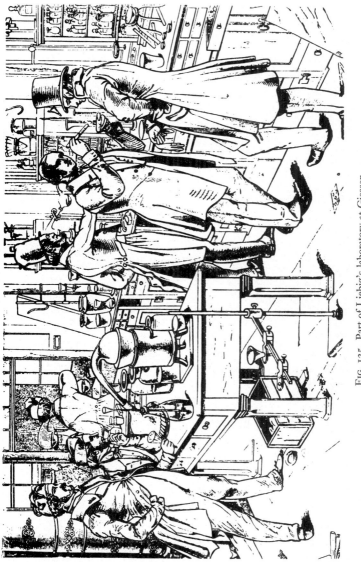

FIG. 125. Part of Liebig's laboratory at Giessen

Reading from left to right, the six persons are: 1, Wyder; 2, F. Varrentrapp (later Director of the Mint); 3, unknown; 4. J. J. Scherer (later Professor of Medicine at Würzburg); 5, E. Boeckmann (later Director of the Fries Ultramarine Works); 6. A. W. Hofmann (Liebig's assistant, later Professor of Chemistry at Berlin)

(Drawing of c. 1840 by W. Trautschold)

published in London (*Animal Chemistry, or Organic Chemistry in its Applications to Physiology and Pathology*). In this important work Liebig discussed the action of oxygen in the process of oxidation in the animal tissues, the nature of the bile, the elements of nutrition in the domestic animals, the composition of the tissues and the part of protein in that composition, the changes which take place in digestion, the composition of calculi, and many other associated problems. Liebig showed that it was not carbon and hydrogen which burned in the body, as had been assumed by Lavoisier, but carbohydrates and fats. The book may be regarded as the first textbook of biochemistry. In it Liebig suggested that the nitrogen in the urine might be used to measure the amount of protein destroyed in the body.

In 1849 Henri Victor Regnault (1810–78) and Jules Reiset (1811–?) of Paris experimented with an animal in a bell-jar of such a type that the carbon dioxide breathed out was absorbed and could therefore be measured; at the same time measured volumes of oxygen were introduced to replace that which the animal used up. This apparatus was probably the first physiological calorimeter. They were therefore easily able to determine the ratio of the carbon dioxide expired to the oxygen inspired. This respiratory quotient (R.Q.), as Pflüger later called it, is a significant ratio which has since then been greatly used. They showed that it varies with the type of food, and that body heat is derived from chemical reactions in the body. They also understood that the consumption of oxygen per unit of body-weight varies enormously in different animals, even though the different species have the same body temperature. For example, the oxygen consumption per unit of body-weight is ten times greater in sparrows than in chickens, and this must be correlated with the fact that relatively to body-weight—or, as we would say, to volume— the sparrow has a much larger surface area, and therefore a much larger cooling surface, than the chicken. This was the first crude expression of the law of surface area. Regnault and Reiset found that the respiratory quotient might vary in the same animal from 0·64 to 1·02; it was constant with the same food, but varied according to the kind of food eaten. It did not depend on the species of animal.

The close of the first period in the study of metabolism was marked by the publication in 1852 of a brilliant work by Friedrich

Heinrich Bidder (1810–94) and Carl Schmidt (1822–94). Bidder was a graduate in medicine who had been a pupil of Johannes Müller, and Schmidt was a chemist who had been trained by Liebig. Both subsequently held chairs at Dorpat, Bidder for thirty-four years and Schmidt for forty-five. Their celebrated book bore the title *Die Verdauungssäfte und der Stoffwechsel* ('The digestive juices and metabolism', 1852). In it they introduced the conception of intermediate metabolism. They also carried farther the suggestion made by Regnault and Reiset, referred to above. Bidder and Schmidt thought that in any animal the extent of the respiration at any time depends on two factors. One of these is a variable, the amount of food undergoing digestion and absorption at that time. The other is a constant for that species; it is determined mainly by the respiration necessary to replace the heat lost by the body, through radiation and conduction, in a fasting animal in a given unit of time. This constant factor was called by Bidder and Schmidt the 'typical respiration', or, as we would now translate their term, the 'typical metabolism'. Much later it became the important factor now referred to as the basal metabolism. They clearly understood that this constant factor could, if numerous experiments were carried out, be accurately determined for different species of animals. Bidder and Schmidt carried out calorimetric experiments, on the lines of Regnault and Reiset, on cats and dogs, and from their data they obtained respiratory quotients comparable with what we now know to be the true values. They also took up Liebig's suggestion that the nitrogen in the urine might be used to measure the amount of protein destroyed in the body. Bidder and Schmidt concluded from their experiments that almost all the nitrogen of protein is split from its combination and carries with it sufficient carbon, hydrogen, and oxygen to form urea, which is excreted in the urine. The remaining parts of these three elements, containing about five-sixths of the total heat value of the protein, are oxidized to carbon dioxide and water, and in the process heat is produced. These results were severely criticized by others, and it was years later before their correctness was established. Bidder and Schmidt also fed meat in excess to a starving cat, and they showed that in these circumstances there is a characteristic increase in metabolism associated with excess of protein in the diet.

They were also interested in the function of bile. By the formation of a fistula they removed the bile from a dog and showed that the digestion and absorption of proteins and carbohydrates proceeded normally. They then gave the dog a weighed quantity of fat, and from the faeces they recovered over half that weight of fatty bodies; putrefaction of unabsorbed fat was proceeding. The role of the bile in the digestion of fat was thus clearly shown.

In the year of publication of this outstanding book (1852) Liebig left Giessen to become professor of chemistry at Munich. In the same year Pettenkofer (p. 231), who for five years had been extra-ordinary professor of medical chemistry at Munich, was promoted to the ordinary chair in that subject. In that year also Carl von Voit (1831–1908), a medical student who had been taking part of his course at Würzburg, returned to complete his studies at Munich. Two years later he graduated in medicine, and he then proceeded to follow an intensive course in science during which he studied chemistry under both Liebig and Pettenkofer. Voit's scientific training was therefore of the highest order. Meanwhile, in the year of his graduation Theodor Ludwig Wilhelm Bischoff (1807–82), who had held chairs of anatomy and physiology at Heidelberg and Giessen, and who was a friend of Liebig and had worked with him, was called to the chair of anatomy and physiology at Munich. He held this chair for twenty-four years (1854–78), during which period he made important contributions to embryology in addition to carrying out much physiological research. A new physiological institute was being built, the director of which was Emil Harless (1820–62), the professor of physiology, and in 1856 Voit entered it as assistant to Bischoff. Four years later Voit was appointed extraordinary pro-fessor of physiology, and in 1863, on the untimely death of Harless, he became ordinary professor of that subject and director of the institute, posts which he held for the next forty-four years.

All modern research on metabolism stems directly from Voit. Of his innumerable pupils several have risen to fame, and of these we have occasion to refer especially to the work of Atwater, Erwin Voit, Rubner, Graham Lusk, and Cathcart. On the European Conti-nent, in Great Britain, and in the United States the direct scientific descent from Liebig and Voit is still active.

When Voit was appointed as assistant in the new physiological institute he at once tackled a problem which was much misunderstood, and which was, moreover, of fundamental importance. Reference has already been made to the experiment of Bidder and Schmidt regarding the elimination of ingested nitrogen in the urine and faeces. During 1857–8 Voit fed weighed quantities of meat to starving dogs and ascertained the amount of nitrogen excreted. He already knew the amount of nitrogen excreted during starvation, and this was assumed to represent the amount of tissue destruction. It was logical to assume also that if this amount of nitrogen was ingested, it would replace that destroyed and there would therefore be a condition of nitrogen equilibrium. Voit found that when the amount of meat equivalent to this amount of nitrogen was given, there was an increase in the amount of nitrogen excreted. As progressively greater quantities of meat were given the excretion of nitrogen at first increased, so that more was excreted than was ingested, and then decreased, until finally a point was reached when the animal was in what he called nitrogen equilibrium. In experiments made many years later Voit showed that this point was reached only when the dog ingested at least two and a half times the amount of protein which it metabolized in starvation. In the early experiments he demonstrated quite clearly that practically all the nitrogen excreted by the body appeared in the urine and faeces, and that every gramme of nitrogen excreted by these channels represents the destruction of 6·25 gramme of protein in the body. Actually the bulk of the nitrogen appears in the urine as urea.

In 1860 Bischoff and Voit published their work *Die Gesetze der Ernährung des Fleischfressers* ('The laws of nutrition in carnivores'). In this book they reviewed the previous work of Voit and others, and from it they calculated that in starvation there is also an elimination of carbon in excess. They considered that this point could be cleared up by estimating not only the nitrogen, but also the carbon, excreted. This involved ascertaining the amount of carbon dioxide breathed out during the period of the experiment. Voit now decided to investigate the metabolism of human subjects. He elicited the help of his friend Pettenkofer, who constructed a chamber large enough to hold a bed or a bicycle ergometer. The chamber was freely ventilated, and the air leaving it could be accurately measured. The amounts of water vapour and carbon dioxide in the air entering and leaving the chamber respectively were determined by calculations from samples frequently taken and analysed. It was therefore an 'open-circuit' apparatus. This 'respiration apparatus' was completed about 1862. Pettenkofer and Voit's first experiment was on a starving man. On one side of their balance sheet they had his weight at the start and the amount of water drunk during the experiment. On the other side they had his weight at the end, the weight of the urine passed, and also the weights of the carbon dioxide and water excreted in the respired air. The difference between the two totals gave the weight of oxygen used up during the experiment. They then analysed the urine and ascertained the total weights of carbon and nitrogen contained in it. From these data they were able to calculate the amount of protein and fat destroyed in the starving man during the experiment. Further, from analysis of protein and fat they calculated the amount of oxygen which would be theoretically required to burn the amounts of those substances which had been destroyed in the body. They found that this oxygen figure agreed closely with that which they had obtained by difference. They concluded that the fasting man supported himself mainly by the combustion of his own protein and fat. They found that the respiratory quotient in this experiment was 0·69.

During the period 1866 to 1873 Pettenkofer and Voit published seven important papers on results obtained using their respiration chamber. They found that during work more fat was burned than during starvation. A carnivorous animal such as a dog could maintain itself on an exclusive protein diet, and if fat were added to such a diet, the fat was nearly all deposited in the body. Carbohydrates, on the other hand, were almost completely consumed. They found also that fat, which burns readily outside the body, is combusted only with difficulty within the body, and that in the case of protein the conditions are reversed.

Voit realized clearly that some method was required to express the value of the proximate principles in terms of energy—preferably in terms of their heat value. In 1860 during a visit to London he acquired a Thomson calorimeter, and two years later he published a paper in which he set out some of his results. However, the real beginning of research on the calorific value of foods was due to the English chemist Sir Edward Frankland (1825–99), who in 1866 gave accurate values for cheese, potatoes, bread, butter, the white and yolk of eggs, and other foodstuffs. This work led to the refinements of the modern bomb calorimeter. By 1873 Pettenkofer and Voit had calculated that 100 grammes of fat are physiologically equivalent to 175 grammes of starch. At a later date (1883) this problem was at Voit's suggestion studied by one of his most brilliant pupils, Max Rubner (1854–1932). He showed that the proximate principles may under certain conditions replace each other in accordance with their caloric values, so that 100 grammes of fat are equivalent to 232 grammes of starch, 234 of cane sugar, and 243 of dried meat. This iso-dynamic law is of great importance in dietetics. Shortly after this in-vestigation Rubner was called to the chair of hygiene at Marburg. He succeeded Koch as the director of the Institute of Hygiene at Berlin, and from 1909 until his retirement in 1922 he filled brilliantly the chair of physiology at Berlin. In addition to his work on metabolism he wrote prolifically on subjects relating to environmental hygiene, the bacterial content of water supplies, and the metabolism of bacteria.

To return to the experiments of Pettenkofer and Voit, in 1866 they showed that active muscular work did not increase protein metabolism even in starvation, and that the metabolism was not proportional to the oxygen supply. They brought out the important conclusion that the absorption of oxygen is not the cause of meta-bolism, although the extent of the metabolism determines the amount of oxygen used. Even at the end of his life Voit had to confess that he did not know the cause of metabolism.

The position about 1885 may be summarized thus. Foodstuffs and excretions could be accurately analysed. The metabolism of many species of animals and of man had been ascertained under various conditions, using a closed-circuit respiration apparatus for animals and the open-circuit apparatus of Pettenkofer and Voit for man. Much was known about the variations produced in the respira-tory quotient by combustion of the different types of foodstuffs. It was realized that when foodstuffs were combusted in the body they produced energy in the form of heat, and, since the end-products were the same, it was assumed that this heat was equivalent to that which they produced when burned in a calorimeter. There was an exception to this assumption. The end-product of the metabolism of protein is urea, and in certain circumstances an excess of carbon. In 1885 Rubner had investigated this matter thoroughly and had concluded that, to obtain the fuel-value of protein in metabolism, the heat-value of the urinary constituents had to be deducted from the heat-value of protein as burned in a calorimeter. In the same year the chemist Friedrich Karl Adolf Stohmann (1832–97) published valuable work on the calorific value of various foods. But it should be emphasized that at this period the heat produced in the animal body during metabolism had not been directly measured.

During the period following 1885 Rubner elucidated four very important principles. Firstly, he applied the heat-values which were commonly accepted for the proximate principles to the data of published experiments on man and animals and showed that the metabolism of the resting individual is proportional to its superficial area. By this law Rubner established the correctness of the deduction of Regnault and Reiset. In these calculations he used the formula for superficial area based on the weight of the individual which had been published by K. Meeh in 1879.

Secondly, Rubner found that the heat-values for closely allied foodstuffs varied slightly. For example, he found that the Calorie value for glucose was 3·755 and for sucrose 4·001. Considering the average composition of a mixed diet, and taking into account the heat-values obtained by various investigations, Rubner suggested the following standard values for the proximate principles: protein, 4·1 Cal.; fat, 9·3 Cal.; carbohydrate, 4·1 Cal.; the value in each case being per gramme of the foodstuff. These values have stood the test of time.

Thirdly, he began in 1885 his investigation of the specific dynamic action of the foodstuffs. It was already known that if protein is given in excess an increase of metabolism results. Rubner's main work on this subject continued until 1902, when he published his book *Die Gesetze des Energieverbrauchs bei der Ernährung* ('The laws of energy utilization in nutrition'). In this work he showed that all the proximate principles increased heat production, in the case of the proteins by as much as a third of their heat-value. This specific dynamic action of the proteins has ever since been important in dietetics.

Fourthly, in 1894 Rubner constructed the first animal calorimeter. This was a chamber in which a dog was kept for a period of twenty-four hours. It was so constructed that the total heat produced by the dog could be measured. The chamber was connected to a respiration apparatus, such as that used by Pettenkofer and Voit (p. 585). The dog's total metabolism was ascertained in the usual way, and from the readings and analysis of the excreta Rubner calculated the total heat evolved by the dog during the twenty-four hours. This calculated figure was compared with the actual value of the heat evolved determined directly by the calorimeter. In the many experiments performed these values were seldom found to differ by more than 1 per cent. These results not only demonstrated the strict applicability to the animal body of the law of the conservation of energy; they also showed that the method of ascertaining the degree of metabolism used by Pettenkofer and Voit was completely justified.

It now became necessary to construct a respiration calorimeter in which the metabolism of a man could be measured, and at the same time the heat evolved by him could be directly measured. Voit had tried to construct such a calorimeter, but the experiments which he made with it were never published. The construction of such an apparatus involved enormous technical difficulties, not least of which was the devising of a means for preventing completely any loss of heat from the chamber in which the experimental subject was confined. The project was tackled in 1892 by Wilbur Olin Atwater (1844–1907), who had been a pupil of Voit and of Rubner, and who was then the occupant of an important post in the United States. Atwater received large financial support from the United States government, and he was associated with the physicist Edward Bennett Rosa (1861–1921), who was largely responsible for the technical perfection of the apparatus. Construction was begun in 1892, lasted several years, and the first description of the apparatus was published in 1897. The associated respiration apparatus was on the open-circuit principle of Pettenkofer and Voit, so that the oxygen used by the subject was not measured directly, but was calculated. With Francis Gano Benedict (1870–1957) Atwater then worked on the construction of a respiration calorimeter of the closed-circuit type in which oxygen was fed into the chamber automatically in quantities exactly sufficient to replace the oxygen used up in respiration. This was effected by means of an electrically operated spirometer. In the very costly apparatus which resulted it was possible to measure very accurately the respiratory and heat exchanges in the subject. Two other calorimeters of this type have since been constructed in New York, one at the Cornell University Medical College and the other at Bellevue Hospital. In the latter it is possible to measure directly the metabolism of patients suffering from various diseases. In all of these calorimeters loss of heat from the chamber is prevented not only by the usual methods of insulation but also by complicated devices. Electric thermo-couples in series between the outer and inner walls register immediately any difference in temperature, and the outer wall is heated or cooled accordingly by electrical devices. The heat produced by the metabolism of the subject is absorbed by water flowing through pipes in the chamber, and by appropriate methods it can be measured.

Another pioneer worker in metabolism was Zuntz (p. 309), a pupil of Pflüger who later occupied the chair of physiology at Berlin. Zuntz was especially interested in metabolism at high altitudes, and about 1888 he perceived that most of the measurements of metabolism of human subjects had been made either while they were starving under experimental conditions, or while they were carrying out some mild form of activity. He appreciated that even mild activity meant expenditure of energy, so that a true picture of what Bidder and Schmidt had called the 'typical respiration' was not obtained. Over a period of thirty years Zuntz measured his own metabolism at intervals, and he showed that it was remarkably constant. He devised a respiration apparatus by means of which the respiratory exchange could be measured with considerable accuracy over short periods. A pupil of Zuntz, Adolf Magnus-Levy (1865–1955), who later held a chair of medicine at Berlin, took the apparatus into the hospital wards in 1893 and was the first to ascertain the 'typical metabolism' in various diseases. He continued making such observations for at least fifteen years. In 1906 Magnus-Levy defined the conditions in which he made his measurements of the metabolism. In order to eliminate the effects of the specific dynamic action of the foodstuffs the determination must be made twelve hours after the last meal. The subject should have taken nothing but water, and during the determination he should be lying down relaxed in a warm atmosphere. The metabolism so determined was called by Magnus-Levy the *Grundumsatz*, and this word was later translated by Lusk and Du Bois as 'basal metabolism'.

Very many direct estimates of the basal metabolism, expressed as Calories per square metre of surface in 24 hours, were made in New York at Cornell and at the Bellevue Hospital by F. G. Benedict, by Lusk and by Eugene Floyd Du Bois (1882–1959), the physiologist and physician of Cornell University. Benedict and others had criticized the accuracy of Meeh's formula for surface area, and as a result Du Bois and his cousin, Delafield Du Bois (1880–), were able to devise by a very ingenious technique the more satisfactory formula which is now widely used. As a result of this work the fundamental facts relating to the basal metabolism were firmly established. The figures for metabolic rates for normal individuals of different ages obtained at that time were slightly lower than those accepted today. The introduction by Haldane of his blood-gas apparatus and the invention of the Douglas bag (p. 307) in 1911 permitted the carrying out of complicated metabolic investigations by the indirect method.

Starvation. Voit made his first important investigation of a prolonged fast in a dog in 1866, and as a result he differentiated between 'circulating protein', available for combustion in the tissues, and 'organized protein', which constitutes the living material of the tissues. Others carried out experiments on fasting animals, but the period of the so-called professional fasting-men began about 1890. In that year Succi was investigated by Luigi Luciani (p. 260), one of the greatest of Italian physiologists, whose work on the results of extirpation of the cerebellum was well known. In 1901 Succi underwent another long fast. In 1893 Cetti was investigated by Immanuel Munk (p. 602) of Berlin, and also by Zuntz. In 1907 Beauté was investigated by Cathcart. Reference is made later to Benedict's fasting experiments in the same year on seven men. In 1915 Benedict experimented on another subject who fasted for thirty-one days. Possibly the longest fast for experimental purposes was that of

Merlatti in Paris (fifty days); but the case is known of a hunger-striker in jail who died on the seventy-fourth day of his fast.

In starvation the behaviour of the proteins is especially interesting. Wilhelm Prausnitz (1861–1933) of Munich and Graz, who had been a pupil of Voit and who later became well known for his writings on hygiene, showed that during the first day of a fast the glycogen stores in the body are mobilized to form sugar, which is combusted. On that day the protein destruction, as shown by the nitrogen elimination, is low, but on the second and subsequent days there is a considerable increase. In 1907 Benedict carried out seventeen experiments on seven men in fasts lasting up to about a week. He showed that where the glycogen stores were low the protein destruction was high even on the first day of the fast. This was the first large investigation carried out in the new modified respiration calorimeter, in which the actual amount of oxygen burned was measured. As a result Benedict was able to calculate not only the amount of protein destroyed on each day, but also the amount of fat and glycogen combusted. The results were given in Benedict's important monograph, *The Influence of Inanition on Metabolism* (1907).

During fasting there is little alteration in the metabolism from day to day. This was first shown by Zuntz and Curt Lehmann in 1893 in their experiments on Cetti during a fast of ten days. There was little variation in the amount of protein, fat, and carbohydrate destroyed, or in the total energy output. In 1915 Benedict carried out another important investigation on a man who fasted for thirty-one days. He showed that during this period there was a reduction of 29 per cent. in the heat production. Erwin Voit (1852–1932), the younger brother and pupil of Carl, showed in 1901 that the amount of protein destruction during starvation depends on the amount of fat in the body. When the supplies of fat are almost used up there is a 'premortal rise' in the protein destruction leading to the death of the animal. In experiments on a dog Lusk and Rudolph John Anderson (1879–) showed in 1917 that the lowered metabolism during a fast does not return at once to its pre-fasting level on feeding; the height of the metabolism is determined by the nutritive condition of the body. This important principle was later confirmed (1926) by Nathaniel Kleitman (1895–) in experiments on the faster Hoelzel, who underwent two fasts of thirty-three and forty days respectively, separated by a month.

Influence of muscular work. Liebig stated categorically that the energy of muscular contraction was derived from the oxidation of muscle tissue, and that therefore muscular exercise must cause an increase in the nitrogen excreted in the urine. This theory was accepted for many years, despite the fact that a very effective demonstration of its erroneousness was made by Adolf Fick (1829–1901). Fick studied at Marburg where he was a pupil of Karl Ludwig. Shortly afterwards he was an assistant to Ludwig at Zurich, and a few years later he succeeded to Ludwig's chair there. From 1868 until his death Fick was professor of physiology at Würzburg, where he built up a distinguished school of that subject. He is especially remembered for his work on the physics of the human organism, on which he wrote a textbook in 1856, for his investigation on the contraction of muscle, on conduction in nerve, work on the special senses, and on intracardiac pressure. He was adept at the invention of instruments used in his investigations. In 1865 Fick and a colleague made an ascent of the Faulhorn in Switzerland. They had had no nitrogenous food for seventeen hours before the start of the ascent. As a result of urine analysis they showed that they had performed at least three times as much work as could be accounted for by the metabolism of protein during the period of the ascent.

In 1866 Pettenkofer and Voit, investigating dogs and a man working an ergostatic wheel, obtained the same result, and four years later Leibig acknowledged that he had been wrong. He now stated that, if the metabolism of muscle increased with mechanical work, a man could, by the exercise of his will, exhaust his entire supply of muscle tissue. Nevertheless, the problem is not so simple as these early researches would seem to indicate. Pflüger, as a result of many experiments by himself and his co-workers, took the attitude that for the production of work the living tissue prefers to use protein when sufficient of that food material is offered to it. That Voit was perhaps not entirely satisfied with his own conclusion is possibly indicated by the fact that on several occasions in later years he gave this problem to several of his assistants or pupils in turn. None of the results was beyond criticism.

The modern period of this investigation was introduced by the important work of Atwater and Benedict (1903), who were able to make direct experiments with the aid of the Atwater-Rosa calorimeter. They concluded that work done by subjects working a stationary bicycle was at the expense of fats and carbohydrates, but not of proteins. About this time the suggestion, based on experiments, was made by Adolf Loewy (1862–1937) that muscular work favours the retention of protein. This would explain the hypertrophy of muscles as a result of exercise. Loewy worked for nearly twenty years in Berlin, and in 1921 he became extraordinary professor of physiology there. He carried out many investigations with Zuntz. In the following year, however, he became director of the Swiss institute for the investigation of the medical problems of high altitudes at Davos. Several other investigators have obtained evidence of increased consumption of protein during muscular work, and Cathcart in 1925 discussed the evidence fully and instanced some of his own experiments in support of this view.

The behaviour of the respiratory quotient during muscular work is a subject of great importance. It was thoroughly investigated in 1913 by Benedict and Cathcart, who employed a professional cyclist. The subject used a stationary bicycle ergometer and rode to the point of exhaustion, which was reached in four hours twenty-two minutes. During this time the rider carried out work equivalent to a cycle-ride of over 100 miles. His respiratory quotient remained virtually unaltered throughout the ride, but after the experiment the value of the R.Q. fell to a figure which indicated that the body glycogen supplies, which had been drawn on during the expenditure of energy, were exhausted. The energy produced by the rider was fairly constant at 600 Calories per hour, which seems to be about the limit of sustained muscular effort for the human subject. After the experiment this professional rider showed for about six hours a significant increase in basal metabolism.

Assuming that the bulk of the energy for muscular work is supplied by fats and carbohydrates, the question arose whether either of these two foodstuffs was superior to the other so far as the efficiency of the body as a machine was concerned. In 1901 Zuntz, as a result of experiments on a human subject, concluded that from this aspect fats and carbohydrates were equally satisfactory. An important investigation on this and similar subjects was published in 1917 by Rudolph John Anderson (p. 591) and Graham Lusk (1866–1932). Lusk studied in Germany and he spent several years in Voit's laboratory. After his return to the United States he held various posts until he was appointed to the chair of physiology at the Cornell University Medical College, New York. His whole active life was devoted to the study of metabolism, especially with the use of the new respiration calorimeters in New York, and some of his investigations are mentioned in this section. In 1906 Lusk published his *The Elements of the Science of Nutrition*, which went through successive editions and reprintings until the fourth edition of 1928. During nearly three decades this great book continued to instruct and inspire all who were devoting themselves seriously to the problems of metabolism.

In their experiments of 1917 Anderson and Lusk used a dog working a treadmill in a respiration calorimeter. Its energy production was determined respectively in starvation, eighteen hours after the ingestion of food, and immediately after the ingestion of a considerable amount of glucose. They showed that the ingestion of glucose allows mechanical work to be performed at the expense of 5 per cent. less energy than when glucose is not taken. By fasting we can reduce the body-weight, the basal metabolism, and the amount of energy required to move the weight of the body, but a given amount of work is carried out only at the expense of the expenditure of a definite amount of energy, which does not vary with the body-weight. Whether this energy is obtained from the consumption of fat and carbohydrates, or whether it is obtained only from the oxidation of body fat in starvation, it is constant.

The relative values of fat and of carbohydrate as sources of muscular energy were investigated in man in 1920 by Krogh (p. 307) and Johannes Lindhard (1870–1947). They showed that when fat alone was burned in the organism about 4·6 Calories of energy had to be liberated in order to produce 1 Calorie of work, whereas with carbohydrate this result was obtained by the liberation of 4·1 Calories of energy. For the production of equivalent amounts of muscular work, therefore, carbohydrate is more efficient than fat.

Protein metabolism. Voit showed in 1869 that absorption of undigested proteins, for example serum protein and uncoagulated egg-albumen, could sometimes take place, but it was soon admitted that such an event could not be the usual method for the absorption of protein. It was then shown that proteins were broken down into peptides, and in 1885 Franz Hofmeister (1850–1922), then at Prague but later a professor at Strasbourg and Würzburg, put forward the theory that immediately after the peptides were absorbed they were converted into protein by the leucocytes in the intestinal wall, and conveyed by them to the tissues. Heidenhain agreed generally with this view, but thought that the active cells were the epithelial cells of the intestine. It was later shown that, even if the leucocytes did perform this function, their numbers were not nearly large enough to deal with the amount of protein ingested during a meal.

The answer to the question had long been partially available, but it had been entirely misunderstood. Kölliker and Müller had in 1856 found the amino-acids leucine and tyrosine in the normal contents of the intestine. They were unable to explain their presence. So also were Kühne (1869) and other scientists who found them present. In 1901 Otto Cohnheim (1873–1953) adopted the theory that these first-stage degeneration products of protein were re-synthesized into protein in the intestinal wall. (Cohnheim, who later adopted the surname Kestner, was the son of the pathologist Julius Cohnheim; he was then at Heidelberg, but later held the chair of physiology at Hamburg.) He always found that the peptides were broken down to simpler products; he discovered a ferment which brought about this breakdown and called it erepsin.

Interest now centred on these simpler products, the amino-acids. Many of these substances had been known for a long time. Cystine was discovered by William Hyde Wollaston (1766–1828) in 1810. Leucine was discovered by Henri Braconnot (1780–1855) in 1820, and in the same year he also discovered glycine. Liebig discovered tyrosine in 1846, and so on. But in 1899 the chemist Emil Fischer (1852–1919) of Berlin began to combine amino-acids to form poly-peptides. By a certain technique he was often able to transform these into substances which were identical with the peptones produced by the natural disintegration of the proteins. Among others who were in this field very active about this period was Albrecht Kossel

(1853–1927) of Berlin, who became professor of physiology successively at Marburg and at Heidelberg; in 1896 he discovered the amino-acid histidine, and in 1910 he was awarded a Nobel Prize for his researches into the chemistry of the cell nucleus. In 1898 Kossel forecast the polypeptide nature of the protein molecule. Gowland Hopkins (p. 611) and Sydney William Cole (1876–1951) jointly discovered tryptophane during the course of their important researches on tryptic digestion and the proteins generally. Emil Abderhalden (1877–1950) of Halle was about this time beginning his long series of researches on the amino-acids.

As a result of this work which we have briefly discussed it now seemed possible that the physiology of protein metabolism might be the physiology of the amino-acids. But there was as yet no proof that amino-acids were absorbed and were present in the blood. The first twelve years of the twentieth century were devoted to this problem, which proved to be extremely difficult since the blood removed the absorbed materials very rapidly. In 1905 Cathcart and John Beresford Leathes (1864–1956), later professor of physiology at Sheffield and the author of an important monograph on the fats, showed that after absorption of protein there was no increase of coagulable protein in the blood. This was evidence against the theory of immediate resynthesis. On the other hand, they obtained much indirect evidence that the simpler products of digestion could be found in the blood. They further showed that during absorption from the intestine nitrogenous material is stored in the liver. In 1906 Howell (p. 545) made the first partially successful attempt to demonstrate the presence of amino-acids in the blood. He drew blood from fasting and fed dogs, enclosed it in collodion sacs, and dialysed it against distilled water. Amino-acids and even more complex substances pass through the membrane. Howell found that a much more definite positive reaction was obtained from the portal blood of well-fed dogs than in the blood from other vessels. The substance obtained was unfortunately of an amorphous nature and could not be identified.

The whole problem was much altered in 1912 when Otto Folin (p. 320), a Swede who was professor of biochemistry at Harvard Medical School, introduced his new micro-methods for the determination of total nitrogen, urea, and ammonia nitrogen. Folin did much work in collaboration with Willey Glover Denis (1879–1929), who about this time was for some years a biochemist at the Massachusetts General Hospital, Boston, but who from 1925 held the chair of biochemistry at Tulane University. By animal experiment Folin and Denis showed in 1912 that when urea, glycine, or egg-albumen was introduced into a ligatured loop of intestine, they entered the blood-stream and accumulated in the muscles. An even more precise technical method was also introduced in 1912 by Donald Dexter van Slyke (1883–), who from 1914 was for nearly thirty-five years chief chemist to the hospital of the Rockefeller Institute for Medical Research. This method enabled him to determine amino-acid nitrogen directly. In his work on protein absorption van Slyke had as a co-worker Gustav Morris Meyer (1875–), who from 1909 also worked as a biochemist at the Rockefeller Institute. In 1912 and the following year van Slyke and Meyer showed that if the amino-acid alanine is injected into the intestine of a fasting dog, the amino-acid nitrogen of the blood is greatly increased. The same result is obtained after a meal of meat. They also confirmed the conclusion of Folin and Denis that the tissues absorb amino-acids very readily.

In all these experiments the conclusion that amino-acids were present in the blood was made from estimations of amino-acid nitrogen. The first actual isolation of individual amino-acids, identified as such, from the blood was made by J. J. Abel (p. 685) and his co-workers in 1913. Abel introduced the ingenious method of vividiffusion, which took advantage of the fact that amino-acids can be dialysed from the blood through a collodion membrane, but overcame the fact that only small quantities of blood could be examined at a time. Abel withdrew blood from an artery of a living animal and passed it through celloidin tubes immersed in saline. The blood then passed to a vein of the animal, so that it was not lost to the body. In this way he gave the proof that amino-acids are present as such in the blood of the living animal.

Meanwhile, much chemical research had been carried out on the composition of the animal and vegetable proteins, and it had been shown that they differed considerably in their amino-acid content. Much of this work was due to Robert Henry Aders Plimmer (1877–

1955) of London, who in 1908 discussed critically the available knowledge in the first edition of his work *The Chemical Constitution of the Proteins*. By the beginning of the twentieth century it had also been repeatedly shown that gelatine alone is not a satisfactory protein. Bischoff and Voit had demonstrated that however much of this substance is ingested, it is always completely burned, usually with some body protein in addition.

This knowledge led to the fundamental experiments of Gowland Hopkins and his co-workers (1906). Hopkins fed mice on a diet in which the sole nitrogenous constituent was casein, the protein of milk, and obtained satisfactory growth. He then substituted zein, the protein of maize, for the casein, and he found that three-quarters of the mice died within twenty days. The addition of the amino-acid tyrosine had no effect, but when tryptophane was added the period of survival was greatly increased. This important work led to the feeding experiments of Osborne and Mendel, and of McCollum (p. 612), by which it was gradually established that certain amino-acids are essential, in that they cannot be synthesized in the body; others are non-essential, in that they can be synthesized. In the same way the proteins were classified into first-class proteins, which contain the essential amino-acids in appropriate proportions; and second-class proteins, in which the proportions are not correct, or from which one or more essential amino-acids are missing.

Theories of protein metabolism. The earliest view which is of historical importance is that of Liebig, who thought that protein was little changed during digestion, and that it then entered the organism and directly replaced the protein wastage of the tissues. In 1867 Voit introduced his theory that after absorption the protein of the food became the 'circulating protein' of the tissue fluids. This 'circulating protein' was easily broken down, and it was used to replace the waste of the living 'tissue protein', which was not readily broken down. As evidence Voit instanced the case of gelatine, which is never converted into tissue protein, but which by its metabolism may serve to spare the wastage of tissue protein. Pflüger, as a result of complex experiments carried out in his laboratory, severely criticized Voit's theory in 1893 and put forward his own theory. Voit had thought that there was no chemical difference between the absorbed protein and the living tissue protein. Pflüger, on the other hand, thought that there was a difference between them. Absorbed food protein was not readily catabolized, but living protein was. Hence the absorbed protein had to be changed into living tissue protein before it could be used for energy purposes by the body. Among the points raised in criticism of Pflüger's theory was the fact that after the ingestion of protein there is a rapid increase in the nitrogen eliminated in the urine. On Pflüger's view this would imply a very rapid process of synthesis and an equally rapid breakdown of tissue protein.

In 1905 Folin put forward the theory that there are two types of protein metabolism, the tissue or endogenous metabolism, and the intermediate or exogenous metabolism. This theory was based on Folin's very numerous analyses of urine, especially on subjects who were respectively on nitrogen-rich and nitrogen-poor diets. He considered that the exogenous metabolism was very variable in quantity and produced in the urine chiefly urea and inorganic sulphates. The endogenous metabolism, on the other hand, was very constant in quantity and produced in the urine chiefly creatinine and neutral sulphur, but also uric acid and ethereal sulphates.

Three years later Rubner put forward a very speculative theory which was largely dependent on his views of the foodstuffs as producers of energy. He thought that after absorption protein was rapidly broken down into a portion containing nitrogen and another portion that was nitrogen-free. During the process of splitting heat was produced which was of no value to the body as a source of energy; it constituted the specific dynamic action of protein. The nitrogen-free part of the protein was used by the body as a source of energy.

Folin's theory was long regarded as the classical theory of protein metabolism. Within recent years it has been modified very materially. It may be noted, however, that the views of Cathcart from a few years after Folin's publication of his theory differed radically from it and were reasonably in accordance with modern views.

Edward Provan Cathcart (1877–1954) graduated at Glasgow, and then went to Buchner's bacteriology department at Munich. While there he studied under Carl Voit. He then spent a year working on chemical pathology in Berlin. After three years at the Lister Institute in London, he returned to Glasgow to take up the lectureship in chemical physiology, which he held for ten years. During this period he worked with Pavlov for five months in Petrograd (1908), so that he participated in the early experiments on conditioned reflexes. Four years later Cathcart spent a year as a research associate at the Carnegie Institution in Boston. Here he worked with F. G. Benedict, and as a result they published their classic monograph on *Muscular Work* (1913), and Cathcart developed a lasting devotion to the study of the energy needs of the body. Apart from four war years as professor of physiology at the London Hospital, the remainder of Cathcart's life was spent in the two physiology chairs at the Institute of Physiology at Glasgow University. As a member of many official councils he exerted a wide influence on research on metabolism, on nutrition, and in the problems of industrial health. Carl Voit was probably the greatest influence in Cathcart's professional life, and the time which he spent in Voit's laboratory inspired most of his future work.

Cathcart's interest in the subject of protein metabolism is possibly first seen in his paper on the composition of the urine during starvation which was published in German in the German biochemical journal in 1907. This investigation, carried out on Beauté the professional faster, was the most complete study of the fasting urine which had appeared. In this investigation he made some very interesting observations on creatine and creatinine. Both substances are normally found in muscle, but the creatinine content is very small compared with that of creatine. Creatine is normally absent from the urine of men, but it is present in the urine of children, and in that of women in certain circumstances. Creatinine, on the other hand, is normally present in the urine, and the amount is constant for the individual and independent of the protein in the food. In the case of the fasting Beauté, however, Cathcart found that the creatinine diminished gradually in the urine throughout the fast. But creatine appeared rapidly in the urine, rose during the next few days, and remained constant to the end of the fast. Folin and Benedict also noticed about the same time the appearance of creatine in the urine during fasting. Cathcart noticed that in his subject the decreased creatinine output was compensated for by the output of creatine. He also made the significant observation that, if the fasting subject was given carbohydrate, the creatine disappeared.

In 1909, as a result of further experimental work, Cathcart extended these observations. He found that the giving of carbohydrate after a fast always caused the creatine to disappear from the urine, but the giving of protein or fat did not. He thought that the appearance of creatine in the urine was due to the absence from the tissues of some substance—viz. carbohydrate—which directly or indirectly caused its retention. He was also of the opinion that the nitrogenous material which was freed by the disintegration of tissue protein was normally reutilized under the influence of carbohydrate. In his view the tissues, like any piece of machinery, were constantly disintegrating into nitrogenous and non-nitrogenous moieties. The latter was combusted, and the nitrogenous part was not excreted in the urine but was reutilized in the form of a very complex molecule containing creatine or one of its precursors. A similar theory had been advanced in 1867 by Ludimar Hermann (1838–1914), of Zurich and Königsberg, the author of a celebrated treatise on physiology, and by others. But none appreciated the part played by creatine or the influence of carbohydrate and fat. Although Cathcart never advanced his views in the form of a theory of protein metabolism, he seems to have approached closer than anyone else of that period to a dynamic conception of the body constituents.

The modern phase was introduced in 1935 with the work of Henry Borsook (1897–), professor of biochemistry at the California Institute of Technology, who, from experiments on the rate of excretion of nitrogen and sulphur, put forward a theory of a continuous intermediate metabolism in which there is a constant interchange between material from the food and material from the tissues. A different and even more valuable approach was made in the same year by Rudolf Schoenheimer (p. 320), formerly biochemist in Aschoff's institute at Freiburg, but then at Columbia University, New York. The chemist Harold Clayton Urey (1893–), also of Columbia, had discovered deuterium (H^2), a stable isotope of hydrogen, three years before, and one of his co-workers now went to Schoenheimer's laboratory. Schoenheimer and various colleagues then used isotopic amino-acids to demonstrate that nitrogen is continuously being exchanged between the various tissues, and the same changes are constantly going on in relation to the fatty acids. By 1940 a very fruitful field of research had been opened up.

Fat metabolism. In 1850 Claude Bernard showed that a solution of butter in ether rapidly developed an acid reaction when it was submitted to the action of the pancreatic juice. In 1851 the chemist Pierre Eugène Marcellin Berthelot (1827–1907) isolated the fatty acids produced during this reaction. This discovery of pancreatic lipase was criticized for many years, but it was later confirmed that this enzyme splits neutral fats in the diet to fatty acids and glycerol. It had long been known that fat is absorbed from the intestine into the lacteals, and it can be recovered from the lymph which flows in the thoracic duct. The sequence of events in the absorption of fat was clearly elucidated as a result of careful research carried out over twenty years by Immanuel Munk (1852–1903), the human and veterinary physiologist of Berlin. In 1880 he showed that if free fatty acids are fed to a dog instead of neutral fat, the lymph in the thoracic duct contains, not fatty acids as might be expected, but neutral fat. He was thus the first to prove that during absorption the free fatty acids are resynthesized to neutral fat. In 1891 Munk and a colleague showed that the same process takes place in man. They were able to obtain valuable evidence from a patient, a girl who had elephantiasis of one leg with a fistulous opening in a dilated lymphatic vessel below the knee. During fasting this fistula discharged clear lymph, but after a meal containing fat it discharged a milky fluid which was indistinguishable from chyle.

Much work on the transport of fat in the blood was done by Walter Ray Bloor (1877–), the biochemist who worked and taught at Harvard, the University of California, and Rochester University. Bloor showed in 1914 that after a dog is fed on fat there is a gradual rise in the fatty acid content of the blood, reaching a maximum six hours after the meal. On the other hand, if large quantities of fat were injected direct into the blood-stream, the excess disappeared within five minutes. Bloor and his co-workers also showed (1922) that the fat in the faeces is not the same fat as is ingested. This confirmed and extended an observation which had been made by Bischoff and Voit in 1860.

Until 1904 very little was known about the manner in which the body effected the oxidation of fatty acids. In that year Franz Knoop (1875–1946), later of Tübingen, published the first statement of his classical theory. Knoop investigated the fate of the phenyl derivatives of the lower fatty acids in the body. He administered to dogs the sodium salts of benzoic, phenylacetic, phenylpropionic, phenyl-butyric, and phenylvaleric acids. The chemical formulae for the last four of these acids can be obtained from that of benzoic acid by adding successively a CH_2 group to the preceding formula. Knoop found that whenever any of these acids was fed to an animal, either hippuric acid or phenaceturic acid appeared in the urine. Hippuric acid is benzoic acid combined with glycine, and phenaceturic acid is phenylacetic acid combined with glycine. When the side-chain of the acid administered had an odd number of carbon atoms hippuric acid always appeared in the urine; whereas if the acid administered had an even number of carbon atoms phenaceturic acid always appeared as the end-product. These results led Knoop to formulate his theory of β-oxidation. According to this theory in the oxidation of fats the carbon atom in the β-position is oxidized and two carbon atoms are dropped from the chain. This theory was confirmed and extended by the important work of Dakin (p. 320). The whole pro-blem has again been extended in recent years by the work of Schoen-heimer and his School.

The metabolism of carbohydrates has been briefly discussed elsewhere in this book.

The interconversion of the proximate principles. The conversion of carbohydrate into fat was first proved indirectly in 1852 by the classical feeding experiments of the agriculturalist Sir John Bennet Lawes (1814–1900), lord of the manor of Rothamsted and founder of the famous research station, and his co-worker, the agricultural chemist Sir Joseph Henry Gilbert (1817–1901) who had been a pupil of Liebig. Two pigs were taken from the same litter. One was killed and its carcass was completely analysed. The other was then fed for a period on weighed quantities of protein, fat, and carbohydrate. It was then also killed and completely analysed. Lawes and Gilbert thus showed that over one-third of the fat synthesized must have been derived from carbohydrate. In 1881 Voit was unable to give a definite proof of the conversion of carbohydrate into fat. But this proof was given by Emmerich Meissl (1855-1905) and Friedrich Strohmer in 1883 as a result of a very careful experiment on a pig. At later dates this conversion was shown by Erwin Voit, Rubner, and others to apply to other animals.

The conversion of protein into carbohydrate was investigated in 1862 by Pettenkofer and Voit. After a meal containing abundant meat they found that a part of the carbon of the protein metabolized was retained in the body. They concluded that this indicated a conversion of protein into fat. The question is, however, not simple. Important experiments were carried out by Lusk and his colleagues in 1912, and from these they concluded that the carbon was retained either in the form of glucose or of glycogen. It is now known that the amino-acids are converted to glucose only after their deamination in the liver. The conclusion of Pettenkofer and Voit referred to above that protein could be converted into fat was challenged by Pflüger, and the problem was accordingly reinvestigated by Max Cremer (1865-1935) who had been a pupil and assistant of Voit. Cremer concluded that a cat which had been starved and then fed on lean meat had stored a portion of the carbon as fat. Lusk and his associates now tested (1922) the theory that, if protein is ingested in excess, the deaminized residues of the amino-acids are converted into glycogen, and when glycogen saturation is reached, fat is formed instead. Lusk concluded that this is what actually takes place.

Normal diets. The first statement regarding the optimum consumption of the proximate principles to be made after the establishment of the study of nutrition on a scientific basis was that of Voit (1881). His standard daily diet, which is still quoted in textbooks of physiology, consisted of protein, 118 gm.; fat, 56 gm.; carbohydrate, 500 gm. This diet contains 2,976 Calories. It should be noted that this diet was advocated before the time when accurate figures for the energy requirements of the human subject were available. They were in fact averages of the figures actually obtained by weighing the food consumed by manual workers. Let us consider first the total energy value of the diet. It was accepted that men doing heavy manual work required a diet containing a much higher energy content. Charles Dayton Woods (1856-1925) and E. R. Mansfield published in 1904 an important study of the diet of the lumbermen

of Maine, and they showed that the average daily diet per man produced 8,083 Calories. This appears to be about the maximum
calorie intake for men engaged in a day-to-day occupation. In 1903
Rubner, using municipal statistics of gross consumption, gave the
average values of diets in the case of four European cities. The
lowest (Königsberg) was 2,394, and the highest (Munich) was
3,014 Calories. In 1903 Atwater reported on the diets of farmers in
the United States, Mexico, and Italy. The average values ranged
from 3,410 to 3,785 Calories. During the First World War much
work was done on this subject. Cathcart and Boyd Orr found that
the average daily expenditure of a recruit was 3,574 Calories in the
British Army. At the outbreak of war the ration of a cavalryman in
the United States Army contained over 8,000 Calories; much of
this was thrown away. John Raymond Murlin (1874–), a colleague
of Lusk who was in charge of such investigations for the United
States Army, did much work on this subject and showed that at a later
stage of the war the average ration per man contained 3,633 Calories.
Atwater and Lusk independently drew up tables of man values,
showing the energy requirements for males and females at different
ages in terms of those of an adult male of average height and weight
considered as unity. More recently it has been customary to add a
quota to allow for waste in cooking and consuming the foodstuffs, and
the daily energy content has therefore been taken as 3,400 Calories.

Voit's figure for protein has been subject to much more serious
criticism. This was based partly on the supposed injurious effect on
the kidneys of excessive protein ingestion, and partly on the actual
protein intake of certain races in various parts of the world. The
strongest criticism came from Russell Henry Chittenden (1856–
1943), who was for forty years professor of physiological chemistry
at Yale University. Chittenden felt that the strain on the body would
be less if the protein requirement could be reduced. He therefore
began an experiment on himself in November 1902. He reduced his
protein intake until in a short time he had cut out breakfast (apart
from a small cup of coffee), and had only a light lunch before a
moderate dinner in the evening. This diet was kept up until 27 June
1904. From careful analysis of the foodstuffs and the urine Chittenden showed that he was maintaining nitrogen equilibrium with a

protein intake of between 30 and 35 gm. of protein per day. In addition he had got rid of various mild rheumatic symptoms. He then carried out similar experiments on his professional colleagues, on soldiers, and on university athletes. To the soldiers he gave a diet containing 50 gm. of protein and 2,500 Calories. He claimed that on this low protein intake all of them maintained their physical efficiency. Chittenden published his results in great detail in 1905 in his much-discussed book, *Physiological Economy in Nutrition.*

These results were criticized among others by Sir James Crichton-Browne (1840–1938) in his book *Parcimony in Nutrition* (1909). Crichton-Browne was an alienist with wide interests, and incidentally it was he who, while he was medical superintendent of the West Riding Asylum, had encouraged Ferrier to carry out his early experiments on cerebral localization (p. 257). Crichton-Browne and others criticized Chittenden's protein allowance mainly on the grounds that in prisons in Great Britain such a protein intake had led to serious malnutrition. In 1912 David McCay (1873–1948) published his work *The Protein Element in Nutrition*, in which he surveyed the diets of the Indian races and showed that those that consumed an ample allowance of animal protein had a good physique. By that time the experiments of Hopkins (p. 598) and others were bearing fruit, and proteins were becoming divided according to their biological value. It was increasingly acknowledged that it was not so much the total protein as the quantities of first-class proteins which mattered. Nevertheless, a few scientists continued to recommend low-protein diets. Among these were Mikkel Hindhede (1862–1945), a Danish physiologist who from 1912 carried out experimental work on this subject for fifteen years.

During the first quarter of the present century much work was done on the theoretical food requirements of the human body, based on experiments involving direct and indirect calorimetry. The science of dietetics was founded on these requirements and on detailed chemical examination of foodstuffs. Among those who have more recently added materially to our knowledge of the composition of foods is Robert Alexander McCance (1898–) of Cambridge and his co-workers. Nevertheless, for some time there was much emphasis on the quantitative aspect of nutrition, and a tendency to ignore the fact that the energy value of a foodstuff is not an exact index of its nutritive value. The discovery of the vitamins also concentrated research on vitamin-containing food. Yet the fact is that in any country at any time people eat primarily to satisfy their hunger, choosing their diet according to taste and what they can afford. It was desirable that dietary studies should be made of the normal diet actually used.

In 1930 Cathcart and his colleagues Mrs. A. M. T. Murray and Margaret Shanks began a series of three important field investigations to ascertain what proportion of the actual foodstuffs consumed by families in this country were made up respectively of the proximate principles; the average total daily calorie intake of individual diets; and the actual kinds of foodstuffs purchased in order to provide these total calories and these amounts of proteins, fats, and carbohydrates. As most of the data which had previously been used were derived from the amounts of food consumed in foreign cities (see p. 605), these investigations broke new ground. During the First World War Randal Mark Kerr M'Donnell (1878–1932), then Viscount Dunluce but later the 12th Earl of Antrim, in collaboration with Major Greenwood (p. 736) had published in 1918 an inquiry of more limited scope in which the population investigated had consisted mainly of munition workers. They had shown that in this population the fat content of the diet was high as compared with the commonly accepted standard.

The first report (1931) of Cathcart and his collaborators related to their investigation of the diets of eighty-six families in St. Andrews, representing a vertical section of the population and including families from all income levels. The authors modified slightly the 'man values' of Atwater and of Lusk. Their main conclusion was that in St. Andrews the consumption of protein and carbohydrate was below, but that of fat much above, the standard values previously widely accepted. In their second report (1932) they carried out a similar investigation in Cardiff and Reading, but in both these cases the inquiries were carried out on horizontal samples of working-class families in these two cities. They again found that the consumption of fat was above the accepted level. Analysis of the average calorie values of the diets consumed showed that 10 per cent. of the calorie intake was derived from proteins, 32 per cent. from fat, and

58 per cent. from carbohydrate. The average daily calorie intake for an adult male was 3,000 Calories. A rather surprising result was that with a rising income the increased intake of fat was greater than that of proteins.

These two studies had been concerned with the content of the diets in terms of proteins, fats, and carbohydrates. Cathcart and his collaborators now used their data obtained in all their investigations to throw light on the actual foods which were purchased by house-wives in St. Andrews, Cardiff, and Reading. They found that in all sections of their populations the amount of tinned or prepared food which was bought was not large, and that in the case of fresh food the waste during preparation and cooking was undoubtedly high. In all three communities the average proportion of the diet repre-sented by protein was surprisingly constant, being 11·03 per cent. in St. Andrews, 10·16 per cent. in Cardiff, and 10·32 per cent. in Reading. On the other hand, there was a surprising variation in the type of food consumed to give these proportions. While 78 per cent. of the people of St. Andrews ate sausages, only 38 per cent. of the Cardiff families ate them. There were very wide variations in the intake of other foodstuffs such as butter, margarine, and oatmeal. A special investigation was made into the calorie-content of the diets of 109 women students in Glasgow, who were found to have an average daily intake of 2,035 Calories. As a result Cathcart suggested that the accepted intake of 3,000 to 3,400 Calories was probably excessive.

In 1920 a report of the Ministry of National Service, which had dealt with the call-up of men for the fighting forces during the First World War, disclosed the fact that a surprisingly large proportion of the young men were unfit for active service because of physical defects. It was some time before the full implications of the detailed results began to influence research, and even longer before the public conscience was fully awakened. Various investigations suggested that poor physique and certain diseases were the direct result of malnutrition. Over a long period McCarrison (p. 527) had been investigating the relation between nutrition and diet in India. By feeding experiments he showed that rats fed on the diet of a certain tribe developed the same types of diseases as were incident to that tribe. A similar investigation in African tribes in Kenya was carried out by (Sir) John Boyd Orr (later, Baron Boyd Orr) (1889–). He showed that a diet rich in carbohydrates but poor in animal proteins, minerals, and vitamins produced bone deformation and pulmonary and intestinal diseases. In 1927 he experimented with additional milk to 1,500 children in seven Scottish towns, and found that there was an increased rate of growth and an improvement in health and vigour.

This important preliminary work led to Lord Boyd Orr's best-known investigation in this field. This was the first attempt to obtain a conspectus of the food position of the country showing the relationship between income, food, and health. The results were published in his *Food Health and Income* (1936), which was produced very cheaply and reached the wide circle of readers for whom it was intended. In this work the population was divided into six income groups, and in discussing the results an optimum standard of food requirements was adopted. It was shown that the diet of the poorest group, comprising over 4 million persons, was on this standard deficient in every constituent. Complete adequacy of diet was not reached until the fourth of the six groups. Detailed examinations were made of the consumption of the main articles of diet in the different groups. It was also shown that in children the improvement in the diet in the lower income groups was accompanied by improvement in health and increased rate of growth. This work had economic and political implications, and it had important applications during the Second World War.

An investigation on a more limited scale was carried out in the early thirties by George Cuthbert Mura M'Gonigle (1888–1939), the medical officer of health of Stockton-on-Tees. The technical aspects were published in 1933, and in 1936 M'Gonigle incorporated them in his well-known book, *Poverty and the Public Health*. During the period after the First World War local authorities had been active in slum clearance and in the rehousing of the inhabitants on new housing estates. In Stockton-on-Tees a half of a large slum area had been cleared and the population rehoused, but it was found that the death-rates and the incidence of certain diseases were higher in the rehoused population than in the population of that part of the slum area which had not been rehoused. As a result of a very detailed investigation M'Gonigle showed that many of these conditions in the rehoused population were due to various degrees of ill-nutrition. He also showed that this was produced by the fact that in their new houses the necessary expenses had increased to such an extent that the inhabitants could not afford the minimum amount of food of the kind which would prevent this malnutrition.

(e) Vitamins and Deficiency Diseases

During the period when Voit and his colleagues were laying the foundations of the science of nutrition it was thought that it would always be possible to construct an artificial diet which would satisfy the needs of the body, and that, provided that the constituents were present in their proper proportions, the problem was purely quantitative. The first to show that all natural diets contained unknown factors was Nicolai Ivanovitch Lunin (1853–1937) working at Basle (1881). He fed mice on an artificial mixture of the constituents of milk (the proteins, fats, carbohydrates, and salts) and found that the mice did not survive. He concluded that a natural food such as milk must also contain small quantities of unknown substances which are necessary for life. This conclusion happened to be purely incidental to the main purpose of Lunin's paper, and its significance was completely missed.

From the earliest times there had been prevalent in the Far East a disease which was characterized by an ascending weakness in the legs with tenderness of the muscles, followed by loss of power in the muscles of the hands and arms. The disease, essentially an acute peripheral neuritis, was later known as beri-beri. The first description of it in Western literature was given by Jacob De Bondt [Bontius] (1598–1631) in his book on Indian medicine (*De medicina Indorum*, 1642). In 1627 Bontius became inspector of surgery at Batavia in the Dutch East Indies, and his account of the diseases which he encountered was seen through the press by his brother after his death. A few years later the disease was again described in his *Observationes medicae* (1652) by Nicolaas Tulp (1593–1674) of Amsterdam. Tulp has a more popular claim to fame in that he is the anatomical demonstrator in Rembrandt's picture *The Anatomy Lesson*. More modern descriptions of the disease brought out the fact that in addition to the neuritic form there occur also the cardiac form, and the 'wet' form in which oedema of the body cavities is common. The first modern account was published by John Grant Malcolmson (?–1844) of Madras in 1835.

About 1880 beri-beri was very prevalent in Japan, and in 1881 Erwin von Baelz (1849–1913) published a description of the Tokyo outbreak. Between 1882 and 1885 Baron Kanehiro Takaki (1849–1915), later director general of the medical department of the Japanese Navy, practically eradicated the disease from that fleet by supplementing the rice diet with fish, vegetables, and meat. Between 1893 and 1897 Christiaan Eijkman (1858–1930), the director of the research laboratory at Batavia, showed that a peripheral neuritis of fowls which closely resembled beri-beri could be produced by feeding them exclusively on a diet of polished rice. Eijkman interpreted these facts in a manner which we now know to be erroneous. His successor Gerrit Grijns (1865–1944) continued with this work, and in 1901 he suggested that both beri-beri and avian polyneuritis were due to absence from the diet of some factor which was present in rice polishings, or in other words that they were 'deficiency diseases'. This suggestion did not immediately bear fruit. But in 1905 William Fletcher (1874–1938) began a feeding experiment in the lunatic asylum at Kuala Lumpur in the Federated Malay States. Fletcher's results, published in 1907, showed clearly that nearly a quarter of those patients who received only polished rice developed beri-beri (half of whom died from the disease), while only two out of 123 patients who received solely unpolished rice developed the disease. Shortly afterwards similar definite results were obtained by Henry Fraser (1873–1930) and (Sir) Ambrose Thomas Stanton (1875–1938) in feeding experiments on healthy labourers in a railroad labour camp in Malaya; their results were published in 1909.

The fact that this disease, and some others such as scurvy and rickets, are really deficiency diseases, due to the absence from the diet of substances which had not yet been isolated, was forcibly stated in 1906 by (Sir) Frederick Gowland Hopkins (1861–1947), and in 1912 he published his important experiments. He fed rats on an artificial mixture of food substances which was theoretically sufficient to maintain growth. When these substances were provided in their crude form growth was indeed maintained. If, however, the substances were provided in a very pure form growth ceased, but continued again normally if a minute amount of milk, in weight less than one twenty-fifth of that of the whole diet, was added to the daily food. In each case the artificial diet contained sufficient calories to maintain growth, and the calories in the milk could not have had any direct effect on nutrition. Eijkman and Gowland Hopkins were jointly awarded a Nobel Prize in 1929.

In 1911 Casimir Funk (1884–), working at the Lister Institute in London, endeavoured to isolate, from the material discarded in the steam-powered mills for polishing rice, a substance which would cure artificial beri-beri in pigeons. He succeeded in obtaining a concentrate which cured in doses as small as 20 milligrammes. It later transpired that Funk's product was not the active constituent in its purest form, but this fact does not detract from his pioneer work. In 1912 Funk discussed the causation of beri-beri, scurvy, and rickets as 'deficiency diseases'. He suggested that these 'accessory food factors', absence of even a minute quantity of which from the diet caused these diseases, should be called 'vitamines' (*vita* implying that they were necessary for life, and *amine* their supposed chemical composition). It was later shown that they were not amines, but the name gradually became accepted, the final e being dropped to avoid the unjustified chemical assumption. This suggestion was made in 1920 by (Sir) Jack Cecil Drummond (1891–1952), who in ways which are outside the scope of this book contributed much to biochemical research, especially on the nature of the vitamins, and who played an important role during the Second World War as the scientific adviser to the Minister of Food.

In 1913 Thomas Burr Osborne (1859–1929) and Lafayette Benedict Mendel (1872–1935), working at Newhaven, Connecticut, showed that butter contains a growth-promoting factor necessary for the development of rats. This was the factor soon to be known as fat-soluble vitamin A. Their paper was received for publication in the same month (June 1913) as another paper by Elmer Verner McCollum (1879–) and Marguerite Davis of Wisconsin, who showed that a similar factor was also abundant in egg-yolk and cod-liver oil. But McCollum and Davis also showed that cow's milk contained (in addition to the fat-soluble growth-promoting factor found in butter), another growth-promoting factor, soluble in water, that was later found widely distributed in foods such as in wheat embryo, the polishings of rice, and yeast. This second factor was soon called vitamin B. Hence, for some years after 1913 it was assumed that the only examples of such accessory food factors were the fat-soluble vitamin A, the water-soluble vitamin B, and the supposed anti-scurvy substance, postulated in the previous year by Funk, and later known as vitamin C. The properties of the anti-neuritic factor which prevented beri-beri were apparently identical with those of vitamin B, and it was assumed that these vitamins were the same substance.

During the First World War the bony deformities resulting from rickets attracted much attention. This disease appears to have existed from quite ancient times, but recognition of the signs as constituting a clinical entity dates only from the mid-seventeenth century. In England it was popularly called 'rickets', and medical writers soon attempted to derive the word from the Greek 'rachites'. There is no doubt that the first medical description of the disease was given by Daniel Whistler (1619–84) in his thesis for the doctorate of medicine at Leyden in 1645. This thesis was published at Leyden in the same year with the title *De morbo puerili Anglorum, quem patrio idiomate indigenae vocant* The Rickets ('On the disease of English children which in their language is called The Rickets'). Whistler, born in Essex, had graduated in Arts at Oxford before he went to Leyden. During the First Dutch War (1652–54) he organized the medical and hospital treatment of the wounded and sick, and his place in the annals of naval medicine is assured. He finally became President of the Royal College of Physicians. His clinical description of rickets is clear and concise, though it probably did not depend greatly on his own observations. Whistler's suggestion of a scientific name for the disease was 'Paedosplanchnosteocaces'.

There was one other brief account of rickets in medical literature —by the Dutchman Arnold Boot (1600?–1653?) who practised in London and Paris—before 1650, when Francis Glisson (p. 123) published his *De rachitide sive morbo puerili, qui vulgo The Rickets dicitur* ('On rachitis or the disease of children which is vulgarly called The Rickets'). This work was based on the observations of a small circle of Glisson's friends, two of whom were to collaborate with him in writing up the material. Having completed his own section Glisson then wrote the sections allocated to his two collaborators, and the book is generally regarded as Glisson's own work. He obviously had first-hand experience of the disease, and though his pathology is dominated by the humoral doctrine, his book must be regarded as the best, though not the first, of the early treatises on rickets. In 1674 Mayow (p. 136) had a section on this disease in his *Tractatus quinque*. In this he made some advances in pathology, but the clinical account is of no importance.

By the middle of the nineteenth century rickets was common in many countries. In treatment cod-liver oil had been used in England in a very few cases as early as 1782, and by the early nineteenth century it was commonly used for this purpose in France, Germany, and Holland. Trousseau (p. 282) thought very highly of it by the middle of the century. By the early years of the twentieth century belief in the virtues of cod-liver oil was unfortunately much less strong. Meanwhile in Glasgow and the industrial areas of the west of Scotland rickets was very common, and the resultant bony deformities led to the pioneer surgical work of Macewen on the bones of the extremities (p. 369). But surgery cannot correct a deformed pelvis, and girls with this deformity often had serious trouble during child-birth in later life.

Around the year 1900 it was commonly held that rickets was a chronic infectious disease, though no organism had been discovered. About that time the theory was put forward that it was due to living conditions which resulted in lack of fresh air, sunlight, and exercise. This theory was due among others to David Paul von Hansemann (1858–1920) of Berlin. The value of sunlight in prevention had been emphasized in 1890 by Theobald Adrian Palm (1848?–1928), but in subsequent work by others this point was not sufficiently understood. In Glasgow active research was carried out during the First World War by Leonard Findlay (1878–1947) and his colleagues, who investigated the importance of social and economic factors, and paid due regard to the virtues of sunlight.

Meanwhile (Sir) Edward Mellanby (1884–1955) of Sheffield had been experimenting with puppies, and by 1918 he was able to produce rickets in them by feeding with diets deficient in a factor found in some animal fats. Mellanby's full report was published in 1921. From these experiments it became clear that rickets was a deficiency disease. Mellanby at that time believed that it was due to lack of fat-soluble vitamin A.

The question was further complicated by the fact that, whatever might be the effect of a suitable diet, the effect of sunlight had been clarified. In 1919 Kurt Huldschinsky (1883–?) of Berlin published his observations which showed that rickets could be cured by the application of artificial sunlight. In order to elucidate the conflicting possibilities (Dame) Harriette Chick (1875–) led a team of workers to Vienna in 1919, and their clinical investigations in that city were continued until 1922. At that period the population of Vienna was suffering severely from the results of under-nutrition during the war, and gross forms of rickets were common. The final report of this team supported both the deficiency theory and the theory that rickets was due to lack of sunlight. They showed that the disease could be cured by sunlight (natural or artificial) or by cod-liver oil, and that any therapeutic procedure adopted must, to be successful, include one of these measures. By 1930 the extensive employment of cod-liver oil and artificial sunlight in the prevention and cure of rickets in the United Kingdom had proved the correctness of these views.

We deal later with the steps by which in 1922 and the few following years it was established that what had been regarded as vitamin A consisted of two separate factors. For one of these the term vitamin A was retained; the other, the antirachitic factor, was termed vitamin D.

Further investigation proved complicated, for the vitamin D itself was found to be a mixture, and over twenty members of the group have now been studied. Thus, vitamin D_1, was soon seen to be a mixture of no importance. Vitamin D_2, the first of the group to be fully investigated, was shown to be a chemical substance and was named calciferol. It is formed by the action of sunlight or ultra-violet light on ergosterol, a chemical substance found only in plants, especially the fungi. Calciferol was first isolated in a pure state independently by German scientists and by Robert Benedict Bourdillon (1889–) and his co-workers in 1931; it has been much used in extremely minute quantities in the treatment and prevention of rickets. Vitamin D_3 is also formed by irradiation, but in this case the process takes place in the animal body. The provitamin (7-dihydrocholesterol) is normally found in the skin, having been formed in the small intestine from the cholesterol derived from the food. Most of the vitamin D_3 required by the body is thus manufactured in the skin, though some foodstuffs contain it already formed. Convincing proof was thus given of the fundamental role which sunlight plays in the prevention of rickets.

During the last thirty years much detailed work has been done on the mode of action of vitamins D_2 and D_3. It has been shown that animals obtain their supplies of vitamin D in two ways, namely, by eating the flesh, containing vitamin D, of other animals, or, more commonly, by the action of sunlight in or on their own skins. In man also the activation of the provitamin appears to occur on the skin. In 1925 Cowell (p. 563) increased the vitamin D content of food by irradiation, and this method has had important commercial applications.

We now turn to the steps which led to the division of the factor originally known as vitamin A. As previously stated, this factor was described in 1913 as a result of experiments which showed that its presence had an effect on growth. In 1917 McCollum and Nina Simmonds (1893–) did further work on this factor, named it fat-soluble A, and showed that its deficiency produced not only retardation of growth but also conjunctivitis and a series of changes in the eyes, collectively known as xerophthalmia, due to progressive keratinization of the cornea. Both these series of results had been described previously, though their significance was not then appreciated. For example, in 1909 Wilhelm Otto Stepp (1882–), a German biochemist, had found that there was some unrecognized factor in fats which was necessary for growth; the addition of pure fats to a fat-free diet did not remedy the deficiency. In the same year Paul Knapp (1874–1954) had found that conjunctivitis resulted when rats were fed on some deficient diets. In 1920 Otto Rosenheim (1871–1955) and Drummond (p. 612) showed that the amount of the pigment carotene contained in plants was directly proportional to their vitamin A activity. This work was confirmed and extended by Katharine Hope Coward (1885–), who later did important work on the standardization of the vitamins.

When Mellanby described the action of the anti-rachitic vitamin he supposed it to be fat-soluble A. But in 1922 E. Margaret Hume of the Lister Institute fed rats on fat-deficient diets and after diseased conditions had appeared she treated the affected rats with ultra-violet rays from a quartz-mercury vapour lamp. She found that those animals suffering from rickets were cured, whereas those with deficient growth or eye-conditions were unaffected. About the same time similar experiments were being carried out by Harry Goldblatt (1891–) and Katharine Marjorie Soames. In 1923 Goldblatt and Sylvester Solomon Zilva found that spinach promoted growth but did not prevent rickets, and that the growth-promoting and the anti-rachitic functions of certain substances, especially cod-liver oil, were destroyed at different rates by varying degrees of heat and oxidation. Two years later Simeon Burt Wolbach (p. 451) and Percy Rogers Howe (1864–1950) demonstrated that the typical changes produced by deficiency of fat-soluble vitamin A consisted in the replacement of various epithelial cells in the body by primitive keratinizing epithelium, and that these changes gave rise to a lowering of the local resistance to infection. In 1926 Mellanby showed in puppies that the protective value of a diet against rickets was not related to its protective value against natural infection. Two years later, the anti-rachitic factor having been termed vitamin D, Mellanby and Harry Norman Green (1902–) studied the anti-infective effects of vitamin A and named it the anti-infective vitamin. The chemical structure of vitamin A was worked out partly by the Swiss, Paul Karrer (1889–), and the pure vitamin in a crystalline form was obtained by Harry Nicholls Holmes (1879–) and Ruth Elizabeth Corbet (1910–) in 1937. The synthesis of vitamin A was effected during the war by workers in several countries; in Great Britain it was synthesized by Sir Ian M. Heilbron (1886–1959) and his co-workers.

The confirmation the deficiency of vitamin A causes various conditions in the human subject, especially diseases of the eyes and skin, was due to many clinical observers. It was also shown, especially by the work of Thomas Moore of Cambridge and his collaborators, in 1931 and the following years, that vitamin A is stored mainly in the liver. One of the earliest symptoms of vitamin A deficiency is transient night-blindness, and the recommendation of liver by the ancient Egyptians and Greeks for the treatment of this condition was thus fully justified by modern discoveries.

Researches on another vitamin, E, are especially associated with the name of Herbert McLean Evans (p. 547) of the University of California. In 1920 it had been shown that rats reared on whole milk grew well but were usually sterile, and the absence of a hypothetical factor essential for reproduction was suggested. In 1922 Evans and Katherine Scott Bishop (1889–) showed that the missing factor, vitamin E, was especially abundant in green leaves and in wheat germ. They then showed that it was fat-soluble, but not identical with any known vitamin. In 1928 Evans and his co-worker, George Oswald Burr (1896–), who later wrote with Evans a monograph on vitamin E, found that young rats suckled by mothers deficient in vitamin E became paralysed, and it was soon shown that some species of animals, if deprived of vitamin E, develop a peculiar enlargement of certain muscles, accompanied by a marked weakness in them. This condition was very similar to the rare disease progressive muscular atropy in man. In 1936 Evans and his co-workers isolated vitamin E from wheat germ. It proved to be a type of alcohol which they named tocopherol. Vitamin E is important in relation to certain diseases of the muscles in man. It also plays a significant role in the problem of sterility, and it has been suggested that the fall in the birth-rate is largely accounted for by the general use of white flour.

The early history of scurvy has already been briefly dealt with. The modern investigation of this condition was introduced accidentally in 1907 by the Scandinavian Axel Holst (1861–1931) and Theodor Christian Brun Frölich (1870–1947). They attempted to produce beri-beri in guinea-pigs by restricting their diets, but the test animals developed scurvy and not beri-beri. After Funk postulated the existence of a vitamin (C) in 1912, many attempts were made to isolate it. Among the most successful of those who worked on this problem was Zilva (p. 617) and his co-workers, and by 1928 they had succeeded in obtaining a powerful concentrated solution, but not the pure vitamin. In the same year Albert Szent-Györgyi (1893–), studying cellular oxidization in Cambridge, isolated from the adrenals a substance which he called hexuronic acid. He did not know that it was really the water-soluble vitamin C. In 1932 W. A. Waugh and Charles Glen King (1896–) isolated vitamin C from lemons and proved it identical with hexuronic acid. In 1933 its name was changed to ascorbic acid, and in 1934 it was synthesized by Walter Norman Haworth (1883–1949), professor of chemistry at Birmingham, who shared a Nobel Prize with Karrer in 1937.

The inter-war years also saw a determined attack on the vitamin B complex. But it was not until 1926 that the belief, generally held since 1913, that this vitamin was a single substance was disproved. In that year Morris Isidore Smith (1887–1951) and E. G. Hendrick in the United States showed that vitamin B consisted of two distinct substances, one of which (the antineuritic factor) was destroyed by heat, whereas the other (the growth-promoting factor) was thermostable. While various names were suggested for these components, in Great Britain the antineuritic factor came to be called vitamin B_1, and growth-promoting factor vitamin B_2.

Vitamin B_1 was isolated in crystalline form from rice polishings by Barend Coenraad Petrus Jansen (1884–) and Willem Frederick Donath (1889–) in 1926. It was isolated from yeast in 1932 by Windaus and his colleagues in Germany. Its chemical structure was worked out by Windaus and by Robert Runnels Williams (1886–) in the United States in 1934 and the following years. Because of the relationship of this vitamin to beri-beri, the name aneurine was proposed for it by Jansen. In the United States the name thiamin was adopted. In 1929 and the following years Sir Rudolph Albert Peters of Oxford worked out the role of aneurine in carbohydrate metabolism (the tricarboxylic acid cycle), and in 1938 Beatrice Mintz (1909–) and Abderhalden (p. 596) independently showed that aneurine checks the formation of cholinesterase at nerve endings. For his work on vitamins Windaus received a Nobel Prize in 1928.

Though vitamin B_1 has not been further simplified, attention was meanwhile directed to vitamin B_2, with the result that it was shown to be a complex. The disease pellagra, characterized by a peculiar exfoliative dermatitis, severe stomatitis and gastro-intestinal disorders, and neurological symptoms often accompanied by insanity, was prevalent in many parts of Europe and America. In the United States Joseph Goldberger (1874–1929) and his co-workers showed in 1914 and later years that pellagra is a deficiency disease. By feeding experiments on human subjects Goldberger showed by 1926 that one of the constituents of the vitamin B complex prevented the serious symptoms of pellagra. In 1937 and the following year Conrad Arnold Elvehjem (1901–) and his colleagues reported that they had cured a similar disease, black tongue, in dogs by nicotinic acid which they had isolated from liver concentrates. Nicotinic acid (niacin) had been known for seventy years, but its pharmacological action had not been suspected. Elvehjem now suggested its use in pellagra, and with his colleagues he published the first report on cases so treated. In 1938 Otto Heinrich Warburg (1883–) published his first reports on the role of the amide of nicotinic acid as a cellular enzyme. But the use of these substances in the treatment of pellagra demonstrated that this is a multiple-deficiency disease which cannot be cured by the administration of this vitamin alone.

From early in the present century atypical outbreaks of what was regarded as pellagra had been described. In 1911 Hugh Stannus Stannus (1877–1957) noted in Nyasaland cases in which the stomatitis did not conform to the usual type, and in which lesions of the genitals were common. Seven years later (Sir) Henry Harold Scott (1874–1956), who subsequently wrote a standard history of tropical diseases, described in Jamaica cases in which these atypical features were accompanied by a peculiar 'central neuritis'. In 1925 Goldberger produced these symptoms experimentally by feeding experiments on human subjects in United States prisons. Within the next ten years other features of what was now regarded as a new syndrome were described.

Meanwhile in Berlin Warburg and Walter Christian had isolated from yeast in 1932 a new yellow enzyme, which they separated into two components, a protein and a pigment. Neither appeared to be active alone. Richard Kuhn (1900–) at Heidelberg then isolated various pigments of this nature from many foodstuffs. That which was shown to produce the syndrome in the human subject was named riboflavin. It is part of the B_2 complex, and it was synthesized by

Kuhn in 1934-5. Kuhn was awarded a Nobel Prize for Chemistry in 1938.

Probably the most important aspect of recent work on the vitamin B_2 complex is that concerned with vitamin B_{12}. In 1849 Addison (p. 284) described a fatal anaemia, later known as pernicious anaemia which produces a typical blood picture. George Hoyt Whipple (1878-) of Rochester, Minnesota, showed in 1925 that raw liver has a marked curative effect on artificially produced 'simple' anaemias in dogs. In 1926 George Richards Minot (1885-1950) and William Parry Murphy (1892-) of Boston, Mass., found that liver cured patients suffering from pernicious anaemia. Then William Bosworth Castle (1897-) of Harvard found in 1929 that meat pre-digested with an artificial gastric juice had no affect on such patients, whereas if normal gastric juice was used the results were good. Hence he thought that the active substances which prevents and cures pernicious anaemia is formed by the combination of an unknown 'intrinsic factor' in gastric juice with an 'extrinsic factor' in the meat; it is stored mainly in the liver. In 1947-8 Mary Shaw Shorb (1907-) introduced the biological assay of liver extracts. In 1948 the anti-pernicious anaemia factor was isolated in Great Britain from liver by Ernest Lester Smith (1904-), and independently in the United States by Edward Lawrence Rickes (1912-) from a mould. It is now produced in the manufacture of streptomycin. This factor was found to be part of the B_2 complex, and was named B_{12}. Its molecule contains both cobalt and a cyanide group, and it is therefore also called cyanocobalamine. It is very effective in the treatment of pernicious anaemia and of its nervous complications.

In 1929 Carl Peter Henrik Dam (1895-) of Copenhagen found that chicks fed on a fat poor diet developed subcutaneous haemorrhages, and that there was an increase in the coagulation time of their blood. Dam, William Douglas McFarlane (1900-) and others established the fact that the condition was due to a deficiency of a fat-soluble vitamin, which Dam named vitamin K, the coagulation vitamin. Workers in different countries, including Dam, Edward A. Doisy (p. 551) in the United States, and Herman James Almquist (1903-), isolated vitamin K in pure form about 1939, and in that year it was synthesized by Louis Frederick Fieser (1899-). In 1940

Doisy and his colleagues isolated vitamin K_2, which has a slightly different composition but produces similar results. The action of vitamin K in accelerating clotting is complex. It is used in the treatment of certain liver diseases marked by a reduced prothrombin content of the blood, and also in haemorrhagic diseases of the new-born. For their work on vitamin K Dam and Doisy shared a Nobel Prize in 1943.

In 1936 Szent-Györgyi postulated the existence of another vitamin, P, deficiency of which led to increased fragility of the capillaries. Despite much work by himself, Zilva (p. 617), Alfred Louis Bacharach (1891–), Cecil Z. Wawra. John Leyden Webb (1914–), and others, the identity and nature of this vitamin has not yet been clearly established.

In addition to the Nobel Prize already mentioned in this section, Warburg was awarded a prize in 1931, and Whipple, Minot, and Murphy received a prize in 1934 for their discoveries relating to the treatment of anaemias with liver. In 1937 Szent-Györgyi received the Nobel Prize for Medicine for his discoveries in connexion with the biological combustion process, especially in relation to vitamin C.

(f) The Function and Diseases of the Heart

Karl Vierordt (p. 313) of Tübingen described in 1855 an instrument called a sphygmograph by which a graphic picture of the pulse at the wrist could be obtained. This instrument was greatly improved in 1860 by Étienne Jules Marey (p. 313), and further improved by the London homoeopath R. E. Dudgeon (p. 313) in 1878. Using these instruments Marey and other workers discovered many fundamental facts about the pulse wave. Marey also devised a polygraph, an instrument by which two short simultaneous records of the wave transmitted by a vein in the neck and of the apex beat of the heart could be obtained side by side on smoked paper. The actual impulse was conducted by the air in a fine tube to a small air-tight drum; the subsequent movement of the skin of the drum activated a fine lever, attached to it, which wrote the graphic record on the moving paper.

In persons suffering from some types of heart disease, and also in normal persons under certain conditions, irregularities of the heart's action are not infrequent. These irregularities had never been studied until 1876, when Marey showed that there is one type in which at varying intervals two beats of the heart succeed one another abnormally rapidly. This condition of extrasystoles was studied experimentally in the frog and in mammals twenty years later.

Meanwhile, a practitioner in Burnley, (Sir) James Mackenzie (1853–1925), had for many years been using various types of sphygmograph and a phlebograph, an instrument which he had devised in 1892 to study the pulse in veins. He found most of these instruments unsatisfactory in that the apparatus was clumsy and unsuited for use in the consulting-room. Further, only a very short tracing could be obtained on the strip of smoked paper, and this might be taken at the very time when the heart's rhythm happened to be normal. Mackenzie therefore invented an ingenious ink-polygraph. By its aid three simultaneous tracings could be made in ink on a long roll of unsmoked paper. With this instrument he was able to correlate pulses in the arteries and veins respectively with the beat of the heart itself. He also shed a flood of light on irregularities of the heart's rhythm, and he was able to distinguish those irregularities which were of no consequence from those which were caused by serious organic disease of the heart. In 1902 Mackenzie published his classical book, *The Study of the Pulse*, in which he gave a full description of his polygraph and its use in clinical work. Six years later he published his large work on *Diseases of the Heart* in which the new attitude to these conditions was fully explained.

This new outlook in the clinical study of heart disease stimulated further physiological researches into the mechanism by which each beat of the heart is initiated and by which it is carried from auricles to ventricles. In 1893 Albert Frank Stanley Kent (1863–1958) and Wilhelm His, Jun. (1863–1934), independently described a small bundle of conducting tissue in the fibrous ring which separates auricles from ventricles. The site of origin of the heart-beat was still unknown; but in 1907 (Sir) Arthur Keith (1866–1953) and Martin William Flack (1882–1931) discovered a small area of tissue in the right auricle which was thought to be the 'pace-maker'. Two years later the correctness of their view was proved by (Sir) Thomas

Lewis (1881–1945) of University College Hospital, London, whose work on the blood-vessels of the skin has been dealt with (p. 560).

There was one type of irregularity of the heart-beat which interested Mackenzie greatly. This was a total irregularity of the rhythm found in the later stages of disease of the mitral valve, probably the commonest of chronic organic heart lesions. It had long been

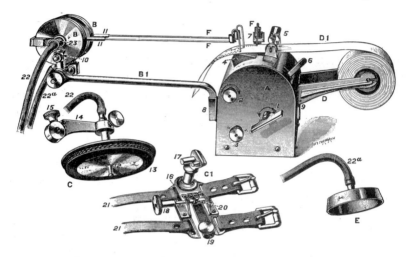

FIG. 126. Mackenzie's ink-polygraph in its original form.

known that in experimental animals the auricles sometimes pass into a state of extremely rapid, irregular, and incomplete contraction. In 1902 Mackenzie recognised that, in the late stages of mitral disease when the pulse was totally irregular, the characteristic wave caused by the contraction of the auricles in a normal tracing from the jugular vein was absent. His explanation happened to be wrong; but the impetus of his work led to the real explanation a few years later. In this condition of auricular fibrillation the muscle-fibres of the auricle contract independently of each other, and at a rate—up to 450 times a minute—which is far greater than can be efficiently conducted to the ventricles. Hence only some impulses get through at irregular intervals, and a complete irregularity of the heart results.

The electrocardiograph, a specialized type of galvanometer which

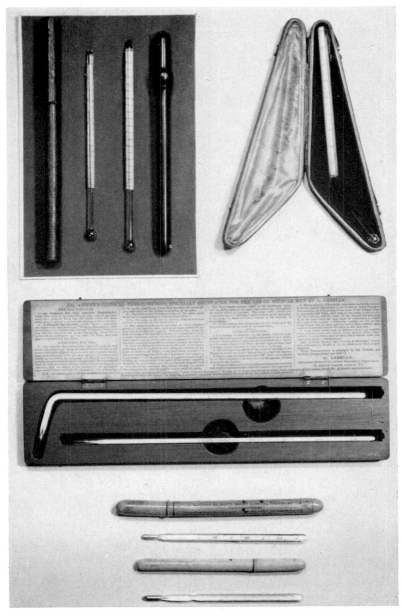

XXI. THE EVOLUTION OF THE CLINICAL THERMOMETER

Above, left, two thermometers of the type described by John Hunter, for observations in animals; *c.* 1800. Above, right, a thermometer of the type used by James Currie (1756–1805) in his cold-water treatment of fevers; *c.* 1800. In centre, two thermometers in case by Maw, Son & Thompson, London, to the design of Sir William Aitken; *c.* 1865. Bottom group, two short clinical thermometers to Allbutt's design, with their cases; *c.* 1870. The upper instrument is the original Allbutt type, made by Harvey & Reynolds, Leeds; the lower instrument was made by Hawksley, London. (Scale, approximately ¼)
(Instruments in the Wellcome Historical Medical Museum)

records the minute electric currents generated by the heart's action and photographs the records, was invented by William Einthoven (1860–1927) of Leyden in 1903. In subsequent years he did much to interpret the records, and in 1924 he received a Nobel Prize. Very important physiological and clinical studies with this complex and expensive instrument were carried out by Sir Thomas Lewis over many years, and in 1911 there appeared the first edition of his *Mechanism and Graphic Registration of the Heart Beat*. In subsequent editions (1920, 1925) it played an increasing role in widening the applications of the method.

Cardiology is indebted to Mackenzie for another important principle. In the hands of Laennec and his disciples (p. 172), and of the Dublin School of physicians, the stethoscope became an important instrument, and great stress was laid on the presence of heart murmurs in assessing the probable course of a cardiac condition. Mackenzie came gradually to the conclusion that in certain heart diseases what really mattered was not the presence of a murmur but the capacity of the heart-muscle to continue to compensate for the disability caused by the abnormal condition of the valves. Despite his insistence on this point, however, medical officers in the very early stages of the First World War were recommending that healthy soldiers who happened to have a type of murmur later recognized as common should be discharged from the army. During the war extensive and important investigations were carried out by Lewis and others on these conditions previously labelled 'disordered action of the heart' (D.A.H.) or 'valvular disease of the heart' (V.D.H.). Lewis explained many of their features by his conception of the effort syndrome (1917).

Angina pectoris and coronary thrombosis have been increasingly emphasized during this century as penalties for the strain of modern life. Angina pectoris, first described by Heberden in 1768 (p. 36), was again described by Parry of Bath (p. 530) in 1799. Early in the present century the coronary theory of its origin held the field. In 1894 Clifford Allbutt put forward the theory that angina pectoris is due to disease of the first part of the aorta. Fourteen years later he discovered that Corrigan (p. 283) had advanced a similar theory in 1837. Allbutt continued to press his views, and in 1915 they were fully set out in his great work on *Diseases of the Arteries, including Angina Pectoris*. In 1923 Mackenzie published a book on angina pectoris in which he attributed the condition to cardiac failure.

Sir Thomas Clifford Allbutt (1836–1925) has claims to be regarded as the most learned and distinguished physician of the last hundred years. Until 1889 he was a physician to the Leeds General Infirmary. On retiring from that strenuous life he was for three years a Commissioner in Lunacy. In 1892 he was called to the regius chair of physic at Cambridge, a post which he filled brilliantly until the day of his death in his ninetieth year. In addition to his work on the arteries he wrote on many clinical subjects, and edited a valuable *System of Medicine* (1896–99). The second edition of this large work, edited in collaboration with his friend and successor in the Cambridge chair, Sir Humphry Davy Rolleston (1862–1944), is still a valuable work of reference. Allbutt was also a wise and learned historian, and his writings on Greek medicine in Rome, on the Middle Ages, and on the Renaissance embody mature wisdom enshrined in dignified prose.

The practitioner of medicine is indebted to Allbutt for his most important instrument. Before 1800 only a very few physicians had ever used a thermometer for clinical purpose. In 1852 (Sir) William Aitkin (1825–92) had a thermometer made for his use, but it was 10 inches long, and was later described by Allbutt as being 'like a short umbrella'. In 1865 Sydney Ringer (p. 315) published observations of the temperature in measles and tuberculosis. The difficulties experienced in using these early instruments were considerable: not only were they clumsy, but they took twenty minutes to register. Nevertheless, from about 1848 Carl Reinhold August Wunderlich (1815–77), the professor of medicine in the University of Leipzig, had been keeping records of the temperature readings in most of his cases. In 1868 he published his great book *Das Verhalten der Eigenwärme in Krankheiten*, which in 1871 appeared in English with the title *On the Temperature in Diseases: a Manual of Medical Thermometry*. This book is one of the great classics of medicine. Wunderlich discussed the use of the instrument, and described fully the course of the pyrexia in very many conditions. But all physicians were not so patient as Wunderlich, and the book's reception and usefulness might well have been much restricted had it not been for Allbutt's action. In 1867 he had made for himself a 'short' clinical thermometer, measuring 6 inches long, which registered its maximum in five minutes. Shortly after he had a thermometer of 3 inches made. This was the prototype of the modern clinical thermometer.

Knowledge of the circulation in both its physiological and its clinical aspects has been much broadened by the work of Carl John Wiggers (1883–), who held the chair of physiology at the Western Reserve University, Cleveland, Ohio, from 1918 until his retirement in 1953. During the whole of this period, and before its start, Wiggers concentrated on the study of the circulation by methods which could also be applied in clinical work. He devised many ingenious instruments, including optical manometers and the Wiggers–Dean Recorder which enabled the oscillations caused by the heart-beat and heart-murmurs to be registered visually.

THE DEVELOPMENT OF MODERN PATHOLOGY

We have dealt at some length with a few of the great physiological advances which transformed the face of medicine. We now glance at some aspects of the development of pathology, and here, at the expense of some repetition, it is necessary to stress certain changes which the science has undergone in the course of time. There was not much science about the work of the founder of morbid anatomy, Antonio di Paolo Benivieni (1443–1502). His posthumous book, *De abditis morborum causis* ('On the hidden causes of diseases'), published in Florence in 1507, contains the clinical records of over 100 cases, on ten of which he performed autopsies. But the book is a record of personal observation, and it is to Benivieni's credit that some of the conditions can be clearly identified from his pathological descriptions. Bonet's *Sepulchretum* (1679) was a compilation of the post-mortem records of others and, though it was a valuable source book in its time, it did not pretend to classify by conditions according to their causes or their main lesions. Some advance in presentation was made by Thomas Bartholin (1616–80), a Dane who held chairs of various subjects in several universities on the Continent. Bartholin was the son of Caspar Bartholin (1585–1629), a famous Danish anatomist, and one of his first works was to produce a new edition of his father's well-known textbook of anatomy. Thomas was later a supporter of Harvey, and he claimed against Rudbeck priority for the discovery of the connexion between the lymphatics and the thoracic duct. His medical writings contain many pathological observations, including cerebral abscess, the pericardium in heart disease, and tumours of the pancreas. Three further early collections, all by Dutchmen, and all unsystematic but influential in their day may be named. Thomas Theodor Kerckring (1640–93) published in 1670 his *Spicilegium anatomicum* in which he described the valvulae conniventes in the intestine. Up till then the post-mortem clots frequently found in the heart were always regarded as pathological structures and were called polyps of the heart. Kerckring was the first to recognize their true nature. In 1688 Steven Blankaart (1650–1702) published his *Anatomia practica*, consisting of accounts of about 200 autopsies. He made some advances in the understanding of tuberculosis and of ovarian cysts. In Amsterdam Frederik Ruysch (p. 516) built up a famous museum of normal and morbid anatomy. He perfected the technique of wax injection for the study of the finer structures of parts, and over many years he illustrated specimens from his museum in a series of atlases. The plates dealing with bone lesions, calculi, and cirrhosis of the liver were outstanding.

The foundations of surgical pathology were laid by Marco Aurelio Severino (1580–1656) of Naples with his *De recondita abscessuum natura* ('On the hidden nature of abscesses', 1632). In it he described swellings of all types, including new growths, granulomas, and buboes. It was the first book to contain illustrations of the lesions.

The important observations of Wepfer (p. 271) and of Lancisi (p. 196) were of a more systematic nature. Raymond Vieussens (p. 245) published in 1705 a work in which he gave the best of the early descriptions of the pathological changes in the heart in mitral stenosis and in aortic insufficiency; he correlated the clinical condition with the autopsy finding, and described the 'water-hammer pulse' of aortic insufficiency, later called after Corrigan (p. 283). Antonio Maria Valsalva (1666-1723) was professor of anatomy at Bologna, and his most illustrious pupil was Morgagni, who edited an edition of his master's work. Valsalva is now best known for his *De aure humana tractatus* ('On the human ear', 1704), in which he gave the first really detailed account of the structure of that organ. But his other writings contain many detailed observations on morbid anatomy, and many others are contained in Morgagni's great book. With the publication of the *De sedibus* of Morgagni (p. 169) we reach the end of one period in the study of morbid anatomy and the beginning of a new and more systematic period.

A generation after Morgagni came one who is not usually regarded as a writer on pathological subjects, but who had the true instinct for the correlation of clinical work with post-mortem findings. This was William Heberden (p. 36), whom Dr. Samuel Johnson called 'Ultimus Romanorum, the last of our learned physicians'. Heberden first described night-blindness (nyctalopia) and the superficial nodes in rheumatic fever. He first differentiated chicken-pox from smallpox. His *Commentarii* (1802, p. 36), the last important medical work to be published in Latin, contained the first complete description of angina pectoris. An autopsy of one of his many cases of this condition showed little but some atheroma of the aorta.

Eduard Sandifort (1742–1814) of Leyden built up a splendid museum of morbid anatomy there, and in 1777 and the following years he published his *Observationes anatomicae-pathologicae*. In this beautifully illustrated work he described and illustrated important lesions such as aortic endocarditis, congenital malformations, and bone lesions. He also made a considerable contribution to our knowledge of inguinal hernia. This second period closes with John Hunter (p. 177), details of whose work in the field of morbid anatomy can now, since the wilful destruction of his notes by Sir Everard Home (1756–1832) after Hunter's death, only be obtained by a close study of the catalogues of his museum. His *Treatise on the Blood, Inflammation, and Gun-shot Wounds* (published posthumously in 1794) contains many notable pathological observations, especially his experimental work on inflammation. If Galen be the founder of experimental pathology, Hunter must be viewed as its modern re-founder. This period closed with Matthew Baillie's *The Morbid Anatomy of some of the most important parts of the Human Body* (1793) (pp. 169–71), and of the accompanying atlas six years later.

Text and atlas constitute the first systematic textbook dealing exclusively with morbid anatomy.

The next period centred almost entirely on France, and especially on the great hospitals of Paris. First in point of time was Pinel. Mention has already been made of his *Nosographie philosophique* (p. 281), which was based on his knowledge of pathological anatomy. On grounds which to him seemed logical, he postulated that similar tissues showed similar lesions, and he had great influence on Bichat and on Laennec.

Corvisart, Pinel's colleague and contemporary, made a very notable contribution to special pathology with his *Essai sur les maladies et les lésions organiques du cœur et des gros vaisseaux* ('Essay on the diseases and organic lesions of the heart and great vessels', 1806). This work contained a very full account of aneurysms, and it is strange that Corvisart did not mention syphilis as a causal factor of this condition. Corvisart's influence was on clinical medicine rather than on morbid anatomy.

Much junior to both these men was Bichat (p. 320), who certainly in his short life gained an enormous experience of autopsies. In his first two works, both published in 1800, the *Traité des membranes en général et diverses membranes en particulier* ('Treatise on membranes [i.e. tissues] in general and of certain membranes in particular') and the *Recherches physiologiques sur la vie et la mort* ('Physiological researches on life and death'), Bichat introduced his theory of the tissues (p. 320), and his general pathological doctrines. In his next work, *Anatomie générale, appliquée à la physiologie et à la médecine* ('General anatomy, applied to physiology and medicine', 1801), Bichat dealt in detail with his view that in disease organs as a whole were not affected, but rather certain individual tissues of which they were formed. His last book, his *Traité d'anatomie descriptive* ('Treatise on descriptive anatomy', 1801–3) is a large work which remained unfinished at his death. Though one must probably accept the fact that Bichat had great influence in directing attention to the tissues as the seat of disease, it must be regretted that he intentionally decided not to use a microscope.

G. L. Bayle (p. 282) was assistant to Corvisart, and though he had an active interest in morbid anatomy in general, his sole book,

Recherches sur la phthisie pulmonaire ('Researches on pulmonary tuberculosis', 1810), deals with the post-mortem records of fifty-four cases of one disease. He distinguished six kinds of phthisis, all of which can now be identified with their modern equivalents.

If the year 1819 stands out as a great landmark in medicine because of the publication of the *De l'auscultation médiate* of Laennec (p. 172), the five years 1825–9 were no less important in the history of pathology. In 1825 P. C. A. Louis published his great book on phthisis (p. 721), and introduced his new approach to the study of disease. In 1826 Laennec published his second edition of his *Auscultation médiate*. In this edition the morbid anatomy of disease of the lungs was dealt with in a revolutionary manner. At one bound this subject became modern, with outstanding accounts of the development of the tubercle through all its stages, and systematic descriptions of infarcts of the lung, emphysema, bronchiectasis, pneumothorax, and other conditions. The terminology introduced by Laennec is still in use today. In 1826 also Pierre Bretonneau (p. 204) of Tours published his monograph on the 'special inflammation' of the throat which he was the first to identify with croup and malignant angina, and to call 'diphthérite' (diphtheria). In 1829 two notable works on typhoid fever were published—Bretonneau's monograph, in which he located the seat of the intestinal lesions in the Peyer's patches, and the larger work of Louis (p. 721).

The subject of pathological anatomy was about to dominate the medical field, and one of the first signs was the foundation of two chairs especially for this subject. The first was established in 1819 at the University of Strasbourg, which was then French. To it was appointed Jean G. C. Frédéric Martin Lobstein (1777–1835), a German from Giessen. He amply justified the choice, and produced a *Traité d'anatomie pathologique* (1829) which was unfinished. He coined the term pathogenesis, and in his view his subject became more related to functional pathology.

The other chair was founded in Paris in 1836. To it was appointed Jean Cruveilhier (1791–1874), a graduate of Paris who had been for a time professor of surgery at Montpellier until he returned to fill the vacant chair of descriptive anatomy in Paris in 1825. While he held this latter post Cruveilhier was also physician to various important Paris hospitals, and he gained very wide experience of morbid anatomy. He believed that a satisfactory atlas of this subject was required, and in 1829 the first part of his *Anatomie pathologique du corps humain* was published. During the next six years successive parts completed the first volume; and in 1835 the second volume began to come out and it was completed in 1842. This, the greatest pathological atlas ever published, contains over 200 lithographs, many in colour, of gross preparations. His aim was to give students standards of comparison. Some of the illustrations of tumours and congenital abnormalities are very fine; and, as might be expected from Cruveilhier's theory, the illustrations of phlebitis are very carefully drawn. The work contains the first description and illustration of disseminated sclerosis and of some other conditions.

While the work was appearing Cruveilhier was developing his theory that morbid changes were always due to morbid secretions into the interstitial tissues. On this theory inflammation was due to a morbid secretion from the capillaries, and was linked with phlebitis, the condition which he thought dominated the whole of pathology. Years later Cruveilhier expounded his theory fully in the five volumes of his *Traité d'anatomie pathologique générale* (1849–64).

Jean Baptiste Bouillaud (1796–1881) of Paris established the relation between the frontal lobes and aphasia. The fact that mitral stenosis is associated with acute rheumatism had been noted by David Pitcairn (1749–1809) of St. Bartholomew's Hospital in 1788, by Edward Jenner in 1789, and by William Charles Wells (1757–1817) of St. Thomas's Hospital in 1812. About 1837 Bouillaud extended these observations.

Meanwhile the leadership in the field of morbid anatomy had passed from France to England, to Ireland, and finally to Germany. In the thirty years following 1826 Bright, Hodgkin, and Addison established at Guy's a name and pathological tradition which still persists (p. 284). The work of the great Dublin physicians has already been described. James Hope (1801–41) studied at Edinburgh and Paris, and became physician to St. George's Hospital, London. He published in 1831 a *Treatise on the Diseases of the Heart and Great Vessels* in which he gave classical descriptions of cardiac asthma and valvular disease, and in which he added to the description of the heart sounds. Hope then turned to pathological anatomy and published *Principles and Illustrations of Morbid Anatomy* (1834), an atlas of coloured lithographs made from his own drawings.

Another atlas was that entitled *Pathological Anatomy. Illustrations of the Elementary Forms of Disease* (1837) by Sir Robert Carswell (1793–1857). Carswell was a Scot who studied medicine at Glasgow and then spent many years studying at Lyons and at Paris, where he was a pupil of P. C. A. Louis. In 1828 he was appointed as the first occupant of the chair of pathological anatomy in the newly established University College, London. Carswell was probably the finest artist of all the professional pathologists. He had just been commissioned to prepare a series of water-colour drawings of diseased structures, and he now returned to Paris to carry out this work. By 1831, when he took up the duties of his chair, he had completed 2,000 drawings. Owing to ill health Carswell resigned his chair in 1840, and became physician to the King of the Belgians. In his great atlas the drawings were selected from his own collection, and he put them upon the stone himself. These coloured lithographs often give remarkably clear pictures of the diseased structures, and his illustrations of pulmonary tuberculosis and of cirrhosis of the liver are especially valuable.

Carswell's work was probably the last great pathological work in English about this time, and the leadership now passed to the German-speaking countries. As has been explained (p. 286), the rise of the New Vienna School associated a great pathologist (Rokitansky) with a great clinician (Skoda). Rokitansky spent the whole of his active life in Vienna, with the enormous resources of the Allgemeines Krankenhaus at his disposal. When he retired from his chair of pathological anatomy he had personally performed well over 30,000 autopsies, and the records of 70,000 were available to him. Rokitansky's greatest work was his *Handbuch der pathologischen Anatomie*, published in three volumes between 1841 and 1846. The second and third volumes, dealing with special pathology, were published before the first volume, dealing with general pathology. Rokitansky in these second and third volumes gave the first description of acute yellow atrophy of the liver, and he greatly improved our conception of pneumonia. He was much interested in congenital malformations, and they are very fully described. In these two volumes there are very few references to microscopical structure. The microscopic observations come in the first volume and it is on a much lower level than the volumes dealing with special pathology. Rokitansky unfortunately attempted to resuscitate a modified form of the humoral theory, at a time when the scientific world was in a ferment at the formulation of the new cell theory in biology. His theories of local 'crases' explained nothing. They were demolished by the young Virchow's incisive attack, and in later editions they disappeared from the book.

At the time when Rokitansky was writing this book the microscope was being increasingly used in pathology. In 1841 John Hughes Bennett (1812–75) started to lecture on histology at Edinburgh University, and part of the course consisted of microscopical demonstrations of morbid histology. He gave such lectures for many years. Hughes Bennett was concerned in one of the first great contributions to pathology. In 1845 he described a case of hypertropy of the spleen and liver, in which he found a gross excess of white corpuscles in the blood. It was the first recognized case of leukaemia. Hughes Bennett thought that death had resulted from 'suppuration of the blood'. Six weeks later Virchow reported a case of 'Weisses Blut' ('white blood') in which he had performed an autopsy, the findings of which he correctly interpreted.

Rudolf Virchow (1821–1902) is the greatest of all pathologists. He had the advantage of studying under Johannes Müller at Berlin, and after graduating he became assistant pathologist at the Charité Hospital. In addition to his autopsy work he carried out intensive microscopical studies. By the time he was twenty-five he was in charge of the pathological work, and in the following year in collaboration with a friend he founded (1847) the journal which still continues under the name of *Virchow's Archiv*. A year later saw his first excursion into active politics, with the result that he was removed from his post. The University of Würzburg seized the chance to appoint him to the first chair of pathological anatomy in Germany. Seven years later he was back in Berlin, the holder of a newly established professorship of pathological anatomy. Here Virchow spent the remainder of his long life, working intensively on his pathological studies, writing innumerable articles, in later life becoming a founder of physical anthropology, and finding time to play a very active political role as a member of the Reichstag, when on more than one occasion he crossed swords with Bismarck himself.

One of Virchow's earliest studies was on thrombosis. He discounted Cruveilhier's theory that phlebitis played a prominent part in the causation of many diseases, and he showed that the prime cause of thrombosis is a slowing of the blood in the vessels. He introduced the concept of embolism, and took a rational view of pyaemia (1846). During his Würzburg period Virchow was building up evidence on the importance of the cell in all vital phenomena. When Schwann originally introduced the cell theory about ten years previously, he thought that new cells arose from a primitive undifferentiated material—the blastema—in which they were embedded. The division of cells by mitosis was not seen until some years later. Rokitansky had adopted Schwann's original views, with the unfortunate result that he attempted to found his whole system of pathology on a substance which did not exist, and on a process—spontaneous generation—which could not be demonstrated. Virchow, with the newer knowledge of cell division at his disposal, took the opposite view, sufficiently summarized in his phrase *Omnis cellula e cellula* ('All cells arise from previously existing cells'). This doctrine formed the basis of the lectures on *Cellularpathologie* which he first published in 1858. This book demolished all humoral theories; it made possible the successful foundation of a systematic, rational pathology; and it opened the door for innumerable new investigations.

Virchow's great doctrine introduced new possibilities in the study of the inflammatory process. In addition, he was the first to distinguish between fatty degeneration and fatty infiltration. He was a pioneer in the field of the degenerations generally. He not only gave the correct interpretation of leukaemia, but very soon afterwards recognised its two types, myeloid and lymphatic. In every way Virchow was an intellectual giant.

About the time of the *Cellularpathologie* various technical developments were taking place which had a profound influence on the progress of morbid histology. The microtome had been invented, and was later much improved by Richard Thoma (1847–1923) and others. Tissue sections of any desired thinness could now be easily obtained. From about 1870 onwards there was also a great development in staining methods. Stains were much improved by, among others, Carl Weigert (1845–1904), who made important studies on tissue degenerations, on embolism and infarction, and on miliary tuberculosis.

Pathological anatomy was now inseparably linked with morbid histology. Special pathology developed in a way that would have delighted Rokitansky, and new light was thrown on many types of lesions. Morbid histology now became a diagnostic aid to the surgeon. Sir James Paget (1814–99) and others wrote important works on surgical pathology. At the same time marked advances were made in the field of general pathology. Mention may be made of the work of Friedrich Daniel von Recklinghausen (1833–1910), who held the Strasbourg chair of pathology for over thirty years. Much of his work dealt with the pathology of bone, with studies on periostitis, bone tumours, osteomalacia, rickets, and also of rare diseases of bone. He made important studies of embolism and infarction, and of haemochromatosis, which he named. His name is associated with multiple neurofibromatosis. He was a worthy product of his master Virchow.

Other pupils of Virchow who made their mark were Edwin Klebs (p. 381) and Georg Eduard Rindfleisch (1836–1908); Cohnheim (p. 353), another pupil, is considered later. Klebs was later better known as a bacteriologist, but his pathological work was also important. Rindfleisch held chairs of pathological anatomy at Zürich and Bonn before he was called to the Würzburg chair in 1874. He was already very well known as a morbid histologist, and his textbook of that subject had by then reached its third edition and had been translated into English. In the next generation must be mentioned the Swiss Ernst Ziegler (1849–1905), who held the chairs of pathological anatomy successively at Zürich, Tübingen, and at Freiburg-im-Breisgau (1889). He did important work on inflammation, the regeneration of tissues, and especially the vessels, on certain aspects of tuberculosis and the pathology of bone. In Great Britain outstanding pathologists were Joseph Coats (1846–99) of Glasgow, W. S. Greenfield (p. 532) of Edinburgh, and Sir Samuel Wilks (p. 285). Coats, a Glasgow graduate, later studied experimental physiology under Karl Ludwig at Leipzig. After six years as pathologist to the Glasgow Royal Infirmary he returned to Germany and studied pathological anatomy with Rindfleisch. On his return he became pathologist to the Western Infirmary at Glasgow. In 1893 the Glasgow chair of pathology was created for him, and on his death he was succeded by Muir (p. 638). Coats published in 1883 a valuable *Manual of Pathology*, which was in its fourth edition when he died. In the United States W. H. Welch (p. 394) was at this time influencing the whole field of pathology and bacteriology.

We pause here to remark that the experimental method has played a very important part in elucidating the problems of general pathology. John Hunter is regarded as the founder of experimental pathology, and towards the middle of the nineteenth century its greatest exponents were Magendie (p. 154) and Claude Bernard (p. 294). Another important early worker was Ludwig Traube (1818–76), a pupil of Purkinje and of Johannes Müller. Traube showed among other things the occurrence of disease of the lungs after section of the vagus nerves. He founded a journal devoted entirely to results obtained by the experimental method. We have already mentioned the very important work of Lister on inflammation (p. 353). Cohnheim (p. 353) occupies a unique place in the history of pathology. Virchow's greatest pupil, he held the chairs of pathology successively at Breslau and at Leipzig. He differed from Virchow's explanation of the source of the cells in inflammation, and he carried out brilliant experimental work which clarified the whole position. These results were published in the two volumes of his *Vorlesungen über allgemeine Pathologie* ('Lectures on general pathology', 1877–80). Ten years later an English translation was published. This book and its translation have continued to enlighten and inspire successive generations of students from many countries. It still reads like a modern textbook, and few modern textbooks fail to mention it.

A relatively fruitful field for experimental pathology is cancer research, and here may be mentioned Katsusaburo Yamagiwa (1863–1930), who was the first to produce tar cancer in rabbits by painting their skins with tar products (1916); Henry Peter George Bayon

(1876–1952), who in 1912 produced epithelial proliferation, probably malignant, by the injection of gasworks tar; and Sir Ernest Laurence Kennaway (1881–1957), of the Royal Cancer Hospital, London, who devoted much of his life to this work. The chemical aspect of pathology was considerably developed in the United States by Harry Gideon Wells (1875–1943), of Chicago, who wrote a pioneer textbook on this subject. Wells also wrote much on the chemical aspects of tuberculosis. In this work he was associated with the pathologist Esmond Ray Long (1890–), the author of a standard history of pathology, who has spent a lifetime on the problems of tuberculosis. Among those chemists who have been active in the field of cancer research is James Wilfred Cook (1900–), whose work with Kennaway on the dibenzanthracene compounds (1932) was very important. The work of Sir Howard Florey is dealt with later (p. 695), and in the sections on the endocrine glands, on neurology, and elsewhere in this book many men are mentioned who in various ways developed experimental pathology.

In conclusion we glance briefly at a very few of the men born since 1860 who have greatly influenced the subsequent development of pathology in general. First in point of time is Eduard Kaufmann (1860–1931), a native of Bonn who held the chair at Basle, and subsequently for twenty years at Göttingen. He did important work on foetal rickets, on the prostate, and on the thyroid. At Freiburg, Ziegler was succeeded by Karl Albert Ludwig Aschoff (1866–1942), on whom fell the mantle of Virchow. Among his innumerable studies may be mentioned his work on appendicitis, on gallstones and jaundice, on suppuration of the kidneys, on thrombosis, and especially his researches on the reticulo-endothelial system (p. 318). Ziegler published the two volumes of his textbook of pathological anatomy in 1881–2, and it had reached its eleventh edition at his death. Kaufmann's textbook of special pathology, also in two volumes, appeared in 1896, and reached its eleventh edition in 1931. Aschoff's great textbook was first published in 1909, and is now in its ninth edition. Ziegler's work is today rather old fashioned; but the books by Kaufmann and Aschoff are still usable and are now among the best things of their kind in German.

In the United Kingdom pride of place goes to Sir Robert Muir

(1865–1959), who for thirty-seven years held the chair of pathology at Glasgow. Muir was in this country for many years the doyen of pathologists, and he filled over twenty chairs with his assistants and former pupils. Besides his distinguished work on problems of immunity and his standard textbook of bacteriology (1897), written in collaboration with James Ritchie (1864–1923), Muir covered the whole field of pathology. Some of his most noteworthy researches dealt with experimental anaemia produced by the injection of haemolytic serum, regenerative changes in the bone marrow as a result of infection, jaundice, regeneration in parenchymatous cells, iron storage in the body, precancerous lesions, and the mode of spread of tumours. His textbook of pathology (1924) has exerted a very wide influence in its successive editions. Arthur Edwin Boycott (1877–1938), of University College, London, did important work on the formation of the blood corpuscles in health and in disease, and the function of the kidney in controlling the volume of the blood. Matthew John Stewart (1885–1957), for many years professor of pathology at Leeds, carried morbid histology to its ultimate limits. With Sir Arthur Frederick Hurst (1879–1944) he was the author of an important work on gastric and duodenal ulcer (1929). In the United States James Ewing (1866–1943) was for many years professor of pathology at Cornell University, New York. He spent most of his life working on tumours, and his *Neoplastic Diseases* (1919) was for many years an indispensable work of reference. Eugene Lindsay Opie (1873–), who held the chair of pathology at St. Louis, did important work on inflammation and on diseases of the pancreas. Later, at the Henry Phipps Institute in Philadelphia, he carried out much important work on the pathology of tuberculosis. We have elsewhere referred to the work of William George MacCallum (1874–1944), of the Johns Hopkins University, on the malaria parasite (p. 461). He also did valuable work on tetany and on diabetes, and his textbook, first published in 1916, was marked by clarity, authority, and beautiful illustrations.

We leave this subject with the statement that the spirit of inquiry is very much alive. As an example of the new works which have appeared in recent years we mention the monumental monograph on the *Pathology of the Cell* (1952) by Sir Gordon Roy Cameron (1899–)

who holds the chair of morbid anatomy at University College Hospital Medical School in the University of London. This work, in the Virchow tradition, is one to which Virchow might well have been pleased to have set his name.

KNOWLEDGE OF THE EYE AND ITS DISORDERS

From an early date the treatment of ailments of the eye has stood somewhat apart from the rest of medical practice. Moreover, the

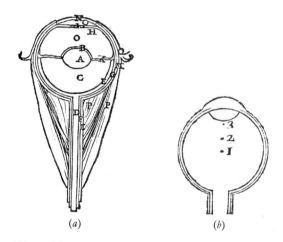

(a)   (b)

Fig. 127. The position of the lens of the eye according to (a) Vesalius, and (b) Fabricius

((a) Vesalius, *Fabrica*, 1543; (b) H. Fabricius, *De visione, voce, auditu*, Venice. 1600)

knowledge of the structure and functions of the parts of the eye has not kept closely parallel with that of other branches of anatomy and physiology.

Knowledge of the position of the lens is of great importance from the historical aspect. Galen thought of the lens as close to the iris. But, as we shall see, the Arabian physicians practised extensively an operation for cataract by which they thought they were displacing opaque matter from its position in front of the lens. It is clear therefore that they must have considered that the lens was situated much farther back in the eye, and in the *Fabrica* of Vesalius (p. 91) it is shown actually in the centre of the organ. In 1601 Fabricius ab

Aquapendente (p. 97) wrote a work on the eye in which he showed the lens in its true position.

Our knowledge of much of the minute structure of the eye was greatly increased by the researches of Sir William Bowman (1816–92), who not only was one of the greatest of British ophthalmologists, but in his earlier years contributed a great deal to our understanding of muscle and of the structure and function of the kidney. In his book *Lectures on the Parts concerned in the Operations on the Eye, and on the Structure of the Retina* (1849) Bowman gave the first comprehensive account of the histology of the tissues of this organ.

Historically, optical errors of the eye were relieved by spectacles before the nature of the defects was understood. The first suggestion for the use of a convex lens for the correction of old sight was made by Roger Bacon (1214?–94). Spectacles were mentioned in a document of 1282, and spectacles with convex lenses were in common use by the middle of the fourteenth century. They were illustrated in miniatures, in sculpture, and later in painting. It may well be that their adoption, by prolonging reading life, had an important effect upon that process of extension of knowledge that is known as the Renaissance. Concave lenses for the relief of near sight came in towards the end of the fifteenth century, but were not widely used till the eighteenth century. A reading glass with a concave lens is shown in the portrait of Leo X painted by Raphael in 1517.

For long there was no means of estimating the amounts of error, whether of old sight, far sight, or near sight, save by trial on the part of the patient himself. Spectacles were a common object of the hawker's trays, and from them the sufferer selected the specimen that suited him best. The first essential improvement in this state of affairs was an elucidation of the mode of action of lenses. The paths of light rays in their passage through a lens were first approximately determined at the beginning of the seventeenth century by the astronomer Kepler (p. 112).

Knowledge of optics was markedly advanced during the seventeenth and eighteenth centuries, notably by Sir Isaac Newton. In the medical field a very notable work was the *Treatise on the Eye: The Manner and Phenomena of Vision* (1759) by William Porterfield. The birth and death dates of Porterfield are unknown. It is certain that he graduated in medicine at Rheims in 1717, and that in 1721 he became a Fellow of The Royal College of Physicians of Edinburgh. In 1724 he was appointed, on the recommendation of the College, professor of the institutes and practice of medicine at Edinburgh University. Monro *primus* had been appointed to his chair of anatomy in 1720. Porterfield resigned his chair within two years after his appointment. Nothing further is known of him except that he published this treatise thirty-three years later. The book is in two volumes and is an excellent summary of contemporary knowledge of the anatomy and physiology of the eye. It also contains many original observations on the anatomy and physiology of the eye. In it Porterfield insisted that the retina is the essential organ of vision, and not the choroid as many had previously held.

Porterfield's work engaged the attention forty years later of one of the most remarkable men who ever applied themselves to medical problems, the Quaker physicist, scholar, and physician Thomas Young (1773–1829). A man of immense learning, he practised medicine for some years and was a physician to St. George's Hospital until his death. He is remembered for his part in deciphering Egyptian hieroglyphics, and he carried out important work on standards of length, on the revision of the *Nautical Almanac*, and on the tides. His work on energy forms the basis of much of modern physics. Young's wave theory of light completely displaced Newton's emission theory, which assumes that light is due to particles of a material substance emitted from a luminous object.

Young was intensely interested in the mechanism of the eye, and in 1801 he read to the Royal Society an important communication on this subject. He carried out difficult experiments on his own eyes, and gave measurements of the length of the eye and of the radius of curvature of the cornea which are remarkably accurate. He then considered the method by which the eye accommodates for near vision, and showed that the result was due to a change, not in the curvature of the cornea or in the length of the eyeball, but in the shape of the lens. At that time the function of the ciliary muscle was unknown, and Young wrongly attributed the power of the lens to change its focus to the action of muscle-fibres in it. He described astigmatism for the first time.

Astigmatic lenses were not contrived till well into the nineteenth century. These cylindrospherical lenses were in fact first prescribed for himself by Sir George Biddell Airy (1801–92), the Astronomer Royal, who discovered that his own eyes were astigmatic. Bifocal lenses appear to have been first made by Benjamin Franklin. Contact glasses were probably first used in 1877 in the treatment of an eye condition. It was not until about 1920 that they were made commercially for the correction of visual defects.

In 1874 Silas Weir Mitchell (p. 185), the distinguished American physician, showed that the eye strain resulting from astigmatism was associated with many nervous conditions. Weir Mitchell's name is familiarly associated with a line of treatment of these conditions. Since his discovery it has been the practice to examine for optical error all sufferers from headache and neurotic symptoms.

The invention of the ophthalmoscope by Helmholtz in 1851 (p. 289) was a most important step in the history of ophthalmology. This instrument not only enabled the physician to observe and classify abnormalities of the retina, but it proved to be invaluable in the measurement of errors of refraction in the eye. Helmholtz himself employed the ophthalmoscope for this purpose, and its use is now standard practice.

The most important advances in the prescribing and fitting of spectacles were carried out by the Dutch ophthalmologist Frans Cornelis Donders (1818–89), who separated errors of refraction from those of accommodation. His book *The Anomalies of Refraction and Accommodation* (1864) was translated into English from his manuscript, and the first edition is in that language. It immediately became a classic. Important also in the advancement of this work was the introduction of sets of standard letters of different sizes, known as test types, for testing the subject's visual acuity. Several workers devised suitable sets, but those introduced by the Dutch ophthalmologist Hermann Snellen (1834–1908) are still in common use.

The operative treatment of the eye is of great antiquity. The most important operative procedure is that for cataract, a condition caused by an opacity of the lens. Couching for cataract, that is depressing the opaque lens, was practised by Alexandrian surgeons in the third century B.C. It is described by Celsus (p. 53) in the first and mentioned by Galen (p. 59) in the second Christian century. In Imperial Roman times there were surgeons who devoted themselves exclusively to cataract operations. These were practised during the Middle Ages by the Arabs and to a less extent by the

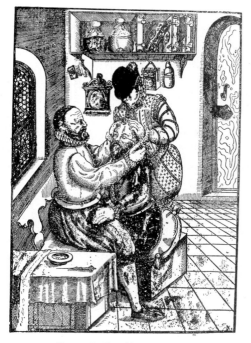

FIG. 128. Couching a cataract

(G. Bartisch, *Ophthalmodouleia. Das ist Augendienst*, Dresden, 1583. Copy, with illustrations roughly coloured by hand, in the Wellcome Historical Medical Library)

Westerns. For the most part the operations were performed by wandering quacks, who were, however, often very skilful. In the sixteenth century operations on the eye began to pass into the hands of recognized medical practitioners.

It should be emphasized, despite the fact that orthodox practitioners shunned the cataract operation, that it was essentially the crux of ophthalmology, and it was to raise a violent storm early in the eighteenth century. From early times cataract had been regarded, not as an opacity of the lens, but as the presence of an opaque substance, an 'inspissated humour', in the 'cataract space' which was supposed to be present between the lens and the iris. Treatment consisted of entering a sharp hooked needle through the cornea or sclerotic into this opaque matter. By manipulating the needle its point broke up the opaque matter and displaced or couched it downwards below the level of the pupil. The fact that Fabricius showed the true position of the lens in 1600 made no difference to this belief.

About 1685 the famous French ophthalmologist Antoine Maître-Jan (1650?–1730) chanced to have two patients whom he 'couched', in each of whom the couched matter was displaced not into the vitreous humour but through the pupil into the anterior chamber of the eye. In each case the couched matter consisted of a thick rounded body, the lens, and not of fragments of opaque membrane. Maître-Jan later examined after their deaths the eyes of persons whom he had couched at some time during their lives, and he confirmed that it was indeed the lens which was affected. All this information Maître-Jan seemed to have kept discreetly to himself. In 1705 a young French physician Michael Brisseau (1670?–1743) discovered the facts anew on a dead soldier and communicated them to the French Academy of Sciences. His report was received with scepticism, even though Maître-Jan made public his observations and gave Brisseau his support. Despite these observations couching continued to be practised. In 1722 Charles de Saint-Yves (1667–1736) attempted to couch a cataract and by mischance he displaced the cataractous body through the pupil into the anterior chamber. He then incised the eye and removed the body. This was the first occasion on which the lens had been removed from a living subject. The credit of giving the correct explanation of the opacity, that is, senile degeneration of the lens, and of inventing the modern cataract operation belongs to Jacques Daviel (1696–1762). In 1748 he published his account of his deliberate operation for removal of the cataractous lens, but it was some years later before he finally decided in favour of this operation rather than that of couching. Over a large range of cases in which he extracted the lens he had only 11 per cent. of failures.

The operation for cataract was not the only one which was

practised. As an example, mention may be made of the operation for enucleation of the eyeball, that is, the complete excision of the eye in the living subject. This operation was first fully described by Georg Bartisch (1535–1605), a travelling practitioner who later became court oculist at the Dresden Court. Bartisch's book, *Ophthalmodouleia. Das ist Augendienst*, was published at Dresden in 1583, and it is the first book on eye conditions written in a vernacular instead of in Latin. Bartisch's rather crude operation for enucleation was practised in cases in which the eye protruded to such an extent as to be hideous. In the nineteenth century this operation was perfected and was practised considerably in cases of injury of one eye in which there was a possibility of the onset of sympathetic ophthalmia in the other eye, a very serious condition. Bartisch's book also dealt with his operation for cataract, and it includes sections on the care of the mouth, teeth, and skin in relation to the eyes. Two years after the appearance of Bartisch's book there was published at Paris a treatise on eye diseases by Jacques Guillemeau (1550–1613), the pupil and son-in-law of Paré (p. 95). This work was entitled *Traité des maladies de l'œil, qui sont en nombre de cent treize, ausquelles il est sujet* ('Treatise on the diseases, one hundred and thirteen in number, to which the eye is subject', 1585). It was written in French, and was the second ophthalmological work to be written in a vernacular.

Advances in the treatment of morbid conditions of the eye were dependent on an accurate knowledge of its pathology. This knowledge began to be available from about the beginning of the nineteenth century, and was much advanced by the work of James Wardrop (1782–1869), who in 1808 and following years published his *Essays on the Morbid Anatomy of the Human Eye*. The importance of his work lay in the fact that he was the first to deal with eye conditions on a strictly anatomical basis. In his work on inflammatory lesions of the cornea he introduced the term keratitis.

A good example of the influence of pathological conceptions on treatment is given by the conditions which had for centuries been included under the term glaucoma. This term was used in Hippocratic times and signified a greenish, or possibly a bluish, discoloration of the pupil. The later Greek physicians differentiated a form of glaucoma which could be cured and one which could not. Then, and until much later times, the word glaucoma probably stood for several conditions which cannot now be definitely identified. But there was a belief that the curable type of glaucoma was really cataract, while the incurable variety was not. In 1622 an English travelling oculist, Richard Banister (1570?–1626), republished an English translation of Guillemeau's book (referred to above) which had long been out of print, and to this he appended a *Breviary* which was based on his own experience. In this small work Banister gave the first clear account of absolute glaucoma, and he recognized that the cardinal sign was not the colour of the pupil but that 'the Eye be growne more solid and hard, then naturally it should be'. Hardness of the eye is not again mentioned in the literature for over a hundred and twenty years, and then very fleetingly. Not until 1830 was it definitely recognized as the distinguishing feature between the blindness due to glaucoma and that due to cataract. The ophthalmoscope finally revealed that the essential cause of glaucoma is an increase of tension in the vitreous humour within the eye. Some forms of glaucoma are certain to lead to complete blindness in the affected eye, and the first step towards satisfactory treatment was the introduction by von Graefe in 1857 of the operation of iridectomy, in which a portion of the iris was removed.

Friedrich Wilhelm Ernst Albrecht von Graefe (1828–70) ushered in the modern era of ophthalmic surgery. He was professor of ophthalmology at Berlin, and he greatly improved the operation for cataract and introduced or improved many other important operations on the eye. He was one of the first to make important clinical observations with the ophthalmoscope, and he showed how the instrument may be made to yield information not only on the condition of the eye itself, but also on the brain and of its membranes, an application which has become of the greatest value in later medical developments. Though he died before the most important work of Pasteur and Lister had become generally accepted, von Graefe was yet practising a system of surgery which was not far from aseptic.

The scientific treatment of strabismus, or squint, is also a product of the nineteenth century. A squint is due to an overaction of one or more of the extrinsic ocular muscles, which thus causes a permanent deviation of the eyeball from its normal axis. The later Greek physicians treated squint by placing over the patient's face a mask with two perforations placed centrally before the eyes. It was argued that the squinting eye, finding its view obstructed, would assume a straight position. By the time of Ambroise Paré this mask was still being recommended. The first person to carry out an operation for the severance of the affected muscle was apparently the Chevalier John Taylor (1703–72). Taylor is commonly regarded as a quack, but he has derived the appellation more from his methods of practising and his mannerisms, diction, and self-advertising than from any lack of education and skill. Actually he studied under Cheselden at St. Thomas's Hospital and later obtained medical qualifications from several Continental universities. He travelled as an itinerant oculist over the whole of the British Isles and in western Europe, and he became oculist to George II. It is possible that in 1738 Taylor cut the tendon of the internal rectus muscle for squint and that he continued with this practice. It was a century later before any other surgeon attempted the operation. In 1839 Johann Friederich Dieffenbach (1792–1847) cut one of the eye muscles for squint, but the results in the hands of others were not very satisfactory. The method of cutting the tendon of the muscle as it lay under the conjunctiva was fully developed by von Graefe in 1853, and it is the basis of all subsequent operations.

An attempt to study the living eye microscopically was made in 1823, and in 1889 Louis de Wecker (1832–1906) devised a microscope for this purpose. Modern instruments depend for their illumination on the slit-lamp, invented by Allvar Gullstrand (1862–1930) of Uppsala. For his important work on the refractory system of the eye, on the shape of the living cornea, and on the nature of the changes of the lens in accommodation, he was awarded a Nobel Prize in 1911.

The theory of colour vision originally advanced by Thomas Young assumes that the retina contains elements in the nerve-endings which are capable of reacting respectively to the three primary (or, as he called them, 'principal') colours, red, green, and violet. All other colours produce reactions in varying degrees in the elements associated with the perception of one or more of these primary colours. The theory was later developed and modified by Helmholtz, who assumed that the primary colours were red, green, and blue. Although there have been other theories in this field, the Young–Helmholtz theory has stood the test of time. An important application of this theory concerns colour-blindness. The account of the first recorded case of this condition was read to the Royal Society in 1777, and the first scientific description was published in 1794 by the chemist John Dalton (1766–1844), who suffered from red-green blindness. In 1837 Ludwig Friederick Wilhelm August Seebeck (1805–49) analysed his cases by getting them to sort coloured paper and glass. A test for colour-vision formerly much used was introduced by Alarik Frithjof Holmgren (1831–97), and consisted of the sorting of strands of wools of standard tints. The theory of colour-vision has been studied by many famous scientists, including Sir John Herschel, James Clerk Maxwell, and Lord Rayleigh.

A further development of ophthalmological practice is that of the manufacture and fitting of artificial eyes. These appliances were probably in use for the living subject in Egyptian times, but they must have been of a very crude character, and their use possibly led to sepsis of the orbit. Paré (p. 95) described artificial eyes of gold and silver, enamelled to represent the natural eye. Glass eyes came much into use in the seventeenth century. The best examples were at first made by the Venetians, and later by the Bohemians and the French. The secrets of the craft were handed on from father to son. About 1835 much improved eyes began to be made in Germany, and that country retained the foremost place until 1933, when, owing to their export being prohibited, Great Britain and the United States were forced to develop other media, including plastics. An artificial eye is not only a cosmetic appliance; its use diminishes the risk of infection in an empty socket. In 1939 there were 350,000 wearers of artificial eyes in the United Kingdom alone, and it is estimated that this figure had risen to nearly a million shortly after the end of the Second World War.

As with most departments of medicine, so also with ophthalmology, the most significant advances during the last generation have been in the direction of prevention rather than cure. Prominent among these measures are, firstly, school inspection with the consequent early detection and isolation of infectious cases of conjunctivitis; secondly, maternity and infant welfare accompanied by prompt notification and treatment of the very dangerous and sight-destroying ophthalmia of the new-born; thirdly, improved light regulation in factories and schools; and, fourthly, adequate provision of spectacles for school children with errors of vision.

The recognition of the infectious character of the very chronic and sight-destroying disease known as trachoma, or granular conjunctivitis, has been of great importance for the public health. The disease is common in the Mediterranean area and by no means rare in slum quarters in the West. A rigid system of inspection of immigrants, together with quarantine combined with treatment, has done much to diminish its ravages in the United States.

THE RISE OF PAEDIATRICS

Although a few of the medical writers of antiquity and the Middle Ages had dealt in some detail with the diseases which especially affected children, the beginnings of paediatrics did not appear until at least the late seventeenth century. Of the classical writers Celsus devoted some space to children's diseases, and he stressed the point that the type of treatment prescribed for adults was not suitable for children. Aretaeus (p. 239) gave a brief list of the diseases to which children were specially subject, and in this he mentioned tetanus. In his treatise on gynaecology Soranus of Ephesus (p. 239) devoted over twenty chapters to the hygiene of infancy and to some of the common diseases of infants. Soranus described one condition which may possibly have been rickets, and another ('seiriasis') which has been variously interpreted as sunstroke, spurious hydrocephalus, or meningitis. He gave a definitive account of the curious custom of 'salting the infant', by powdering it with powdered soda-ash, which had been practised for centuries before his time, and which continued to be practised until at least the fifteenth century.

The first work on children's diseases to appear after the invention of printing was *De infantium aegritudinibus et remediis* ('Children's diseases and their treatment', Padua, 1472) of Paolo Bagellardo (?–1492). It was mainly a compilation from the Arabian writers, but it went through three editions. In 1545 there was published in London, as an appendix to another book, a small treatise entitled the *Boke of Children*. The author, Thomas Phaer (?–1560), seems to have been born at Norwich about 1510. (His name is also spelt Faier, Phayre, and in many other variants.) He was also a lawyer of some distinction, and the author of an early, and possibly then best known, translation of a great part of Virgil's *Aeneid* into English. The paediatric work makes available the practice of the older writers, but adds nothing new. Hieronymus Mercurialis (1530–1606), professor of medicine at Bologna and later at Pisa, published in 1583 his *De morbis puerorum* ('On diseases of children'). He had already published a number of books which were important in their time, including a well-known work on ancient gymnastics (1569). His book on paediatrics was prepared by one of his students from his lecture notes. Although based on the writings of the classical authors, it embodies many original views of minor importance. In the seventeenth century the most popular work on paediatrics was the *De morbis acutis infantum* ('On the acute diseases of infants', 1689) of the Englishman Walter Harris (1647–1732). Between its publication in 1689 and 1742 this book passed through eighteen editions in several languages, including three separate English translations. It is not a comprehensive treatise, but a plea for the use of his own method of treatment. As a follower of Franciscus Sylvius (p. 142) Harris believed that many children's diseases are due to the collection of acids in the body. Treatment should therefore consist of the frequent administration of alkalis. His 'Testaceous Medicines' included chalk, cuttle-fish, egg-shells, coral, pearls, and especially oyster-shells, powdered and given suspended in syrup.

The eighteenth century was marked by the publication of several progressive books on children's diseases. The *Essay upon Nursing, and the Management of Children, from their Birth to three Years of Age* was sent to one of the Governors of the Foundling Hospital in London, and was published anonymously by the Committee of that Hospital in 1748. A second anonymous edition followed in the same year, but the third edition bore the name of the author, William Cadogan (1711–97). Cadogan, a Londoner, studied at Oxford and Leyden, and practised in London for many years. He became physician to the Foundling Hospital in 1754. He was also the author of a *Dissertation on the Gout* (1771). His book on children is merely a small tract, but it contains much wisdom and went through at least ten editions. Cadogan criticized the custom, very common at that time, of overloading an infant with clothing and wraps. He was a strong advocate of breast feeding and of a rational choice of food, and he criticized heavily the practice of baby-farming. About the same time there was published at Stockholm (1765) a book on paediatrics which had appeared during the previous year as a series of papers presented to the Swedish Academy of Sciences. Its author was Nils Rosén von Rosenstein (1706–73), the distinguished professor of medicine and colleague of Linnaeus at the University of Uppsala. Rosen's book deals largely with observations made in his own day, and it is specially strong on the management of infants. In his numerous descriptions of individual diseases he is obviously drawing on his own experience. This book was a definite forward step towards the establishment of paediatrics as a speciality.

During the eighteenth century two further important works appeared in Britain. George Armstrong (1720–89), then practising in London, published in 1767 the first edition of his book *An Essay on the Diseases most fatal to Infants*, which in the third edition (1777) was expanded to deal also with older children. Armstrong experimented with different drugs in the treatment of certain diseases. He was the first to use increased muscular irritability as a test for toxaemia, he established the familial nature of congenital pyloric stenosis, and he may have observed cases of poliomyelitis. This book, the establishment of his Dispensary (p. 655), and his teaching of doctors in it, have established him as the founder of modern paediatrics. Some years after this third edition there was published *A Treatise on the Diseases of Children* (1784) by Michael Underwood (1736–1820) of London, who was then specializing in obstetrics, gynaecology, and children's diseases. The first edition was a small work in one volume. The third edition was of two volumes, and the fourth consisted of three volumes. The book passed through at least seventeen editions, and remained a standard work for sixty years. It contained the first published descriptions of several diseases, including sclerema and malignant familial jaundice in the new-born.

In his fourth edition (1799) he discussed the diagnosis and importance of congenital heart disease in children. This discussion was all the more remarkable because at that time little was known of the pathology of these conditions, Auenbrugger's method of percussion was little practised, and Laennec was still a medical student.

Underwood retired from practice in 1801, and to the nineteenth century he bequeathed the fourth edition of his book. With this edition, marked by accurate observation, clear description, and the introduction of sections on the chemistry of milk, paediatrics became modern. In 1804 William Heberden, the Younger (1767–1845), the son of the elder Heberden (p. 36), published his *Morborum puerilium epitome* ('Epitome of children's diseases') which was written in an epigrammatic style and contained much excellent clinical observation in small compass. About this time (1802–8) John Cheyne (p. 535) published a series of essays on individual diseases of children, including one on acute hydrocephalus. After that Cheyne settled in Dublin, where he built up a great reputation. In 1818 he published the first description of the pathological findings in a patient who had shown the type of breathing later known as Cheyne–Stokes respiration (p. 283).

In 1848 there appeared the first edition of the work on paediatrics which in much of the English-speaking world was to supplant Underwood's treatise. This was the *Lectures on the Diseases of Infancy and Childhood* by Charles West (1816–98). West was a physician to several London hospitals, and these lectures were delivered at the Middlesex Hospital. They were based on the fully kept case notes of 600 of the 14,000 children whom West had examined. The book reached a sixth edition. West's other great claim to fame is discussed later.

Paediatrics as a specialty was now becoming established in several countries. In France Charles Michel Billard (1800–32) published in 1828 his *Traité des maladies des enfans nouveau-nés et à la mamelle* ('Treatise on the diseases of infants and sucklings'), in which, as a result of many autopsies carried out by himself, he correlated the post-mortem and clinical findings and introduced a much more scientific system of classification. Possibly the greatest French work of the century on this subject was the *Traité clinique et pratique des maladies des enfants* ('Clinical and practical treatise on diseases of children') by Frédéric Rilliet (1814–61) and Antoine Charles Ernest Barthez (1811–91), the three volumes of which were published between 1838 and 1843. In subsequent editions the individual case histories gradually disappeared, and the modern form of a medical treatise was introduced. Eugène Bouchut (1818–91) of Paris was one of the first to use the ophthalmoscope in the diagnosis of nervous diseases, and he was the author of a large and very successful work on paediatrics (1845). Meanwhile, Trousseau (p. 282) had published the equivalent of a treatise on children's diseases as an integral part of his great work on internal medicine.

In German-speaking countries interest in diseases of children was equally active. Of many outstanding men we mention two. Eduard Heinrich Henoch (1820–1910) was in charge of paediatric work at the Charité at Berlin, and he is now best remembered for his description of the abdominal type of purpura which bears his name (1874). His attitude to children's diseases is essentially modern, as is seen in the published form of his lectures, which first appeared in 1861 and went through eleven editions. Carl A. C. J. Gerhardt (1833–1902) held clinical chairs at Jena, Würzburg, and Berlin, and was also well known as a general physician. As an indication of the extent to which paediatrics had developed by the fourth quarter of the nineteenth century, it may be noted that Gerhardt edited a great collaborative German treatise on paediatrics (*Handbuch der Kinderkrankheiten*) which appeared in sixteen volumes between 1877 and 1893.

In the United States the growth of paediatrics ran somewhat parallel to its growth in the United Kingdom. Charles Delucena Meigs (1792–1869) made many interesting observations on disease in children, including cases of sudden death due to 'heart-clot' or embolism (1849). In the following year Meigs published his *Observations on Certain Diseases of Young Children*, a work showing many features of clinical interest; for example, he compares the chemical composition of human milk and cow's milk, and concludes that the higher casein content of cow's milk accounts for the frequency of digestive disturbances in artificially fed children. But in the publication of a textbook Meigs had already been forestalled by his son John Forsyth

Meigs (1818–82), who at the age of thirty published his work on the diseases of children. It went through four editions. A third bearer of the name, Arthur Vincent Meigs (1850–1912), was a pioneer in the chemical analysis of human and cow's milk, and he wrote an important book on that subject (1885).

Perhaps the most distinguished of the older American paediatricians was Abraham Jacobi (1830–1919). Jacobi was born in Germany and graduated at Bonn in 1851. He was then detained in fortresses because of his supposed revolutionary activities. After two years he escaped to England, and reached New York in 1853. Seven years later he was appointed to the first chair of paediatrics in the New York Medical College—with the facilities afforded by a new paediatric clinic. Jacobi wrote extensively on paediatrics, and he was one of the first to recommend the boiling of milk used for infant feeding. In 1885 a successful method of intubation of the larynx for continued obstruction—as in diphtheria—was introduced by Joseph P. O'Dwyer (1841–98) of New York. Jacobi adopted this method in preference to tracheotomy, of which he had had an extensive experience. Of more recent American paediatricians mention may be made of Luther Emmett Holt (1855–1924), who worked with various chemists on the metabolism of young children. Holt's treatise on the diseases of infancy and childhood (1896) went through many editions.

Elsewhere in this present book there are references to men who have carried out research on individual diseases of children, such as Glisson, Sydenham, Jenner, Robert Whytt, Bretonneau, Heine and Medin, and Leonard Findlay. Among those remembered eponymously for their descriptions of new diseases are Sir Thomas Barlow (1845–1945), who gave an excellent description of infantile scurvy in 1883; and Sir George Frederic Still (1868–1941), who in 1896 described chronic articular rheumatism in children. Among others who have written extensively on children's diseases, including famous textbooks, are John Thomson (1856–1926) of Edinburgh, and his pupil Sir Robert Hutchison (1871–1960) of the London Hospital.

Children's hospitals. Foundling hospitals were established on the continent of Europe from an early date. That at Milan was founded in 787, and many other cities followed in later centuries. In London

Captain Thomas Coram (1668?–1751) obtained in 1739 a charter for the establishment of The Foundling Hospital, and it was founded two years later. Children's hospitals arose not so much from these institutions as from the Dispensary for the Infant Poor established in London by George Armstrong in 1769. The term 'Infant Poor'

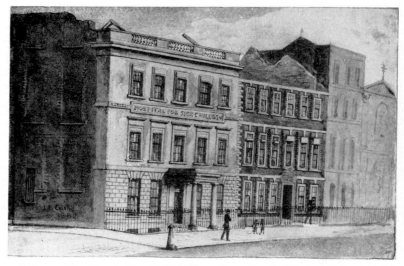

Fig. 129. The Hospital for Sick Children, Great Ormond Street, London, in the house formerly occupied by Dr. Richard Mead
(Water-colour drawing of 1882 by J. P. Emslie in the Wellcome Historical Medical Museum)

referred to children up to twelve years. This was the first institution of its type in the world, and soon after its establishment Armstrong visualized that it might be transformed into a hospital for in-patient treatment. The Dispensary was very successful; but subscribers were few, and for many years Armstrong bore nearly the whole of the expense of running it. It ceased to exist for this reason about 1783. In 1816 John Bunnell Davis (1780–1824) founded a similar dispensary in London, and in the following year he published an inquiry into the high rate of infantile mortality in London and elsewhere. This work led ultimately to the beginnings of voluntary health visitors for the instruction of mothers in the care of their infants. His dispensary was later removed to Waterloo Bridge Road, and ultimately became the Royal Waterloo Hospital for Children and

Women. Before this took place there was an interlude which led to the founding of one of the most famous of all children's hospitals.

The Waterloo Dispensary was extended by similar institutions built close by, and about 1850 Charles West tried to convert these institutions into a true in-patient hospital for children. The attempt failed, and West then carried out a very extensive investigation of children's hospitals in many parts of Europe. In 1852 he established the Hospital for Sick Children in the house at 49 Great Ormond Street which had formerly been occupied by Richard Mead (p. 200) and which had housed his famous museum and library (Fig. 129). In addition to acting as chief physician West organized much of the administration of the hospital, and contributed to its upkeep. The hospital has been enlarged and rebuilt on several occasions, and has long been the headquarters of paediatric teaching in Great Britain. In the United States the first children's hospital was established in New York in 1854.

Orthopaedics. A few remarks may not be out of place here on this subject, especially as it affected children. The subject of orthopaedics arose out of the desire of Nicolas André (1658–1742) to prevent deformities in children. André was professor of medicine at Paris, and at the age of eighty he introduced this subject. Two years later he had coined its name, had developed it considerably, and had published a two-volume treatise on it. This work was entitled *L'orthopédie ou l'art de prévenir et de corriger dans les enfans les difformités du corps* ('Orthopaedics, or the art of preventing and correcting bodily deformities in children', 1741). Within a comparatively short time the new methods had passed into the hands of the surgeon, and the main questions centred round the methods by which bone is formed. Feeding experiments with the dye madder were carried out on animals by the French scientist Henri Louis Duhamel du Monceau (1700–82), and he showed that only certain portions of their bones were stained by the dye. He concluded from the distribution of the stained areas that bone is formed by the periosteum. John Hunter claimed that in bone formation two processes are going on simultaneously, namely deposition of bone and absorption of bone. In many ways Hunter emphasized the great lesson that complete rest of the part is the most effective healer.

Especially important was the work of Jacques Mathieu Delpech (1777-1832) of Montpellier, who has been justly described as the real founder of the specialty. Before his time the tendo Achillis had been cut for the cure of club-foot, but the results had been bad. Delpech performed the operation in 1816, and he developed the procedure into a very useful method, applicable to the contractures of other muscles. Delpech held the chair of surgery at Montpellier, and he established between that city and Toulouse a fine hospital devoted to his orthopaedic work. In 1828 he published *L'orthomorphie*, in which his methods were fully discussed. Dupuytren (p. 184) played a part in the development of orthopaedics, though his interests were much wider. A certain type of fracture of the fibula and a contracture of the fascia of the palm of the hand still bear his name. He was the first to treat wry-neck by division of the sternomastoid muscle. A little later Duchenne (p. 273) was striving to conserve muscles by electrical treatment, and his ideas were adopted by some of his surgical friends. The conservative principle was dignified by the weight of authority when adopted by Sir Benjamin Collins Brodie (1783-1862), an expert on bones and joints. As president of the Royal College of Surgeons he had much influence on younger men. Some years later John Hilton (1804-78) of Guy's Hospital was teaching that the surgeon's main function was to remove any tissue which might impede the restorative powers of nature. His *Rest and Pain* (1863) contains lessons which are timeless, and it is a book which is still much read today.

The method of tendon division still had many supporters, and among these was Georg Friedrich Ludwig Stromeyer (1804-76) who studied in Germany and Great Britain. After years of disappointment Stromeyer had, at the age of twenty-nine years, a case of club-foot successfully cured by subcutaneous tenotomy. Three years later he had divided the tendons by this method in nearly 700 cases.

The founder of orthopaedic surgery in Great Britain was William John Little (1810-94). He had himself a club-foot, and Stromeyer divided the tendon with a successful result. Little then determined to specialize in orthopaedics, and in 1838 he founded the Orthopaedic Hospital in London. His book, *On the Nature and Treatment of the Deformities of the Human Frame* (1853), was the first British treatise on the subject. Little is known for his description of the type of spastic paralysis of infants which bears his name.

Orthopaedics was further greatly developed by the very ingenious methods of Hugh Owen Thomas (1834–91), the son of a bone-setter in Liverpool. Thomas studied medicine at Edinburgh, under Syme and J. Y. Simpson, at London and at Paris. He devised the Thomas's splint and other mechanical appliances called after him. Thomas taught his nephew (Sir) Robert Jones (1857–1933), who greatly developed the modern methods of tendon transplantation and bone grafting. In the United States the greatest of the early followers of orthopaedic surgery were Philip Syng Physick (p. 351), the professor of surgery in the University of Pennsylvania, and Henry Jacob Bigelow (1818–90) of Boston.

While these figures were passing across the stage the controversy regarding the growth of bone and articular cartilege still continued. In the latter sphere excellent work was done by Peter Redfern (1821–1912) of Aberdeen. He showed that the cells of articular cartilege act differently from osteoblasts, and that it is never repaired by its own tissue. Reference has been made to the lengthy experiments of Macewen of Glasgow on the growth of bone (p. 368). He was convinced that bone arose, not from the periosteum, but from bone itself. In 1880 he put his conviction to a crucial test. He then saw a boy of five years who, two years previously, had had a severe osteo-myelitis of the humerus; except for small portions of bone at the upper and lower extremities of the bone, the whole shaft had been resected, and the arm was useless. Macewen removed wedges of bone from the tibiae of boys suffering from rachitic deformities and transplanted them into the space formerly occupied by the shaft of the patient's humerus. Most of the grafts were devoid of periosteum, but they grew and formed a new shaft. Thirty years later the patient had a useful arm, and the humerus had almost doubled its length.

THE TEETH AND THEIR DISEASES

The symptom which until recent years most urgently drove an individual to consult a dentist or doctor about a carious tooth was pain. Though other methods for the relief of pain are now commonly employed, the final method is to extract the offending tooth, and this practice has been in use from quite early times. There are references to tooth-extraction in the Greek medical writers, but Hippocrates assumed that only loose teeth could be extracted. The Arabian writers also referred to extraction, and Abulcasis (p. 76) gave the first illustrations of dental instruments.

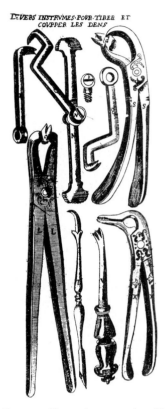

DIVERS INSTRVMES·POVR·TIRER ET COVPPER LES DENS

We have, however, considerable knowledge of dental instruments used from the fifteenth century onwards. The pelican, so called from its supposed resemblance to a pelican's beak, was used to lever the tooth out of its socket. In its simplest form it consisted of a straight shaft with an enlargement called a bolster at one end, and hinged to its centre one end of a shank, the other end of which was curved to form a claw. The lengths of the shank and shaft were such that, when the shank was folded along the shaft, the claw projected over the bolster. In use the bolster was placed at the root of the affected tooth, or of an adjacent tooth, and the claw was then folded over the affected tooth. On forcible depression of the shaft the bolster acted as a fulcrum and the tooth was

FIG. 130. Sixteenth-century dental instruments. Three different types of extraction forceps, three pelicans, and two elevators are shown

(J. Guillemeau, Œuvres de chirurgie, Rouen, 1649)

levered out. The use of the pelican must have caused much damage to the tissues. Another instrument for extraction was the dental key, or English key. It was about the size of an ordinary corkscrew, and consisted of a metal shaft with a transverse handle at one end. At the other end was a bolster, together with a hinged claw which could move in a plane at right angles to the axis of the shaft. The bolster

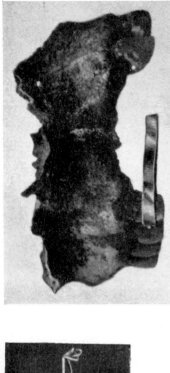

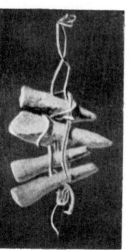

(a)

(c)

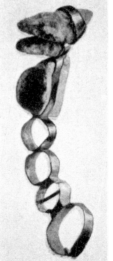

(b)

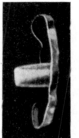

(d)

FIG. 131. Early artificial teeth

(a) Greek prosthetic appliance (Archaeological Museum, Athens);
(b) Etruscan appliance, *in situ* in upper jaw (Museum of University of Ghent);
(c) Etruscan appliance supporting three artificial teeth (Civic Museum of Corneto);
(d) Roman appliance, with gold crown for lower incisor.

(a, b, c, d, from Guerini, *History of Dentistry*)

was placed against the root of the tooth, and the claw was then hinged over its crown. A forcible turn of the handle then extracted the tooth. The English key was first mentioned about 1740 and was in common use until at least 1860. An instrument used especially for extracting

Figure des Dents artificielles.

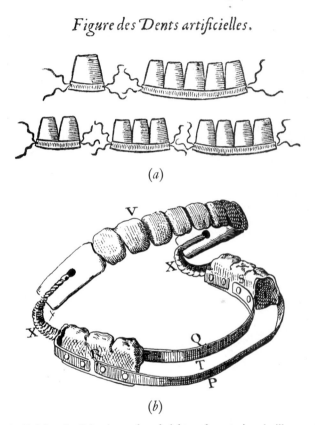

(a)

(b)

FIG. 132. Artificial teeth of the sixteenth and eighteenth centuries. As illustrated (a) by Ambroise Paré (*Œuvres*, 1575); (b) by Fauchard (*Chirurgien dentiste*, 1746)

stumps was the dental elevator, in use from Arabian times onwards. It consisted essentially of a short, pointed shaft which was used to lever out the stump.

The forceps is the instrument which is now used for tooth extraction, and in its evolution it has undergone many changes in design (Fig. 130). It was illustrated by Abulcasis (p. 76). From the sixteenth century onwards several different types were used, each designated by the supposed resemblance of the blades to the beak of a particular bird. The modern form of the forceps is due largely to (Sir) John Tomes (1815–95), who invented the various types in 1839–40 while he was a house-surgeon at the Middlesex Hospital. Tomes did valuable work on the structure of the teeth; and he was mainly responsible for the introduction of the licence in dentistry in 1858, and for the founding of the Odontological Society.

From early times attempts have been made to provide artificial teeth to replace those lost naturally or extracted. The earliest fixed denture of which we have knowledge was found in a Phoenician grave at Sidon; the four substitute teeth were strung together and fitted to the adjacent teeth with gold wire. Many Etruscan fixed dentures have also been discovered. As substitutes for the missing teeth the Etruscans used human teeth or artificial teeth carved from ox teeth. Each substitute tooth was surrounded at its base by a gold ring, and these were soldered together and to two other rings which surrounded the two adjacent natural teeth. These Phoenician and Etruscan specimens are the earliest examples of gold bridges. Paré described the use of artificial teeth carved from bone or hippopotamus or walrus ivory, and Jacques Guillemeau (p. 646) was the first to recommend artificial teeth made from inorganic materials; his recipe included white coral and pearls.

Removable dentures were greatly improved by Pierre Fauchard (1678–1761), whose remarkable work *Le chirurgien dentiste, ou traité des dents* ('The surgeon dentist, or treatise of the teeth', 1728), was the first book to be devoted entirely to the subject and to cover it in all its aspects. Fauchard did not make an impression of the mouth when he was constructing a denture. A piece of bone or ivory was roughly carved to the required shape; then the teeth were carved in it, and the denture was worked on until it fitted the mouth. These dentures were usually kept in position by means of springs. Fauchard also employed the artificial crown. The natural crown of the tooth was removed, the pulp cavity was filled with lead, and into it the artificial crown was fixed by a pin or a dowel.

Improvements in the manufacture of individual artificial teeth took place especially in the first half of the nineteenth century. It

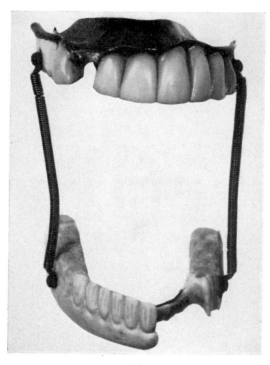

(*a*)

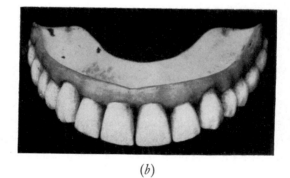

(*b*)

FIG. 133. Early dentures of the nineteenth century
(*a*) upper and lower dentures with springs;
(*b*) upper denture, base of ivory, with teeth pegged in
(*a* and *b* in the Wellcome Historical Medical Museum)

was found that food and the fluids of the mouth acted on natural and ivory teeth and produced an unpleasant smell and taste. As a result of the collaboration of two Frenchmen, the apothecary Duchâteau and the dentist Nicolas Dubois de Chémant (1753–1824), complete dentures of porcelain were first produced in 1788. A generation later the Neapolitan Giuseppangelo Fonzi (1768–1840), who was then practising dentistry in Paris, experimented with different porcelain mixtures and by 1808 he had succeeded in making individual teeth of that material. Each tooth had a platinum hook fixed in it to facilitate the attachment of the tooth to a separate base-plate. There were many technical difficulties, but by 1840 the manufacture of porcelain teeth had been perfected. Two years previously Claudius Ash had introduced the tube tooth which in a modified form is still in use. The original type had a small tube of a precious metal fused in its centre, and this tube could easily be fitted over a projecting pivot in a root or in a base.

The history of the dental crown provides an example of a change in popularity which is due partly to fashion and partly to scientific principles. Fauchard (p. 663) was one of the first to fit crowns to individual teeth successfully. In the year of the second edition of Fauchard's book (1746), Claude Mouton (?–1786) described a gold crown, which was fixed into the root by a pin. A later development was a shell of gold which fitted like a cap over the remaining part of the natural tooth. The final stage was a gold crown cast from a wax mould. About 1850 the 'banded crown' appeared, the crown being encircled by a gold band which served as an additional method of fixing it to the root. By joining together by a gold bar two teeth thus crowned, a support was provided for artificial teeth attached to the bar. This is the principle of the crown and bridge work first used by Fauchard. It had a remarkable vogue after the introduction of porcelain teeth about 1840.

During the first decade of the twentieth century extensive investigations were carried out by William Hunter (1861–1937) of Charing Cross Hospital, London, into the constitutional effects of dental sepsis, especially the production of pernicious anaemia. As a result the crown, and particularly crown and bridge work, began to fall into disfavour.

Nowadays all this is avoided by the removable denture, but this has developed slowly. Reference has already been made to the work of Fauchard and others (p. 663). The problem involves the choice of a substance which will take an accurate impression of the mouth,

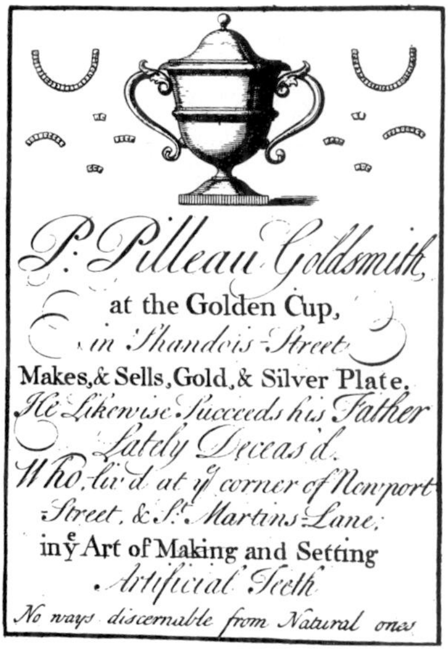

FIG. 134. Trade-card of Pezé Pilleau, goldsmith and maker of artificial teeth. (In the collection of Sir Ambrose Heal)

and the development of a material for a base which will be strong, easily worked, and not eroded by the acids in the mouth. About 1733 the goldsmith Pezé Pilleau (*fl.* 1715–55) used wax for taking impressions. Pilleau has been stated to have been a Frenchman, but he seems to have been an Englishman who carried on his trade of goldsmith and maker of artificial teeth at the Golden Cup on the Paved Stones in Chandos Street, Westminster, from 1719 to at least 1755. Fig. 134 is an example of his trade-card, which is also interesting as regards Pilleau's father, another Pezé, who carried on the same trade. In 1746 Philip Pfaff (1716–80), the dentist to Frederick the Great of Prussia, used wax in the taking of impressions. Plaster of Paris for impressions came to be widely used after 1844, but its disadvantages led to the introduction of the first compound material thirteen years later. At the present time the compounds used for taking impressions consist of colloids such as agar-agar, mixed with waxes and synthetic resins.

The first moderately satisfactory material used for the manufacture of the base of the denture was gold. Though strong and not subject to erosion, it was not easily worked and fixing individual teeth to the gold base was tedious. We have already mentioned that by 1788 Dubois de Chémant was making complete dentures of porcelain—the teeth and the dental base or plate which was fitted into the mouth were all of one piece. Fonzi's manufacture of single teeth of porcelain (1808) stimulated a search for a suitable base to carry them. During the early nineteenth century various materials were used as bases for dentures, such as a type of gum tried in France, and a 'silver paste' which was an amalgam of silver and mercury. In 1847 Edwin Truman (1809–1905) used gutta-percha as a base for dentures. Three years later tortoise-shell was introduced as a base, and then celluloid. In 1855 Charles Goodyear (1800–60) obtained a patent for vulcanite as a base, and its use later became general. Collodion was also used about this time, and about 1870 celluloid began to have a vogue which lasted until the end of the century.

It will be seen that the provision of a suitable material for a base presented very great difficulties. Shortly after the First World War the use of synthetic resins became common. These materials are grouped into two types, the thermo-plastic resins and the thermo-setting resins. The former do not undergo a chemical change during the processing, while the latter do. The first of the thermo-plastics, celluloid, was also the first to be used extensively for the making of dentures. This substance, hard at ordinary temperatures, becomes plastic on heating and can be moulded to the required shape. As the heating does not bring about a chemical change, the process of heating and remoulding can be repeated. Of the thermo-setting resins bakelite was most widely used for artificial dentures. It had, however, certain disadvantages. In 1935 polymerized acrylic resin (methyl methacrylate) was first used for this purpose and has generally been found very satisfactory.

Having dealt briefly with the history of radical dentistry, that is, the replacement of unsound teeth by artificial teeth, we now deal with conservative dentistry, or the methods used to arrest caries in individual teeth. Hollow teeth seem to have been filled by crude methods from very early times, but the practice aimed rather at the rounding off of rough edges and corners than at the arrest of the carious process. Celsus (p. 53) mentions this practice, and it would seem that wax, resin, and gold foil were thus used about that time. Joannes Arculanus (*fl.* fifteenth cent.) probably used gold foil extensively for this purpose. It is not very clear when the carious cavity was first cleaned out before it was filled. In the Middle Ages the cautery was probably used to prevent further decay; and Fabricius ab Aquapendente (p. 97) used a drill, followed by the instillation of a strong acid and the cautery, and finally filled the cleaned cavity with gold leaf. Guillemeau's (p. 646) paste was used not only for the preparation of artificial teeth but also for the filling of cavities.

With Pierre Fauchard (p. 663) a new stage was reached in the treatment of caries. His book suggests the master, familiar with every professional detail, who had put to the test all known methods. In dealing with a carious cavity Fauchard first cleaned out the carious matter, and he describes in detail the instruments which he used. Pain was treated by the application of oil of cinnamon. The cavity was filled with tin, lead, or gold, with a preference for tin. The metal in thin foil was inserted into the cavity in very small portions with specially designed pluggers.

The use of an amalgam of mercury and silver, plastic when prepared and setting later to a crystalline mass, has given rise to controversy. This 'silver paste' was probably first devised in France in 1826, but first extensively used by Joseph Murphy of London eleven years later. It was later found to be subject to changes of temperature and other external conditions, but it took over forty years to produce more satisfactory amalgams, due to the work of Thomas Fletcher, Sir John Tomes (p. 662), and Sir Charles Sissmore Tomes (1846–1928) in England, and of Josiah Foster Flagg (1789–1853) and Greene Vardiman Black (1836–1915) in the United States. Research had long been done on the use of solid fillings for cavities. When more accurate methods of taking impressions of cavities were introduced it was found possible to fill these by cast inlays of gold, and porcelain was also used for this purpose. Much work was also done on the introduction of silicate compounds for plastic fillings.

In recent times there has been considerable controversy about the best method of preparing a carious cavity. Fauchard certainly recognized that it was essential to remove all the decayed matter from the wall of the cavity. For this purpose he used hand instruments and also a simple drill twisted by the fingers alternately right and left. Fauchard describes the use of the jeweller's bow-drill, but this was in the manufacture of artificial teeth and it was practically unused in dentistry. Charles Merry of St. Louis invented about 1850 a hand-drill driven by a toothed wheel. Eight years later he improved the instrument by fitting to it a flexible shaft, consisting of a close-coiled spiral wire, an appliance which had been invented in 1829 by the Scottish engineer James Nasmyth (1808–90), who later became famous for his steam-hammer. The improved Merry drill was therefore the forerunner of the modern dental engine. In 1870 a foot-operated engine on the same principle appeared, and in 1908 electric power was first used to operate the flexible cable. A further advance in the preparation of the cavity was the recognition of the fact that before the filling was introduced the cavity had to be rendered quite dry. A sheet of rubber shaped to surround the tooth (1864) was the first step in this direction. The problem was not easy, but in recent years great progress has been made by the use of rolls of gauze to isolate the tooth, and by the final drying of the cavity with hot air.

The cause of dental caries has been one of the most discussed subjects in the history of dentistry. From Babylonian times at least it was believed that small worms in the decayed tooth caused the decay. The Roman writer Scribonius Largus (*fl.* A.D. 40) advised for this condition fumigation of the tooth with the vapour produced by casting hyoscyamus seeds on burning charcoal. It was asserted that the worms would be seen falling out of the teeth. An identical method was recommended by Guy de Chauliac (p. 83) many centuries later. Doubts about the correctness of this view arose in the sixteenth century, but Fauchard in 1706 is said to have finally overthrown it. Nevertheless this erroneous view continued to be expressed for some years.

John Hunter (p. 177) is usually regarded as one of the founders of modern scientific dentistry because of two of his books. These were *The Natural History of the Human Teeth* (1771), and *A Practical Treatise on the Diseases of the Teeth* (1778), in which he discussed appliances for malocclusion. Hunter concluded that the carious process starts on the surface of the tooth and not in its interior, and that the process is especially liable to be found where food particles tend to lodge. This view was completely substantiated by Levi Spear Parmly, an American dentist working in London. Parmly examined thousands of teeth taken from the bodies of those who had fallen in battle, and he showed (1820) that the initial aperture in the enamel is so minute as to escape attention unless it is looked for deliberately. The search for micro-organisms of disease included the study of dental caries, but it was soon shown that there was no particular micro-organism responsible, and that the carious process is conditioned by other factors. Clinical and experimental investigations by (Lady) May Mellanby showed that the onset of caries is determined partly by deficiency of certain substances in the diet, especially salts of calcium and phosphorus and certain vitamins, and that a part is also played by the structure of the tooth, which is determined largely by the diet in the developmental period. The recent researches on this complex subject are beyond the scope of this book.

During the last fifty years the condition of the teeth of the community has been vastly improved. Three factors have contributed to this. First, artificial dentures were greatly improved, and made more freely available, as a result of the assistance given, at first by the National Health Insurance Act of 1911, and more recently under the National Health Service Act, 1946. Preventive dentistry was given a great impetus by the establishment of school dental clinics, beginning in 1912. Thirdly, the mouths of many children were greatly improved by developments in the practice of orthodontics. John Hunter wrote much on dental irregularities, but the first book devoted exclusively to irregularities of the teeth was published by Charles Gaine of Bath in 1858. In 1880 the distinguished American dentist Norman William Kingsley (1829–1913) published his book entitled *Oral Deformities*, a comprehensive treatise which is generally regarded as having laid the foundations of the subject. Another prominent American worker was John Nutting Farrar (1839–1913), who developed the mechanical appliances which were considered necessary to correct malposition of the teeth. The modern practice of orthodontics was founded by Edward Hartley Angle (1855–1930), who in 1900 gave the first specialized course in the subject. Angle headed the movement against the indiscriminate extraction of permanent teeth for the correction of faulty natural dentures, and his work also led to considerable simplification in the corrective appliances which were then in use.

THE STUDY AND USE OF THE NATURAL DRUGS

(a) The History of the Pharmacopoeias

The modern pharmacopoeias are a strange mixture of the ancient and the modern, and in no other branch of medicine is the force of tradition so clearly seen. A pharmacopoeia is a list of drugs prepared for a certain group of physicians, or a certain hospital, city, or country. The drugs contained in the list are chosen by agreement and are supposed to be accepted as valuable by the majority of those who use them. In the later pharmacopoeias there is given under the name of each drug a description of the source from which the crude drug is obtained, approved methods of preparation and testing, and the standard dose. From the earliest times it was intended that drug-lists should serve as guides, not only for the physicians who prescribed the drugs but also for the apothecaries or pharmacists who made up the prescriptions. We have referred to the medical papyri, to the great treatise on materia medica by Dioscorides and to the drugs of Galen (pp. 53, 59). In the fifteenth century certain treatises on drugs were written in Italy, but these had no official standing. The most important of these books was the Commentary on the works of Dioscorides by Pietro Andrea Mattioli (1501–77) of Siena. Mattioli practised in several cities and was later personal physician to the Emperor Maximilian II. This book introduced the plants of Dioscorides to the sixteenth-century Italians. It was first published in 1544 and went through many editions.

In 1498 the first pharmacopoeia in the modern sense was published in Florence as the *Nuovo Receptario Composito* ('The New Compound Dispensatory'), the first edition of the *Ricettario Fiorentino* ('The Florentine Dispensatory'), which was made the official and obligatory guide for the apothecaries of Florence. Other Italian cities soon published their own official pharmacopoeias—Mantua in 1559, Bologna in 1574, Rome in 1580, and Venice in 1618—but on the rest of the Continent pharmacopoeias did not appear until later.

In England a proposal for an official pharmacopoeia had been made by the College of Physicians in 1585, but publication was long delayed. Among those active in the final stages of its preparation was Sir Theodore Turquet de Mayerne (1573-1655), court physician to the Early Stuarts, who was responsible for the inclusion of certain chemical remedies which had been recommended by Paracelsus (p. 100) and others. Eventually the *Pharmacopoeia Londinensis* was published in May 1618, but was withdrawn and a revised edition issued in December of the same year. This, though really a new pharmacopoeia, is generally referred to as the second edition of the First London Pharmacopoeia. It was superseded by the Second London Pharmacopoeia in 1650. The Fourth London Pharmacopoeia (first edition, 1721) is interesting because in it an attempt was made to omit the many superstitious and disgusting remedies that had been officially recognized for more than a century. The Tenth—and last—London Pharmacopoeia appeared in 1851. Several editions of each of these pharmacopoeias were issued. Meanwhile the highly successful and internationally known *Pharmacopoeia Edinburgensis* appeared in 1699. Of the various Edinburgh Pharmacopoeias some fifteen editions in all were published. The less well known Dublin Pharmacopoeia was first issued in 1807.

In 1858 the Medical Act created the General Medical Council, one of the duties of which was to compile an official pharmacopoeia for the whole of the United Kingdom, to supersede the three current Pharmacopoeias. This was to be called *The British Pharmacopoeia*, and the first edition of the first British Pharmacopoeia was published in 1864. The Pharmacopoeia is prepared for the General Medical Council by a Pharmacopoeia Commission of experts. The fifth British Pharmacopoeia was first published in 1914 and remained in force until 1932. The sixth British Pharmacopoeia was published in 1932, the seventh in 1948, the eighth in 1953, and the ninth in 1958. The different intervals between successive publications will be noted. The General Medical Council prepares and issues the British Pharmacopoeia under the authority of various Medical Acts, now consolidated by the Medical Act, 1956. By this Act the Council is empowered to cause to be published new editions of the British Pharmacopoeia at such intervals as they may determine. The Sub-Committee of the Committee of Civil Research had recommended that ten years would be a suitable interval between successive issues; but in 1947 the General Council, on the recommendation of its Pharmacopoeia Commission, resolved that from 1948 the normal interval should be five years, and that during each of the intervals an addendum should be published. In 1955 therefore an Addendum to the eighth Pharmacopoeia was published. The period 1914–58 has seen great changes in the materia medica; and in studying the history of drugs since the First World War it is desirable to consider the fifth British Pharmacopoeia in some detail. It contained about 140 crude vegetable drugs, and it is interesting to note that of these roughly a third were known and used by the time of Galen; another third were added during the Middle Ages and after the discovery of America; and the remainder were eighteenth- and nineteenth-century additions.

For example, acacia, aniseed, castor-oil, coriander, juniper, myrrh, poppy, and turpentine are all mentioned in the Egyptian medical papyri. The Egyptians used also some mineral remedies which are still employed, such as alum, copper salts, sodium carbonate and bicarbonate, sulphur, and possibly some arsenical compounds. Assyrian medical tablets refer to most of the Egyptian drugs as well as to others such as almond oil and liquorice. Early Indian medicine had a very extensive materia medica, and *Cannabis indica* ('hashish' or Indian hemp), cardamoms, colocynth, cassia, and datura were all introduced from India. It is possible that mercury preparations were also of Indian origin.

The medical herb lore of the Greeks comes to us chiefly from Dioscorides (p. 53), who mentions about 500 plants, some of which are still used, but others are now unidentifiable. Besides the Egyptian, Assyrian, and Indian drugs mentioned above, these included aloes, ammoniacum, chamomile, cinnamon, cloves, crocus, dill, hyoscyamus, linseed, liquorice, male fern, mustard, pome-granate, rhubarb, rosemary, scammony, sesame, squill, stavesacre, tragacanth, and valerian. The Arabians derived their pharmacopoeia direct from the Greeks, but they also added many new drugs such as belladonna, caraway, cubebs, dandelion, nutmeg, and senna. Of drugs introduced from America we have already discussed cinchona and ipecacuanha; others were arachis (ground-nut) oil, cascara sagrada, capsicum, catechu, copaiba, guaiac, and jalap. Of the many additions made in the eighteenth and nineteenth centuries, few were important, though these included podophyllum from America, and digitalis (p. 683). A notable addition which was made in the early nineteenth century was the drastic purgative, croton oil, brought from India about 1812.

The sixth, seventh, eighth and ninth British Pharmacopoeias (1932–58) have successively eliminated many of these crude veget-able drugs, but they have also introduced many synthetic drugs to which reference will be made later. About eighty-five of these vegetable drugs which were officially used in the 1920's have now been eliminated, and about fifty still remain. Among those drugs which no longer appear are ammoniacum, asafetida, cajuput, canna-bis indica, cantharides, cassia, catechu, chamomile, colocynth, copaiba, croton oil, cubebs, guaiac, jalap, juniper, East Indian kino, mustard, myrrh, scammony, serpentaria, spearmint, squill, staves-acre, and valerian. The deletions from the ninth (1958) Pharmacopoeia in this category include clove, creosote, fennel, lavender oil, nut-meg, and quassia.

As the British Pharmacopoeia is an official work on the preparation and standards of drugs which are in current use, it must necessarily include only those substances concerning the reliability of which there can be no doubt. But new drugs or preparations which have passed laboratory tests have to be used in the treatment of disease in human patients before their efficacy and usefulness can be thoroughly established. In 1903 the Council of the Pharmaceutical Society of Great Britain decided that there was a need for a work of reference which would include not only official drugs but also drugs which have not yet become official, together with some drugs which were still used although excluded from the current British

Pharmacopoeia. As a result the First British Pharmaceutical Codex was prepared and was published in 1907. The Codex was subsequently revised and reissued in 1911, 1923, 1934, 1949, 1954, and 1959. Drugs included in it but not in the British Pharmacopoeia are labelled 'B.P.C.'.

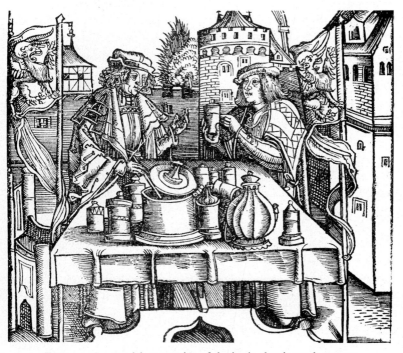

FIG. 135. Ceremonial preparation of theriac in the sixteenth century
(H. von Braunschweig, *Liber de arte distillandi*, Strasbourg, 1512)

In former times a vast number of drugs were habitually employed by physicians, and they were often given in very complicated prescriptions. The most remarkable example of this practice was the use of the remedy known as theriac. The first description of the preparation of this remedy was in verse and was dedicated to the Emperor Nero. It was supposed to be a sovereign remedy against all poisons, and it was credited as effective against most other ailments. In early periods of its existence it contained about sixty different ingredients, of which the flesh of the viper was the most

important. In the Renaissance period it was prepared under ceremonial conditions in the presence of civic and medical dignitaries
(Fig. 135). In English literature theriac was first mentioned in 1124,
and references to it are frequent in Chaucer and Milton. The
number of ingredients always remained large, and the remedy was
very widely used. When Claude Bernard was an apprentice apothecary about 1830, he was warned by his master not to throw away any
remedy which he had spoiled in making up a prescription; the result
of his bad technique was to be kept, as it could always be used in
making theriac.

For centuries physicians were prone to write long and complicated prescriptions on the principle of a blunderbuss. 'Polypharmacy', the prescribing of complex mixtures of drugs, is a vice
from which medicine has now in large part freed itself. The number
of drugs given by scientific physicians is far fewer than it was. For
this there are several reasons. Firstly, many drugs were found
useless for the purpose for which they were administered, and were
at times even dangerous. Secondly, since attention has been drawn
to the active principles of drugs rather than to the crude natural
drugs, it has been seen that, in fact, many of the drugs that were
being given were merely duplicates one of another, and that often
the administration of the active principle itself was more effective
and more reliable than that of the source from which it was obtained.

(b) *Contents of a Modern Pharmacopoeia*

The reader may ask what is the general nature of the drugs administered by scientific physicians today. The question is not easy
to answer. Despite all the simplification and elimination of recent
years, the current editions of standard works on materia medica
and pharmacology divide the officially used drugs into about fifty
different classes. We must be content with some comments on a few
of the commoner and more widely used classes of drugs.

The group of inorganic and organic acids used to be considered
to act by a simple chemical reaction in the stomach, but it is now
known that they are rapidly converted into salts, and that after
absorption their main function is to affect the alkali content of the
blood. This in turn leads to a complex chain of reactions. The

fifth British Pharmacopoeia contained numerous inorganic and organic acids, many of which were not primarily used for their acid properties. Deletions of the common inorganic acids have been heavy. Sulphuric and sulphurous acids went out early; nitric is now deleted in the ninth British Pharmacopoeia, and only hydrochloric acid remains. The carbonates and bicarbonates of the alkali and alkaline earth metals are used to neutralize acidity and they then act by a simple chemical reaction. Other salts of these metals are used for various purposes; for instance, the iodides to increase secretion as expectorants, and the bromides as soporifics. Salts of the remaining metals contribute about the same number of drugs to the eighth as to the fifth British Pharmacopoeia, but it is true to say that some are now much less used than formerly. For instance, lead when taken internally is a cumulative poison, and it is no longer thus used in treatment. Antimony, formerly so popular and reputedly effective as to have been the subject of a book entitled *The Triumphal Chariot of Antimony*, is now practically only used in the treatment of certain protozoal diseases. On the other hand, iron is an essential constituent of haemoglobin, the oxygen-carrying pigment of the blood. It is important in the treatment of anaemia; but recent research has shown that it is dependent for its effect on the presence of a minute trace of copper. In the ninth British Pharmacopoeia this process of removing further salts of the heavy metals has been carried a stage farther. Notable deletions are mercuric chloride, and also mercurous chloride (calomel) which was so extensively given until recent years.

A word may be said about the purgatives, which as a group are amongst the oldest drugs in the pharmacopoeia. The only commonly employed mineral purgative now remaining is magnesium sulphate (Epsom salts), and the only synthetic organic purgative in general use is phenolphthalein. The purgatives act in different ways, and they also vary in the time necessary to produce their effects. Of the drastic purgatives—colocynth, croton oil, jalap, podophyllum, and scammony—the only one which remains in the pharmacopoeia is podophyllum, and it is now used almost only externally for other purposes.

From the historical aspect two very interesting groups of remedies are the vegetable bitters and the volatile, or essential, oils. The simple bitters act on the nerves of taste and produce an increased flow of saliva and gastric juice. If given before food they act as general tonics and appetizers. Thirty years ago the physician had a choice of at least eleven different official drugs of this class, but nowadays only about six of the most effective are used. The volatile oils are complex mixtures. They are obtained from plants by distillation, and they include all the substances which can be thus obtained without damaging the plants. They impart the characteristic odour to some species of plants, and the oils of cinnamon, ginger, and peppermint are used to give a pleasant taste to medicines. Certain other oils were formerly used to give a medicine an unpleasant taste, the resultant effect being psychological. The essential oils used in medicine have other mild effects. They cause the eructation of gas from the stomach, and are thus used in the treatment of children. Some of them also have a mild effect on the secretion of the bronchi and of the kidneys. Individual brands of liqueurs owe their peculiar flavours to essential oils. These substances have been distilled from the time of the Late Middle Ages, and it was to them that the large number of plant remedies which were formerly in use owed their reputed efficacy. The chemical investigation of these essential oils is very difficult, and much of our knowledge of them is due to the work of Frederick Belding Power (1853–1927). Only in the present century was it realized that many essential oils are highly dangerous, and their elimination led to a notable reduction of the vegetable remedies in the official pharmacopoeia. Less than half a dozen essential oils still remain in the pharmacopoeia.

A class of drugs that has in recent years shown a notable increase in numbers is that of the synthetic organic compounds (that is, substances which do not occur in Nature and are produced entirely from inorganic sources). Of some ninety of these drugs which occur in the eighth, but not in the fifth, British Pharmacopoeia, about 20 per cent. are represented by the chemotherapeutic remedies (pp. 687 ff.), and more than a further 30 per cent. are anaesthetics, hypnotics, and other drugs acting on the nervous system. The remaining drugs are used for various purposes, including the treatment of parasitic and skin conditions. Some are disinfectants, and others are used for special radiological examinations. The five years since 1953 have seen an enormous production of new synthetic drugs, of which of course only some have justified their existence. Nevertheless, sixteen of these synthetic drugs were added in the Addendum of 1955, and a further fifty-six are included in the ninth British Pharmacopoeia (1958). The number of new synthetic drugs added to the official Pharmacopoeia in this period 1953–8, and not subsequently deleted, is therefore seventy-two; and the synthetic drugs in the British Pharmacopoeia has now reached the impressive total of over 160.

It is interesting to note the almost complete change in the character of the official preparations, as a result of which many of the old-fashioned tinctures and mixtures have become obsolete. Many of them were excluded from the sixth Pharmacopoeia, when the number of these preparations fell by over a hundred. Further deletions occurred from the seventh and eighth Pharmacopoeias, but the numbers have been partially made up by the inclusion of about 150 compressed tablets and prepared injections.

We have already referred to the hormones (p. 519), the vaccines and antitoxins (pp. 409 ff.), and the vitamins (pp. 610 ff.), and we now proceed to discuss at greater length the active principles derived from the crude vegetable drugs.

(c) *Active Principles: Alkaloids and Glycosides*

One of the things that separates the practice of medicine of our time from that of previous ages is our power to give drugs in 'pure' form. This means not only that we can secure drugs without adulteration, but also that the active substances in drugs can be chemically isolated and given without admixture. Most drugs used in medicine are, in fact, of vegetable origin. The possibility of giving them in chemically pure form depends upon the discovery, early in the nineteenth century, that plants owe their poisonous and remedial properties to small quantities of active principles, which are susceptible of chemical extraction and isolation. Thus the science that deals with the action and nature of drugs, pharmacology, really took its rise about 140 years ago, though many had experimented with drugs at an earlier date.

The group of active principles consists almost entirely of the alkaloids. It also contains a few important glycosides and several other substances.

By alkaloid is understood a nitrogenous substance, usually of vegetable origin, which forms salts with acids. The alkaloids are mainly obtained from the dicotyledonous plants. Generally they occur in nature in combination with plant acids such as citric or tartaric acid. The alkaloid group contains some of the most important drugs that we possess. Among them are morphine, strychnine, cocaine, atropine, and quinine. Their chemical structure is usually complicated, and in consequence attempts to synthesize them have not met in the past with much success. It has, however, been possible to prepare a few modifications of the naturally occurring alkaloids by means of comparatively simple chemical processes.

The investigation of the alkaloids began with the nineteenth century. Alkaloids were isolated from opium by the Parisian apothecary Charles Louis Derosne (1780–1846) in 1803. He failed, however, to recognize the nature of morphine, which was first grasped in 1805 by the German, Friedrich Wilhelm Adam Sertürner (1783–1841). Their work, however, attracted but little notice until attention was drawn to it by the French chemist Joseph Louis Gay-Lussac (1778–1850), in 1817. The result was the concentration of much scientific ability on the alkaloids.

The man who had possibly the greatest influence on this search for the active principles of drugs was François Magendie (p. 154), the teacher of Claude Bernard (p. 294). Magendie has been rightly called the Father of Experimental Pharmacology. In 1809 he carried out the first experiments ever made with the arrow-poison of the Javanese. The active constituent of this substance was later shown to be strychnine, and Magendie's experiments went far to elucidate its mode of action. Two years later he made some very important experiments on the mechanics of vomiting, and on the action of certain emetics in producing it. In 1817, along with Pierre Joseph Pelletier (1788–1842), Magendie returned to this work and experimented with different species of the plant ipecacuanha. They showed that the emetic properties of this plant are due to a substance which they named emetine. They were unable to isolate the alkaloid in a pure form, and since then it has been shown that their emetine was a mixture of at least three other alkaloids.

Pelletier now became associated with Joseph Bienaimé Caventou (1795–1877). Between 1818 and 1820 they isolated from cinchona the alkaloids quinine and cinchonine, and from nux vomica the alkaloids strychnine and brucine. In 1821 Friedlieb Ferdinand Runge (1795–1867) isolated caffeine from the coffee bean, and in the following year this alkaloid was independently isolated by Pelletier, Caventou, and Pierre Jean Robiquet (1780–1840). Pelletier in collaboration with the great chemist Jean Baptiste André Dumas (1800–84) made a quantitative examination of several alkaloids in 1823, and they isolated narceine in 1832 and thebaine in 1833. In 1819 Rudolph Brandes (1795–1842) isolated atropine in an impure state, and shortly afterwards it was isolated in a pure state by Philipp Lorenz Geiger (1785–1836), who isolated also hyoscyamine and aconitine.

Magendie's reaction to the early discoveries of Pelletier and Caventou was of great importance. In 1821 he published a pocket formulary for the use of practising physicians. This work bore the title *Formulaire pour la préparation et l'emploi de plusieurs nouveaux médicamens, telsque la noix vomique, la morphine, l'acide prussique, la strychnine, la vératrine, les alcalis des quinquinas, l'émetine, l'iode* ('Formulary for the preparation and use of several new drugs, such as nux vomica, morphine, prussic acid, strychnine, veratrine, the cinchona alkaloids, emetine, iodine'.) Magendie was the first to use alkaloids in the treatment of disease, and this book deals almost entirely with the clinical use of the new remedies.

In the thirties and forties of the nineteenth century Liebig, who had developed his doctrine of radicles (p. 238), attempted to determine the formula of alkaloids. He was soon followed by Wöhler. Since then an immense amount of work has been done in investigating the chemical nature and physiological action of alkaloids. The general result has been to reveal the fact that each alkaloid-yielding plant contains not one but a number of alkaloids. Those from the same plant often have similar but not identical action upon the animal body. The differences in physiological action of allied alkaloids have occupied much of the attention of pharmacologists. The accurate knowledge of these differences has made possible a far greater finesse in the administration of alkaloid drugs than was previously possible. Some alkaloids can be prepared synthetically, but the process is mostly of theoretical rather than practical importance. Our knowledge of the chemical importance of these substances is much indebted to the researches of Thomas Anderson Henry (1873–1958), whose standard work on *The Plant Alkaloids* (1913) passed through many editions. The ninth British Pharmacopoeia has entries on twenty-one alkaloids, two of which—colchicine and reserpine—have been added since the 1955 revision.

That Nature still holds surprises in relation to the alkaloids is shown by the recent history of ergot. Ergot is a fungus which sometimes develops on the ears of rye, and during the Middle Ages there were a number of outbreaks of *ignis sacer* (sacred fire), a disease characterized by an inflammation of the skin similar in appearance to erysipelas. It was caused by eating bread made from ergot-infected rye. Even today chronic ergot poisoning is not unknown in Europe, and is characterized by a chronic gangrene of the extremities leading to loss of the fingers and toes. A liquid extract of ergot causes strong contractions of the muscles of the pregnant uterus. It was first used to hasten labour in the sixteenth century, and since then it has been a constant obstetric aid and is given also to prevent uterine bleeding. Ergot seems to have been first analysed in 1816 but no active constituent was discovered. In 1830 it was supposed that the active principle had been isolated; it was named ergotine. By 1875 three other supposed alkaloids had been isolated, one of which, ergotinine, was long held to be the active substance. In 1906 the alkaloid ergotoxine was isolated by George Barger (p. 527), Francis Howard Carr (1874–), and (Sir) Henry Dale (p. 555), and this was the real beginning of the pharmacological investigation of the drug. However, no direct comparisons were made of its action compared with that of extracts of ergot, and until 1920, when ergotamine was isolated by Karl Spiro (1867–1932) and Arthur Stoll (1887–), ergotoxine was generally accepted as the active principle. Methods were now devised for the assessment of the potency of ergotoxine and ergotamine, and in doing so it was found that extracts of ergot prepared according to the official formula of the British Pharmacopoeia contained neither of them. This curious fact led to the first scientific assessment of the potency of these ergot extracts in 1932. It was conclusively demonstrated that they were very powerful, and the inference was that they contained still another active principle which had not then been isolated. Three years later the alkaloid ergometrine, which appears to be almost wholly responsible for the action of ergot, was isolated by Harold Ward Dudley (p. 546) and John Chassar Moir (1900–). The story of ergot illustrates well the difficulty of pharmacological investigation.

The glycosides are an ill-defined group which have in common the property of yielding a sugar-like substance—usually glucose itself—as a result of certain chemical processes. They are mostly of vegetable origin and the history of their investigation has been parallel with that of the alkaloids. Glycosides are generally crystalline solids which are soluble in water. The first glycoside to be isolated was salicin, which was obtained from willows in an impure state in 1825 and in a pure form in 1829. It is the active principle of the very ancient remedy for rheumatism, oil of wintergreen. Salicylic acid was introduced into internal medicine in 1874, when a process was developed for producing it synthetically on a commercial scale, and its derivative, aspirin, in 1899. Both drugs are of great importance, and many other derivatives of salicylic acid are in use. These derivatives can be prepared synthetically, and the synthetic products are in use in medicine.

Of all the glycoside-yielding plants, perhaps medically the most important is the foxglove, *Digitalis purpurea*. The use of the plant was known to some of the medieval herbalists, and is, moreover, recommended in the German and English printed herbals of the sixteenth and seventeenth centuries. Foxglove is mentioned as a folk remedy in George Eliot's *Silas Marner*, the story of which refers to a period round about 1750 before the Industrial Revolution, 'when the spinning-wheels still hummed busily in the farm-houses'. It was introduced into scientific medicine in 1785 by William Withering (1741–99) of Birmingham in his *Account of the Foxglove*, which gives details of numerous cases treated with it.

Digitalis long resisted attempts to extract an active principle, but since the seventies it has yielded a series of glycosides. Some of these have been shown to be of no practical importance. The glycoside digitoxin was isolated from digitalis by Oswald

Schmiedeberg in 1874, and it could long claim to be the most active of these glycosides. When the tincture of digitalis is used in the treatment of cardiac conditions, it is liable to give toxic symptoms unless the dosage is carefully regulated. For this reason it fell into disfavour during the late nineteenth century, and it was due to Sir James Mackenzie (p. 623) that the use of this very valuable drug was revived. But digitalis tinctures have the disadvantage that they vary greatly in the quantity of the active principles which they contain. Search for these active glycosides was now intensified. At the present time the most valuable in the domain of treatment is digoxin, a chemically pure glycoside obtained only from another species of the genus, *Digitalis lanata*. The time when heart disease will be treated only with chemically pure active principles is rapidly approaching.

(*d*) *Pharmacology, the Scientific Investigation of Drug Action*

The science of pharmacology arose early in the nineteenth century, and from the middle until near the end of that century the investigation of the physiological action of drugs was mainly in German hands. The greatest of the early teachers was Rudolf Buchheim (1820–79), who was professor of pharmacology at Dorpat (now Tartu), where he established a pharmacological laboratory in 1849, and later at Giessen. His textbook first appeared in 1856. Another prominent scientific exponent of pharmacology was Carl Binz (1832–1913), who founded a pharmacological institute at Bonn in 1869. Binz's lectures were translated into English in 1895, and they had a profound influence in the English-speaking world. Perhaps the greatest of the German pharmacologists was Johann Ernst Oswald Schmiedeberg (1838–1921), a pupil of Buchheim, who held the chair of pharmacology at Strasbourg for nearly fifty years. Schmiedeberg published in 1883 the first edition of his very famous textbook, and he trained many of the well-known pharmacologists of the next generation.

Pharmacological laboratories were established much later in the English-speaking world than in Germany. As a house physician at Edinburgh (Sir) Thomas Lauder Brunton (1844–1916) had under his care a severe case of angina pectoris, together with several milder cases. From physiological experiments which he had seen his friend

Arthur Gamgee (1841–1909) perform with amyl nitrite Brunton thought that inhalation of this volatile substance would relieve the severe pain and the arterial tension of angina. His hopes were fully realized, and this new and useful drug was later included in the pharmacopoeia. About 1873, when Brunton was a lecturer at St. Bartholomew's Hospital in London, he transformed a small scullery into the first pharmacological laboratory in the United Kingdom. Although Brunton, in association with colleagues and students, carried on experiments there for years, this small laboratory could hardly rank as a department of pharmacology. In 1885 Brunton published the first edition of his large textbook of pharmacology and materia medica. The first 500 pages of this very large book form an independent treatise on experimental pharmacology, and the work had a wide influence.

Two of Schmiedeberg's pupils became pharmacologists of the first rank. John Jacob Abel (1857–1938), a native of Cleveland, Ohio, studied at the University of Michigan and at many European universities, including a long period under Schmiedeberg. In 1891 he became the first occupant of the newly established chair of pharmacology at Ann Arbor. This was the first pharmacological laboratory to be founded in America. In 1893 Abel was called to the new chair at Johns Hopkins University, Baltimore, and he was succeeded at Ann Arbor by Arthur Robertson Cushny (1866–1926), a Scot who was then an assistant to Schmiedeberg. The first real department of pharmacology in Great Britain was established at University College, London, in 1905, and Cushny was appointed as the first occupant of the chair. He later became professor of materia medica at Edinburgh. Cushny wrote a celebrated textbook, and he spent most of his active life on research work connected with digitalis, the heart, and circulation, and on the mode of action of drugs which increase the secretion of urine. Since the First World War much attention has been paid to the nature of the action by which drugs affect individual cells of the body, and in this research the work of Alfred Joseph Clark (1885–1941), who also held the chair of materia medica at Edinburgh, has been especially important.

Improvements have been made not only in the drugs themselves but also in modes of administration. The ancient methods of inunction and inhalation, as well as other older methods, have been greatly elaborated in modern times, and are now of wider application than they were. No advance of this order compares in importance with the introduction of the hypodermic method of administering drugs. This is done by means of a hollow needle attached to a small syringe. By means of this instrument test reagents can be injected into the sub-

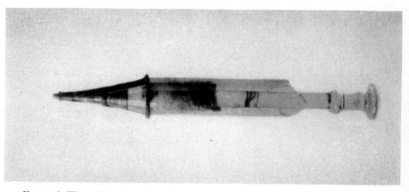

FIG. 136. The original hypodermic syringe invented and used by Alexander Wood
(Museum of the Royal College of Surgeons, Edinburgh)

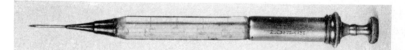

FIG. 137. Hypodermic syringe by Coxeter, London, c. 1860
(In the Wellcome Historical Medical Museum)

stance of the skin (as in the Schick test for susceptibility to diphtheria), or drugs into the superficial tissues below the skin (hypodermic or subcutaneous injection). A drug administered by this method acts more swiftly and under better control than if given by mouth.

There has been much confusion over the so-called 'invention of the hypodermic syringe', long stated to be due to the French surgeon Charles Gabriel Pravaz (1791–1853) in 1853. We now know that Pravaz never administered a drug to a patient by the hypodermic route, and also that he never claimed to have invented any particular type of syringe. He did inject certain substances into the veins of animals for the experimental production of coagulation of the blood in the vessels, but the apparatus which he used was not a hypodermic syringe. In any case, injection of substances through hollow tubes into the veins had been practised for nearly two centuries.

The first to use the hypodermic method of administering a drug was Alexander Wood (1817–84) of Edinburgh (1853). Wood used a type of syringe and hollow needle which was already used for other purposes, but he seems to have modified the cutting-point of the needle to make it suitable for hypodermic injection. Wood's first results were published in 1855, and four years later Charles Hunter (1835–78), a London surgeon, used the method advocated by Wood and attempted to claim it as his own. Hunter's writings did much to popularize the hypodermic method. In a word, it may be said that there was no 'invention' of the hypodermic syringe. The essence of the discovery lay in the introduction of the hypodermic method by Alexander Wood.

CHEMOTHERAPY AND ALLIED METHODS OF TREATMENT

During the twentieth century the outlook on drug treatment has been modified by the success obtained in the *specific* treatment of certain diseases, that is to say, treatment by remedies which strike at a particular disease and no other. Until 1910 scientific medicine recognized very few specific remedies. It had been ascertained that cinchona owes its value in malaria to the alkaloid quinine which acts as a specific exterminator of the malaria parasites and not simply as a remedy for fever in general. It had also been ascertained that ipecacuanha owes its value in tropical dysentery to the alkaloid emetine, which acts similarly as a specific exterminator of the protozoal organisms which are the infective agents. Quinine and its allied alkaloids and emetine and its allied alkaloids were, except mercury for syphilis, practically the only specifics the value of which had been scientifically proved.

The word 'chemotherapy' is associated particularly with the twentieth century. It was not, however, a new word, for it was certainly used in a Wittenberg thesis in 1785. The term was re-coined by Paul Ehrlich (1854–1915) of Frankfort-on-Main about 1905. Eight years before this he had carried out most important research on diphtheria antitoxin, and he had also formulated his 'side-chain theory' (p. 413). He was therefore much impressed by the fact that an antibody in the blood, which has been produced by the body in response to the presence of a certain micro-organism, is specific for that organism and is highly effective in killing it. Further, although such an antibody is highly lethal for the organism, it is quite harmless to the subject who harbours it. Here are ideal remedies provided by Nature herself. Ehrlich compared these antibodies to magic bullets which flew straight to their mark and injured nothing else. It was with all this in mind that Ehrlich set out on his new quest. His problem was to find a chemical substance which would be specific for a particular organism and completely non-injurious for its host. This is an ideal which has only recently been achieved, and for practical purposes the problem was to find a chemical substance which would be as lethal as possible for a particular organism and as little injurious as possible for its host.

Ehrlich therefore conceived chemotherapy as the discovery of synthetic chemical substances acting specifically on disease-producing micro-organisms in the body. For a long time after his discovery of salvarsan (p. 689) all chemotherapeutic substances were specific, in the sense that they acted only on one kind of micro-organism, and, with certain exceptions, synthetic, in the sense that they were not substances which occurred naturally but were built up in the laboratory from inorganic chemical substances. Since Ehrlich's time the meaning of the term 'chemotherapy' has changed considerably. Since the discovery of the sulphonamides (p. 692) chemotherapeutic remedies have no longer been strictly specific, and since the introduction of the antibiotics (p. 693) some are not synthetic products.

The earliest uses of drugs employed to destroy pathogenic organisms in the body were the action of mercury in syphilis, which had been known since 1495, and of quinine, used in malaria since about 1630.

When Ehrlich began the study of chemotherapy observers had long known that certain aniline dyes have a special affinity for certain cells or organisms. Indeed the affinity of certain of the dyes for certain bacteria had made possible the work of Koch on tuberculosis and on other diseases. As far back as the seventies and eighties much work had been done on the subject, and the action of these dyes had interested a large variety of investigators. Ehrlich had studied the biological action of the dye methylene blue for many years, and in 1891 he administered it to a malaria patient under the care of Paul Guttmann (1834–93). Ehrlich considered that benefit resulted. This was the first practical application of 'chemotherapy' (using the word in Ehrlich's sense). He now proceeded to test this and other synthetic aniline dyes in laboratory infections with malaria parasites and trypanosomes.

(a) Protozoal and Spirochaetal Diseases

At this point Ehrlich's interest was diverted from the aniline dyes to the organic compounds of arsenic by the discovery at the Liverpool School of Tropical Medicine that a synthetic organic arsenic compound known as atoxyl was more effective in dealing with experimental infections with trypanosomes in certain animals than was inorganic arsenic. Ehrlich confirmed this, but found that, if the dose was too low, the trypanosomes rapidly developed a resistance to the drug. He therefore began to modify atoxyl in the hope of forming a compound which would kill all the trypanosomes in the body with one dose, so that none would remain to develop drug resistance. Ehrlich had working under him a small team of expert chemists, and they set out to synthesize successive modifications of this basic organic arsenical. As each compound was synthesized it was tested for its efficiency in killing trypanosomes in animals. Ehrlich was a genius who practised the most heterodox chemical methods. In 1907 some of his chemists left him because their practice was too orthodox, but Alfred Bertheim remained with him to make the great discovery.

In 1905, two years before this quarrel, the protozoal parasite which causes syphilis had been discovered by Fritz Richard Schaudinn (p. 394) and Paul Erich Hoffmann (p. 395). This thread-like, undulating organism was named the *Spirochaeta pallida*, but it has now been renamed the *Treponema pallidum*. By 1907 Ehrlich had synthesized and tested over 600 arsenic compounds. No. 418 in this series proved very effective in the treatment of laboratory infections with trypanosomes, but No. 606 had been reported by one of his assistants as being inactive against the *Treponema pallidum*. In

1909 the Japanese bacteriologist Sahachiro Hata (1873–1938) came as assistant to Ehrlich. Hata was expert at the transmission of syphilis to rabbits, and Ehrlich set him the task of retesting the whole series of his synthetic preparations for their action on the *Treponema* in the animal body. As a result it was established that a mistake had previously

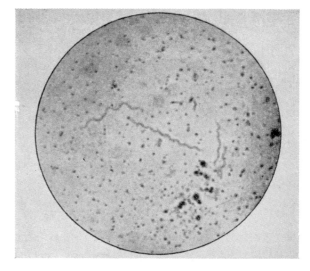

FIG. 138. The first illustration of the causal organism of syphilis, *Spirochaeta pallida*. The spirochaetes are seen as wavy and cork-screw-like forms (Schaudinn and Hoffmann, *Act. a. d. Kaiserl. Ges. Amt.*, 1905, xxii)

been made, and that 606 was very active. It was named 'Salvarsan', and in 1911 it was first used in the treatment of human syphilis.

Salvarsan revolutionized the treatment of syphilis, but it was soon found that it had certain disadvantages. It is only sparingly soluble, and the required dose must be injected in a large quantity of solvent. For these reasons Ehrlich later introduced 914 (neosalvarsan, now called neoarsphenamine), and since then other variants have been synthesized and used. Ehrlich was awarded a Nobel Prize in 1908.

In 1920 the pharmaceutical firm of Bayer synthesized a substance, named by them Bayer 205, which proved to be of great value in the treatment of human trypanosomiasis. Since then it has been revealed that it is a complex derivative of urea and naphthaleine, and it is included in the official pharmacopoeia under the name of suramin.

About the mid-1920's the only chemotherapeutic substances which were effective were mercury, quinine and its alkaloids, emetine, salvarsan and its variants, and Bayer 205. Their mode of action was not understood, and it is interesting to glance at the difficulties which the pharmacologist encountered.

Quinine at that time was—and indeed still is—regarded as a general protoplasmic poison, and it was thought to have a selective affinity for malaria parasites in the blood. But the phrase 'general protoplasmic poison' was, even in the 1920's, regarded as vague and rather meaningless. For example, it was realized that in laboratory experiments outside the body quinine is no more active in killing the malaria parasite than other substances which are quite useless for this purpose in animal experiments. Even more significant was the fact that, in order to kill the parasites *in vitro* in laboratory experiments, ten times the concentration of quinine is necessary than exists in the blood of a human malaria patient after he has received full doses of quinine. This fact suggested that the action in the body was not a direct killing of the parasites in the blood, but a change which was produced in the body tissues which prevented the further development of the parasites. At that time it was suggested that this effect made the red blood corpuscles resistant to the entry of the parasites. It should be said that the mode of action of quinine and its related alkaloids in the human body is still uncertain. Opinion now inclines to the view that the continued development of the parasites in the blood (asexual cycle) depends on an unknown enzyme, and that the quinine interferes with the action of this enzyme.

During the First World War the Germans became apprehensive lest their supplies of quinine from the Dutch East Indies should be cut off. Ample supplies of quinine are of course vital for the conduct of any military campaign in tropical or sub-tropical countries. The Germans went back to the observations of Ehrlich and Guttmann in 1891 (p. 688), and attempted to modify the design of the molecules of methylene blue before trying other lines. By 1926 they had synthesized the active substance named plasmochin, and in 1933 they had produced the dye atebrin, now known as mepacrine, in the search for which 12,000 compounds were synthesized and tested. By the outbreak of the Second World War the Germans had synthesized the drug now known as chloroquin. During this war the Anglo-American cause was confronted, after the Japanese invasion of Java, with the same difficulties, and most intensive research was carried out to produce new anti-malarials. In the United Kingdom the drug paludrine was synthesized at the 4,888th attempt, and chloroguanide was synthesized in the United States. Some of these new compounds have been found to be very effective against the sexual forms of the parasite (crescent forms), and in the hands of British workers their use has led to the discovery of hitherto unsuspected stages in the life-cycle of the malarial parasite.

Similar difficulties have been met with in interpreting the pharmacological action of the organic arsenical compounds in the treatment of syphilis and trypanosomiasis. As a result of his extended work on the biological reactions of the aniline dyes, Ehrlich felt convinced that these dyes, in their pharmacological effects, acted upon certain parts of the individual cell. From work on certain venoms which he carried out quite early in his career he developed his famous side-chain theory, which, very briefly, implies that the individual cell bears a number of 'receptors' for which certain side-chains in the drug have a selective chemical affinity. This theory is still of some importance in immunology. When Ehrlich began to develop his chemotherapeutic remedies, he applied this theory to their action, and was led to believe that theoretically a drug could be found which would kill off all the organisms in the body without in any way affecting the body-cells. It was discovered later, however, that cultures of the organisms of syphilis, trypanosomiasis, and certain other diseases continue to thrive almost normally *in vitro* in laboratory experiments when exposed to concentrations of salvarsan much greater than any that could possibly be produced in animals and man. The reaction which occurs during the treatment of the disease cannot therefore be a direct chemical combination between the drug and some essential constituent of the parasite. From other evidence it is now held that the complex organic arsenical does not act as such, but that it is reduced in the body to a simpler form. The whole mechanism is, however, still rather obscure.

(b) *Bacterial Infections*

For about a quarter of a century the known chemotherapeutic drugs were effective only against protozoal parasites or the organism of syphilis. Although many compounds, including some new synthetic dyes, had been tried for years against the much commoner bacterial diseases of temperate climates—the cocci and bacilli— no success had been obtained. However, in 1935, Gerhard Domagk (1895–) published his experiments with prontosil red, one of these new dyes, and showed that it would protect mice which had been artificially infected with streptococci. French workers confirmed the observation at once and showed that the effectiveness of prontosil red was due to the fact that it was converted in the body into sulphanilamide, a member of a group of chemical substances known as the sulphonamides. It was shown that drugs of this group, although only feebly disinfectant *in vitro*, produced a remarkable protective action *in vivo*, and were especially valuable in the treatment of diseases which had always been found to be very grave. Efforts were then made to synthesize new sulphonamides which would be even more effective than sulphanilamide, and hundreds of new products were made and tested. Most were discarded, but of the compounds which still survive are sulphanilamide, sulphathiazole, sulphadiazine, and M. & B. 693. Domagk was awarded a Nobel Prize in 1939.

When the sulphonamides are administered to a patient or an animal infected with a certain micro-organism, they do not kill the bacteria but they so alter the metabolism of the bacteria that they are prevented from multiplying. Thus they can be dealt with by the normal defensive mechanisms of the body. These drugs have been found to be very effective in erysipelas, puerperal fever and other diseases due to streptococci, and also in pneumonia, meningitis, gonorrhoea, and certain infective diseases of the bowel and urinary tract. Their use is not infrequently followed by complications, but their greatest disadvantage is that the infecting bacilli sometimes become resistant to them. When drug-resistance to a particular sulphonamide has once developed it is permanent.

(c) *The Antibiotics*

The greatest contribution to the science of medical treatment made in the twentieth century is the development of the antibiotics. The word 'antibiosis' was introduced at the end of the nineteenth century to indicate antagonism between one organism and another. From the time of Pasteur onwards various bacteriologists had studied

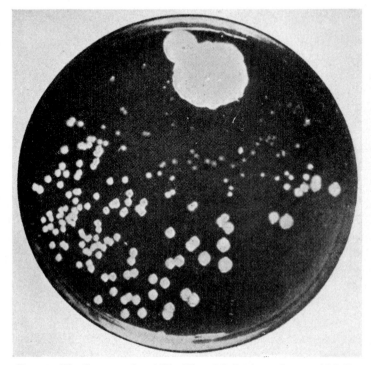

FIG. 139. The discovery of penicillin. The original culture plate on which Sir Alexander Fleming observed the lytic effect of the mould *Penicillium notatum* on the growth of colonies of other organisms
(Fleming, *Brit. J. Exp. Path.*, 1929)

the inhibitory effect of certain organisms which are normally present in the soil, but none of these observations led to any practical result.

In 1928 Sir Alexander Fleming (1881–1955), professor of bacteriology at St. Mary's Hospital in London, found that a mould had gained access to a culture plate (Fig. 139) on which he had been growing colonies of a common coccus. He noted that the colonies in the neighbourhood of the mould, which previously had been developing normally, were now showing signs of dissolution. Since this was an unusual phenomenon, the mould was isolated in pure culture and was later identified as *Penicillium notatum*. Fleming later showed that this mould produces in the culture fluid a substance which strongly inhibits the growth of the causative organisms of certain common infectious diseases. Fleming named the active substance penicillin. He tabulated the organisms which are sensitive to it, and he showed that its toxicity for animals is very low. Fleming failed to concentrate penicillin, but he continued to use the crude culture fluid containing it for bacteriological purposes in his laboratory.

Between 1930 and 1932 Harold Raistrick (1890–), professor of biochemistry at the London School of Hygiene and Tropical Medicine, and his co-workers worked on this mould, and they found that the penicillin could be extracted from the culture fluid but that in the process much of the penicillin was destroyed.

After the discovery of the sulphonamides in 1935 the medical profession became chemotherapeutically minded. Under this stimulus Sir Howard Walter Florey (1898–) and Ernst Boris Chain (1906–) at Oxford decided that it would be worth while to attempt the formidable task of concentrating penicillin. This they ultimately effected and a stable solid product suitable for therapeutic use was obtained. The results of many animal experiments carried out by Florey and Chain and published in 1940 showed that penicillin was probably the most effective chemotherapeutic drug known, and moreover was relatively non-toxic. The results of trials on a small number of human subjects were published in 1941.

It was obvious that penicillin would be of enormous importance in the Allied war-effort, but the problem was to produce it in quantity. The Oxford workers established a small factory in their laboratory, and the penicillin produced there was used for further experimental work and for the treatment of selected cases. The Oxford workers now went to the United States, which were not then at war, and laid their data before the authorities. As a result commercial production on a large scale was started in America, and at a later date the United Kingdom was able to add her quota to the enormous amounts of penicillin which were then being used. It was found that, under differing conditions of culture, different products were obtained, and that these were all organic acids of closely related chemical constitution. In 1944 a Conference called by the League of Nations Health Organization recommended that the International Unit should be defined in terms of a pure preparation of the crystalline sodium salt of penicillin G (benzyl penicillin). At that time several structural formulae had been proposed for the penicillin group, and subsequently one of them (known as the beta-lactam formula) has obtained general recognition. For their work in the discovery and therapeutic development of penicillin, Fleming, Florey, and Chain were jointly awarded a Nobel Prize in 1945.

The penicillins are very effective against most types of pus-forming cocci, and against the pneumococcus, gonococcus, meningococcus, diphtheria bacillus, and the bacilli of anthrax and tetanus. They are also very active against the *Treponema pallidum*, and it is possible that they may soon supplant the organic arsenicals entirely in the treatment of syphilis.

Penicillin is only one of many antibiotics which are giving good service in medicine. Attempts to utilize the antagonism between certain bacteria, or between certain moulds and bacteria, have been carried on for at least seventy years. The results of the study of antagonism between bacteria and other bacteria have on the whole been disappointing. Many efforts were made to utilize practically the bacteriophage phenomenon of Twort and d'Herelle (p. 406), and various lysogenic factors were tested. The most systematic studies in this field have been those of René Jules Dubos (1901–), who as a young man migrated from France to the United States and who has long been on the staff of the Rockefeller Institute for Medical Research. The work of Dubos on the general life and metabolism of the bacterial cell is well known. In the field of antibiotics he was especially interested in organisms having a lytic action on the pathogenic cocci. He adopted the principle that, if samples of soil were infected with these organisms, antagonistic bacteria would appear in the soil and could be isolated. Acting on this principle Dubos isolated in 1939 a motile bacterium belonging to the genus *Tyrothrix* which had the power of destroying these test cocci. From this bacterium Dubos was able to prepare the substance tyrocidine, which had some effect when tested clinically.

Research on the antagonism between fungi and moulds on the one hand, and certain bacteria on the other, has been more remunerative. In 1940 Selman Abraham Waksman (1888–), who has worked with various colleagues on these problems, had his first success. A Russian who migrated to the United States as a young man, Waksman became a distinguished soil microbiologist. In that year, working with H. B. Woodruff, he discovered a new species of actinomyces, and from it they isolated an active antibiotic which they called actinomycin. This substance was markedly lethal to bacteria, but it proved to be very toxic and was therefore not tried clinically. In 1944 Waksman discovered another new species of this fungus to which the name *Streptomyces griseus* was later given. From this he isolated the antibiotic streptomycin. This substance is very active against certain organisms, especially the tubercle bacillus, and its toxicity is relatively low. Streptomycin was first tried out on a large scale in tuberculosis by another migrant to the United States. This was William Hugh Feldman (1892–), who was born in Glasgow, was taken to America as a young child, and became professor of comparative pathology at the Mayo Foundation in the University of Minnesota. The administration of streptomycin in tuberculosis is liable to be followed by the appearance of strains of the bacillus which are resistant to the drug. Feldman has been prominent in research which has partially overcome this drawback. Combined in a course of treatment with para-aminosalicylic acid (PAS) and isonicotinic acid hydrazide (isoniazid), streptomycin has revolutionized the prognosis in pulmonary tuberculosis. For his outstanding work in the field of antibiotics Waksman received a Nobel Prize in 1952.

Another antibiotic, chloramphenicol, which is of relatively simple constitution compared with other antibiotics, was first isolated from a mould in 1947, and was synthesized two years later. It is the first antibiotic which has so far been synthesized. It is valuable in the treatment of certain diseases, such as typhoid and typhus fevers, which do not react to penicillin. Aureomycin was first obtained from a mould in 1948. It is a mixture of the hydrochlorides of several organic bases, and is very valuable in the treatment of pneumonia. It seems certain that these are only the forerunners of others, and that these very valuable methods of treatment will soon be greatly extended.

BLOOD TRANSFUSION

As a practical therapeutic method blood transfusion is almost entirely a product of the last thirty-five years, but the fundamental procedure has a long and interesting history. From prehistoric times the blood was known to be essential to life, and there are references in the Roman poets to attempts at rejuvenation by drawing off the patient's blood and replacing it by magical substances. An effort was made to rejuvenate Pope Innocent VIII by getting him to drink the blood of three youths, who were killed in order to provide it. Harvey never attempted transfusion of blood, and the procedure could not have been contemplated on a scientific basis before the discovery of the circulation.

Blood transfusion was made practicable by the work of (Sir) Christopher Wren (1632–1723), the most celebrated of British architects, who was also a distinguished natural philosopher and an Original Fellow of the Royal Society. In 1657 Wren injected various medicinal fluids into the veins of animals, thus producing vomiting, purging, intoxication, and other conditions according to the nature of the substance injected. Physicians were thus familiarized with the practicability of injecting fluids into the veins. The Royal Society, shortly after its foundation, became interested in the subject, and in 1665 John Wilkins (1614–72), the leading spirit in the foundation of the Society, drew off into a bladder blood from the vena cava of a dog and then injected it through a brass tube into the femoral vein of a bitch, which apparently showed no ill effects. This was probably the first indirect transfusion of blood from one animal to another.

The first direct transfusion of blood (1666) from an artery of one animal into a vein of another was performed by another early Fellow of the Royal Society, Richard Lower (1631–91). Lower first used quills to connect the two vessels, but later he used fine silver tubes.

So far no one had tried to inject blood into a vessel of a human subject, but it was inevitable that the attempt would soon be made. Jean Baptiste Denys (c. 1625–1704) carried out preliminary experiments on animals, and then on 15 June 1667 he transfused a boy of 15 years with blood from an artery of a lamb. Five months later Lower and a colleague made a direct transfusion in London from a sheep to a man, and three weeks later they gave the same man another transfusion without ill effects. In the following year (1668) one of the patients transfused by Denys died. The patient's widow brought an action against Denys, but it was ultimately established that the death was due to arsenic administered by the widow herself. Nevertheless, the repercussions of the case were wide, and in no country was blood transfusion again attempted until the early nineteenth century.

The first really successful transfusion for therapeutic purposes was performed by James Blundell (1790–1877), physician and obstetrician to Guy's Hospital. By many experiments on animals he established the fact that blood from one species of animal is incompatible with the blood from another; he therefore rightly decided that for the transfusion of human subjects human blood must be used. In 1818 he carried out a transfusion in a patient suffering from an incurable disease; the blood was drawn from several of Blundell's assistants, and a syringe was used to transfer it from donor to recipient. Blundell repeated this experiment in nineteen hopeless cases, and in 1829 he first tried it on a patient who had a faint chance of recovery. A woman suffering from post-partum haemorrhage was transfused with 8 oz. of blood drawn from the arm of Blundell's assistant. The operation took three hours and was completely successful. Blundell was already experiencing difficulties owing to coagulation, and he later invented two special pieces of apparatus to enable the blood to be transfused from the donor to the recipient with the minimum of physical interference.

Successful direct transfusions from donor to patient were also carried out by James Hobson Aveling (1828–92). In 1863 he invented a portable transfusion outfit, and he carried it about in his pocket for nine years before he met with a suitable case. The result was very satisfactory, and he had other successful cases. During the Franco-Prussian War a number of direct transfusions were carried out using a portable apparatus which did not involve the use of an anticoagulant.

Now that transfusion had been shown to be a practicable method, the real difficulties were studied. The most obvious was the tendency of the donor's blood to coagulate before it reached the recipient's circulation. Sodium phosphate was first used as an anticoagulant about 1869. Defibrinated blood—that is, blood from which the fibrin has been removed by a mechanical method—had been employed much earlier for other purposes, and defibrination was now used to prevent coagulation in transfusions. The method was in use until quite recent times, but it has the disadvantage of removing most of the valuable constituents of the blood. Other substances were also tried, and finally in 1914 sodium citrate in a certain concentration was shown to be a very effective anticoagulant provided that not more than a total of 5 gm. of citrate was administered.

A typical complication of transfusion was early met with. It was found that in certain cases the transfusion was followed by an unexpectedly rapid destruction of the red cells of the transfused blood in the recipient's circulation, or by destruction of the recipient's own red cells. The liberation of proteins and other substances by the lysis of the red cells produced in the recipient haemolytic shock which was often fatal. There were other complications, but this allergic manifestation was the most noteworthy.

In 1900 Karl Landsteiner (1868–1943) showed that when the red blood cells of one individual were mixed with the blood serum from another individual, clumping together of the cells (agglutination) sometimes occurred. Following up these observations he and others showed that all human subjects could be divided into four groups according to the presence of two complex agglutinating substances, A and B. The red cells of the individuals tested might contain one (A), the other (B), both (AB), or neither (O) of these antigens. This is known as the ABO grouping. Many years later it was shown as a result of extensive examinations that human populations could be divided into groups in the following proportions:

Group A   41·8 per cent.
Group B   8·6 per cent.
Group AB   3·0 per cent.
Group O   46·6 per cent.

It is beyond our scope to explain the significance of these groups and their sub-groups in the prevention of haemolytic reactions after transfusion. It is sufficient to say that for a recipient belonging to a certain group, the transfusion must be carried out with blood from a donor of an appropriate group. Landsteiner was awarded a Nobel Prize in 1930. For many years Group O was regarded as a ' universal donor ', since it was claimed that blood of this group could be given to a recipient in any group. It is now known that haemolytic reactions do sometimes follow transfusion with Group O blood, but blood from a ' universal donor ' is still important in emergencies.

In 1940 Landsteiner and a colleague inoculated a rabbit with red cells from the blood of a rhesus monkey. The serum of the rabbit developed specific agglutinating substances which reacted with the red cells of a large proportion (85 per cent.) of human subjects. It was also shown that this reaction had no relation to the ABO grouping. This Rh-grouping, as it is usually called, has an important place in the technique of transfusion. Further, it has been shown that this Rh-factor is responsible for haemolytic diseases in the new-born, and for this reason special precautions are now used in transfusing women patients of child-bearing age. During the Second World War transfusion became a common practice in obstetrics, and the discovery of the Rh-factor was just in time to prevent disastrous consequences as a result of transfusion with blood which from the aspect of this factor was incompatible. The presence of certain other groups of antigens, such as the Kell, the MNS, and the P, are also of some practical importance in transfusion.

Transfusion of blood was formerly an individual operation; a suitable donor, often a relative, was chosen for each patient. During the First World War some successful attempts were made to store blood, but there were no further attempts until the Spanish Civil War. Early in the Second World War the practice was actively developed, and blood banks of stored blood were instituted. In the United Kingdom, between the wars, arrangements for individual transfusions were carried out by the British Red Cross Society, and especially its London Blood Transfusion Service. The collection and storage of blood is now in the hands of the National Transfusion Service.

THE REVOLUTION IN NURSING

The thirteenth century saw a great increase in the number of the secular orders. A notable order was the Third Order of St. Francis, whose members, both men and women, wore the habit of the order but did not take vows or live in community. The main work of these Tertiaries was often nursing. The other orders also formed secular branches, the members of which took up nursing; and, in addition, certain famous hospitals had regular orders of nuns who undertook the nursing. Such were the Augustinian Sisters of the Hôtel-Dieu of Paris, who were certainly active in the thirteenth century. The sisters spent their whole lives in the hospital, except when they went into the city as visiting nurses.

In the sixteenth century a number of religious orders which were almost exclusively connected with nursing were founded on the Continent. Most important of these were the Sisters of Charity founded by St. Vincent de Paul (1576–1660). The sisters were first formed into an order in 1634 under their Sister Superior, Mlle Le Gras, and their spiritual training was undertaken by St. Vincent. These sisters may take annual but not perpetual vows. They are now the largest Roman Catholic nursing sisterhood in existence.

The dissolution of the monasteries in England began in 1535, and resulted in a serious lack of accommodation and attention for the sick who could not be treated at home. The Royal Hospitals, founded by Edward VI, had to be staffed with ignorant and inexperienced women, and as time went on matters did not improve. Even the spate of hospital building in London which began in 1740 did not lead to any improvement in the type of nurses employed. The trouble lay partly in the fact that nursing was not a profession. No standard of character or of education was demanded of any woman who wished to become a nurse, and no training was provided anywhere. There was a complete lack of incentive to progress.

The reader may gain some insight into the life of a nurse from the conditions that prevailed until beyond the middle of the nineteenth century at a very good and well-managed English provincial hospital, the Radcliffe Infirmary at Oxford. The salary of a nurse was £5 a year. There was no distinction between a nurse and a domestic servant. One nurse only was the allowance for a ward of seventeen patients. A nurse's day began at 6 a.m. The wards were cleaned till 7, when a bell was rung and each nurse had to bring down her ashes and sift them under the direction of the porter, who then gave her coals for the day. She took breakfast with the patients, who helped her, so far as they were able, with the ward work. At 2 p.m. she went to the servants' hall, where she had her dinner in company with the servants on daily hire. During the dinner the ward was left in charge of a patient. After dinner she took away a plate of meat and vegetables for her supper. For the night there was normally only one nurse for the whole hospital of about 100 beds. There were no regular holidays, and the nurse was never allowed to leave the hospital before 6 p.m. The practice of nurses receiving gratuities from patients continued till 1870 and even beyond. Those patients who wished to secure a nurse's early attention for their dressings gave tips, those who did not frequently had to wait.

What sort of woman could such a system produce? That some nurses at least were kind and skilful, even under such conditions, is a fact, and is pleasing evidence of the natural goodness and wisdom that reside in the human heart. Many, however, can have been no better than Sairey Gamp and Betsy Prig.

The first important reform in Protestant countries began in Germany, through the influence of Elizabeth Fry (p. 190). In 1822 Theodor Fliedner (1800–64), the young pastor of the church at Kaiserswerth, a little town on the Rhine near Düsseldorf, visited England and was much impressed by Elizabeth's teaching and example. Returning to his charge, he devoted himself to the spiritual and physical care of gaol-birds. In 1833 he and his devoted wife Friederike (1800–42) opened a refuge for discharged female convicts. From them the couple turned their attention to the sick poor. The conception of an organized body of specially trained women crossed their minds. In 1836 they opened a small hospital.

At this hospital six young women of the most spotless character were induced to serve as 'Deaconesses'. It was their duty to perform all the tasks of the hospital in rotation. The physicians who attended the hospital gave them instruction. The Kaiserswerth idea rapidly spread and the Kaiserswerth Deaconesses became and remain an important order, which is still occupied in good works in many parts of the world. The conception of the order is different from that of most religious orders in that the members make no attempt to withdraw from the world, and marriage is not forbidden to them.

Moreover, the duties of the Kaiserswerth Deaconesses are rather different from and more varied than those of a sick-nurse. They include teaching, both secular and religious, nursing, household duties, management of children and convalescents. In 1865 a preparatory school for probationers was opened.

In England Anglican orders of a somewhat similar character were formed in the forties and fifties. In 1840 Elizabeth Fry visited Kaiserswerth and, inspired by what she saw, she founded in the same year a small society of nurses, the Institute of Nursing Sisters, to work among the poor. Training consisted in the individual sisters going daily to Guy's Hospital for a few months, where they picked up what knowledge the untrained ward nurses were disposed to give them. Several local societies of Sisters of Mercy were also formed. In 1848 the St. John's House Nurses were formed, and, working from their house in Fitzroy Square, their activities were soon extended. They were trained in three of the London teaching hospitals. St. John's House took over the whole of the nursing in King's College Hospital from 1856 to 1885, and a similar body, the All Saints Sisterhood, was responsible for the whole of the nursing at University College Hospital from 1862 to 1899. These organizations thus played a very active part in the hospital nursing of the Metropolis.

The second important reform of nursing was due to the determination and drive of Florence Nightingale (1820–1910). A lady of good birth and education, she was drawn to nursing as early as 1844. In 1846 she heard about the Kaiserswerth Deaconesses through an annual report, and in 1850 she spent a fortnight at Kaiserswerth. In the following year she went through a regular course of training at Kaiserswerth for three months. She was profoundly impressed by the extremely high character of the Deaconesses, most of whom were peasant women. In 1853 she became the superintendent of the Establishment for Gentlewomen during Illness in Upper Harley Street, but her ambition still was to train nurses. Shortly afterwards she accepted the post of Superintendent of Nurses at King's College Hospital, but an event happened which prevented her from ever taking up her duties. This was the outbreak of the Crimean War in March 1854.

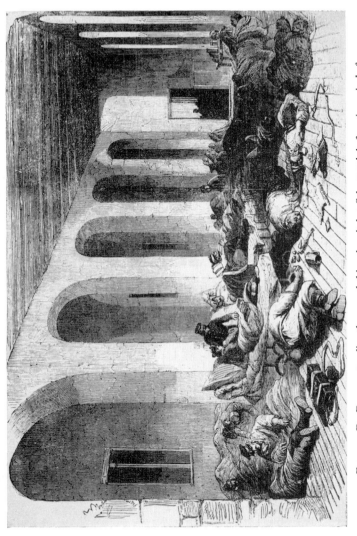

Fig. 140. Dr. Durgan attending the wounded in a hospital at Sebastopol, before the arrival of Florence Nightingale

(Woodcut after E. A. Goodall, for *The Illustrated London News*, 1854)

Rumours of the lack of treatment of the sick and wounded from the battlefields soon reached London, and these were confirmed by the brilliant reports of the special correspondent of *The Times*, which began to be published in October. He reported that there were in the hospitals neither surgeons, dressers, nurses, nor the commonest appliances of a workhouse sick ward. Though there were no women nurses at all in the British Army, the French had the help of women from their religious orders. Very soon *The Times* was demanding that the British Army should have Sisters of Charity. Florence Nightingale wrote immediately to the wife of her friend Sidney Herbert (later Lord Herbert of Lee), the Secretary at War, offering her services. Her letter crossed his letter to her asking that she should organize a staff of women nurses for service in Scutari. The party was quickly collected, and consisted of ten Roman Catholic Sisters, eight Anglican Sisters, six St. John's House Nurses, and fourteen from various hospitals. Each member was selected personally by Florence Nightingale. This inclusion of women in the services of the British Army was an innovation, and led to much acrimonious discussion. Throughout the whole of her period of service Florence Nightingale had active opposition from senior members of the Services, but she earned the love and respect of the many men whose lives she saved by her administrative action and the nursing efficiency of her subordinates. The Battle of Inkerman was fought on the day after the arrival of the party at Scutari, and the four British hospitals were immediately flooded with wounded men lying in their uniforms 'stiff with gore and covered with filth'. The first thing that Florence Nightingale requisitioned was three hundred scrubbing brushes, for the hospitals were in a deplorably insanitary state. It was at this period that she was touring the hospitals all day and writing reports and letters during much of the night. It was then, too, that she earned the name of The Lady with the Lamp. Touring the hospitals was in itself a task, since there were four miles of beds, not more than eighteen inches apart. At the end of the war she had a staff of 125 nurses. She also did very valuable work in connexion with the provision of meals in the hospitals, in the arrangements for the washing of clothes and bedding, and in the provision of comforts for the soldiers. The war ended in February 1856, but

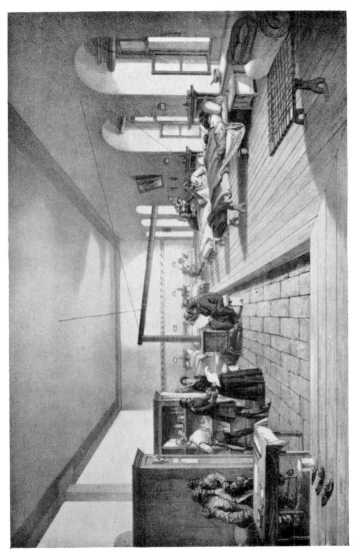

FIG. 141. A hospital ward at Scutari, showing the improved conditions effected by Florence Nightingale

(Lithograph by E. Walker after W. Simpson)

she was not able to return home until August. She was then received as a national heroine.

On her return Florence Nightingale was at once immersed in long-term policy relating to the treatment of sick and wounded soldiers. In 1857 a Royal Commission on the Health of the Army was appointed. It was unthinkable at that time that any woman should be appointed on such an official body; but Sidney Herbert and other leading members were constantly in touch with her, and hers was the unseen hand which guided most of the deliberations of the Commission.

Before the war ended a public fund was opened to enable Florence Nightingale to carry on her reform of nursing under peace conditions. Owing to her activities in connexion with the Royal Commission and to the state of her health, she was forced to abandon the opportunity of founding her own institution and to work through an existing hospital. St. Thomas's Hospital was chosen, and the Nightingale School started its work there in 1860. The matron of the hospital at this time worked under the general guidance of Florence Nightingale, and she remained Superintendent of the School for twenty-seven years. Briefly, suitable candidates were accepted for training as probationers for one year; they then joined the hospital staff for a further two years, after which they were considered as competent to take over any nursing post. The Nightingale School was the model for the many other schools which were developed in other hospitals, and throughout her life Florence Nightingale kept in the closest touch with its activities and its pupils.

Florence Nightingale was a woman of the most powerful will and an admirable organizer and administrator. Her system of nursing contained many new features, not quite all of which have stood the test of time. That nursing rapidly and steadily improved from the moment she was in authority cannot at all be doubted. Looking back, it is apparent that the immediate success of her methods was due to three main factors. First was her capacity to secure women of high character and good social position to accept positions of responsibility. Second was her removal of the control of the nursing staff entirely from the hands of men into those of women. Third was her insistence on the necessity for a thorough training in the theory and practice of nursing. She saw clearly that, in order to succeed, nursing had to become a profession. Her influence soon passed across the Atlantic, and she was associated with the United States Sanitary Commission and the women who took charge of army nursing during the American Civil War.

While Florence Nightingale was reforming nursing, her contemporary, Mary Carpenter (1807–77), was applying herself to the kindred task of looking after neglected children, establishing reformatory and industrial schools and improving the position of Indian women. She obtained a large measure of public support and exercised considerable influence in America, which she visited in 1873. Many other distinguished and devoted women worked on similar lines.

Among the indirect results of the activity of Florence Nightingale was the establishment at Geneva in 1864 of the International Red Cross Committee, the branches of which have done good service in many wars and have been no less useful in peace.

Florence Nightingale opposed anything in the way of State Registration of nurses. Concentrating on a high ideal of competence and character for the nurse, she failed to grasp some of the secondary effects of her own scheme. A large nursing service is now a necessity in every civilized country as a result of her efforts and example. Having regard to human imperfections, we can as little hope that every woman who nurses will be a born nurse, devoted to her task, as that every doctor or teacher will have a natural vocation for his work. In an imperfect world mankind must protect itself against the incompetent and the unfit. Registration is a way—doubtless an imperfect way—of doing this. The first law to enforce the registration of nurses was passed in New Zealand in 1901. Certain States of the U.S.A. followed fairly soon after, but by the outbreak of the First World War only relatively few countries had adopted such legislation. A Nurses Registration Act became law in Great Britain in 1919.

Since the beginning of a system of approved training for nurses there have been many changes and developments in training and in working conditions. The most important have been a reduction of the number of hours worked weekly by the student or trained nurse, the provision of semi-skilled assistance, and a broadening of the theoretical basis of the nurse's studies. In the early days nurses worked very long hours, and it is only within the last fifteen years that a definite improvement has been effected in this direction. In most British hospitals an attempt is made to reduce the working hours to 96 per fortnight. From early times nurses have had associated with them subsidiary workers who relieved them of some of the drudgery. As early as 1908 a suggestion was made that there should be two grades of nurses in British hospitals, and by 1930 both grades were commonly employed in large hospitals. By an Act of 1943 the assistant nurse was recognized, and authority was given to the General Nursing Council to approve schools for training, to control examinations, and to supervise the Roll of Assistant Nurses. Student nurses preparing for their examinations for State Registration now have to take theoretical courses which cover not only nursing subjects proper, but also elementary courses in the basic scientific and medical subjects, and also in those social subjects which will later be of use to them as units in a complex modern society.

The present century has also seen the development of specialization in the nursing service. It has for long been possible for a girl to be trained in a branch of nursing, for example, in the nursing of fevers, or tuberculosis, or sick children, without taking a full training in a general hospital. After qualification a fully trained nurse may take the special course of study for the Health Visitor's Certificate, or for other branches of public health work. Again, a trained nurse may decide to specialize in the training of others, and for this purpose she is now almost obliged to take the Sister Tutor Diploma or the Diploma in Nursing instituted by two English universities. In the United States the provision of advanced university instruction in nursing has proceeded farther than it has in any other country.

COLLECTIVE MEDICAL DATA

(a) *Demography and vital statistics*

We now deal with matters relating not to individual patients but to large groups of individuals, both sick and healthy. Before doing so we would point out that the methods which we discuss revealed long ago that the number of persons living on this planet was increasing. The rate of increase differs in different countries and the fact that the population of the world as a whole is increasing at an accelerated rate is due partly to the improvement in medical methods and in public health measures during the last hundred years. Hence the population problem has become important not only to medical men, who have had much to do with its production, but also to every citizen.

In the world as a whole the size of the population is determined by the relationship between births and deaths. If there is an excess of births over deaths the world population increases. In any particular country the size of the population is also affected by the extent of migration. So far as the Western countries were concerned there does not appear to have been any population problem until medical science began to deal effectively with the great epidemic diseases such as smallpox and malaria from the beginning of the nineteenth century onwards. From the later part of that century medicine also played an increasingly important role in disturbing the ratio by effecting a decline in infantile mortality.

The countries of the world can be divided roughly into two classes. There are firstly those countries, such as the United Kingdom, for which reliable figures for the size and age- and sex-constitution of the population are available; and secondly those countries for which only estimates of the size of the population can be obtained. At the present time over two-thirds of the inhabitants of the world are enumerated by effective censuses.

In 1845 the population of the world was estimated as 1,009 millions. In 1928 the world population was approximately 1,900 millions, and in 1940 the estimate was 2,170 millions. At the present time the populations of many Eastern countries are increasing very rapidly.

In any civilized community accurate data on the size of the population, of the community as a whole and of its constituent parts, are required for many official purposes, including the calculation of rates for births, deaths, and the incidence of various diseases. The study of human populations by statistical methods is now known as

Demography. It deals with the number of persons living, being born, and dying in a particular country, and also in its constituent urban and rural areas. It includes also the study of data dealing with social conditions such as housing and wealth.

Domesday Book (1086) was an early though imperfect example of such a study, and in 1662 John Graunt urged the establishment of a government department for the collection of such data (p. 180). The first complete census of any country appears to be that made in Sweden in 1749, and a complete census was also made in Spain in 1798. In the United Kingdom a Private Bill for taking an annual census passed through the House of Commons in 1753, but it was thrown out by the Lords.

During the late eighteenth century the population of Europe was apparently increasing rapidly, as also were the prices of the necessities of life. In 1798 the Rev. Thomas Robert Malthus (1766–1834) published anonymously a work entitled *An Essay on the Principle of Population, as it affects the Future Improvement of Society*, in which he argued that population, when unchecked, increases 'in a geometrical ratio', whereas the means of subsistence increase only 'in an arithmetical ratio'. Malthus argued that the increase of population, if unchecked, would soon outrun the means of subsistence, and that under ordinary conditions Nature imposed two main checks on an increase of population, the most important constituents of which were man's fear of the results of contracting early marriages and a high infant mortality. Malthus's theory was not new, but it was elegantly and popularly expressed, especially in his enlarged second edition (1803). In 1822 Francis Place (1771–1854) openly advocated birth control for the checking of an excessive increase in the population, and from him dates the recognition of the fact that this practice is a more effective check than the bar to early marriage.

As a result of the Population Act of 1800 the First Census of Great Britain was made on 10 March 1801, and from then onward a Census was made at ten-year intervals, the Fourteenth Census in 1931. Because of the war there was no Census in 1941, and the decennial Censuses were resumed in 1951.

The material for the Censuses of 1801, 1811, 1821, and 1831 was provided largely by the overseers of the poor and the parish priests, and the names, ages, and marital states of individuals were not compulsorily obtained. By an Act of 1836 the General Register Office was set up in London and a Registrar General was appointed. To him was transferred the organization of the 1841 Census, and the whole country was divided into 2,193 registration districts, each in the charge of a District Registrar, and each divided into enumeration districts. For the first time a schedule was distributed to each householder, and he was directed, under penalty, to complete the schedule on the appointed Census Day. In this 1841 Census details were obtained regarding the name, age, marital condition, place of birth, and nature of work of every member of the population. In succeeding Censuses a few further questions were asked. In 1891 and 1911 especially further important questions were asked regarding accommodation, and in 1911 questions relating to fertility were first asked. The complete reports for the 1911 Census extend to sixteen folio volumes. The scope of the 1951 Census is wider than that of any of its predecessors.

The particulars given in the various Census volumes are very numerous, and include the population of every administrative district in England and Wales, divided by ages and sexes. Occupations and habitations are dealt with very fully. In the medical field the most valuable information is the age and sex constitution of the population. As a brief indication of the changes in the population since 1801, the data of Fig. 142 are abbreviated from a table given by the Registrar General. This table shows that the rate of increase in the population reached its maximum about 1820. Since then, although the population increased, the rate of increase declined steadily until 1911–21, when, as a result of factors arising out of the First World War, the decline became marked.

It is with these figures for the country as a whole, or the corresponding population figures for constituent parts of the country, that all rates—for births, marriages, deaths, and individual diseases —are calculated. Accurate results will be given where the rates required relate to a Census Year. For intercensal years the intercensal population—an estimate calculated and published by the Registrar General for every administrative area in the country—is used.

Fig. 142. *England and Wales: Population, 1801–1951*

Census year	Population			Decennial rate of increase per cent. of population			No. of females to 1,000 males
	Persons	Males	Females	Persons	Males	Females	
1801	8,892,536	4,254,735	4,637,801	..	..	..	1,057
1811	10,164,256	4,873,605	5,290,651	14·00	14·24	13·78	1,054
1821	12,000,236	5,850,319	6,149,917	18·06	20·03	16·23	1,036
1831	13,896,797	6,771,196	7,125,601	15·80	15·73	15·86	1,040
1841	15,914,148	7,777,586	8,136,562	14·27	14·39	14·15	1,046
1851	17,927,609	8,781,225	9,146,384	12·65	12·68	12·62	1,042
1861	20,066,224	9,776,259	10,289,965	11·90	11·30	12·47	1,053
1871	22,712,266	11,058,934	11,653,332	13·21	13·14	13·27	1,054
1881	25,974,439	12,639,902	13,334,537	14·36	14·29	14·42	1,055
1891	29,002,525	14,052,901	14,949,624	11·65	11·17	12·11	1,064
1901	32,527,843	15,728,613	16,799,230	12·17	11·94	12·39	1,068
1911	36,070,492	17,445,608	18,624,884	10·89	10·91	10·86	1,068
1921	37,886,699	18,075,239	19,811,460	4·93	3·53	6·24	1,096
1931	39,952,377	19,133,010	20,819,367	5·53	5·94	5·16	1,088
1951	43,744,924	21,024,187	22,720,737	4·65	4·84	4·48	1,081

Vital registration. Sweden is regarded as the birthplace of official vital statistics, since a law was passed there in 1748 requiring the authorities of each parish to complete yearly a statement showing the number of baptisms, weddings, and deaths which had occurred in the parish during the year.

The English Act of 1836 not only established the General Register Office and the post of Registrar General, but it also prescribed the forms to be used for the registration of births, deaths, and marriages. Registration was to be carried out by the District Registrars, who transmitted the information to the central office. Registration was at first optional, but by the Births and Deaths Registration Act of 1874 it became compulsory, and by an Act of 1926 still-births also became compulsorily registrable.

In the First Annual Report of the Registrar General (1839) Dr. William Farr (p. 717) pointed out that in the death certificates which had been received during that first year the same disease had sometimes been denoted by three or four different terms, and each term had been applied to as many diseases. Vague names had been used, and complications had been registered as the cause of death instead of the primary diseases which caused them. Farr called for a uniform statistical nomenclature of diseases. Examples of ill-defined names for fatal diseases are debility in infancy, senility in old age, and the indefinite term membranous croup for the more scientific term diphtheria. At the First Statistical Congress, held in Brussels in 1853, Farr and Jacob Marc d'Espine (1806–60) of Geneva were therefore invited to draw up a classification of diseases for international use. Their International List of the Causes of Death has since been often revised, Adolphe Louise Jacques Bertillon (1851–1922) having been specially active here. The number of possible names for diseases runs to many thousands, and the purpose of the International List is to enable vital statisticians in different countries to classify the recorded causes of death in about 200 manageable groups. Medical men are also encouraged to use only names of diseases which are acceptable at least on a national classification, and to this end an official book, *The Nomenclature of Diseases*, drawn up by a Committee appointed by the Royal College of Physicians of London, was first published in 1869 and has since been frequently revised. When a medical practitioner fills in a cause of death which is unacceptable, the Registrar General communicates with him in an attempt to elucidate the diagnosis. In these ways the accuracy of death statistics has been much improved throughout the years.

Soon after the foundation of these official death statistics the matter of the very high mortality rate in the first five years of life was also tackled. In the Second Report of the Registrar General (1840) Farr showed that the best measure of the mortality of children under 1 year of age is obtained by expressing the result as the number of deaths per 1,000 live births. This is termed the infantile mortality rate.

The rise of the English public health movement in the middle of the nineteenth century, and the obligatory appointment of the first medical officers of health in 1856, led to a demand for a new type of official statistics. Conway Evans (1830–92), the Medical Officer of Health for the Strand District of London, undertook to prepare for the newly formed Metropolitan Association of Medical Officers of Health (later the Society of Medical Officers of Health) a weekly return of sickness which the General Board of Health undertook to print and distribute. The return dealt with new cases of illness in persons receiving in- and out-relief and also in persons admitted for treatment to several public institutions. The named diseases included all the common infectious fevers. Evans carried on this work unaided until the end of 1857, and a volume of returns was published covering the period 4 April 1857 to 2 January 1858. After that the Central Government refused to bear the cost of printing, and this pioneer effort ceased.

During the next twenty years medical officers repeatedly complained that their work was handicapped by lack of knowledge of infectious diseases in their areas. A compromise was reached by allowing local authorities, by means of Local Acts, to make infectious diseases compulsorily notifiable in their areas. The first town to promote such a Local Act was Bolton (1877), and other towns followed. In 1889 the Infectious Diseases (Notification) Act was passed. This was an adoptive Act, and infectious diseases were compulsorily notifiable in all areas which had adopted it. This anomalous position was rectified in 1899, when infectious diseases became compulsorily notifiable throughout the country.

Notification of an infectious disease is made to the medical officer of health by the doctor who is treating the patient. It is the duty of the medical officer of health to take whatever action he considers desirable to prevent the spread of the disease and to ensure that the patient is receiving satisfactory treatment, including proper isolation if considered desirable. The medical officer of health must also transmit weekly to the Ministry of Health a statement of all infectious illnesses which have occurred in his area during the previous week. Compulsory notification has provided over the years a mass of data which has been invaluable in the study of individual diseases, and of the biology of infectious diseases in general.

For over eighty years the annual national statistics were published in the form of an *Annual Report of the Registrar General*, folio volumes issued yearly. Since 1920 the data for each year are published in three octavo volumes entitled *The Registrar General's Statistical Review of England and Wales for the Year* [—]. Two of the volumes contain the tables, medical and civil respectively, and the third volume is a very detailed commentary by the Registrar General on the tables and the deductions which can be made from them. The Registrar General also issues weekly and quarterly returns of the incidence of infectious diseases in all the main administrative areas. Changes in the diagnosis, which are sometimes necessary after the notification has been made, are allowed for by the Registrar General in his quarterly and annual figures.

The first Registrar General was Thomas Henry Lister (1800–42), known also as a novelist and dramatist. He was succeeded in 1842 by George Graham (1801–88), a very able administrator who held the office for thirty-seven years.

The founder of vital statistics, William Farr (1807–83), studied medicine in Paris and London and then settled in practice in the Metropolis. In 1837 he contributed the article on vital statistics to the collaborative work, *A Statistical Account of the British Empire*, planned and edited by a famous economist. This article was probably the foundation of vital statistics, and largely because of it Farr was appointed in the following year to the new post of Compiler of Abstracts in the office of the Registrar General. To the First Report of the Registrar General (1839) he contributed a valuable report on deaths. This was the first of the long series of contributions made by him in the Registrar General's Reports, and as time passed he virtually wrote the annual report. He worked in the Registrar General's office for over forty years, and although the great efficiency of the department was due to Graham, Farr's research work was so important and widely known that in other countries he was often thought to be the Registrar General.

Farr ranged over the whole field of vital statistics and himself introduced many new lines of investigation. In the First Report (1839) he laid down the classification of deaths which was used officially thereafter. On many occasions he dealt with the mortality in different occupations, and he showed that the best measure of the ' sanitary condition ' of an area is given by the death-rate for children under five. Perhaps more than any other person Farr provided the basic material, and justifiable deductions from it, which was used by the great English sanitary reformers of the mid-nineteenth century. As Sir John Simon (p. 219) wrote, Farr was 'a master of the methods by which arithmetic is made argumentative'.

The population of England and Wales since 1801 is given in Fig. 142. It can be shown that until the twentieth century there was no very remarkable change in the proportions of the population at different ages. Until about 1875 the trend of the birth-rate in Great Britain was upwards, and from about 1900 until 1940 it was slightly downwards. The cumulative result of this and of other factors was to change the proportional age distribution, so that there are relatively fewer individuals below 20 years, and relatively more aged

FIG. 143. *Population of Great Britian by age-groups, 1891 and 1947*

	1891		1947	
Ages	*Thousands*	*Per cent. of total*	*Thousands*	*Per cent. of total*
0–19	14,974	45	13,672	28
20–39	9,990	30	14,666	30
40–59	5,603	17	12,507	26
60 and over	2,462	7	7,343	15
Total	33,028	100	48,188	100

over 60. We are now confronted, therefore, with an ageing population. These facts are shown in the table (Fig.143) and graphically in Fig. 144. In the inter-war years it was feared that the falling birth-rate in Great Britain might be due to a decrease in fertility. Population experts asserted that the damage was already done, and that, while the population would increase slowly for some years, it would thereafter show a gradual but continuous decline. In 1944 a Royal Commission on Population was appointed, and in its main report (1949) it emphasized that one of the root causes of the problem is the question whether the population as a whole thinks it worth while to produce sufficient children to reproduce itself. Nevertheless, in discussing the population growth revealed by the 1951 Census, the Registrar General stressed that so far there was no sign of any tapering away of the successive increments of growth such as would normally be expected to herald the early approach of an ultimate population maximum.

Some of the main vital statistics for England and Wales since the beginning of compulsory registration are given in Fig. 145. It is seen

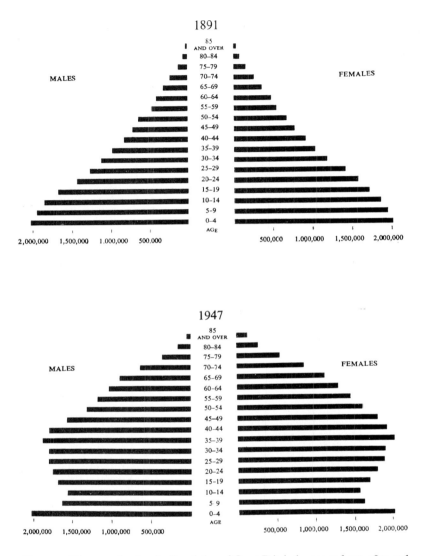

FIG. 144. Diagrams showing the Population of Great Britain by age and sex, 1891 and 1947.
(Reproduced from the *Royal Commission on Population Report*, H.M.S.O., 1949)

that the fall in the birth-rate is in fact compensated by a marked
decline in the general death-rate, owing to improvements in medical
treatment and in the standard of living. But the fall in the birth-rate
and the decline in the death-rate act at opposite ends of the scale.

FIG. 145. *Vital Statistics of England and Wales, 1876–1955*

Period	Birth-rate per 1,000 living	Crude death-rate per 1,000 living	Infant mortality rate per 1,000 births	Maternal mortality rate per 1,000 births*	Crude death-rates per million living				
					Respiratory diseases (excluding phthisis)	Tuberculosis (all forms)	Tuberculosis (respiratory)	Heart disease†	Cancer
1876–1880	35·3	20·8	145	..	3,956	..	2,041	..	..
1881–1885	33·5	19·4	139 ⎫	5·01	3,716	..	1,831	..	..
1886–1890	31·4	18·9	145 ⎭		3,768	..	1,636	1,564	..
1891–1895	30·5	18·7	151 ⎫	5·36	3,723	..	1,462	1,555	..
1896–1900	29·3	17·7	156 ⎭		3,098	1,907	1,324	1,517	801
1901–1905	28·2	16·0	138	4·27	2,771	1,584	1,218	1,450	867
1906–1910	26·3	14·7	117	3·74	2,544	1,567	1,107	1,422	940
1911–1915	23·6	14·3	110	4·03	2,452	1,419	1,051	1,492	1,056
1916–1920	20·1	14·4	90	4·12	2,603	1,462	1,124	1,562	1,190
1921–1925	19·9	12·1	76	3·90	2,053	1,082	857	1,537	1,270
1926–1930	16·7	12·1	68	4·27	1,716	943	770	2,028	1,411
1931–1935	15·0	12·0	62	4·32	1,351	807	672	2,658	1,534
1936–1940	14·7	12·5	55	3·26	1,710	658	551	2,970	1,625
1941–1945	15·9	12·8	50	2·26	1,523	660	548	3,202	1,869
1946–1950	18·0	11·8	36	1·09	1,299	487	421	3,462	1,868
1951–1955	15·2	11·7	27	0·73	1,377	216	191	3,761	1,944

* These rates are given per 1,000 live births up to and including 1927. From 1928
onwards they are given per 1,000 total (i.e. live and still) births.

† Owing to changes in the constitution of the groups which together make up 'heart
disease', the official rates for this condition from 1950 onwards are not directly comparable with the rates for the preceding years. The rates used in the calculation of this
table for the years 1950 to 1955 inclusive are adjusted in order to make them comparable
with the rates for the earlier periods. We are indebted to Dr. W. P. D. Logan, Chief
Medical Statistician of the General Register Office, for suggesting the classes suitable
for inclusion.

While there may not be much change in the total number of persons
living, the numbers at the early ages are progressively diminished,
while those at the upper age limits are progressively increased. But
the former result is itself counterbalanced by the very marked fall
in the infant mortality rate arising from the action of maternity and

child-welfare schemes and of general public health measures. Despite the actual increase in numbers of aged persons there has been a marked and progressive decline in deaths from respiratory diseases of all forms, including those types of pneumonia and bronchitis which were formerly a fruitful cause of death in old persons. Heart disease and cancer have both shown a marked and disturbing increase, the former during the last thirty years and the latter during the last fifty. Part at least of the increased number of deaths caused by diseases of the heart is attributable to angina pectoris, coronary disease (disease of the arteries which supply the heart itself), and similar conditions affecting the heart-muscle which seem to be an expression of the increasing strain of modern life.

(*b*) *Biometry and medical statistics*

We now turn to the application of arithmetic to small groups of cases—such as are met with in medical research—instead of to large populations.

'*The Numerical Method*'. This was the method of describing medical facts based on the conviction that clinical acumen depended entirely on observation. It was introduced by Pierre Charles Alexandre Louis (1787–1872), who spent six of his early years studying pulmonary tuberculosis ('phthisis') and typhoid fever. He kept detailed records of the presence or absence of nearly all possible symptoms and signs in those patients; and after death he noted the condition of all the organs and tissues in the body. Louis published his *Recherches anatomico-pathologiques sur la phthisie* ('Anatomico-pathological researches on phthisis') in 1825. It is based on 123 cases, with post-mortem findings in 50. His work on typhoid fever (1829) is based on 138 cases, with post-mortem findings in 50.

Louis gave actual figures for the number of cases in which the different conditions were found, and he seldom gave his findings in the form of percentages. The result is that his figures can still be used for statistical work, though he embodied his numerical statements in the text instead of setting them out in the form of tables, as we would do nowadays.

Although a society was founded in Paris, with Louis as perpetual president and British and American physicians among its members, to develop Louis's practices, the Numerical Method was on the whole not well received in the country of its origin. The French physicians were interested in individual patients, while Louis was more interested in the science of medicine. He conceived that, if his own observations were repeated many times in the same way by others, the cumulative result might be a forward step. He certainly appreciated that some of his numerical results were due to the pathological processes present, while others were due merely to chance. There were mathematicians in France at that time who could have helped him to separate one group from the other, to test his deductions, but they were never constrained to direct their energies to medical problems. The result was that after a long interval the initiative passed to Great Britain, and it was mainly in London that the science of Medical Statistics had its brilliant origin and early development.

Probability and the normal curve. The type of problem with which Louis had to deal is one which is almost inseparable from medical research nowadays. Until almost the present century physicians judged their results by a process of intuitive reasoning derived from long experience. Then the method of tabulating results numerically began to become fashionable, giving data of the type provided by Louis, but in a more easily readable form. This method gave greater accuracy, but it introduced difficulties which had until then been appreciated by few.

Let us put the problem in its simplest possible form. Suppose that a physician treats 10 patients suffering from a certain disease by a method recognized as acceptable, and all of them die; and suppose he treats his next 10 patients suffering from that disease by a new drug, and all of them recover. In that case the physician will have some grounds for believing that the new drug is very effective. This deduction will be strengthened if he gets a similar result with the next 10 patients treated. But supposing in his third sample of 10 patients so treated he has only 2 recoveries, an element of doubt may enter his mind, and if he goes on having only moderate success with further samples, he may think that his earlier favourable results were due at least in part to chance.

It need hardly be said that in practice it would be astonishing if any new method of treatment produced such an enormous improvement in results. The nearest approach might be the action of penicillin and other antibiotics in certain diseases. What would be much more likely to happen would be events such as the following: A physician treats by a recognized method 10 patients suffering from a certain disease, and he gets 4 recoveries and 6 deaths. He continues to treat samples of 10 patients by this method, and on an average he gets 4 recoveries and 6 deaths. He then treats 10 patients with a new drug, and he has 5 recoveries and 5 deaths. On continuing to treat samples of 10 patients with this drug, he finds that his recoveries per sample are usually 5, and never more than 6. Does the new drug really exercise a beneficial effect, or is the slight numerical improvement due to the action of chance?

Problems of this type can be answered by repeating the samples indefinitely where the two possible occurrences are not the recovery or death of a patient, but the occurrence of a head or a tail in the toss of a coin. But in clinical medicine, and often in laboratory work, we cannot go on multiplying our samples indefinitely. We must take the material which comes to hand, carry out the test and obtain a numerical expression of the result, and we must then apply to this result some statistical test to determine whether it may possibly have been due to chance.

It can be shown that, if the physician is dealing with a disease in which recognized methods produce, say, 50 per cent. of recoveries, then if he treats an infinite number of cases, and if the actual number of recoveries are plotted on a graph, the resultant curve will be symmetrical and in shape somewhat like an inverted bell (Fig. 146). No matter what the nature of the material with which we are working, the usual curve representing it will be expressed by a complicated equation containing two constants, two independent variables, a number (n) which is given by the data, and a quantity (σ) which is characteristic of the distribution under investigation. This is the *normal curve*, and its spread is determined by this quantity σ, known as the standard deviation.

It can also be shown that in any distribution of this type only about 5 per cent. of the observations will differ from the mean by as much as or more than twice the standard deviation, and in the same way that only about 0·27 per cent. of the observations differ from the mean by as much as or more than three times the standard deviation. It is conventionally assumed that values which differ from the mean value by as much as twice the standard deviation are unlikely to occur by chance alone, and that values three times greater than the standard deviation are very unlikely to do so. In such cases we assume that some factor other than chance—such as a new type of treatment—is responsible for the improvement.

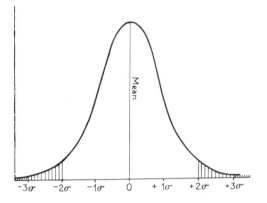

FIG. 146. The normal curve, showing the proportions of observations which deviate from the mean by as much as or more than twice and thrice the standard deviation respectively.

In any distribution arising as a result of our experimental trials, what we are interested in is whether the proportion of the observations which fall outside the limits of twice and thrice the standard deviation as measured from the mean of the observations is substantially greater as compared with the corresponding proportion of the theoretical distribution which most nearly represents our series. In most cases that theoretical distribution is the normal curve, and Fig. 146 illustrates that what we are really concerned with are the areas formed by the tails of the curve.

The areas under the normal curve between the vertical representing the mean and a vertical at any other point on the X-axis have been calculated from the curve and are given in tables of the probability integral. The normal curve can thus be employed rapidly to give the 'significance' of experimental results. It is also very usefully employed to calculate the theoretical class frequencies corresponding to the observed class frequencies of observations arranged in classes of ascending magnitude. This is a common method of arranging statistical data for the purpose of computation.

It should be said that similar arguments apply when the probabilities of death or recovery are not equal, but certain modifications have to be introduced in the methods used.

The 'normal curve of error', as it was formerly called, was discovered in 1733 by Abraham de Moivre (p. 180), and published as a second supplement (now very scarce) to his *Miscellanea analytica*, the original edition of which was published in 1730. De Moivre, a Frenchman who spent most of his life in London, discovered the curve as the result of his interest in the mathematics of games of chance. His work on the normal curve was long overlooked, and the discovery has been attributed to Pierre Simon Laplace (p. 166) and to Karl Friedrich Gauss (1777–1855), both of whom added to the mathematical theory of the curve.

In 1837 Quetelet (p. 181) became interested in statistics, and his work was published as *Lettres sur la théorie des probabilités* (1846). One letter, on the application of statistics in medicine, is a plea for accurate observation and recording of results; it contains nothing of importance. The significant part of Quetelet's book is the extensive series of notes. In these Quetelet gave the first applications of the normal curve to biological observations, his two examples being the chest measurements of soldiers in Scottish regiments, and the height of French conscripts.

In 1869 (Sir) Francis Galton (1822–1911) published his *Hereditary Genius*, a landmark in the history of biology, heredity, and of statistics. Basing his work on these two examples by Quetelet of the 'law of deviation from an average' (i.e. the normal curve), Galton used the curve for the elucidation of mental characters, and thereafter he constantly attempted to improve the method. To Galton more than to anyone else is due the scientific application of statistical methods.

Correlation. Correlation refers to the extent to which two series of events or characters vary concomitantly, one in relation to the other. In order to obtain a measure of this relationship, the two events or characters must be related in pairs. The correlation coefficient expresses the degree of relationship between the different variables in the form of a single numerical quantity.

Although the word correlation had been used by Georges Léopold Chrétien Frédéric Cuvier (p. 236), Galton was the first to use it in a sense which seemed to indicate that the relationship between two different characters in the same individual was quantitative (1869). Six years later he made his first successful attack on the problem from the quantitative aspect. This early work was on the lines of regression (or 'reversion', as he then called it). It was not until 1888 that he realized that, by measuring each character in terms of its own variability as a unit, the slope of the regression line was a measure of the correlation coefficient. In *Natural Inheritance* (1889) he developed the new principles from a practical aspect; he published the first correlation table and introduced the symbol r for the correlation coefficient.

The 'chi-square test'. The leading exponent of Galton's ideas was Karl Pearson (1857–1936), mathematician and pioneer in the new science of biometry at University College, London. His *Grammar of Science* (1892) was a very important criticism of the current methods and philosophy of science. He was mainly responsible for the foundation of the journal *Biometrika* (1901) dealing with statistical methods especially in their relation to biometry and heredity, and alone or in collaboration he edited it for thirty-five years.

In 1900 Pearson introduced the χ^2 ('chi-square') test for the significance of the differences between a series of proportions. This test is especially valuable in medical research, in which, for example, the comparison is made between the efficiencies of two methods of treatment by expressing the results in tabular form. An apparent superiority of one method, as expressed by the figures, might be due to chance, and the 'chi-square' test is a convenient method of ascertaining the probability of this being the case.

The technique of small samples. The arithmetical mean of a series of observations is one of the fundamental qualities used in many statistical calculations. When the number of observations is greater than 15, no difficulty arises. In 1908 'Student' (William Sealy

Gosset, 1876–1937) published a very important paper on the probable error of the mean in which he introduced the test now known as Student's t. This test was later developed to embrace the significance of means of small samples (say, less than 15 observations per sample). The most eminent statistician of this generation is Sir Ronald Aylmer Fisher (1890–), who more than anyone else has developed the statistical technique of small samples based on Student's work, and who has evolved his z test which is of great value in testing the significance of correlation coefficients and for other purposes. In medical research the number of observations is often very limited, and the small-sample technique is therefore especially useful.

The design of experiments. Medical statistics, like statistics applied to any other human activity, will not give more information than is contained in the data. The most expert statistician cannot make a silk purse out of a sow's ear. Correct methods and arithmetical accuracy are not only useless but may well be misleading if the material to which they are applied is not appropriate. It was realized long ago that in biological experiments it was often desirable to set up control experiments, in which all the physical conditions were kept the same as those of the main series, except that the factor which was being tested was omitted from the control series. Modern medical and biological research demands even more elaborate measures to ensure the absence of the influence of chance, and to secure data which can be treated adequately by statistical methods. Much of this work derives from the investigations of Fisher, as set out especially in his book on *The Design of Experiments* (1935). Fisher emphasized that, where a number of factors have to be taken into consideration, it is waste of time and energy to carry out experiments to test only one factor at a time. The experiments should be designed to test four or five factors at once. In agricultural research this principle has worked well, but it is not clear that it is equally satisfactory in medical research.

(c) Epidemiology

Infectious diseases cannot be studied scientifically as crowd-phenomena without adequate data. The science of epidemiology is therefore a product of the last hundred years, and especially of the last fifty.

Hippocrates was the first to show a genuine interest in the prevalence of infectious diseases. The first half of *Airs Waters Places* is the Hippocratic treatise on endemic diseases. It sets out the diseases associated with different climatic conditions and with different places—presumably in the island of Thasos. The two books which really form one treatise known as *Epidemics I and III* give forty-two clinical case histories, and discuss the four 'Constitutions' with the epidemic diseases prevalent in each. These Constitutions were not seasons of the year, but varying periods of time presumably occurring in different years. Mumps and malaria can be clearly recognized in these descriptions. But Hippocrates, the master of observation and concise clinical description, is sparing in his numerical statements. When he says that 'many fell victims to quotidians', we cannot even guess what he meant by 'many'. The non-arithmetical form of epidemiological literature was fixed by Hippocrates for two thousand years.

Galen created a medical philosophy which explained all diseases as the interaction of the constitutions, the temperament of the individual, and factors such as nutrition, occupation, and exercise which influence his resistance. These theories were accepted blindly for over fourteen centuries.

Sydenham (p. 110) harked back to the Constitutions of Hippocrates. He divided the fevers which were rife in London into stationary and intercurrent fevers. He believed that different years have different 'constitutions', which depend upon 'certain hidden and inexplicable changes within the bowels of the earth'. The 'epidemic constitution' of any year determined its endemic (stationary) fevers, and the prevailing stationary fever had an effect on any epidemics in that year. If in a certain year smallpox was endemic and an epidemic of measles occurred, then all the measles patients would show features peculiar to smallpox.

Sydenham's doctrine must not be dismissed off-hand. Neglected for three centuries, it attained much significance in the twentieth. During the First World War there were serious outbreaks of cerebrospinal fever in troops and civilians. In 1917 a new disease, encephalitis lethargica ('sleepy sickness'), broke out in Vienna and spread over Europe. In 1918–19 there was an enormous pandemic of influenza. For years after the war there was excessive prevalence of poliomyelitis, encephalitis lethargica, and of a type of encephalitis which was a complication of common infectious diseases. To explain this complex phenomenon the most important theories are that a new virus, active especially in nervous tissue, was at work; or alternatively that, owing to unknown factors, the virus of the primary infection had taken on certain characteristics which sometimes made it attack the central nervous system. To cover such occurrences Sir William Heaton Hamer (1862–1936) and his followers revived a variant of Sydenham's doctrine which in the future may well be resurrected in some modified form.

For two centuries after Sydenham there was no study of epidemiology worthy of the name. Discussion of the mode of spread of epidemics was futile, since no one, until the brilliant effort of John Snow (p. 345), recognized the importance of field epidemiology.

During these two centuries, barren from the epidemiological aspect, a theory of great antiquity continued to exercise a restraining influence. This was the theory of the miasmata, those subtle exhalations from the bowels of the earth or arising from the air which were supposed to be the cause of epidemics. It is true that Fracastor had postulated a *contagium vivum*, but it is also the case that epidemiologically speaking he had little influence during this period. There were miasmatists and contagionists, and there was an interminable war between them. But in practice the measures adopted to control infectious diseases were based on the theory of contagion; and as late as the close of the nineteenth century, when, as in the case of plague, known principles of infection based on knowledge of the life-history of the specific parasite failed to explain the facts, even the contagionists sought refuge in the miasmatic theory.

A noteworthy attempt to dispel the miasmatic fog was made by Jakob Henle (p. 321), who later became a famous anatomist. In 1840 Henle published an essay entitled *Von den Miasmen und Kontagien* ('On miasmata and contagion'). In this work he divided epidemic diseases into three groups. The first group—due to miasma

—consisted only of the disease malaria. In his second group—which included most of the common infectious diseases—he held that the original beginning of the disease was due to a miasma; but thereafter a living parasite developed in the human body, multiplied, and spread the disease to others by infection. In his third group—which included syphilis and scabies—contagion alone was involved in the spread. It was not until the bacteria of many of the common infectious diseases had been discovered, and the life histories of some of the pathogenic protozoa had been worked out, that Henle's essay came to be appreciated at its true value. It laid down clearly the principles of the specific origin of infectious diseases.

Asiatic cholera first reached the United Kingdom in October 1831. In 1831–2, 1848–9, and 1853–4 it caused very deadly outbreaks there, and smaller outbreaks in 1868 and 1893. Even as late as 1832 the current view was that the disease was a visitation of Divine Providence on sinners, and many practitioners did not even consider that it was communicable from one person to another. At the close of the 1848–9 epidemic John Snow suggested, in a short essay, that material from the excreta of cholera patients was accidentally swallowed by healthy persons and in them multiplied itself. He considered that cholera was spread by the accidental emptying of sewers, bearing infected excreta, into the drinking water of the community. In London most of the cholera deaths had occurred in a district which obtained its drinking water from the Thames where that river was most polluted by sewage. Snow also suggested that contaminated water could be purified by filtration through sand and gravel, or by allowing it to stand in reservoirs. These simple preventive measures were completely rational and could hardly be bettered today. Yet they were proposed over thirty years before the discovery of the causative organism of cholera (p. 391).

At the close of the 1854 epidemic of cholera in Great Britain there occurred the famous incident of the Broad Street pump. In a very small area in Central London over 500 cholera deaths occurred in ten days. As a result of a house-to-house inquiry Snow showed that only those who obtained their drinking water from the Broad Street pump had contracted cholera. He advised removal of the pump-handle, and a few days after this was done new cases ceased. It can now be shown that the outbreak had already subsided, but for generations the incident served as a salutary reminder. A few months later Snow published a revised edition of his short essay, now grown to a substantial book. It included his most important contribution to epidemiology, namely the results of his investigations into the source of the drinking water used by every house south of the Thames in which a case of cholera had occurred. It is a field epidemiological investigation on the grandest scale.

Typhoid fever. What Snow did for cholera, William Budd (1811–80) of Bristol did for typhoid fever. His work should have made it obvious that this disease is spread by the ingestion of infected material from a patient, and that defective sewers are the most likely cause of infection of the water supply. But it was difficult to exclude other hypothetical causes, and Budd's doctrines were never accepted by Murchison, who had more experience of typhoid fever than any other physician in the country. Charles Murchison (1830–79) graduated in medicine at Edinburgh, studied thereafter in Dublin and Paris, served for over two years in the Bengal army of the East India Company, and then settled in London, where he held a succession of important posts in the London teaching hospitals. These posts, and his long connexion with the London Fever Hospital, gave him unrivalled opportunities for the study of fevers. His *Treatise on the Continued Fevers of Great Britain* (1862) dealt mainly with typhus, typhoid, and remittent fever, and is still valuable from the clinical aspect. But on the subject of etiology it is dogmatic; and even in the second edition (1873) Murchison continued to oppose the new doctrines.

Infection and immunity. The discovery of the specific organisms of certain infectious diseases (pp. 390–5)—suggested long before by Fracastor (p. 105)—apparently provided the key. Injection of the organism into susceptible laboratory animals, or accidental infection of a laboratory worker, produced the disease. If the animal, or the individual, did not contract the disease, it was assumed that the dose had been too small. Then the theory of immunity to the particular organism had to be taken into account. The effects of immunity have perhaps been most fully worked out in the case of diphtheria (p. 434). Further difficulties in explaining the facts led to consideration of the manner in which the organisms were transmitted from sick to healthy individuals. It will be seen that these three aspects of the problem are neatly covered by the parable of the Sower: the study of the particular organism being represented by the Seed, the immunity or resistance of the body to it being represented by the Soil, and the method of transfer of the organism by the Sowing. Very extensive research on these lines has led to a widening of our outlook on infectious diseases—and also to further problems.

In this brief summary of the development of epidemiological thought no attention will be given to change of views regarding the behaviour of individual diseases, but something will now be said of the broad principles of behaviour of epidemic diseases in general.

William Farr was the first to note that the rise, decline, and fall of an epidemic is an orderly phenomenon. If the number of cases occurring in successive small time-intervals—usually weeks—are plotted, a fairly smooth curve can often be drawn through the points representing the weekly incidences. Farr conceived that this orderliness might be described in mathematical language, and in the Second Report of the Registrar General (1840) he used the weekly cases of smallpox which had just been epidemic. He found that the mathematical expression which most closely described the observed facts was the equation of the normal curve. Although Farr stated that he would pursue this matter further, it was not until twenty-seven years later that he was induced almost by accident to return to the subject. In 1867 cattle plague was very serious, and in Parliament a member made the statement that unless some effective action was taken, all the cattle in the country would be destroyed. Farr then modified slightly his previous mathematical method and applied it to the data for the epidemic up to that time. In a letter to the public press he pointed out that on the basis of the course of the epidemic, his prediction was that it would terminate within a certain stated time. His prediction later proved to be approximately accurate.

It might be thought that the epidemiological tool which Farr had thus forged would have soon been used in the investigation of epidemics, and especially in the prediction of their further course after their origin. But in fact, for two main reasons, few such attempts were made. There were very few medical men who had the necessary mathematical and statistical ability to follow Farr. Further, it was soon evident that many outbreaks did not follow a pattern which could be adequately described by the normal curve. It was stated earlier that this curve is symmetrical, the ascending and descending limbs being of equal steepness. But in many seasonal epidemics the ascending limb rises more steeply than in the normal curve, while the descending limb falls away more slowly; that is, the outbreak is of an explosive type, reaches its maximum rapidly, and then gradually declines. This type of curve is seen especially in outbreaks due to infected water-supplies, such as typhoid or cholera (Fig.147). Once the water has become infected, the organisms multiply rapidly, and infected water reaches a large number of consumers almost at the same time. On the other hand, in certain outbreaks of other diseases the rise to the maximum is gradual, and the decline is rapid.

It was not until early in the present century that a further tool was devised which was capable of being adapted to such varied data. Karl Pearson then described six types of frequency curves, and for each he derived the appropriate mathematical equation. These curves were first extensively employed in epidemiological work by John Brownlee (1867–1927), a founder of scientific epidemiology. Pearson's curves are applicable to many epidemics which are— mathematically speaking—of a simple nature and have only one peak; and they have been satisfactorily fitted to the existing data for historic outbreaks, such as the first epidemic of cholera in the United Kingdom (Fig. 147). But when the outbreak reaches its maximum, begins to decline, and then shows one or more phases of recrudescence, more complicated modern methods have to be used.

These studies of the epidemic wave emphasized the dictum that, in epidemics as in other phenomena, Nature tends to work to a pattern, varied as a result of circumstances and environment.

It was assumed quite early in the bacteriological era that disease-producing organisms possessed two essential characters, infectivity and virulence, and experimental proofs of this assumption multiplied as time passed. Infectivity is the property possessed by an organism of producing disease in an individual to whose tissues it has gained access. (It is not the power of spreading to other individuals; for the spread is not brought about by active movement on the part of the organism. It is produced by physical or biological agents, such as water, food, direct contact, or lice in the case of typhus.) If infectivity is high, then the organism is fairly certain to produce the disease in a non-immune person to whom it has been transferred.

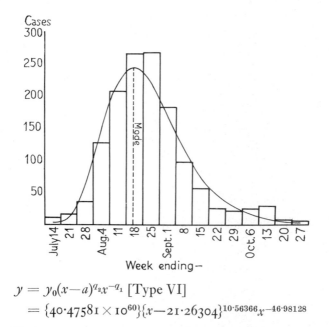

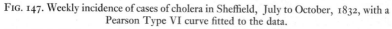

$$y = y_0(x-a)^{q_2}x^{-q_1} \ [\text{Type VI}]$$
$$= \{40 \cdot 47581 \times 10^{60}\}\{x - 21 \cdot 26304\}^{10 \cdot 56366}x^{-46 \cdot 98128}$$

FIG. 147. Weekly incidence of cases of cholera in Sheffield, July to October, 1832, with a Pearson Type VI curve fitted to the data.

(From E. A. Underwood, *Proc. Roy. Soc. Med.*, 1934–5, xxviii (Sect. Hist. Med.), 5–18)

Virulence on the other hand is a measure of the gravity of the disease produced when the organism has infected an individual. A very virulent organism may cause death; an organism of low virulence may cause little disturbance of health.

It was soon recognized that these two properties of an organism do not go hand in hand. A particular organism may have great infectivity and cause a large outbreak; but the virulence may be low and there may be few deaths. On the contrary, cases may be few, but deaths and severe cases may be relatively numerous. To take an example of these features spread over a short period, we may cite the enormous pandemic of influenza which afflicted practically the whole world during 1918–19. In the first wave, which occurred in June and July 1918, cases were very numerous and acute, but the disease was generally not of a fatal type. It showed the usual features of epidemic influenza. In the second wave in October and November, cases were again numerous; but the disease was now very grave, and in about a fifth of the cases the patients showed a pulmonary condition which killed in a few hours. The features of the third wave, in February 1919, resembled those of the second wave. During the whole pandemic there was an alteration of the age grouping usually associated with influenza; the disease was now especially fatal in youths and young adults.

To take an example of the behaviour of a disease spread over a long period, we may repeat that scarlet fever has changed its type on several occasions. Sydenham referred to it as *hoc nomen morbi*—a name but scarcely a disease. By the end of the eighteenth century it had become quite a serious disease; then again it became mild. But after 1830 the virulence of scarlet fever increased, and in the third quarter of the nineteenth century it was the chief cause of death among the infectious diseases of childhood.

A few epidemiologists of the early twentieth century were very interested in the phenomenon of the epidemic wave, and one problem which demanded solution was the reason why an epidemic ceases spontaneously. There are at least two possible explanations. As the epidemic proceeds the infectivity of the organism may gradually diminish until the spread of the organism finally ceases to establish sufficient cases to carry on the epidemic. The other main possibility is that, assuming that one attack of the disease is followed by at least temporary immunity to a second attack, as the epidemic proceeds the number of susceptible persons ultimately becomes insufficient to carry on the infection. In many epidemics of limited extent it is obvious to a qualified epidemiologist, without the application of complicated methods, that the decline of the epidemic could not have been due to an exhaustion of the susceptible population at risk. (It is sometimes surprising how many children pass through a measles epidemic without contracting the disease.)

In these circumstances the supposition is that the epidemic has been terminated by a decline in the infectivity of the organism. But in other epidemics the facts are not so clear, and mathematical methods are required to illumine the problem. It was Brownlee's merit to have been the first to demonstrate that an epidemic is a biological phenomenon which is, mathematically speaking, a function of the infectivity or invasiveness of the causative organism—a function, be it said, which is not static but which is constantly varying throughout the epidemic wave. To various aspects of this problem Major Greenwood (1880–1949) made contributions of lasting value.

Greenwood did physiological research for five years at the London Hospital, trained as a statistician under Karl Pearson (p. 726), and held two pioneer statistical posts before he was appointed to the chair of epidemiology and vital statistics at the newly founded London School of Hygiene and Tropical Medicine (1926). There for nearly twenty years his witty and penetrating lectures, adorned by apt quotations drawn from his wide reading, stimulated in his postgraduate students a spirit of inquiry. Greenwood's early writings dealt with many subjects, especially the hours of work, the dietaries, and the health of industrial workers, accident proneness in factories, and the epidemiology of plague in India. He was also concerned in an attempt to extract some statistical conclusions from the enormous mass of data left in the wake of the 1918 influenza pandemic. His later papers in *Biometrika*, the *Journal of Hygiene*, and elsewhere, deal especially with the statistical measure of infectiousness, and other theoretical aspects of infection and its consequences. His general approach to his subject in all its aspects is perhaps most comprehensively set out in his Herter Lectures, *Epidemiology, Historical and Experimental* (1932). (His important work in the experimental field is discussed briefly below.) Greenwood's much larger book, *Epidemics and Crowd-diseases* (1935), is the most unorthodox and literary of textbooks, and will remain an enduring memorial to the man.

In tropical countries the communicable diseases commonly encountered often require for their propagation the services of an intermediate host. Malaria is a good example. In these circumstances we are dealing not only with factors which influence the parasite and the human host, together or individually, but also with the same or other factors which influence the intermediate host. The scientific elucidation of an epidemic of this type is therefore much more complex. It was to explain such conditions that Sir Ronald Ross (p. 460) evolved a mathematical method which was suggestive for further work.

Another type of problem which greatly interested these early twentieth-century epidemiologists was that of the periodicity of diseases. This problem is in a way an extension of the problem of the termination of an epidemic, but the results have been more difficult to appraise. A common example of a disease with a regular periodicity is measles. It was shown that in many cities in this country epidemics of measles succeeded each other at intervals of roughly 97 weeks. Brownlee, Herbert Edward Soper (1865–1930), and a few others worked on this problem, and there was some evidence that biological factors were responsible. It is, however, yet too early to dogmatize, and the theory of the exhaustion of susceptibles in this disease still claims much support.

Experimental epidemiology. It will be obvious that epidemiological research of this nature requires peculiar gifts, and in execution concentrated thought. John Hunter once wrote to his old pupil, Edward Jenner, the famous question: 'But why think? Why not try the experiment?' Would it be possible to solve some of these difficult epidemiological problems by the experimental method? Anyone who had such an inclination would be faced at once with a problem largely outside his control, viz. the raising of a sufficient number of volunteers. During the war the treatment of the skin disease scabies, which is due to the burrowing of the itch mite in the skin, was greatly improved by the assistance of volunteers who allowed research workers to give them the disease, but, while the results were *therapeutically* of great value, they were *epidemiologically* insignificant. For the experimental investigation of a common infectious disease a great number of volunteers would be required, and for this and other reasons no one would make the attempt.

It is, however, possible to use mice for such experiments. In the case of mice kept in captivity, a month in the life of an individual mouse is equivalent to about two and a half years of human life. Herds of mice can therefore be observed over, in their chronology, long periods without the expenditure of more than a decade or two in the lives of their human observers. The herds can be subjected to infection by certain viruses and bacteria which cause typical epidemic infections in mouse herds, while being non-pathogenic for human beings. Many of the mice which die can be subjected to post-mortem examination: only many and not all, because up to a third of the mice in a sick herd are the victims of cannibalism on the part of their stronger, or less ethical, brothers. Further, the effects of artificial immunization of immigrants to the herd on the reactions of the herd itself can be scrutinized in a manner hardly possible in human populations.

These mice experiments were initiated by William Whiteman Carlton Topley (1886–1944) who, after five fruitful years as professor of bacteriology at Manchester, was called in 1927 to the chair of that subject in the London School of Hygiene and Tropical Medicine. This experimental epidemiology is Topley's greatest claim to fame; but another magnificent achievement was his *Principles of Bacteriology and Immunity* (1929), written in collaboration with Graham Selby Wilson (1895–). About 1921 Topley began these experiments, and they were continued without interruption for at least fifteen years. The mice were kept under ideal conditions, in cages cleaned out and sterilized daily, and were 'sumptuously fed'. Everything possible was done to exclude extraneous infections. The experiments were planned from the epidemiological aspect by, and later discussed fully in collaboration with, Major Greenwood and Austin Bradford Hill (1897–). During the investigation nearly 200,000 mice were used. These experiments tended to show that, once an infection has been introduced into a herd, it does not normally die out while there are sufficient survivors to keep it going. The 'survival of the fittest' partly accounts for the fact that certain mice will pass apparently unaffected through a long outbreak. But a more important role is probably played by an increase in natural immunization, due to their constantly receiving small doses of the infecting organism. As in human communities, the population exposed to risk of the infection is essentially in a state of unstable equilibrium, varying states of immunity in individuals causing subtle changes in the mass immunity of the herd. These experiments gave a fine demonstration of the effects of immigration—the introduction of new arrivals into the herd. It is obvious that the introduction of infected animals will necessarily cause an epidemic or a flare-up of an existing outbreak. But more remarkable is the fact that the introduction of perfectly healthy animals also keeps the infection alive.

A detailed study of the results on the herd of immunizing individual mice artificially against the infecting organism was an important aspect of this long-term investigation by Topley, Greenwood, and their colleagues. It was to be expected that the level of immunity attained naturally by unimmunized mice which survived throughout an epidemic would be very high, and this was found to be the case. It was also found that by means of artificial immunization the resistance of mice which were just entering the herd could be in-increased to a level almost as high as these survivors. It has long been known that in outbreaks of epidemic diseases there may be three degrees of infection. In infection of the first degree the process is so virulent that the patient dies before he has either the time or the ability to develop immunity; this is called a lethal infection. In infection of the second degree—which in many diseases, but not all, constitutes the bulk of the infections—the virulence of the organism is not so high, or the resistance of the patient is greater, and he recovers. In the process of recovery he develops some degree of immunity to the organism. This is a sub-lethal infection. In infection of the third degree the virulence of the organism is so low, or the resistance of the patient is so great, that no clinical symptoms develop; the patient has not had an attack of the disease, but he may infect others. The slight infection with the organism—latent infection—is often sufficient to give the patient a substantial degree of immunity, or to boost up an already existing low degree of immunity to a higher level.

These long-term mice experiments showed that sub-lethal or latent infection is the process by which a herd of mice develops natural immunity to an organism. Detailed observations were made on the changes which took place in the level of this immunity under various conditions. It is very probable that in the human herd natural immunity is produced by the same factors. The experiments also showed that after an epidemic wave had subsided changes in the constitution of the population gradually occurred; this led to a slow increase in the number of susceptible mice, and when a certain concentration was reached, another wave was liable to occur. In 1906 Hamer (p. 729) showed that in human communities a measles epidemic is followed by a gradual accumulation of susceptible individuals, so that a point is ultimately reached when another epidemic wave begins. These mice experiments have tended to confirm Hamer's theory.

Shortly after the commencement of these London experiments Leslie Tillotson Webster (1894–1943) and his colleagues in the United States began somewhat similar experiments on fowls and rabbits. The approach was, however, that of a study of the effects of infection on individual animals rather than on the herd. Webster's work was also important from the genetic aspect, since he attempted to breed strains resistant to infection.

Historical epidemiology. Perhaps more than any other investigators of biological phenomena, the philosophic epidemiologist—as opposed to the field worker—cannot divorce himself from consideration of events long past. He must therefore lean partly on the historians of epidemics. Of these one of the earliest was John Caius (1510–73) of Norwich, who studied at Cambridge. In 1539 he went to Padua, where he lectured on Greek and also studied medicine and was a pupil of Vesalius. After graduating M.D. at Padua he toured Italy, Germany, and France in search of manuscripts of Hippocrates and Galen. Caius later lectured on anatomy in London for twenty years. He was one of the greatest of the humanists and the most distinguished physician in England before Harvey. He is now chiefly remembered as the refounder of his old Cambridge college, Gonville Hall, under the name of Gonville and Caius. In 1552 Caius published *A Boke or Counseill against the Sweate or Sweatyng Sicknesse.*

The sweating sickness (English sweat, *sudor Anglicus*) first appeared in London on 19 September 1485. The illness attacked with dramatic suddenness, giving rise to fever, headache, general pains, and profuse sweating. Death was common and often took place within six hours. It was a disease of the rich rather than of the poor.

On four further occasions this mysterious disease—which may have been a type of influenza—recurred in England in 1508, 1517, 1528, and 1551. In his book Caius described all the outbreaks, but his historical data are not very sound.

The real founder of historical epidemiology was Justus Friedrich Karl Hecker (1795–1850) of Berlin. His best-known works are his essays on the Black Death (1832), the Dancing Mania (1832), and the English Sweat (1834). These were translated into English with the title *The Epidemics of the Middle Ages* (1846), to which book a reprint of the essay by Caius on the English sweat was added as an appendix.

Later historians of epidemics include Heinrich Haeser (1811–84), who in 1845 published in one volume the first edition of his history of medicine, in which much space was devoted to epidemic diseases. In the second edition the work was published in two volumes, of which the second was devoted entirely to epidemics. In the three-volume third edition the much enlarged third volume (1882) constituted a monumental *Geschichte der epidemischen Krankheiten* ('History of epidemic diseases'). Meanwhile, in 1859 August Hirsch (1817–94) published the first volume of the first edition of his *Handbuch der historisch-geographischen Pathologie* (*Handbook of Geographical and Historical Pathology*), and twenty years later the first volume of the greatly enlarged second edition was published. The three volumes of this work give the history of diseases, including epidemic diseases, of the whole world from the earliest times. Hirsch's work was translated into English by Charles Creighton (1847–1927), who later published his own great work on *The History of Epidemics in Britain* (1891–4). Despite his rather heterodox views on certain modern subjects, in this field Creighton was unrivalled. It is a pleasure to end this book with some mention of this man, who has been rightly described as the greatest British medical scholar of the nineteenth century.

EPILOGUE

WE have now traced briefly various advances in medicine through the ages, and we have seen how different sciences have played their parts in the alleviation of suffering. We have seen also how the consideration of disease as a whole, and of the health of peoples as a whole, has brought about a new attitude to the treatment of disease. Health is a public asset, and its promotion has now been recognized as a public duty. There are undeniable disadvantages in placing officers of the State in control of the personal liberties of its citizens, but in matters of health the advantages on the whole outweigh the disadvantages. Only a pessimist or a reactionary could deny the gains to humanity resulting from the passing of preventive measures from private into public hands.

When this book was first published thirty years ago, organized public health measures had been compulsorily applicable to England and Wales as an administrative whole for about seventy years. At first largely environmental and designed to prevent the spread of infection by curtailment of the movements of infected individuals, official public health soon provided sufferers from infectious diseases with free treatment in isolation hospitals. After a long interval it was realized that the effective treatment of certain conditions was the best method of preventing the onset of other diseases. The Central Government, through the local authorities, therefore assumed a modified responsibility for the treatment of a limited number of diseases.

All this work, however, left untreated the mass of illnesses which afflict the human race. The individual who developed a major acute disease could get treatment, free or at reduced cost, in a hospital financed by voluntary subscriptions. But the beds were limited in number, and they had to be reserved for fairly serious conditions. Most of the time of a general practitioner is spent in treating minor and chronic illnesses, sufferers from which were rarely admitted to hospitals, or if admitted, only for short periods. The practitioner had to be paid for his services, and for the wage-earner illness meant medical fees together with loss of wages. To provide funds to meet such double misfortunes medical clubs and approved societies were formed; and in the United Kingdom a new principle was formally adopted as a national policy when the National Health Insurance Act was passed in 1911. The State then assumed the responsibility for ensuring that the wage-earner did lay aside sufficient money for his treatment when he was ill, and there was an implied undertaking on the part of the wage-earner that he would seek medical treatment in the event of illness.

Great as were the benefits conferred by the National Health Insurance Act, it did not go far enough. Wives and younger children were largely excluded from its benefits. It was essentially a financial Act, concerned with the cost, and not the quality, of the treatment provided. From before the outbreak of the Second World War there was criticism of the lack of provision for treatment of conditions common in old age, for the restoration of full physical capacity after illness, and for the treatment of chronic disease in general. Such matters were referred to as 'social medicine', a term which really implied an extension of the work already done under the older name of 'public health'. The term 'social medicine' has perhaps already outlived its usefulness. It was also suggested that the State should consider measures for the improvement of the hospital services, for the amelioration of the conditions under which the general practitioner worked, and for the provision of medical treatment, free or at reduced cost, for all members of the community. The Beveridge Report (1942) was a step towards the fulfilment of this end. The National Health Service Act (1946) was the legislative measure which almost at a stroke changed not only the face of medicine but also the lives and conditions of many who practised it.

There is another side of the picture which we must bear in mind. The advances in medicine and the resulting advantages have depended entirely on the application of the rational method of observation and experiment. To control Nature we must above all things understand Nature. The amount of labour and ingenuity now devoted to the investigation of Nature is seldom appreciated even by men of science. Some conception of the very rapid growth of scientific literature in modern times may be obtained from an account of one attempt to record it. In 1867 the Royal Society issued in six volumes a catalogue of the titles of all scientific papers published in any language between 1800 and 1863. Two new volumes, covering the titles of papers published between 1864 and 1873, appeared soon after the latter date. But four additional volumes bringing the work up to 1883 were not published until 1902. At that date there was thus a lag of twenty years. For the seventeen years 1884–1900 seven volumes were required, and it took more than ten years to publish them. No supplements have since been published dealing with the literature since 1900, and it is unlikely that this or any similar project will ever be completed.

Anyone who attempts to compile a list of the titles of papers dealing with medicine and the medical sciences is met by similar difficulties. Manuscript lists of medical writings existed long before the invention of printing, and as early as 1506 a small medical bibliography was printed. From then until about 1800 several important bibliographies were published in each succeeding century. Each of these had naturally to deal with more books than its predecessor. Most of these bibliographies listed only medical books. But meanwhile the medical journal had made its appearance, and much valuable material remained unnoticed because there was no guide to the articles which such journals contained. Between 1793 and 1797 a new bibliography was published in eight volumes. It dealt with books and journal articles and was supposed to be complete to 1793. But in the meantime the literature had increased so rapidly that it took four further volumes to cover the work published between 1794 and 1797. Of the succeeding 'complete' bibliographies the only one which we need mention is the *Index-Catalogue of the Surgeon-General's Library*—now called the National Medical Library—at Washington. This work set out to list books and also important journal articles. The first large volume was published in 1880 and the sixteenth and final volume in 1895. But the work was then complete only to 1880, so a second series of volumes, to cover the following fifteen years, was commenced. Twenty-one volumes were necessary to do this, and twenty years were required to publish them. This second series was followed by a third, and that by a fourth, the last volume of which, dealing with the letter M, was recently published. But the work—which had been called America's greatest gift to medicine—was by then so much behind that it was decided to discontinue the whole project. Meanwhile, other indexes had appeared; without setting out to be cumulative from the start, these did attempt to give the titles of all the articles in several thousand medical and scientific journals which had been published in the year previous to the publication of each volume.

The crux of the problem is the rapid multiplication of medical and scientific journals. In 1800 the number of journals devoted to both these branches of knowledge was 910. By 1866 it was more than 14,000; by 1901 the number was nearly 60,000; by 1908 it was more than 70,000, and since then there have been further great increases. Considering only journals devoted to medicine or the strictly related sciences, similar developments are found. At the present time about 5,000 medical journals are regularly published throughout the world. Of this enormous number the largest medical library in the United Kingdom takes regularly about 2,000. Only a mere fraction of this vast output is of any permanent value for the advancement of medicine. Many otherwise worthless articles may have some local value, or may help to disseminate to selected audiences the results of the researches of others. But the greater the output of such articles, the more difficult it is to index them in such a way that they will not waste the time of serious workers.

It is not merely the enormous bulk of writings on science and medicine that forms the main deterrent to the general comprehension of its principles. Probably since at least the eighteenth century the mass of scientific detail has been beyond the grasp of any one mind. But in tracing the long course of rational medicine to its debouchment in our own time, we find an entirely new situation. In approaching our own age we have found increasing difficulty in discussing rational medicine as a single channel of thought. It spreads into a delta which tends to diverge ever wider, though still the many mouths may inosculate. This diffusion, brought about by increasing specialization, cannot go on indefinitely without defeating the objects for which specialism arose.

One result of the great increase in knowledge of the causes and treatment of disease experienced during the last fifty years has been a significant change in the power, the outlook, and the experience of the individual medical practitioner. During the second half of the nineteenth century the general practitioner was the backbone of the profession. The practitioner who treated our great-grandparents, and perhaps our parents, had in his consulting-room, as it were, the mantle of Hippocrates—if he was wise enough and skilful enough to wear it. In those days the general practitioner, especially in country districts, was often a wise counsellor to his patients. But the increasing need of specialized knowledge, such as that provided by bacteriology and radiology, soon created races of specialists. On the Continent this specialization began earlier and went farther than in the United Kingdom. Even here it became difficult for the practitioner to appear wise and dogmatic when faced with, for example, a doubtful case of diphtheria, for the parents soon realized that if a swab was taken from the child's throat, its examination might settle the diagnosis and the treatment. The mere microscopic examination of the swab might give the diagnosis, and this an enlightened and enthusiastic practitioner could do. But soon after the advent of Koch it was recognized that cultural examination of the organisms in the swab would often be needed, and there were few practitioners who would attempt that. This was a legitimate type of specialism, and the doctor who made use of it diminished neither his knowledge nor his relations with his patients. Legitimate also was the general physician who had had wide experience in medical—in contra-distinction to surgical—cases. In consulting him the practitioner widened his own knowledge, and was encouraged in his own natural tendency to study the patient as a sick man and not to concentrate merely on his disease.

Less praiseworthy perhaps, but not on that account without his place and purpose, is that type of specialist who takes for his province not a sick man, but some part of his body or even a particular disease. This statement must be read with caution. For example, no one would deny the good results obtained in the treatment of tuberculosis by physicians who had specialized in such work. But even thirty years ago there were many who thought his realm was too narrow, and that he should deal with all diseases of the lungs and not one particular disease. The correctness of this view has been shown by the success achieved since the adoption of the wider role under the National Health Service. Nevertheless, the increase of medical specialties is rightly regarded with concern in certain quarters, and warning has been given that the disappearance of the general consulting physician would be a grave blow to the progress of clinical medicine.

The harnessing of more scientific methods and investigations to the practice of medicine has increased the value and extent of clinical observations, and has made the average general practitioner more skilled and more competent to deal with his patients. But this view must only be adopted with certain reservations. The great increase in hospitalization during the present century has made it less easy for the practitioner to follow his patient through the whole course of the illness. Admission of his patient to hospital has diminished his potential experience. Formerly his working day was spent almost entirely in the practice of his profession, with occasional interludes when he attended medical societies to discuss his cases and those of his colleagues. In less than half a century much of this has changed. The National Health Insurance Act thrust on the general practitioner the burden of filling up forms for each patient. The National Health Service Act has multiplied this responsibility many times, and the practitioners, formerly free agents, have now to negotiate with the government for their remuneration. The general practitioner now sends so many of his patients to clinics and hospitals that his surgery is sometimes simply a clearing house. The future will decide whether in the long run the combination of these conditions will increase his knowledge, experience, and interest.

All things considered, there is no doubt that modern medicine, from the patient's point of view, is a very much more powerful instrument than the medicine of even half a century ago. This increase in the power of medicine is conditioned by a philosophical basis. Disease and death were once thought to be Acts of God, but they are now known to be brought about, or determined, by natural causes which obey known natural laws. This is scientific determinism. Increase in the detailed knowledge of Nature has widened the conception of the Reign of Law. Much of the work of men of science in general, and of medical men in particular, is done in a spirit which implies that these predetermined laws are universal and are wholly beyond ourselves. There is even a school that claims our very thinking as but a seeming, and that we do but behave as though we thought. Three centuries ago Descartes conceived that the animal might be treated as a machine. If man be but an animal, consequences are entailed from which Descartes shrank, for the watchword of his philosophy was *Cogito ergo sum* (I think, therefore I am). A new school, the work of which has been at times intimately bound up with the progress of medicine, would abandon this basic doctrine of the father of modern philosophy, who is also the founder of physiology as a separate discipline.

It is not our task to discuss the philosophic background of modern science, or of modern medicine. Yet we would point out that, though the principle of complete scientific determinism has served very well for scientists in explaining, at least to themselves, the basis on which their experiments have been founded in the past, it has been acceptable to but a few philosophers, and of late to even fewer. Before any philosophical system can be accepted as applicable to science as a whole, the unity of science must be accepted. There is a subtle difference between the apple, just fallen at Newton's feet, and that apple a moment before its fall, still attached by its stalk to its parent tree, still capable of organic growth and of the many processes which cumulatively constitute, but do not entirely explain, the phenomena of life. *E nihilo, nihil fit* is as true of the living world as it is of inanimate nature. Despite the triumphs of organic chemistry, as a result of which more and more substances which formerly appeared to be produced only in the body of the living organism were synthesized in the laboratory, a stage was reached when chemists despaired of producing a living organism. In this impasse the study of the viruses during the last few decades opened a new field, and seemed to bring closer together the most minute living organisms and the large molecules of certain proteins. Yet the mechanist has still failed to pass the crucial test of producing, from dead inorganic or organic material, a living organism capable of growth, disintegration and repair of its own tissues, predetermined reaction to stimuli and, the final criterion, the ability to reproduce itself down the corridors of time.

Much has been written on the role of mind in relation to the body. This problem is perhaps outside our scope, and our remarks will be brief. From a practical aspect we would mention the progress made in the study of psychosomatic diseases; conditions such as peptic ulcer of the stomach and duodenum, where the pathological condition of the tissues of the diseased organ is supposed to be produced, or at least influenced, by mental strain. Further investigation will no doubt add to the list of such diseases; but their total will probably remain small as compared with the number of diseases in the causation of which, so far as we know at present, the mind exerts no influence.

It may be argued that if we knew the full philosophical implications of the relations between mind and body, a synthesis of our whole knowledge of science—and *ipso facto* of its medical implications—would be possible. Though this is admittedly a legitimate field of inquiry, we must point out that most of the advances which are mentioned in this book were made as a result of observation or experiment, or both. It is doubtful whether the work of those who made them would have been in any way modified if they had had at the back of their minds any synthesis of natural knowledge in its philosophical implications. The same may be said of the great advances of modern times. In his conception of the processes of disease the pathologist bases his work on Virchow's cellular pathology, which was itself due to careful observation. The most outstanding modern advance in diagnosis, the discovery and use of X-rays, was due to a purely physical investigation of very limited scope. In the realm of treatment the first chemotherapeutic drugs resulted from a series of detailed chemical syntheses, while the first antibiotic was discovered by a process of pure observation.

It is not the function of the historian to deal with the present or the future. But since this book is essentially an 'introduction to medical principles', it may be justifiable to take stock of the results achieved in recent years, and to indicate possible trends.

A significant development in this period has been the increasing application of current biological principles to many aspects of medicine. While formerly it was sufficient to understand the minute chemical structure of living things, it was obvious that the ultimate chemical analysis brought us no nearer to an explanation of what made these chemical substances into a living organism. Modern research is veering to an electrodynamic conception. This regards the relationship which the chemical elements in protoplasm bear to each other as an electromagnetic system. Consideration of the structure and arrangement of the molecules of living things is an approach which promises to yield important results.

Aristotle suggested that the change from inanimate to living matter is so gradual that possibly no clear line of division can be drawn. His wisdom has again become evident in recent years as a result of a vast amount of work on the viruses. Scientists are still unable to agree on the fundamental nature of the viruses. Chemists and physicists who work with them only incidentally consider that they are chemical molecules; while those whose work is entirely in the field of the viruses and their pathogenic effects tend to consider them as organisms. Good arguments can be put forward on both sides. These lowly organisms—or whatever they may be—still hold secrets which are of fundamental importance not only to medicine but also to biology.

The triumphs of antibiotics have been followed by certain difficulties which are not likely to become less as time passes. It is now well known that certain strains of organisms are unfortunately resistant to the action of antibiotics. During a successful course of treatment with a certain antibiotic, a few resistant organisms may multiply rapidly and offset the destruction of all the other strains. Several theories have been advanced to explain this unfortunate phenomenon. For example, there is some evidence that the drug actually produces a mutation in the organism, as a result of which strains are produced which differ in their metabolic processes from the parent strains. Whatever the explanation, it appears that it may involve the science of genetics, the great problems of which have hardly been mentioned in this book.

In the field of pathology similar tendencies are making themselves felt. The behaviour of the cell in the diseased state is now being studied in some laboratories with a thoroughness which would have delighted Virchow, and, apart altogether from the problem of cancer, significant results are emerging. There is some evidence that diseases now generally described as psychosomatic are really due to an inherent quality in the protoplasm of the affected cells. If this be the case, the suggested influence of the mind must be regarded as highly problematical. During the last thirty years the conception of some diseases has been so much changed as almost to place them in an entirely different classificatory grouping. Pernicious anaemia is a case in point. Formerly regarded as one of the most clear-cut of blood diseases, it always presented a very typical blood picture when a film of blood was examined microscopically. Also typical were the peculiar yellowish colour of the skin, the enlargement of the spleen, and the organic lesions of the central nervous system. Nowadays, owing to much earlier diagnosis and the efficacy of treatment by cyanocobalamine, this clinical picture is rarely seen. A provisional diagnosis is now made by examination of the bone marrow and the gastric juice. Absence of hydrochloric acid from the gastric juice, along with certain typical changes in the cells of the bone marrow, is very suggestive, but the diagnosis of pernicious anaemia may only be clinched by the patient's reaction to the administration of cyanocobalamine.

During the present century certain problems have been solved by the methods of experimental pathology. These methods are now widely used by specialists, and in no field have they been put to greater use than in cancer research. From the early days of the development of bacteriology attempts had been made to establish some micro-organism as the cause of cancer. But in spite of the considerable amount of work done in this field, it is now considered that no such relationship has yet been shown to exist between bacteria or viruses and any malignant tumour. Greater success, however, has attended investigations into the production of cancer by certain chemical substances, the carcinogens. The causal connexion between soot and a well-recognized cancer of the skin in chimney-sweeps had been recognized as long ago as the late eighteenth century. But it was not until 1915 that two Japanese pathologists succeeded in producing cancer artificially in rabbits by repeatedly painting their ears with tar. Coal-tar is a complex substance, and research was carried on actively in an attempt to discover in it a pure carcinogenetic compound. The first of such pure compounds was isolated in 1932 by British workers, who had to use 2 tons of pitch in order to obtain 7 gm. of the compound. These advances were followed by the synthesis of compounds for the purpose of testing their carcinogenetic effect. A further interesting development of the use of synthetic carcinogens is the demonstration that one of these substances, when injected into mice, produces a cancer of the stomach .

It is now over twenty years since a relationship was demonstrated between the activity of the sexual glands and the development of certain types of malignant disease. Injection of hormones of the ovary produced spontaneous cancer of the breast in mice. The mechanism of this process is too complex for discussion here, but the conception has some important practical applications which will be mentioned later.

Diagnosis was revolutionized by the invention of the stethoscope and again by the discovery of X-rays. In this generation it has been further advanced by some quite unexpected developments. Nearly twenty years ago a research worker succeeded in passing a soft rubber tube up a vein in his arm until its tip entered the right atrium of his heart. This procedure, cardiac catheterization, has been much developed and is now used to gauge the pressure in various veins and in the chambers of the heart before an operation for valvular disease. Injection into the arteries of substances opaque to X-rays, angiography, is now used to ascertain the condition of certain arteries, especially those in the brain. Mention has already been made of the use of the electroencephalograph in epilepsy and of the diagnostic use of radioactive isotopes.

Since the Second World War a new branch of medical treatment has arisen—gerontology, or the care and management of the aged. This was due partly to the fact that, as the result of relative ageing of the population, there were large numbers of old people who had no proper homes and who often suffered from incapacitating chronic illnesses. Intensive study has been made of the physiology of old age, and of certain diseases which are commonly encountered among the aged. The psychology of the aged has also been approached from new angles. Further, administrative measures have been introduced to improve the social and domestic amenities of old people. Despite this work, the problem of the aged is still one of the most important in medicine.

Since the war much work has been done on chronic rheumatism and allied diseases. New methods of treatment have been tried, and some—including advances in physical medicine—have been proved effective. There have also been significant advances in the treatment of certain forms of cancer by hormones. In 1889 it was shown that castration of the male hedgehog reduced the size of its prostate gland. Forty years later it was shown that a similar reduction in the size of the prostate could be effected by the injection of ovarian extracts. Since then such extracts have been used in the treatment of cancer of the prostate, and the results have certainly been encouraging. Radioisotopes are being used increasingly in treatment, especially in overactivity of the thyroid gland, in malignant disease of the thyroid, and in the treatment of certain diseases of the blood.

Surgery has also experienced its own revolution. Over twenty years ago a great surgeon said that surgery had been made safe for the patient and that the problem was to make the patient safe for surgery. This has involved a study of the effects of various operations on the patient's circulatory, respiratory, and excretory systems, and also a study of his metabolism These measures, with the great advances made in anaesthesia during and since the Second World War, have made surgical operations very different from what they were thirty years ago. Revolutionary advances have been made, especially in the surgery of the heart, and operations on that organ are now commonly performed which would have been considered impossible even twenty years ago.

We do not intend to attempt to draw up a balance-sheet of modern medicine, but something may be said about certain conditions which are still proving refractory to research. No certain method has yet been found of aborting the common cold. The treatment of chronic bronchitis still takes up much space in a text-book of medicine. This indicates that there is no uniformly success-ful method of treatment; but it should be remembered that many factors may be involved in causing the condition. Bronchial asthma is another disease which has not yet been conquered. The factors which cause this disease and those which precipitate attacks are also complex, but modern methods have been fairly successful in treating both the disease and the attacks. In its ordinary forms influenza is nowadays adequately dealt with. But after an interval a malignant type may be met with, and this may give rise to difficulties in treatment. We are powerless to modify the prevailing type of the disease.

Of diseases of the circulatory system, hypertension is probably the most important. The basic condition in this disease is thickening of the walls of the arteries leading to an increase in blood-pressure. This may ultimately lead to diseases of the heart, the brain, or the kidneys. Within recent years many new drugs have been used to reduce the blood-pressure. Though the prospect for the patient is now greatly improved, the causes of the changes in the arteries are not yet understood. In the treatment of the cerebral complications of hypertension, such as apoplexy, important advances in treatment are scarcely to be expected; but the improvements in the treatment of hypertension may lessen the incidence of these cerebral complications. Although advances have been made in the treatment of the leukaemias, some types still resist treatment. Certain nervous diseases, such as disseminated sclerosis, present very peculiar and still unsolved difficulties, and the treatment of the muscular dystrophies has not shown much advance.

Cancer still presents an enormous problem. Though the cause is not yet understood, it will be appreciated from what was said previously that definite advances have been made. So far as the patient is concerned, it can at least be said that nowadays cancer in some organs of the body is curable provided that it is diagnosed and effectively treated at an early stage.

Research in medicine and the allied sciences has now become so complex that more and more it lies within the province of research workers acting together in research groups. This is because the methods employed are often very complicated, so that it is more efficient to get the members of a small team—all of whom probably specialize in different aspects of the work—to carry out different stages of the process. But it should not be thought that all research necessarily involves teams of workers and expensive procedures. Of the great advances made in the last sixty years, the following are examples of those made in each case by one or two men, sometimes at little cost: X-rays by Röntgen; the electrocardiograph by Einthoven; penicillin by Fleming; insulin by Banting and Best. Nor can it be said that many of these great discoveries in medicine led to any fundamental change in the Laws of Nature. Though sometimes involving extensive research and very original conceptions, they were essentially observational and not synthetic discoveries; but this fact does not diminish their value to humanity. It is dangerous to apply to medical research the same criteria which are applicable to general research in the sciences.

Reference was made previously to the enormous bulk of medical writing at the present day. Not all the papers published deal directly with research. Many are reports of interesting cases, and many others are the texts of lectures which, while themselves containing no account of new research, summarize and expand recent work. Even when such communications are excluded there remains a substantial body of papers dealing with original research. These papers vary greatly in quality and accuracy, and only a few report work of first-rate importance. Yet it should not be assumed that the others are value-less. Some of these researches have been undertaken in order to close gaps in a line of research which may be exercising many workers in different parts of the world. Other papers report research which has possibly miscarried from the original intentions of those who carried it out. To avoid fruitless repetition by other research workers, all these researches must be reported, and the reports must be detailed if they are to be of any value. When the whole problem has been solved these papers will be forgotten, but until that event happens they may be of considerable use to all who work in that particular field.

No man can forecast the advances in medical thought and practice which will be made in the future. That there will be advances is certain. It is also certain that, however great the advances, they will not prevent each of us dying when his time comes. They will have done much if they enable each man and woman to live free from organic disease to a ripe old age.

Medicine cannot give immortality, but it should enable us all to live out our full lives. Death, coming in due and not undue time, is shorn of much of his sharpness when it can be said of everyone,

'Thou shalt come to thy grave in a full age, like as a shock of corn cometh in in his season.' (Job v. 26.)

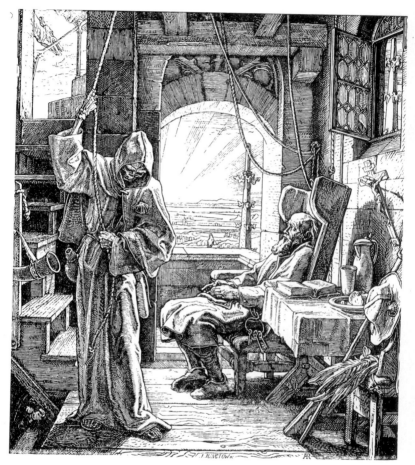

Friendly Death

(From a drawing, c. 1844, by Alfred Rethel)

NOBEL PRIZEWINNERS

THIS list includes only those prizewinners whose discoveries bear a relation to Medicine. Prizewinners not already mentioned in the text are marked with an asterisk. The class in which the prize was awarded is designated as follows: (P) Physics; (C) Chemistry; (PM) Physiology and Medicine. Phrases quoted are from the official citations.

1901 W. C. RÖNTGEN (P): 'in recognition of the extraordinary services he has rendered by the discovery of the remarkable rays which have subsequently been called after him'.

1901 EMIL VON BEHRING (PM): 'for his work on serum therapy, especially its application against diphtheria'.

1902 EMIL FISCHER (C): for work on the structure of the sugars. Fischer's work on the structure of the proteins, though in progress, had not advanced sufficiently to be mentioned in the award.

1902 RONALD ROSS (PM): 'for his work on malaria'.

1903 H. A. BECQUEREL / PIERRE CURIE / MARIE S. CURIE (P), shared: Becquerel for the discovery of spontaneous radioactivity; the Curies for their joint work concerning radiation phenomena.

1903 NIELS R. FINSEN (PM): for 'his contribution to the treatment of diseases, especially *lupus vulgaris*, with concentrated light-rays'.

1904 I. P. PAVLOV (PM): for 'his work on the physiology of digestion'.

1905 ROBERT KOCH (PM): 'for his investigations and discoveries in regard to tuberculosis'.

1906 CAMILLO GOLGI / S. RAMÓN Y CAJAL (PM), shared: each for 'his work on the structure of the nervous system'.

1907 ALPHONSE LAVERAN (PM): for 'his work regarding the role played by protozoa in causing diseases'.

1908 PAUL EHRLICH / ELIE METCHNIKOFF (PM), shared: each 'in recognition of his work on immunity'.

1909 THEODOR KOCHER (PM): 'for his works on the physiology, pathology and surgery of the thyroid gland'.

1910 ALBRECHT KOSSEL (PM): for 'the contributions to the chemistry of the cell which he had made through his work on proteins, including the nucleic substances'.

1911 MARIE S. CURIE (C): for her work on the chemistry of radioactive elements.

1911 A. GULLSTRAND (PM): 'for his work on the dioptrics of the eye'.

1912 *ALEXIS CARREL (PM): for 'his work on vascular suture and the transplantation of blood-vessels and organs'.

1913 CHARLES RICHET (PM): 'in recognition of his work on anaphylaxis'.

1914 *ROBERT BÁRÁNY (PM): 'for his work on the physiology and pathology of the vestibular apparatus'.

1919 JULES BORDET (PM): 'for his discoveries in regard to immunity'.

1920 AUGUST KROGH (PM): 'for his discovery of the capillary motor regulating mechanism'.

1922 { A. V. HILL O. MEYERHOF } (PM), shared. Hill 'for his discovery relating to the production of heat in muscles'; Meyerhof 'for his discovery of the fixed relationship between the consumption of oxygen and the metabolism of lactic acid in muscle'.

1923 { F. G. BANTING J. J. R. MACLEOD } (PM), shared: 'for their discovery of insulin' (but see pp. 554–5).

1924 W. EINTHOVEN (PM): 'for his discovery of the mechanism of the electrocardiogram'.

1926 *JOHANNES FIBIGER (PM): 'for his discovery of the *Spiroptera* carcinoma'.

1927 J. WAGNER-JAUREGG (PM): 'for his discovery of the therapeutic value of malaria inoculation in the treatment of *dementia paralytica*'.

1928 ADOLF WINDAUS (C): for 'his researches into the constitution of the sterols and their connexion with the vitamins'.

1928 CHARLES NICOLLE (PM): 'for his work on typhus fever'.

1929 { C. EIJKMAN F. GOWLAND HOPKINS } (PM), shared: Eijkman 'for his discovery of the anti-neuritic vitamin'; Hopkins 'for his discovery of the growth-stimulating vitamins'.

1930 K. LANDSTEINER (PM): 'for his discovery of the human blood groups'.

1931 O. WARBURG (PM): 'for his discovery of the nature and mode of action of the respiratory enzyme'.

1932 { C. S. SHERRINGTON E. D. ADRIAN } (PM), shared: 'for their discoveries regarding the function of the neuron'.

1933 *T. HUNT MORGAN (PM): 'for his discoveries concerning the function of the chromosome in the transmission of heredity'.

1934 H. C. UREY (C): for the discovery of heavy hydrogen.

1934 { G. R. MINOT W. P. MURPHY G. H. WHIPPLE } (PM), shared: 'for their discoveries concerning the treatment of the anaemias with liver'.

1935*HANS SPEMANN (PM): 'for his discovery of the organizer effect in embryonic development'.

1936 { H. H. DALE } (PM), shared: 'for their discoveries relating to the { OTTO LOEWI } chemical transmission of nerve impulses'.

1937 { W. N. HAWORTH } (C), shared: Haworth 'for his researches into { PAUL KARRER } the constitution of carbohydrates and vitamin C'; Karrer 'for his researches into the constitution of carotenoids, flavins and vitamins A and B_2'.

1937 A. SZENT-GYÖRGYI (PM): 'for his discoveries in connexion with the biological combustion process, with special reference to vitamin C and the catalysis of fumaric acid'.

1938 RICHARD KUHN (C): 'for his work on carotenoids and vitamins'.

1938 *CORNEILLE HEYMANS (PM): 'for his discovery of the role of the carotid sinus and aortic mechanisms in the regulation of respiration'.

1939 { A. BUTENANDT } (C), shared: Butenandt 'for his work on sex hor- { L. RUZICKA } mones'; Ruzicka 'for his work on polymethylenes and higher terpenes'.

1939 G. DOMAGK (PM): 'for his discovery of the antibacterial effects of prontosil'.

1943 *G. DE HEVESY (C): 'for his work on the use of isotopes as tracer elements in researches on chemical processes'.

1943 { HENRIK DAM } (PM), shared: Dam 'for his discovery of vitamin { E. A. DOISY } K'; Doisy 'for his discovery of the chemical nature of vitamin K'.

1944 { E. J. ERLANGER } (PM), shared: 'for their discoveries regarding the { H. S. GASSER } highly differentiated functions of single nerve fibres'.

1945 { A. FLEMING } (PM), shared: 'for the discovery of penicillin and { H. W. FLOREY } its curative value in a number of infectious { E. B. CHAIN } diseases'.

1946 { *J. B. SUMNER } (C), shared: Sumner 'for his discovery that { *J. H. NORTHROP } enzymes can be crystallized'; Northrop and { W. M. STANLEY } Stanley 'for their preparations of enzymes and virus proteins in a pure form'.

1946 *H. J. MULLER (PM): 'for his discovery of the production of mutations by means of X-ray irradiation'.

1947 { CARL F. CORI } (PM), shared: the Coris 'for their discovery of { GERTY T. CORI } how glycogen is catalytically converted'; { B. A. HOUSSAY } Houssay 'for his discovery of the part played by the hormone of the anterior pituitary lobe in the metabolism of sugar'.

1948 P. H. MÜLLER (PM): 'for his discovery of the high efficacy of DDT as a contact poison against several arthropods'.

1949 {*W. R. HESS / A. C. DE EGAS MONIZ} (PM), shared: Hess 'for his discovery of the functional organization of the interbrain as a co-ordinator of the activities of the internal organs'; Egas Moniz 'for his discovery of the value of prefrontal leucotomy in certain psychoses'.

1950 {PHILIP S. HENCH / EDWARD C. KENDALL / TADEUS REICHSTEIN} (PM), shared: for their work on the treatment of rheumatoid arthritis with cortisone and A.C.T.H.

1951 MAX THEILER (PM): for his work on yellow fever.

1952 S. A. WAKSMAN (PM): for his discovery of streptomycin.

1953 {*H. A. KREBS / *F. A. LIPMANN} (PM), shared: Krebs for his discovery of the citric acid cycle in the metabolism of carbohydrates; Lipmann for his work on co-enzyme A.

1954 {*JOHN F. ENDERS / *FREDERICK C. ROBBINS / *THOMAS H. WELLER} (PM), shared: for their discovery of the ability of the poliomyelitis virus to grow in cultures of different tissues.

1955 *VINCENT DU VIGNEAUD (C): for his synthesis of oxytocin and other hormones of the posterior pituitary.

1955 *HUGO THEORELL (PM): for his studies on haemoglobin, cytochromes, and the oxidation chain in living tissues.

1956 {*WERNER FORSSMANN / *ANDRÉ F. COURNAND / *DICKINSON W. RICHARDS} (PM), shared: for their work on cardiac catheterization.

1957 *ALEXANDER TODD (C): for his work on nucleotides and the nucleotide co-enzyme.

1957 *DANIEL BOVET (PM): for his synthesis of antihistaminic compounds and of certain muscle relaxants.

1958 *F. SANGER (C): for his elucidation of the chemical structure of the insulin molecule.

1958 {*G. W. BEADLE / *E. L. TATUM / *J. LEDERBERG} (PM), shared: for their researches on the mechanism by which the chromosomes in the cell nucleus transmit inherited characters.

1959 {*SEVERO OCHOA / *ARTHUR KORNBERG} (PM), shared: for their artificial synthesis of nucleic acids by means of enzymes.

1960 {F. M. BURNET / *P. B. MEDAWAR} (PM), shared: for their work on acquired immunological tolerance.

SELECT LIST OF REFERENCE MATERIAL

THIS list is intentionally neither comprehensive nor bibliographical. Its aim is to give brief particulars of publications, mainly in English, French, or German, which should be found useful by students, arranged, apart from the introductory general sections, to correspond to the various sections of this book. It deals only with those subjects discussed in the text. In order to save space titles of books are sometimes abbreviated, and titles of papers are frequently abbreviated, or altered to give a concise indication of their contents.

General omissions from the list are as follows:

(*a*) Works mentioned in the text. Exceptions to this general rule include some translations and collected editions; also a very few works previously mentioned in the text which are given in this list on account of the historical material contained in them.

(*b*) The publications of the New Sydenham Society. These are very important for the study of nineteenth-century work; but as the foreign works of which they are translations are mentioned in the text, they are, with very few exceptions, omitted from this list.

(*c*) Relatively few biographies are included; those which are included usually contain material relative to the researches carried out by the subjects of the biographies.

(*d*) Bibliographical and iconographical works, and works relating to the cultural, artistic, or satirical aspects of medical history.

The *Ciba Zeitschrift* and the *Ciba Symposia* contain numerous valuable short articles and reviews which are relevant to the contents of this book. To have included even a selection of these would have expanded the list inordinately, and they are therefore entirely omitted. The student should become familiar with the contents of these works.

Details of many of the works mentioned in the text, but not included in this list, are given in Garrison and Morton's *Medical Bibliography* (2nd ed., London, 1954), which should be constantly consulted.

In order to save space the following abbreviations are used for the titles of some publications frequently cited in the list:

A.M.H.   *Annals of Medical History*
Ann. Sci.   *Annals of Science*
B.H.M.   *Bulletin of the History of Medicine*
B.M.J.   *British Medical Journal*
J.H.M.   *Journal of the History of Medicine and Allied Sciences*
P.R.S.M. *Proceedings of the Royal Society of Medicine*
            Unless otherwise stated the page references are to the pages of the proceedings of the Section of the History of Medicine
S.M. & H. *Science Medicine and History* (see p. 764)

A. GENERAL

General Histories of Medicine

(*a*) *Comprehensive Histories published since* 1925:

ACKERKNECHT, E. H. *A short history of medicine*. New York, 1955.
CASTIGLIONI, A. *A history of medicine*. Trans. and ed. E. B. Krumbhaar. New York, 1947.
DIEPGEN, P. *Geschichte der Medizin*. 2 vols. (in 3). Berlin, 1949–55.
GARRISON, F. H. *An introduction to the history of medicine*. 4th ed. Phila. and London, 1929.

GOTFREDSEN, E. *Medicinens historie.* Copenhagen, 1950. (In Danish.)
GUTHRIE, D. *A history of medicine.* London, 1945.
LAIGNEL-LAVASTINE, M. (ed.). *Histoire générale de la médecine, de la pharmacie, de l'art dentaire.* 3 vols. Paris, 1936–49.
MAJOR, R. H. *A history of medicine.* 2 vols. Springfield and Oxford, 1954.
METTLER, CECILIA C. *History of medicine.* Phila. and Toronto, 1947.
MEYER-STEINEG, T., and SUDHOFF, K. *Geschichte der Medizin im Überblick.* 4th ed. (by B. von Hagen). Jena, 1950.
PAZZINI, A. *Storia della medicina.* 2 vols. Milan, 1947.
SIGERIST, H. E. *A history of medicine.* New York, vol. i, 1951; vol. ii, 1961.

(*b*) *Older Histories, now classical:*

DAREMBERG, C. *Histoire des sciences médicales.* 2 vols. Paris, 1870. (Of interest especially for Greek medicine.)
HAESER, H. *Lehrbuch der Geschichte der Medicin und der epidemischen Krankheiten.* 3rd ed. 3 vols. Jena, 1875–82. (The third volume of this enlarged edition is still a standard work on the history of infectious diseases.)
NEUBURGER, M., and PAGEL, J. (eds.). Puschmann's *Handbuch der Geschichte der Medizin.* 3 vols. Jena, 1902–5. (Still the most comprehensive treatise on all aspects of the subject up to the date of publication.)
NEUBURGER, M. *History of medicine.* Trans. E. Playfair. Vol. i, and vol. ii, pt. i (all published). London, 1910–25. (This uncompleted work extends to the Middle Ages. Especially valuable for Neuburger's views on the Classical Period.)

(*c*) *Other General Histories, medicine in individual countries, techniques, &c.:*

ARTELT, W. *Einführung in die Medizinhistorik.* Stuttgart, 1949.
BAAS, J. H. *Outlines of the history of medicine.* Rev. ed., trans. H. E. Handerson. New York, 1889.
BOUCHUT, E. *Histoire de la médecine et des doctrines médicales.* 2 vols. Paris, 1873.
BUCK, A. H. *The growth of medicine* [to *c.* 1800]. New Haven, 1917.
—— *The dawn of modern medicine.* New Haven, 1920.
CASTIGLIONI, A. *Italian medicine.* (Clio Medica.) New York, 1932.
CHAPLIN, A. *Medicine in England during the reign of George III.* London, 1919.
CLENDENING, L. *Source book of medical history.* New York, 1942.
COMRIE, J. D. *History of Scottish medicine.* 2nd ed. 2 vols. London, 1932.
CUMSTON, C. G. *An introduction to the history of medicine.* London, 1926.
DIEPGEN, P. *Geschichte der Medizin* (Sammlung Göschen). 5 vols. Berlin and Leipzig, 1913–28.
FLEETWOOD, J. *History of medicine in Ireland.* Dublin, 1951.
GALDSTON, I. *Progress in medicine: a critical review of the last hundred years.* New York, 1940.
GANTT, W. HORSLEY. *Russian medicine.* (Clio Medica.) New York, 1937.
HABERLING, W. *German medicine.* Trans. J. Freund. (Clio Medica.) New York, 1934.
HEAGERTY, J. J. *Four centuries of medical history in Canada.* 2 vols. Bristol, 1928.
HIRSCH, A. *Geschichte der medicinischen Wissenschaften in Deutschland.* Munich and Leipzig, 1893.
HOWELL, W. B. *Medicine in Canada.* (Clio Medica.) New York, 1933.
LAIGNEL-LAVASTINE, M., and MOLINERY, R. *French medicine.* Trans. E. B. Krumbhaar. (Clio Medica.) New York, 1934.
LAIN ENTRALGO, P. *Historia de la medicina.* Barcelona and Madrid, 1954.
—— *La historia clínica.* Madrid, 1940.
MAJOR, R. H. *Classic descriptions of disease.* Springfield, 1932.
MOORE, Sir N. *The history of the study of medicine in the British Isles.* Oxford, 1908.

OSLER, Sir W. *The evolution of modern medicine.* New Haven, 1921.
PACKARD, F. R. *History of medicine in the United States.* 2 vols. New York, 1931.
POWER, Sir D'ARCY. *Medicine in the British Isles.* (Clio Medica.) New York, 1930.
ROBINSON, V. *The story of medicine.* New York, 1931; reprinted 1943.
SHRYOCK, R. H. *The development of modern medicine. An interpretation of the social and scientific factors involved.* London, 1948.
SIGERIST, H. E. *Man and medicine.* London, 1932.
—— *Great doctors.* London, 1933. (Important not only from the biographical but also from the historical standpoint. A second edition in German was published in 1954.)
—— *American medicine.* New York, 1934.
STUBBS, S. G. B., and BLIGH, E. W. *Sixty centuries of health and physick.* London, [1931].
SUDHOFF, K. *Kurzes Handbuch der Geschichte der Medizin.* Berlin, 1922.
WITHINGTON, E. T. *Medical history from the earliest times.* London, 1894.
WUNDERLICH, C. A. *Geschichte der Medizin.* Stuttgart, 1859.

Biographical Material

Study of biographical points frequently necessitates the use of a large specialized library. Reference to the national biographies, such as the *D.N.B.* and the *Allgemeine deutsche Biographie*, is essential. The following list contains only a few suggestions which may be useful in relation to better-known persons. Easily accessible information on about 200 famous medical men, with references, will be found in the individual biographies by E. A. Underwood in *Chambers's Encyclopaedia*.

BAILEY, H., and BISHOP, W. J. *Notable names in medicine and surgery.* London, 1944 and later eds.
BAYLE, A. L. J., and THILLAYE, A. J. *Biographie médicale par ordre chronologique.* 2 vols. Paris, 1840–1. Also ed. of 1855.
BETTANY, G. T. *Eminent doctors.* 2 vols. London, [1885].
BUESS, H. *Schweizer Ärzte als Forscher, Entdecker und Erfinder.* Basel, 1946.
FUETER, E. *Grosse Schweizer Forscher.* Zurich, 1939.
KELLY, H. A., and BURRAGE, W. L. *Dictionary of American medical biography.* New York, 1928.
MACMICHAEL, W. *The gold-headed cane.* London, 1827. Several later editions, the last published in London in 1953.
MUNK, W. *The roll of the Royal College of Physicians of London.* 2nd ed. 3 vols. London, 1878. A fourth vol., compiled by G. H. Brown and covering the period 1826–1925, appeared in 1955.
OSLER, Sir W. *An Alabama student and other biographical essays.* London, 1908.
Plarr's Lives of the Fellows of the Royal College of Surgeons of England. Revised by Sir D'Arcy Power, W. G. Spencer, and G. E. Gask. 2 vols. Bristol, 1930. Supplement, covering period 1930–51, by Power and W. R. LeFanu, 1953.
POWER, Sir D'ARCY (ed.). *British masters of medicine.* London, 1936.
RICHARDSON, Sir B. W. *Disciples of Aesculapius.* 2 vols. London, 1900.
SIGERIST, H. E. *Great doctors.* London, 1933.
WICKERSHEIMER, E. *Dictionnaire biographique des médecins en France au moyen âge.* 2 vols. Paris, 1936.

Collective Works and Selected Writings

Contributions to medical and biological research dedicated to Sir William Osler. 2 vols. New York, 1919.
COPE, Sir Z. (ed.). *Sidelights on the history of medicine.* London, 1957. (A selection of papers originally published in the *P.R.S.M.*)

Festschrift zum 80. Geburtstag Max Neuburgers (ed. E. Berghoff). Vienna, 1948.
POWER, Sir D'ARCY. *Selected writings, 1877–1930.* Oxford, 1931.
POYNTER, F. N. L. (ed.). *The history and philosophy of knowledge of the brain and its functions.* Oxford, 1958.
SIGERIST, H. E. *On the history of medicine* [Selected papers]. New York, 1960.
—— *On the sociology of medicine* [Selected papers]. New York, 1960.
SINGER, C. (ed.). *Studies in the history and method of science.* 2 vols. Oxford, 1917–21.
—— and SIGERIST, H. E. (eds.). *Essays on the history of medicine presented to Karl Sudhoff.* London and Zürich, 1924.
UNDERWOOD, E. A. (ed.). *Science medicine and history. Essays . . . in honour of Charles Singer.* 2 vols. London, 1953. [*S.M. & H.*]

General Histories of Science

CLAGETT, M. *Greek science in antiquity.* London, 1957.
CROMBIE, A. C. *Augustine to Galileo. The history of science, 400–1650.* London, 1957.
DAUMAS, M. (ed.). *Histoire de la science.* (Encyclopédie de la Pléiade.) Paris, 1957.
HALL, A. R. *The Scientific Revolution, 1500–1800.* London, 1954.
PLEDGE, H. T. *Science since 1500.* 2nd ed. London, 1959.
SARTON, G. *Introduction to the history of science.* 3 vols. (in 5). Baltimore, 1927–48.
—— *Horus. A guide to the history of science.* Waltham, Mass., 1952.
—— *A history of science.* London and Camb., Mass. Vol. i, 1953; vol. ii, 1959.
SINGER, C. *A short history of scientific ideas to 1900.* Oxford, 1959.
TATON, R. (ed.). *La science antique et médiévale (des origines à 1450).* Paris, 1957.
TAYLOR, F. SHERWOOD. *A short history of science.* London, [1939].
WIGHTMAN, W. P. D. *The growth of scientific ideas.* Edinb. and London, 1950.
WOLF, A. *A history of science, technology, and philosophy in the 16th & 17th centuries.* 2nd ed., revised by D. McKie. London, 1950.
—— *A history of science, technology, and philosophy in the eighteenth century.* 2nd ed., revised by D. McKie. London, 1952.

Reference works on, and histories of, subjects

Anatomy

CHOULANT, L. *History and bibliography of anatomic illustration.* Trans. M. Frank, with additional essays by Garrison, Frank, Streeter, and Singer. New York, 1945.
CORNER, G. W. *Anatomy.* (Clio Medica.) New York, 1930.
DOBSON, JESSIE. *Anatomical eponyms.* London, 1946.
HUNTER, R. H. *A short history of anatomy.* 2nd ed. London, 1931.
PORTAL, P. *Histoire de l'anatomie et de la chirurgie.* 6 vols. Paris, 1770–3.
PREMUDA, L. *Storia dell'iconografia anatomica.* Milan, [1957].
SINCLAIR, H. M., and ROBB-SMITH, A. H. T. *A short history of anatomical teaching at Oxford.* Oxford, 1950.
SINGER, C. *The evolution of anatomy.* London, 1925.
—— How medicine became anatomical. *B.M.J.*, 1954, ii, 1499–1503.
STEUDEL, J. 'Zur Geschichte der anatomischen Nomenklatur'. *Deut. Med. Wchnsch.*, 1956, lxxxi, 1572–4.

Biology

COLE, F. J. *A history of comparative anatomy.* London, 1944.
DAWES, B. *A hundred years of biology.* London, 1952.
GREEN, J. REYNOLDS. *A history of botany, 1860–1900.* (A continuation of Sachs.) Oxford, 1909.
NORDENSKIÖLD, E. *The history of biology.* Trans. L. B. Eyre. London, 1929.
SACHS, J. VON. *History of botany (1530–1860).* Trans. and rev. Oxford, 1906.

SINGER, C. *A history of biology.* 3rd ed. London and New York, 1959.

Chemistry

FINDLAY, A. *A hundred years of chemistry.* 2nd ed. London, 1948.
MEYER, E. VON. *A history of chemistry.* Trans. McGowan. 3rd ed. London, 1906.
PARTINGTON, J. R. *A short history of chemistry.* 3rd ed. London, 1957.
STILLMAN, J. M. *The story of early chemistry.* New York, 1924.

Embryology

DE BEER, Sir G. *Embryos and ancestors.* 3rd ed. Oxford, 1958.
HERRLINGER, R. Earliest embryological illustrations. *Ztsch. Anat.*, 1951, cxvi, 1–13.
MEYER, A. W. *An analysis of the* De Generatione Animalium *of William Harvey.* Stanford and Oxford, 1936.
—— *The rise of embryology.* Stanford and London, 1939.
NEEDHAM, J. *A history of embryology.* 2nd ed., asstd. by A. Hughes. Cambridge, 1959.

Materia Medica, Pharmacy, Pharmacology

BERENDES, J. *Geschichte der Pharmazie.* Leipzig, 1898.
BUESS, H. *Die historischen Grundlagen der intravenosen Injektion.* Aarau, 1946.
FLÜCKIGER, F. A., and HANBURY, D. *Pharmacographia. A history of the principal drugs of vegetable origin.* London, 1874.
KREMERS, E., and URDANG, G. *History of pharmacy.* 2nd ed. Phila., 1951.
LAUDER BRUNTON, Sir T. *A text-book of pharmacology, therapeutics and materia medica.* London, 1885.
PEREIRA, J. *The elements of materia medica.* 4th ed. 2 vols. (in 3). London, 1854–7.
REUTTER DE ROSEMONT, L. *Histoire de la pharmacie.* 2 vols. Paris, 1931–2.
WARING, E. J. *Bibliotheca therapeutica.* 2 vols. London, 1878–9.
WOOTTON, A. C. *Chronicles of pharmacy.* 2 vols. London, 1910.

Medicine

BETT, W. R. (ed.). *The history and conquest of common diseases.* Norman, Oklahoma, 1954.
DELAUNAY, P. 'L'évolution médicale [en France] du XVIe au XXe siècle'. *Bull. Soc. franç. d'hist. méd.*, 1928, xxii, 17–56.
MOORE, Sir N. *The history of the study of medicine in the British Isles.* Oxford, 1908.
OSLER, Sir W. *The principles and practice of medicine.* New York, 1892 (and later editions).
POWER, Sir D'ARCY. *Medicine in the British Isles.* (Clio Medica.) New York, 1930.
ROLLESTON, Sir H. *Internal medicine.* (Clio Medica.) New York, 1930.

Pathology

FLOREY, Sir H. (ed.). *General pathology.* 2nd ed. London, 1958.
GOLDSCHMID, E. *Entwicklung und Bibliographie der pathologisch-anatomischen Abbildung.* Leipzig, 1925.
KRUMBHAAR, E. B. *Pathology.* (Clio Medica.) New York, 1937.
LONG, E. R. *A history of pathology.* London, 1928.
—— *Selected readings in pathology.* Springfield and Baltimore, 1929. 2nd ed., 1961.
WRIGHT, G. PAYLING. *An introduction to pathology.* 3rd ed. London, 1958.

Physics

CAJORI, F. *A history of physics.* Rev. ed. New York, 1938.

Physiology

BAYLISS, Sir W. M. *Principles of general physiology.* London, 1915 (and later editions).
BEST, C. H., and TAYLOR, N. B. *The physiological basis of medical practice.* London, 1937 (and later editions).

Davson, H. *General physiology.* 2nd ed. London, 1959.

Foster, Sir M. *A text book of physiology.* London, 1877 (and later editions).

—— *Lectures on the history of physiology during the sixteenth, seventeenth and eighteenth centuries.* Cambridge, 1901.

Fulton, J. F. *Selected readings in the history of physiology.* Springfield, 1930.

—— *Physiology.* (Clio Medica.) New York, 1931.

Franklin, K. J. *A short history of physiology.* 2nd ed. London, 1949.

Rothschuh, K. E. *Geschichte der Physiologie.* Berlin, 1953.

Schäfer, E. A. (ed.). *Textbook of physiology.* 2 vols. Edinb. and London, 1898–1900.

—— *History of the Physiological Society.* London, 1927.

Starling, E. H. *Principles of human physiology.* London, 1912 (and later editions by Sir C. Lovatt Evans).

Stirling, W. *Some apostles of physiology.* London, 1902.

Underwood, E. A. Johann Gottfried von Berger (1659–1736) of Wittenberg and his text-book of physiology (1701). *S.M. & H.,* ii, 141–72.

Wright, Samson. *Applied physiology.* London, 1926 (and later editions).

Surgery

Billings, J. S. The history and literature of surgery, in F. S. Dennis, *System of surgery,* Phila., vol. i, 1895, 17–144.

Brunn, W. von. *Kurze Geschichte der Chirurgie.* Berlin, 1928.

Gaujot, G., and Spillmann, E. *Arsenal de la chirurgie contemporaine.* 2 vols. Paris, 1867–72.

Leonardo, R. A. *History of surgery.* New York, 1943.

Meyerson, Åke. *Studier i Serafimerlasarettets instrumentsamling.* Stockholm, 1952.

Miles, A. *The Edinburgh School of Surgery before Lister.* London, 1918.

Møller-Christensen, V. *The history of the forceps.* Copenhagen and London, 1938.

Parker, G. *The early history of surgery in Great Britain.* London, 1920.

Power, Sir D'Arcy. *A short history of surgery.* London, 1933.

Scultetus, J. *Armamentarium chirurgicum,* ed. J. B. Lamzweerde. Amsterdam, 1672.

Sudhoff, K. *Beiträge zur Geschichte der Chirurgie im Mittelalter.* 2 pts. Leipzig, 1914–18.

Thompson, C. J. S. *The history and evolution of surgical instruments.* New York, 1942.

Wall, C. *History of the Surgeons' Company, 1745–1800.* London, 1937.

B. INDIVIDUAL SECTIONS

Prehistoric medicine (pp. 1–3):

Lucas-Championnière, J. *Trépanation néolithique.* Paris, 1912.

Moodie, R. L. *Paleopathology.* Urbana, Ill., 1923.

—— *The antiquity of disease.* Chicago, 1923.

Parry, T. Wilson. The prehistoric trephined skulls of Great Britain. *P.R.S.M.,* 1920–1, xiv, 27–42.

—— Trephination of the living skull in prehistoric times. *B.M.J.,* 1923, i, 457–60.

Ruffer, Sir M. A. *Studies in the palaeopathology of Egypt.* Chicago, 1921.

Sigerist, H. E. *History,* vol. i.

Underwood, E. A. Introduction to *Prehistoric man in health and sickness.* London, 1951.

Ancient Egypt (pp. 3–9):

Breasted, J. H. *The Edwin Smith Surgical Papyrus.* 2 vols. Chicago, 1930.

Ebbell, B. *The Papyrus Ebers.* Copenhagen and Oxford, 1937.

ELLIOT SMITH, G. The most ancient splints. *B.M.J.*, 1908, i, 732–4.
—— and DAWSON, W. R. *Egyptian mummies*. London, 1924.
GARDINER, Sir A. *Egypt of the Pharaohs*. Oxford, 1961.
GLANVILLE, S. R. K. (ed.). *The legacy of Egypt*. Oxford, 1942.
GRAPOW, H. *Grundriss der Medizin der alten Ägypter*. Berlin. (Especially vol. i, 'Anatomie und Physiologie' (1954); vol. ii, 'Von den medizinischen Texten' (1955); vol. iii, 'Kranker, Krankheiten und Arzt' (1956)).
JAYNE, W. A. *The healing gods of ancient civilizations*. New Haven, 1925.
KRAUSE, A. C. Ancient Egyptian ophthalmology. *B.H.M.*, 1933, i, 258–76.
LEAKE, C. D. *The Old Egyptian medical papyri*. Kansas, 1952.
—— LARKEY, S. V., and LUTZ, H. F. The management of fractures according to the Hearst Medical Papyrus. *S.M. & H.*, i, 61–74.
LEFEBVRE, G. *La médecine égyptienne de l'époque pharaonique*. Paris, 1956.
LUCAS, A. *Ancient Egyptian materials & industries*. 3rd ed. London, 1948.
PARTINGTON, J. R. *Origins and development of applied chemistry*. London, 1935.
RANKE, H. Medicine and surgery in Ancient Egypt. *B.H.M.*, 1933, i, 237–57.
SIGERIST, *History*, vol. i.
WATERMANN, R. *Bilder aus dem Lande des Ptah und Imhotep*. Cologne, 1958.

Assyria and Babylonia (pp. 9–15):

CONTENAU, G. *La médecine en Assyrie et en Babylonie*. Paris, 1938.
DAWSON, W. R. *The beginnings, Egypt & Assyria*. (Clio Medica.) New York, 1930.
HOMMEL, E. 'Zur Geschichte der Anatomie im alten Orient'. *Arch. Gesch. Med.*, 1919, xi, 177–82.
JASTROW, M. *Aspects of religious belief and practice in Babylonia and Assyria*. New York and London, 1911.
—— The medicine of the Babylonians and Assyrians. *P.R.S.M.*, 1913–14, vii, 109–76.
—— Babylonian-Assyrian medicine. *A.M.H.*, 1917–18, i, 231–57.
OEFELE, F. VON. 'Keilschriftmedicin'. *Abh. Gesch. Med.*, iii, Breslau, 1902.
—— Babylonian medical textbooks. *J. Amer. Orient. Soc.*, 1917, xxxvii, 250–6.
SIGERIST, *History*, vol. i.
TEMKIN, O. Recent publications on Egyptian and Babylonian medicine. *B.H.M.*, 1936, iv, 247–56, 341–7.
THOMPSON, R. CAMPBELL. *The devils and evil spirits of Babylonia*. 2 vols. London, 1903–4.
—— *The Assyrian herbal*. London, 1924.
—— Assyrian medical texts. *P.R.S.M.*, 1923–4, xvii, 1–34; 1925–6, xix, 29–78.

Greek Medicine (pp. 16–66):
(a) *General works:*

BROCK, A. J. *Greek medicine*. London, 1929.
DAREMBERG, C. *La médecine, histoire et doctrines*. Paris, 1865.
—— *La médecine dans Homère*. Paris, 1865.
DIELS, H. *Die Fragmente der Vorsokratiker*. 5th ed. by W. Kranz. Berlin, 1934–8.
EDELSTEIN, L. 'Die Geschichte der Sektion in der Antike'. *Quell. u. Stud. z. Gesch. Med.*, 1933, iii, pt. ii.
FARRINGTON, B. *Greek science and its meaning for us*. 2 vols. Harmondsworth, 1944–9.
JONES, W. H. S. *The medical writings of Anonymus Londinensis*. Cambridge, 1947.
LIVINGSTONE, Sir R. (ed.). *The legacy of Greece*. Oxford, 1921.
LUND, F. B. *Greek medicine*. (Clio Medica.) New York, 1936.
MEYER-STEINEG, T. *Chirurgische Instrumente des Altertums*. Jena, 1912.
MILNE, J. S. *Surgical instruments in Greek and Roman times*. Oxford, 1907.

Oxford Classical Dictionary, especially arts. on Anatomy, Physiology, Medicine, Surgery, Hippocrates, Galen.

SIGERIST, H. E. 'Alkmaion von Kroton und die Anfänge der europäischen Physiologie'. *Schweiz. Med. Wchnsch.*, 1952, lxxxii, 964–5; and his *History*, vol. ii.

SINGER, *Studies*, vols. i and ii.

SINGER, C. *Greek biology & Greek medicine*. Oxford, 1922.

TAYLOR, H. O. *Greek biology and medicine*. London, 1922.

WELLMANN, M. 'Alkmaion von Kroton'. *Archeion*, 1929, xi, 156–69.

(*b*) *Temple medicine* (pp. 16–27):

EDELSTEIN, E. J. and L. *Asclepius, a collection and interpretation of the testimonies*. 2 vols. Baltimore, 1945.

FRITZ, K. VON. Asclepius: a review. *J.H.M.*, 1947, ii, 110–16.

GASK, G. E. The cult of Aesculapius and the origin of Hippocratic medicine. *A.M.H.*, 1939, 3rd. ser. i, 128–57.

HAMILTON, MARY. *Incubation or the cure of disease in pagan temples and Christian churches*. St. Andrews and London, 1906.

HERZOG, R. *Die Wunderheilungen von Epidauros*. Leipzig, 1931.

D'IRSAY, S. The cult of Asklepios. *B.H.M.*, 1935, iii, 451–82.

KERÉNYI, C. *Asklepios, archetypal image of the Physician's existence*. London, 1960.

ROUSE, W. H. D. *Greek votive offerings*. Cambridge, 1902.

(*c*) *Cos, Cnidos, and Hippocrates* (pp. 27–41):

EDELSTEIN, L. Development of Greek anatomy. *B.H.M.*, 1935, iii, 235–48.

—— Greek medicine in its relation to religion and magic. *B.H.M.*, 1937, v, 201–46.

—— The genuine works of Hippocrates. *B.H.M.*, 1939, vii, 236–48.

—— *The Hippocratic Oath*. Baltimore, 1943.

GASK, G. E. Cyrene, Cos and Cnidos. *A.M.H.*, 1940, 3rd. ser. ii, 15–21.

HEIDEL, W. A. *Hippocratic medicine*. New York, 1941.

HIPPOCRATES. Trans. Jones and Withington. (Loeb Classical Library.)

ILBERG, J. 'Die Aerzteschule von Knidos'. *Ber. d. Königl. Sächs. Akad. d. Wissensch., Phil.-hist. Kl.*, Leipzig, 1924, lxxvi, pt. iii.

JONES, W. H. S. *Malaria and Greek history*. Manchester, 1909.

—— *The doctor's oath*. Cambridge, 1924.

—— *Hippocrates and the Corpus Hippocraticum*. London, 1945.

—— *Philosophy and medicine in Ancient Greece*. Baltimore, 1946.

LARKEY, S. V. The Hippocratic Oath in Elizabethan England. *B.H.M.*, 1936, iv, 201–19.

LESKY, ERNA. 'Die Samentheorien in der hippokratischen Schriftensammlung', in *Neuburger Festschrift* (see p. 764), pp. 302–7.

MUCH, H. *Hippokrates der Grosse*. Stuttgart and Berlin, 1926.

POHLENZ, M. *Hippokrates und die Begründung der wissenschaftlichen Medizin*. Berlin, 1938.

SIGERIST, H. E. Notes and comments on Hippocrates. *B.H.M.*, 1934, ii, 190–214.

SINGER, C. On Francis Adams, translator of Hippocrates. *B.H.M.*, 1942, xii, 1–17.

SOUQUES, A. 'La douleur dans les livres hippocratiques'. *Bull. Soc. franç. d'hist. méd.*, 1937, xxxi, 209–44, 279–309; 1938, xxxii, 178–86, 222–42; 1939, xxxiii, 37–48, 131–44.

SUDHOFF, K. *Kos und Knidos*. Munich, 1927.

TEMKIN, O. 'Der systematische Zusammenhang im Corpus Hippokraticum'. *Kyklos*, 1928, i, 9–43.

—— 'Geschichte des Hippokratismus im ausgehenden Altertum'. *Kyklos*, 1932, iv, 1–80.

(*d*) *Aristotle* (pp. 41–47):

JAEGER, W. *Diokles von Karystos*. Berlin, 1938.
—— *Aristotle, fundamentals of the history of his development*. (Trans. R. Robinson.) 2nd ed. Oxford, 1948.
LONES, T. E. *Aristotle's researches in natural science*. London, 1912.
OGLE, W. Introduction to his translation of 'On the Parts of Animals', London, 1882.
PLATT, A. Aristotle on the heart, in Singer, *Studies*, vol. ii (see p. 764).
ROSS, Sir W. D. *Aristotle*. 3rd ed. London, 1937.

(*e*) *Alexandrian School* (pp. 48–51):

DOBSON, J. F. Herophilus. *P.R.S.M.*, 1924–5, xviii, 19–32.
—— Erasistratus. *P.R.S.M.*, 1926–7, xx, 21–28.
GASK, G. E. School of Alexandria. *A.M.H.*, 1940, 3rd ser. ii, 383–92.
MARX, K. F. H. *Herophilus*. Carlsruhe and Baden, 1838.
NEUBURGER, M. *History*, vol. i (see p. 762).
WELLMANN, M. Erasistratos. Art. in A. Pauly and G. Wissowa, *Real-Encyclop. d. klass. Altertumswissensch.*, vi, 333.

(*f*) *Greek Medicine in Rome* (pp. 51–59):

ALBERT, M. *Les médecins grecs à Rome*. Paris, 1894.
ALLBUTT, Sir T. C. *Greek medicine in Rome*. London, 1921.
BAILEY, C. (ed.). *The legacy of Rome*. Oxford, 1923.
BURN, A. R. 'Hic breve vivitur. A study of the expectation of life in the Roman Empire.' *Past & Present*, 1953, Nov., No. iv, 1–31.
CASTIGLIONI, A. Celsus as a historian of medicine. *B.H.M.*, 1940, viii, 857–73.
CELSUS. Trans. W. G. Spencer. (Loeb Classical Library.)
DAREMBERG, *Hist. sci. med.* (see p. 762), vol. i.
DRABKIN, I. E. Soranus and his system. *B.H.M.*, 1951, xxv, 503–18.
FRONTINUS. *Water supply of the city of Rome*. (Trans. Herschel.) Boston, Mass., 1899.
GASK, G. E. The school of medicine in Rome. *A.M.H.*, 1941, 3rd ser. iii, 524–9.
—— and TODD, J. The origin of hospitals. *S.M. & H.*, i, 122–30.
ILBERG, J. *Celsus und die Medizin in Rom*. Leipzig, 1907.
LEAKE, C. D. Roman architectural hygiene. *A.M.H.*, 1930, 2nd ser. ii, 135–63.
MEYER-STEINEG, T. *Das medizinische System der Methodiker*. Jena, 1916.
SINGER, C. Science under the Roman Empire, in his *From magic to science*, London, 1928, pp. 1–58.
SPENCER, W. G. Celsus' De medicina. *P.R.S.M.*, 1925–6, xix, 129–39.
TEMKIN, O. Celsus On Medicine and ancient medical sects. *B.H.M.*, 1935, iii, 249–64.
WELLMANN, M. *Die pneumatische Schule bis auf Archigenes*. Berlin, 1895.
—— *A. Cornelius Celsus, eine Quellenuntersuchung*. Berlin, 1913.

(*g*) *Galen and later writers* (pp. 59–66):

ARETAEUS. Extant works, trans. F. Adams. London, 1856.
FLEMING, D. Galen on the motions of the blood. *Isis*, 1955, xlvi, 14–21.
FRANKLIN, K. J. The foetal cardio-vascular apparatus, from Galen to Harvey. *Ann. Sci.*, 1941, v, 57–90.
GALEN. *On the natural faculties*. Trans. A. J. Brock. (Loeb Classical Library.)
GREEN, R. M. *A translation of Galen's Hygiene*. Springfield, 1951.
MEYER-STEINEG, T. On Galen's physiology. *Arch. Gesch. Med.*, 1912, v, 172–224.
PAULUS AEGINETA. *Works*, trans. F. Adams. 3 vols. London, 1844–7.
PRENDERGAST, J. S. Galen on the vascular system. *P.R.S.M.*, 1927–8, xxi, 79–87.
—— The background of Galen's life and activities. *P.R.S.M.*, 1929–30, xxiii, 53–70.
SARTON, G. *Galen of Pergamon*. Kansas, 1954.

SINGER, C. *Galen On anatomical procedures*. London, 1956.
—— *Galen as a modern*. *P.R.S.M.*, 1948–9, xlii, 563–70.
—— *Galen's elementary course on bones*. *P.R.S.M.*, 1952, xlv, 25–34.
TEMKIN, O. *On Galen's pneumatology*. *Gesnerus*, 1951, viii, 180–9.
WALSH, J. J. *Galen on the recurrent laryngeal nerve*. *A.M.H.*, 1926, viii, 176–84.
—— *Galen's writings*. Five papers in *A.M.H.*, 1934–9.
WALZER, R. *Galen On medical experience*. London, 1944.

Byzantium, the Dark Ages, Salerno (pp. 67–73):
BAYON, H. P. *The Masters of Salerno; the origins of professional medical practice*. *S.M.&H.*, i, 203–19.
Caelius Aurelianus, On acute diseases and on chronic diseases. Ed. and trans. I. E. Drabkin. Chicago, 1950.
CAPPARONI, P. *Magistri Salernitani nondum cogniti*. London, 1923.
CORNER, G. W. *Rise of medicine at Salerno*. *A.M.H.*, 1931, 2nd ser. iii, 1–16.
GIACOSA, P. *Magistri Salernitani nondum editi*. 2 vols. Turin, 1901.
GRATTAN, J. H. G., and SINGER, C. *Anglo-Saxon magic and medicine*. London, 1952.
GUNTHER, R. T. *The Greek Herbal of Dioscorides*. Oxford, 1934.
KRISTELLER, P. O. *The School of Salerno*. *B.H.M.*, 1945, xvii, 138–94.
PAYNE, J. F. *English medicine in the Anglo-Saxon times*. Oxford, 1904.
School of Salernum. Trans. Sir J. Harington. With a history of the School by F. R. Packard and a note by F. H. Garrison. New York, 1920.
SIGERIST, H. E. *Studien und Texte zur frühmittelalterlichen Rezeptliteratur*. Leipzig, 1923.
—— A *Salernitan student's surgical notebook*. *B.H.M.*, 1943, xiv, 505–16.
SINGER, C. *The medical literature of the Dark Ages*. *P.R.S.M.*, 1916–17, x, 107–60.
—— *The herbal in antiquity*. *J. Hellenic Studies*, 1927, xlvii, 1–52. (See also Singer, *From magic to science*.)
—— and D. *An unrecognized Anglo-Saxon medical text*. *A.M.H.*, 1921, iii, 136–49.
—— —— *The origin of the medical school of Salerno*, in Singer and Sigerist, *Essays presented to Sudhoff* (see p. 764).
—— —— *The School of Salerno*. *History*, 1925–6, x, 242–6. (See also Singer, *From magic to science*.)
SORANUS. *Gynaecology*. Trans. Temkin *et al.* Baltimore, 1956.
STEUDEL, J. 'Beiträge der Schule von Salerno zur anatomischen Nomenklatur'. *Atti del XIV congr. internaz. di storia della medicina, Roma-Salerno*. (Reprint.)

Arabian Medicine (pp. 73–76):
BROWNE, E. G. *Arabian medicine*. Cambridge, 1921.
CAMPBELL, D. *Arabian medicine*. 2 vols. London, 1926.
ELGOOD, C. *Medicine in Persia*. (Clio Medica.) New York, 1934.
—— *A medical history of Persia*. Cambridge, 1951.
GRUNER, O. C. *A treatise on the Canon of Medicine of Avicenna*. London, 1930.
MEYERHOF, M. Art. on Science and Medicine in *The legacy of Islam*, ed. Sir T. Arnold and A. Guillaume, Oxford, 1931.
MIELI, A. *La science arabe*. Leyden, 1938.
WÜSTENFELD, F. *Geschichte der arabischen Aerzte*. Göttingen, 1840.

The Middle Ages (pp. 76–87):
(*a*) *General works*:
CRUMP, C. G., and JACOB, E. F. (eds.). *The legacy of the Middle Ages*. Oxford, 1926.
DIEPGEN, P. 'Die Bedeutung des Mittelalters für den Fortschritt in der Medizin', in Singer and Sigerist, *Essays presented to Sudhoff* (see p. 764).

HASKINS, C. H. *Studies in the history of mediaeval science.* 2nd ed. Camb., Mass., 1927.
PREVITÉ-ORTON, C. W. *The shorter Cambridge medieval history.* 2 vols. Cambridge, 1952.
TAYLOR, H. O. *The mediaeval mind.* 4th ed. 2 vols. London, 1938.
THORNDIKE, L. *Medieval Europe, its development & civilization.* London, 1920.
—— *A history of magic and experimental science.* 8 vols. New York, 1923–58.

(*b*) *Universities*:

D'IRSAY, S. *Histoire des universités françaises et étrangères.* 2 vols. Paris, 1933–5.
KAUFMANN, G. *Geschichte der deutschen Universitäten.* 2 vols. Reprint, Graz, 1958.
RASHDALL, H. *The universities of Europe in the Middle Ages.* Rev. ed. by F. M. Powicke and A. B. Emden. 3 vols. Oxford, 1936.
WICKERSHEIMER, E. Origins of the Faculty of Medicine at Paris. *Bull. Soc. franç. d'hist. méd.,* 1914, xiii, 249–60.
—— *Commentaires de la Faculté de Médicine de l'Université de Paris (1395–1516): Préface et introduction.* Paris, 1915.

(*c*) *Medicine and science*:

ALLBUTT, Sir T. C. *Science and mediaeval thought.* London, 1901.
—— *The historical relations of medicine and surgery to the end of the sixteenth century.* London, 1905.
ARTELT, W. 'Die ältesten Nachrichten über die Sektion im mittelalterlichen Abendland'. *Abh. Gesch. Med. und Naturwiss.,* 1940.
COOPER, S. The Medical School of Montpellier in the 14th cent. *A.M.H.,* 1930, 2nd ser. ii, 164–95.
CORNER, G. W. *Anatomical texts of the earlier Middle Ages.* Washington, 1927.
CROMBIE, A. C. *Augustine to Galileo* (see p. 764).
FLEMMING, P. The medical aspects of the medieval monastery in England. *P.R.S.M.,* 1928–9, xxii, 25–36.
FLETCHER, G. R. J. St. Isidor of Seville and his book on medicine. *P.R.S.M.,* 1918–19, xii, 70–95.
GORDON, B. L. *Medieval and Renaissance medicine.* New York, 1959.
GUY DE CHAULIAC. *La Grande Chirurgie.* Ed. E. Nicaise. Paris, 1890.
KIBRE, PEARL. Hippocratic writings in the Middle Ages. *B.H.M.,* 1945, xviii, 371–412.
MACKINNEY, L. C. *Early medieval medicine.* Baltimore, 1937.
MØLLER-CHRISTENSEN, V. *Bone changes in leprosy.* Copenhagen, 1961.
RIESMAN, D. *The story of medicine in the Middle Ages.* New York, 1935.
ROBIN, P. A. *The old physiology in English literature.* London, 1911.
SINGER, C. (trans.). *The Fasciculus Medicinae of Johannes de Ketham.* Milan, 1924.
—— (trans. and ed.). *The Fasciculo di Medicina Venice 1493.* Florence, 1925.
SUDHOFF, K. *Ein Beitrag zur Geschichte der Anatomie im Mittelalter.* Leipzig, 1908.
THEODORIC. *Surgery.* Trans. E. Campbell and J. Colton. 2 vols. New York, 1955–60.
THORNDIKE, L. (ed.). *The Herbal of Rufinus.* Chicago, 1946.
WICKERSHEIMER, E. The first dissections at the Faculty of Medicine at Paris. *Bull. Soc. de l'hist. de Paris et de l'Ile-de-France,* 1910, xxxvii, 159–69.
—— *Anatomies de Mondino dei Luzzi et de Guido de Vigevano.* Paris, 1926.

The Renaissance (pp. 88–*c.* 111):

(*a*) *General works*:

ALLBUTT, Sir T. C. *The historical relations of medicine and surgery to the end of the sixteenth century.* London, 1905.
CASTIGLIONI, A. The medical school at Padua and the renaissance of medicine. *A.M.H.,* 1935, 2nd ser. vii, 214–27.

MacNalty, Sir A. S. The Renaissance, and its influence on English medicine, surgery, and public health. *B.M.J.*, 1945, ii, 755–9.
Newman, G. *A century of medicine at Padua.* London, [1921].
Taylor, H. O. *Thought and expression in the sixteenth century.* 2 vols. New York, 1920.
Wickersheimer, C. A. E. *La médecine et les médecins en France à l'époque de ia Renaissance.* 2 vols. Paris, 1906.

(*b*) *Anatomy and surgery*:

Adelmann, H. B. *The embryological treatises of Hieronymus Fabricius of Aquapendente.* Ithaca, N.Y., 1942.
Belt, E. *Leonardo the anatomist.* Kansas, 1955.
Berengar da Carpi, Isagogae Breves. Trans. L. R. Lind. Chicago, 1959.
Castiglioni, A. *The renaissance of medicine in Italy.* Baltimore, 1934.
Clark, W. E. Le Gros. Berengario of Carpi. *St. Thomas's Hosp. Gaz.*, 1929–31, xxxii, 110–21.
Cushing, H. *Bio-bibliography of Andreas Vesalius.* New York, 1943.
Eriksson, R. (ed.). *Andreas Vesalius' first public anatomy at Bologna, 1540.* Uppsala and Stockholm, 1959.
Farrington, B. (trans.). The preface of Vesalius to the *Fabrica*, 1543. *P.R.S.M.*, 1931–2, xxv, 39–48.
Fischer, H. 'Leonardo als Physiologe'. *Gesnerus*, 1952, ix, 81–123.
Gnudi, M. T., and Webster, J. P. *The life and times of Gaspare Tagliacozzi.* New York, 1950.
Keele, K. D. *Leonardo da Vinci on the movement of the heart and blood.* London, 1952.
Lind, L. R. (trans.). *The Epitome of Andreas Vesalius.* New York, 1949.
MacCurdy, E. *The notebooks of Leonardo da Vinci.* 2 vols. London, 1938.
McMurrich, J. P. *Leonardo da Vinci the anatomist.* Baltimore, 1930.
O'Malley, C. D. Andreas Vesalius, Count Palatine. *J.H.M.*, 1954, ix, 196-223.
—— and Saunders, J. B. de C. M. *Leonardo da Vinci on the human body.* New York, 1952.
—— —— Andreas Vesalius, Imperial Physician. *S.M. & H.*, i, 386–400.
Packard, F. R. *The life and times of Ambroise Paré.* New York, 1921.
Paget, S. *Ambroise Paré and his times.* London, 1897.
Paré. *Œuvres complètes* (ed. Malgaigne). 3 vols. Paris, 1840–1.
—— *The Apologie and Treatise* (ed. G. Keynes). London, 1951.
—— *The case reports and autopsy records of Ambroise Paré* (trans. W. B. Hamby). Springfield, 1960.
Putti, V. *Berengario da Carpi.* Bologna, 1937.
Roth, M. *Andreas Vesalius Bruxellensis.* Berlin, 1892.
Saunders, J. B. de C. M., and O'Malley, C. D. (trans.). *Andreas Vesalius Bruxellensis: The Blood-letting Letter of 1539.* New York, 1948.
—— (trans. and ed.). *The illustrations from the works of Andreas Vesalius.* Cleveland and New York, 1950.
Singer, C. A study in early Renaissance anatomy. The Anothomia of Hieronymo Manfredi (1490), in Singer, *Studies*, i, 79–164 (see p. 764).
—— *The evolution of anatomy.* London, 1925.
—— *Vesalius on the human brain.* London, 1952.
—— Some Galenic and animal sources of Vesalius. *J.H.M.*, 1946, i, 6–24.
—— and Rabin, C. *A prelude to modern science . . . the Tabulae Anatomicae Sex of Vesalius.* Cambridge, 1946.
Singer, D. W. *Selections from the Works of Ambroise Paré.* London, 1924.
Steudel, J. 'Vesals Reform der anatomischen Nomenklatur'. *Ztsch. Anat. u. Entwicklungsgesch.*, 1942–3, cxii, 675–81.

STRAUS, W. L., Jr., and TEMKIN, O. Vesalius and the problem of variability. *B.H.M.*, 1943, xiv, 609–33.

(*c*) *Concepts of disease, medicine, syphilis:*

ARBER, AGNES. *Herbals, their origin and evolution.* Rev. ed. Cambridge, 1938.
BLOCH, I. *Der Ursprung der Syphilis.* 2 pts. Jena, 1901–11.
COPEMAN, W. S. C. *Doctors and disease in Tudor times.* London, 1960.
FRACASTOR, *De contagione.* Trans. W. C. Wright. New York and London, 1930.
—— *Syphilis or the French Disease.* Trans. H. Wynne-Finch. London, 1935.
HOLCOMB, R. C. *Who gave the world syphilis?* New York, 1937.
—— The antiquity of congenital syphilis. *B.H.M.*, 1941, x, 148–77.
JACOBS, J. *Paracelsus. Selected writings.* London, 1951.
JEANSELME, A. E. *Histoire de la syphilis.* Paris, 1931.
MUNGER, R. S. Guaiacum, the holy wood. *J.H.M.*, 1949, iv, 196–229.
OSLER, Sir W. *Thomas Linacre.* Cambridge, 1908.
PAGEL, W. *Paracelsus. An introduction to Philosophical Medicine in the era of the Renaissance.* Basel, 1958.
PROKSCH, J. K. *Die Litteratur über die venerischen Krankheiten.* 5 vols. Bonn, 1889–1900.
—— *Die Geschichte der venerischen Krankheiten.* 2 vols. Bonn, 1895–1900.
PUSEY, W. A. *The history and epidemiology of syphilis.* Springfield, 1933.
ROLLESTON, Sir H. *Internal medicine.* (Clio Medica.) New York, 1930.
SHERRINGTON, Sir C. *The endeavour of Jean Fernel.* Cambridge, 1946.
SIGERIST, H. E. Paracelsus after 400 years, in *The March of Medicine*, 1941, pp. 28–51.
—— Laudanum in the works of Paracelsus. *B.H.M.*, 1941, ix, 530–44.
SINGER, C. and D. W. *The development of the doctrine of Contagium Vivum, 1500–1750.* [Privately printed.] 1913.
—— —— The scientific position of Girolamo Fracastoro. *A.M.H.*, 1917, i, 1–34.
STODDART, A. M. *The life of Paracelsus.* London, 1911.
SUDHOFF, K. *Aus der Frühgeschichte der Syphilis.* Leipzig, 1912.
—— 'Mal Franzoso in Italien in der ersten Hälfte des 15. Jahrh.', in *Zur historischen Biologie der Krankheitserreger*, Giessen, 1912, 5 Heft.
—— and SINGER, C. *The earliest printed literature on syphilis.* Florence, 1925.
WILLIAMS, H. U. The origin and antiquity of syphilis. *Arch. Path.*, 1932, xiii, 779–814, 931–83.

The first physical synthesis (pp. 111–15):

ARMITAGE, A. *Sun, Stand Thou Still: The life and work of Copernicus.* New York, 1947.
BAUMGARDT, CAROLA. *Johannes Kepler.* London, 1952.
FAHIE, J. J. *Galileo, his life and work.* London, 1903.
—— The scientific works of Galileo, in Singer, *Studies*, ii, 206–84 (see p. 764).
SINGER, D. W. *Giordano Bruno, his life and thought.* New York, 1950.

Physiology in the seventeenth century (pp. 115–23):

BASTHOLM, E. *The history of muscle physiology* [to Haller]. Copenhagen, 1950.
BAYON, H. P. William Harvey: his precursors, opponents and successors. *Ann. Sci.*, 1938, iii, 59–118, 435–56; 1939, iv, 65–106, 329–89.
—— Allusions to a 'circulation' of the blood in MSS. anterior to 'De motu cordis' 1628. *P.R.S.M.*, 1938–9, xxxii, 37–43.
—— The significance of the demonstration of the Harveian circulation by experimental tests. *Isis*, 1941, xxxiii, 443–53.
—— Harvey's application of biological experiment, clinical observation, and comparative anatomy to the problems of generation. *J.H.M.*, 1947, ii, 51–96.

BITTAR, E. E. A study of Ibn Nafīs. *B.H.M.*, 1955, xxix, 352–68, 429–47.

CASTIGLIONI, A. *La vita e l'opera di Santorio Santorio.* Bologna and Trieste, 1920.

CHAUVOIS, L. *William Harvey: His life and times; his discoveries; his method.* London, 1957.

COHEN, Sir H. Harvey and the scientific method. *B.M.J.*, 1950, ii, 1405–10.

COPPOLA, E. D. The discovery of the pulmonary circulation. *B.H.M.*, 1957, xxxi, 44–77.

CURTIS, J. G. *Harvey's views on the use of the circulation of the blood.* New York, 1915.

DALTON, J. C. *Doctrines of the circulation.* Phila., 1884.

FLEMING, D. William Harvey and the pulmonary circulation. *Isis*, 1955, xlvi, 319–27.

FLOURENS, P. *Histoire de la découverte de la circulation du sang.* 2nd ed. Paris, 1857.

FOSTER, Sir M. *Lectures on the history of physiology.* Cambridge, 1901.

FRANKLIN, K. J. Valves in veins: an historical survey. *P.R.S.M.*, 1927–8, xxi, 1–33.

—— (trans.). *De venarum ostiolis 1603 of Hieronymus Fabricus of Aquapendente.* Springfield and Baltimore, 1933.

—— William Harvey—a speculative note. *Gesnerus*, 1948, v, 70–74.

GOTFREDSEN, E. The reception of Harvey's doctrine in Denmark. *Acta Med. Scandinav.*, 1952, cxlii, Supp. (Papers dedicated to Erik Warburg), 75–86.

—— Some relations between British and Danish medicine in the 17th and 18th centuries. *J.H.M.*, 1953, viii, 46–55.

HARVEY, W. *Praelectiones anatomiae universalis.* London, 1886.

—— *Movement of the heart and blood.* Trans. K. J. Franklin. London, 1957.

—— *The circulation of the blood.* Trans. K. J. Franklin. London, 1958.

—— *De motu locali animalium.* Trans. Gweneth Whitteridge. Cambridge, 1959.

IZQUIERDO, J. J. *Harvey, iniciador del metodo experimental.* Mexico, 1936.

—— A new view of Servetus on the circulation. *B.H.M.*, 1937, v, 914–32.

KEITH, Sir A. Harvey as an anatomist. *Lancet*, 1928, i, 999–1000.

KEYNES, Sir G. *The personality of William Harvey.* Cambridge, 1949.

—— *Harvey through John Aubrey's eyes.* London, 1958. (Reprinted from the *Lancet* with additions.)

LANGDON-BROWN, Sir W. *Some chapters in Cambridge medical history.* Cambridge, 1946.

MACKALL, L. L. Servetus notes, in *Contributions dedicated to Osler*, ii, 767–77.

—— A manuscript of the 'Christianismi Restitutio' of Servetus, placing the discovery of the pulmonary circulation anterior to 1546. *P.R.S.M.*, 1923–4, xvii, 35–38.

MACNALTY, Sir A. S. William Harvey: his influence on public health. *Roy. Soc. Health J.*, 1957, lxxvii, 324–37.

MAJOR, R. H. Santorio Santorio. *A.M.H.*, 1938, 2nd ser. x, 369–81.

MALLOCH, A. *William Harvey.* New York, 1929.

MEYERHOF, M. 'Ibn an-Nafīs und seine Theorie des Lungenkreislaufs'. *Quell. u. Stud. z. Gesch. Med.*, 1933, iv, 37–88.

—— Ibn an-Nafīs and his theory of the lesser circulation. *Isis*, 1935, xxiii, 100–20.

O'MALLEY, C. D. *Michael Servetus. A translation of his geographical, medical and astrological writings.* Phila. and London, 1953.

PAGEL, W. Religious motives in the medical biology of the 17th century. *B.H.M.*, 1935, iii, 97–128, 213–31, 265–312.

—— 'Circulatio'—its unusual connotations and Harvey's philosophy, in *Neuburger Festschrift* (see p. 764), 358–62.

—— The reaction to Aristotle in seventeenth-century biological thought. *S.M. & H.*, i, 489–509.

POWER, Sir D'ARCY. *William Harvey.* London, 1897.

ROLLESTON, Sir H. The reception of Harvey's doctrine, in Singer and Sigerist, *Essays presented to Sudhoff* (see p. 764).

SINGER, C. *The discovery of the circulation of the blood.* London, 1922.
TAYLOR, F. SHERWOOD. The origin of the thermometer. *Ann. Sci.*, 1941–7, v, 129–56.
TEMKIN, O. Was Servetus influenced by Ibn an-Nafîs? *B.H.M.*, 1940, viii, 731–4.
TRUETA, J. The contribution of Servetus to the scientific development of the Renais-
    sance. *B.M.J.*, 1954, ii, 507–10.
WILLIS, R. *William Harvey.* London, 1878.
YOUNG, J. F. Malpighi's 'De Pulmonibus'. *P.R.S.M.*, 1929–30, xxiii, 1–11.

The Classical Microscopists (pp. 124–35):
CLAY, R. S., and COURT, T. H. *The history of the microscope.* London, 1932.
DOBELL, C. *Antony van Leeuwenhoek and his 'Little Animals'.* London, 1932.
'ESPINASSE, MARGARET. *Robert Hooke.* London, 1956.
GUNTHER, R. T. *Early science in Oxford.* Vol. xiii [facsimile ed. of Hooke's *Micro-
    graphia*, 1665]. Oxford, 1938.
MIALL, L. C. *The early naturalists, their lives and work (1530–1789).* London, 1912.
ROOSEBOOM, M. *Microscopium.* Leyden, 1956.
SINGER, C. Notes on the early history of microscopy. *P.R.S.M.*, 1913–14, vii, 247–79.
—— The dawn of microscopical discovery. *J. Roy. Micros. Soc.*, 1915, 3rd ser. xxxv,
    317–40.

From alchemy to chemistry (pp. 135–7):
HOLMYARD, E. J. *Alchemy.* Harmondsworth, 1957.
MORE, L. T. *The life and works of the Hon. Robert Boyle.* New York and London, 1944.
READ, J. *Prelude to chemistry.* 2nd ed. London, 1939.
TAYLOR, F. SHERWOOD. *The alchemists, founders of modern chemistry.* New York, 1951.
TEMKIN, O. Medicine and Graeco-Arabic alchemy. *B.H.M.*, 1955, xxix, 134–53.

Scientific societies (p. 136):
ANDRADE, E. N. DA C. *A brief history of the Royal Society.* London, 1960.
LYONS, Sir H. *The Royal Society, 1660–1940.* Cambridge, 1944.
McKIE, D. The origins and foundation of the Royal Society. *Notes & Records Roy.
    Soc. Lond.*, 1960, xv, 1–37.
ORNSTEIN, M. *The rôle of scientific societies in the seventeenth century.* 3rd ed. Chicago,
    1938.
SPRAT, T. *History of the Royal Society.* New ed. by J. I. Cope and H. W. Jones.
    St. Louis and London, 1959.
WELD, C. R. *A history of the Royal Society.* 2 vols. London, 1848.

The Medical Theorists (pp. 137–44) *and Sydenham* (pp. 110–11):
BALZ, A. G. A. *Descartes and the modern mind.* New Haven, 1952.
CAPPARONI, P. 'Sulla patria di G. A. Borelli'. *Riv. stor. sci. med. e nat.*, 1931, xxii,
    53–63.
COMRIE, J. D. *Selected works of Thomas Sydenham.* London, 1922.
DELAUNAY, P. 'L'évolution philosophique et médicale du biomécanicisme'. *Progrès
    méd.* (Paris), 1927, liv, 1289–93, 1337–42, 1347–52, 1369–78, 1383–4.
HOFFMANN, K. F. On Borelli. *Wien. Med. Wchnsch.*, 1930, lxxx, 190.
MARTIN, R. C. C. *Descartes médecin.* Thèse de Paris, 1924, no. 248.
NEWMAN, Sir G. *Thomas Sydenham, reformer of English medicine.* London, 1924.
PAGEL, W. *J. B. van Helmont. Einführung in die philosophische Medizin des Barock.*
    Berlin, 1930.
—— Helmont, Leibnitz, Stahl. *Arch. Gesch. Med.*, 1931, xxiv, 19–59.
[——] On the 300th anniversary of the death of van Helmont. *B.M.J.*, 1945, i, 59.
—— Van Helmont on gastric digestion. *B.H.M.*, 1956, xxx, 524–36.
—— The position of Harvey and van Helmont in the history of European thought.
    J.H.M., 1958, xiii, 186–99.

PAYNE, J. F. *Thomas Sydenham*. London, 1900.
SCOTT, J. F. *The scientific work of René Descartes*. London, 1952.
STRUNZ, F. *J. B. van Helmont*. Leipzig and Vienna, 1907.
SYDENHAM. *Works*, trans. G. R. Latham. 2 vols. London, 1848–50.

The Reign of Law (pp. 145–47):
MORE, L. T. *Isaac Newton, a biography*. New York and London, 1934.

Clinical teaching and medical systems (pp. 147–50):
COHEN, E. Boerhaave and chemistry. *Janus* (Leyden), 1918, xxiii, 223–90.
COMRIE, J. D. On Cullen. *Edinb. Med. J.*, 1925, N.S. xxxii, 17–30.
FISCHER, I. [On Stahl.] *Wien. Med. Wchnsch.*, 1934, lxxxiv, 560–1.
HUNGER, F. W. T. 'Boerhaave comme Naturaliste'. *Janus* (Leyden), 1918, xxiii, 347–57.
JOHNSON, SAMUEL. Life of Boerhaave.
LEERSUM, E. C. VAN. Hermann Boerhaave. *Janus* (Leyden), 1918, xxiii, 195–206.
NEUBURGER, M. 'Boerhaave's Einfluss auf die Entwicklung der Medizin in Oesterreich'. *Janus* (Leyden), 1918, xxiii, 215–22.
RICHARDSON, Sir B. W. Arts. on Boerhaave, John Brown, and Cullen, in his *Disciples of Aesculapius*, 1900, i, 95–107, 245–61; ii, 439–60.
STAPLES, F. Cullen's place in the history of medicine. *New York Med. J.*, 1897, lxv, 689–91.
THOMSON, J. *An account of the life, lectures, and writings of William Cullen*. 2 vols. Edinb. and London, 1832–59.

Anatomy; the Edinburgh School (pp. 150–1):
COMRIE, J. D. *Hist. Scottish medicine* (see p. 762).
COPE, Sir Z. *William Cheselden*. Edinb. and London, 1953.
RICHARDSON, Sir B. W. Arts. on Cheselden and Monro *primus*, in his *Disciples of Aesculapius*, 1900, i, 128–42; ii, 425–38.

Physiological advances (pp. 151–61):
For this section, see especially Foster, *Hist. Physiol.* (1901). For Bell and Magendie, see under later section on *Nervous system*.
BEAUMONT, W. *Experiments and observations on the gastric juice*. Facsimile of the original ed. of 1833. Cambridge, Mass., 1929.
BURGET, G. E. Spallanzani. *A.M.H.*, 1924, vi, 177–84.
CLARK-KENNEDY, A. E. *Stephen Hales*. Cambridge, 1929.
CUMMINS, B. Spallanzani. *Sci. Progress*, 1916–17, xi, 236–45.
FRANCHINI, G. Spallanzani. *A.M.H.*, 1930, 2nd. ser. ii, 56–62.
GALVANI, L. *Commentary on the effects of electricity on muscular motion*. Trans. M. G. Foley, with introduction and notes by I. B. Cohen. Norwalk, Conn., 1953.
HALLER, A. VON. 'A dissertation on the senible and irritable parts of animals'. With introduction by O. Temkin. *B.H.M.*, 1936, iv, 651–99.
HINTZSCHE, E. 'Albrecht Hallers anatomische Arbeit in Basel und Bern'. *Ztsch. Anat. u. Entwicklungsgesch.*, 1941, cxi, 452–60.
KLOTZ, O. Albrecht von Haller. *A.M.H.*, 1936, 2nd ser. viii, 10–26.
KRONECKER, H. 'Haller redivivus'. *Mitteil. d. Naturf. Gesellsch. in Bern* (1902), 1903, 203–26.
M'KENDRICK, J. G. Spallanzani. *B.M.J.*, 1891, ii, 888–92.
MILLER, GENEVIEVE. *William Beaumont's formative years*. New York, 1946.
REED, C. B. Albrecht von Haller. *Bull. Soc. Med. Hist. Chicago*, 1911–16, i, 23a–46a [i.e. 259–82].

The nature of the air (pp. 161–8):

AYKROYD, W. R. *Three philosophers* (Lavoisier, Priestley, Cavendish). London, 1935.

DUVEEN, D. I., and KLICKSTEIN, H. S. Lavoisier's contributions to medicine and public health. *B.H.M.*, 1955, xxix, 164–79.

GOTCH, F. *Two Oxford physiologists* (Lower and Mayow). Oxford, 1908.

GRIMAUX, E. *Lavoisier, 1743–1794.* Paris, 1888.

HARTOG, Sir P. The newer views of Priestley and Lavoisier. *Ann. Sci.*, 1941–7, v, 1–56.

McKIE, D. *Antoine Lavoisier, the father of modern chemistry.* London, 1935.

—— *Antoine Lavoisier, scientist, economist, social reformer.* London, 1952.

—— Fire and the Flamma Vitalis: Boyle, Hooke and Mayow. *S.M. & H.*, i, 469–88.

PATTERSON, T. S. John Mayow in contemporary setting; respiration and combustion. *Isis*, 1931, xv, 47–96, 504–46.

RAMSAY, Sir W. *The gases of the atmosphere.* London, 1896.

—— *The life and letters of Joseph Black.* London, 1918.

UNDERWOOD, E. A. Lavoisier and the history of respiration. *P.R.S.M.*, 1943–4, xxxvii, 9–24.

Morbid anatomy (pp. 168–71), see later section on *Modern pathology* (p. 791)

Clinical methods and instruments (pp. 171–4):

DOCK, G. Auenbrugger and the history of percussion. *Michigan Alumnus*, 1898, (reprint).

—— Rozière de la Chassagne and the early history of percussion of the thorax. *A.M.H.*, 1935, 2nd ser. vii, 438–50.

HALE-WHITE, Sir W. The history of percussion and auscultation. *Lancet*, 1924, i, 263–5.

HOYLE, CLIFFORD. The life and discoveries of Laennec. *Brompton Hosp. Repts.*, 1944, xiii, 137–50.

KORNS, H. M. The history of physical diagnosis. *A.M.H.*, 1939, 3rd ser. i, 50–67.

LAENNEC, R. T. H. *Selected passages from De l'auscultation médiate.* Trans. Sir W. Hale-White. London, 1923.

MAUCLAIRE, M. 'Description des tubercules osseux, articulaires et ganglionaires dans les manuscrits de Laennec'. *Bull. Soc. franç. d'hist. méd.*, 1927, xxi, 112–17.

MIDDLETON, W. S. The history of physical diagnosis. *A.M.H.*, 1924, vi, 426–52.

MITCHELL, S. WEIR. The early history of instrumental precision in medicine. *Trans. Congr. Amer. Phys. and Surg.*, 1891, ii, 159–98.

NEUBURGER, M. John Floyer's pioneer work. *B.H.M.*, 1948, xxii, 208–12.

ROUXEAU, A. *Laennec avant 1806.* Paris, 1912.

—— *Laennec après 1806.* Paris, 1920.

SIGERIST, H. E. (ed.). On percussion of the chest, being a translation of Auenbrugger's original treatise by John Forbes, M.D. London, 1824. *B.H.M.*, 1936, iv, 373–403.

UNDERWOOD, E. A. The training of Laennec. *Brit. J. Dis. Chest*, 1959, liii, 109–12, 121–4.

WALSH, J. J. Auenbrugger, in his *Makers of modern medicine*, 2nd ed., New York, 1910.

WEBB, G. B. *Laennec, a memoir.* New York, 1928.

WILLIAMS, T. Laennec and the evolution of the stethoscope. *B.M.J.*, 1907, ii, 6–8.

Obstetrics and surgery in the eighteenth century (pp. 174–9):

DOBSON, JESSIE. *William Clift.* London, 1954.

FISCHER, G. *Chirurgie vor 100 Jahren. Historische Studie.* Leipzig, 1876.

HUNTER, J. *Works*, ed. Palmer. 4 vols. and atlas of plates. London, 1837.

JOHNSTONE, R. W. *William Smellie.* Edinb. and London, 1952.

KOUWER, B. J. Hendrik van Deventer. *Janus* (Leyden), 1912, xvii, 425–42, 506–24.

MATHER, G. R. *Two great Scotsmen, the brothers William and John Hunter.* Glasgow, 1893.
OPPENHEIMER, JANE M. *New aspects of John and William Hunter.* London, 1946.
PAGET, S. *John Hunter.* London, 1897.
PEACHEY, G. C. *A memoir of William & John Hunter.* Plymouth, 1924.
RADCLIFFE, W. *The secret instrument* [the Chamberlen forceps]. London, 1947.
TURNER, G. GREY. *The Hunterian Museum, yesterday and to-morrow.* London, 1946.

Vital statistics (pp. 179–81), see pp. 794-5
Military, naval and prison medicine and medical reforms (pp. 181–91):
ABRAHAM, J. JOHNSTON. *Lettsom, his life, times, friends and descendants.* London, 1938.
ALLISON, R. S. *Sea diseases.* London, 1943.
BROCKBANK, E. M. *The foundation of provincial medical education in England and of the Manchester School in particular.* Manchester, 1936.
DUKES, C. E. London medical societies in the 18th century. *P.R.S.M.*, 1959–60, liii, 19–26.
DUNCAN, A. *Memorials of the Faculty of Physicians and Surgeons of Glasgow.* Glasgow, 1896.
FOX, R. HINGSTON. *Dr. John Fothergill and his friends.* London, 1919.
GARRISON, F. H. *Notes on the history of military medicine.* Washington, 1922.
KEEVIL, J. J. *Medicine and the Navy* [to 1714]. 2 vols. Edinb. and London, 1957–8.
Lind's Treatise on Scurvy, ed. C. P. Stewart and D. Guthrie. Edinb., 1953.
POYNTER, F. N. L. *Selected writings of William Clowes, 1544–1604.* London, 1948.
RICHARDSON, Sir B. W. Arts. on Benjamin Rush and Richard Wiseman in his *Disciples of Aesculapius*, 1900, i, 62–75, 158–75.
RODDIS, L. H. *James Lind.* New York, 1950.
—— *A short history of nautical medicine.* New York and London, 1941.
SINGER, C. William Gilbert. *J. Roy. Naval Med. Service*, 1916, ii, 494–510.
SINGER, D. W. Sir John Pringle and his circle. *Ann. Sci.*, 1948–50, vi, 127–80, 229–61.
UNDERWOOD, E. A. Naval medicine in the ages of Elizabeth and James. *Ann. Roy. Coll. Surg. Eng.*, 1947, i, 115–36.

The Industrial Revolution, communal disease (pp. 191–8):
BAUMGARTNER, L., and RAMSEY, E. M. J. P. Frank and his 'System'. *A.M.H.*, 1933, 2nd ser. v, 525–32; 1934, vi, 69–90.
FRANK, J. P. See in Sigerist, *Great doctors (v.a.)*, and *Landmarks in the history of hygiene.*
LEROY, M. *Histoire des idées sociales en France.* Paris, 1946.
LESKY, E. J. P. Frank as organiser of medical education. *Arch. Gesch. Med.*, 1955, xxxix, 1–29.
MEIKLEJOHN, A. *The life, work and times of Charles Turner Thackrah.* Edinb. and London, 1957.
RAMAZZINI, *De morbis artificum* (*Diseases of workers*). Ed. and trans. W. C. Wright. Chicago, 1940.
ROSEN, G. *The history of miners' diseases.* New York, 1943.
SHRYOCK, R. H. *The development of modern medicine: an interpretation of the social and scientific factors involved.* New York and London, 1947.
SIGERIST, H. E. Historical background of industrial and occupational diseases. *Bull. N. York Acad. Med.*, 1936, 2nd ser. xii, 597–609.
TRAILL, H. D., and MANN, J. S. (eds.). *Social England.* 6 vols. London, 1901–4.
TREVELYAN, G. M. *English social history.* 3rd ed. London, 1946.

Epidemic disease (pp. 198–204):
BARON, J. *The life of Edward Jenner.* 2 vols. London, 1838.

DREWITT, F. D. *The life of Edward Jenner.* 2nd ed. London, 1931.
GOODALL, E. W. *A short history of the epidemic infectious diseases.* London, 1934.
HALSBAND, R. *The life of Lady Mary Wortley Montagu.* Oxford, 1956.
KLEBS, A. C. The historic evolution of variolation. *Bull. Johns Hopkins Hosp.*, 1913, xxiv, 69–83.
MILLER, GENEVIEVE. *The adoption of inoculation for smallpox in England and France.* Phila., 1957.
ROLLESTON, J. D. *The history of the acute exanthemata.* London, 1937.
—— Bretonneau: his life and work. *P.R.S.M.*, 1924–5, xviii, 1–12.
UNDERWOOD, E. A. Edward Jenner. *B.M.J.*, 1949, i, 881–4.
—— Introduction to *Catalogue of Jenner Exhibition* (Wellcome). London, 1949.
—— Jenner, Waterhouse and the introduction of vaccination to the U.S.A. *Nature,* 1949, clxiii, 823–8.

Preventive medicine (pp. 208–28; 231–6)

BROCKINGTON, C. FRASER. *A short history of public health.* London, 1956.
—— *Medical officers of health, 1848 to 1855: an essay in local history.* London, 1957.
BUDIN, P. *The nursling. The feeding and hygiene of premature & full-term infants.* Trans. W. J. Maloney. London, 1907.
DELMEGE, J. A. *Towards national health, or health and hygiene in England from Roman to Victorian times.* London, 1931.
DRAKE, T. G. H. Infant feeding in England and in France from 1750 to 1800. *Amer. J. Dis. Child.*, 1930, xxxix, 1049–61.
—— Infant welfare laws in France in the 18th century. *A.M.H.*, 1935, 2nd ser. vii, 49–61.
FINER, S. E. *The life and times of Sir Edwin Chadwick.* London, 1952.
FISCHER, A. *Geschichte des deutschen Gesundheitswesens.* 2 vols. Berlin, 1933.
FRAZER, W. M. *Duncan of Liverpool . . . the work of Dr. W. H. Duncan.* London, 1947.
—— *A history of English public health, 1834–1939.* London, 1950.
LEWIS, R. A. *Edwin Chadwick and the public health movement, 1832–54.* London, 1952.
McCLEARY, G. F. *The maternity and child welfare movement.* London, 1935.
McCRACKEN, I. E. How Sir John Simon entered the public health service. *Med. Officer*, 1948, lxxx, 157–8.
McCURRICH, H. J. *The treatment of the sick poor of this country.* London, 1929.
MacNALTY, Sir A. S. *The history of state medicine in England.* London, 1948.
NEWMAN, Sir G. *The building of a nation's health.* London, 1939.
NEWSHOLME, Sir A. *Evolution of preventive medicine.* London, 1927.
—— *Fifty years in public health.* London, 1935.
—— *The last thirty years in public health.* London, 1936.
RICHARDSON, Sir B. W. *The health of nations. A review of the works of Edwin Chadwick.* 2 vols. London, 1887.
ROSEN, G. *A history of public health.* New York, 1958.
SIGERIST, H. E. *Landmarks in the history of hygiene.* London, 1956.
SIMON, Sir J. *Public health reports.* 2 vols. London, 1887.
—— *English sanitary institutions.* 2nd ed. London, 1897.
THORNE-THORNE, Sir R. *On the progress of preventive medicine during the Victorian Era.* London, 1888.
UNDERWOOD, E. A. The field workers in the English public health movement, 1847–1875. *Bull. Soc. Med. Hist. Chicago*, 1948, vi, 31–48.
—— The centenary of British public health. *B.M.J.*, 1948, i, 890–2.
—— The quest for child health—the historical beginnings. *Rept. Ann. Conference Nat. Assoc. for Maternity and Child Welfare*, 1951, pp. 3–10.
WALKER, M. E. M. *Pioneers of public health.* Edinb., 1930.

WILLIAMS, J. H. HARLEY. *A century of public health in Britain, 1832–1929.* London, 1932.
WILLIAMS, R. C. *The United States Public Health Service, 1798–1950.* Washington, D.C., 1951.

Tuberculosis (pp. 228–31, and later sections on tuberculosis):
BROWN, LAWRASON. *The story of clinical pulmonary tuberculosis.* Baltimore, 1941.
BURKE, R. M. *An historical chronology of tuberculosis.* 2nd ed. Springfield and Baltimore, 1955.
CUMMINS, S. LYLE. *Tuberculosis in history.* London, 1949.
FLICK, L. F. *Development of our knowledge of tuberculosis.* Phila., 1925.
KAYNE, G. G. *The control of tuberculosis in England, past and present.* London, 1937.
—— PAGEL, W. and O'SHAUGHNESSY, L. *Pulmonary tuberculosis.* London, 1939, and later editions.
KIDD, P. The doctrine of consumption in Harvey's time and to-day. *Lancet,* 1918, ii, 543–6, 582–5.
—— Forty years in the history of tuberculosis. *Lancet,* 1922, ii, 1207–13.
LONG, E. R. Jean Fernel's conception of tuberculosis. *S.M. & H.,* i, 401–7.
MEACHEN, G. N. *A short history of tuberculosis.* London, 1936.
PAGEL, W. Humoral pathology, a lingering anachronism in the history of tuberculosis. *B.H.M.,* 1955, xxix, 299–308.
PIÉRY, M., and ROSHEM, J. *Histoire de la tuberculose.* Paris, 1931.
VARRIER-JONES. *Papers of a pioneer, Sir Pendrill Varrier-Jones.* Ed. P. Fraser. London, [1943].
WEBB, G. B. *Tuberculosis.* (Clio Medica.) New York, 1936.
YOUNG, Sir R. A. Clinical aspects of tuberculosis and diseases of the chest, 1906–56. *Brit. J. Tuberc. and Dis. Chest,* 1956, l, 23–32.

Anatomy and embryology, nineteenth century (pp. 236–7):
KEEN, W. W. *The early history of practical anatomy.* Phila., 1874. (Reprinted in his *Addresses and other papers,* Phila. and London, 1905.)
See also works by Meyer and Needham in general section on *Anatomy* (p. 764).

Chemical physiology, nineteenth century (pp. 237–8):
MCKIE, D. Wöhler's 'synthetic' urea and the rejection of vitalism. *Nature,* 1944, cliii, 608–10.
SHENSTONE, W. A. *Justus von Liebig, his life and work.* London, 1895.
VOLHARD, J. *Justus von Liebig.* 2 vols. Leipzig, 1909.

Nervous system and neurology (pp. 239–80):
(*a*) *General works:*
GARRISON, F. H. History of neurology, in C. L. Dana, *Textbook of nervous diseases,* 10th ed., New York, 1925, xv–lvi.
GUTHRIE, L. G. *The history of neurology* (FitzPatrick Lecture, 1908). London, 1921.
HAYMAKER, W. (ed.). *The founders of neurology.* Springfield, 1953.
RIESE, W. *A history of neurology.* New York, 1959.

(*b*) *Anatomy and physiology* (pp. 241–50):
BAST, T. H. Karl Fredrick Burdach. *A.M.H.,* 1928, x, 34–46.
BELL, Sir C. *Idea of a new anatomy of the brain.* London, [1811]. Reprinted in *Medical Classics,* 1936, i. 105–20.
CANNON, DOROTHY F. *Explorer of the human brain . . . Ramón y Cajal.* New York, 1949.
DAWSON, W. R. (ed.). *Sir Grafton Elliot Smith. A biographical record.* London, 1938.

DEJERINE, J., and DEJERINE-KLUMPKE, A. *Anatomie des centres nerveux.* 2 vols. Paris, 1895–1901.

FULTON, J. F. *Physiology of the nervous system.* 3rd ed. London, 1949.

GOLDSCHMID, E. Heinrich Quincke. *Schweiz. Med. Wchnsch.*, 1945, lxxv, 973–7.

GORDON-TAYLOR, Sir G., and WALLS, E. W. *Sir Charles Bell, his life and times.* Edinb. and London, 1958.

KEITH, Sir A., *et al.* The position of Sir C. Bell among anatomists. *Lancet*, 1911, i, 290–3, 470, 542, 614–15, 697, 764–5, 835–6, 901–2, 1032, 1718–19.

KISCH, B. Valentin, Gruby, Remak, Auerbach. *Trans. Amer. Philos. Soc.*, 1954, N.S. xliv, pt. ii, 139–317.

LEVINSON, A. Domenico Cotugno. *A.M.H.*, 1936, 2nd ser. viii, 1–9.

—— *Cerebrospinal fluid in health and disease.* 3rd ed. London, 1929.

NEUBURGER, M. *Die historische Entwicklung der experimentellen Gehirn- und Rückenmarksphysiologie vor Flourens.* Stuttgart, 1897.

OLMSTED, J. M. D. *François Magendie.* New York, 1944.

SINGER, C. Brain dissection before Vesalius. *J.H.M.*, 1956, xi, 261–74.

SYMONDS, Sir C. The circle of Willis (Harveian Oration). *B.M.J.*, 1955, i, 119–24.

VIETS, H. R. Domenico Cotugno's description of the cerebrospinal fluid. *B.H.M.*, 1935, iii, 701–38.

WILLIAMS, HARLEY. *Don Quixote of the microscope; an interpretation of Ramón y Cajal.* London, 1954.

(c) *Reflex action* (pp. 250–4):

CLARK-KENNEDY, A. E. *Stephen Hales* (see p. 776).

FEARING, F. *Reflex action, a study in the history of physiological psychology.* Baltimore, 1930.

FULTON, J. F. *Muscular contraction and the reflex control of movement.* Baltimore, 1926.

JEFFERSON, Sir G. Marshall Hall, the grasp reflex and the diastaltic spinal cord. *S.M. & H.*, ii, 303–20.

LIDDELL, E. G. T. *The discovery of reflexes.* Oxford, 1960.

Memoirs of Marshall Hall, by his widow. London, 1861.

(d) *Cerebral localization* (pp. 254–60):

FERRIER, Sir D. *The functions of the brain.* London, 1876.

HUGHLINGS JACKSON, J. *Selected writings.* Ed. J. Taylor. 2 vols. London, 1931–2.

OLMSTED, J. M. D. Pierre Flourens. *S.M. & H.*, ii, 290–302.

RIESE, W., and HOFF, E. C. History of doctrine of cerebral localization. *J.H.M.*, 1950, v, 50–71; 1951, vi, 439–70.

TEMKIN, O. Gall and the Phrenological Movement. *B.H.M.*, 1947, xxi, 275–321.

—— The neurology of Gall and Spurzheim. *S.M. & H.*, ii, 282–9.

WALSHE, Sir F. M. R. On the mode of representation of movements in the motor cortex. *Brain*, 1943, lxvi, 104–39.

—— On the contribution of clinical study to the physiology of the cerebral motor cortex. (Victor Horsley Lecture.) Edinb., 1947.

—— *Critical studies in neurology.* Edinb., 1948.

—— The contribution of clinical observation to cerebral physiology. *Proc. Roy. Soc. Lond.* (B), 1954, cxlii, 208–24.

(e) *Autonomic nervous system* (pp. 260–3):

FULTON, J. F. Edward Selleck Hare and the syndrome of paralysis of the cervical sympathetic. *P.R.S.M.*, 1929–30, xxiii, 152–7.

GASKELL, W. H. *The involuntary nervous system.* London, 1916.

KROGH, A. *The anatomy and physiology of the capillaries.* 2nd ed. New Haven, 1929.
LANGDON-BROWN, Sir W. Gaskell and the Cambridge Medical School. *P.R.S.M.*, 1939–40, xxxiii, 1–12.
LAIGNEL-LAVASTINE, M. 'Note sur l'histoire du sympathique'. *Bull. Soc. franç. d'hist. méd.*, 1923, xvii, 401–6.
LANGLEY, J. N. *The autonomic nervous system.* Cambridge, 1921.
OLMSTED, J. M. D. *Charles-Édouard Brown-Séquard.* Baltimore, 1946.
VIETS, H. R. John Newport Langley. *Boston Med. Surg. J.*, 1925, cxciii, 1040.

(f) Sherrington and nervous integration (pp. 263–6):
COHEN OF BIRKENHEAD, Lord. *Sherrington, physiologist, philosopher and poet.* Liverpool, 1958.
DENNY-BROWN, D. The Sherrington School of Physiology. *J. Neurophysiol.*, 1957, xx, 543–8.
FULTON, J. F. Sherrington's impact on neurophysiology. *B.M.J.*, 1947, ii, 807–10.
SHERRINGTON Sir C. *The integrative action of the nervous system.* New York, 1906. Reprint, with a new foreword, Cambridge, 1947.
—— *Selected writings.* Compiled and ed. D. Denny-Brown. London, 1939.

(g) Pavlov and conditioned reflexes (pp. 266–9):
PAVLOV, I. P. *Conditioned reflexes. An investigation of the physiological activity of the cerebral cortex.* Trans. and ed. G. V. Anrep. London, 1927.
—— *Lectures on conditioned reflexes.* Trans. Gantt and Volborth. New York, 1928.

(h) Sensory perception and sensory disturbances (pp. 269–71):
HEAD, Sir H., *et al. Studies in neurology.* 2 vols. London, 1920.
KEELE, K. D. *Anatomies of pain.* London, 1957.
WOOLLARD, H. *Recent advances in anatomy.* London, 1927.

(i) Neuropathology and clinical neurology (pp. 271–80):
BALLANCE, Sir C. *A glimpse into the history of the surgery of the brain.* London, 1922.
BONIN, G. VON (ed.). *Some papers on the cerebral cortex.* Trans. from Fr. and Ger. Springfield, 1960. [Includes also papers in Eng. by Hughlings Jackson and Sherrington.]
CRITCHLEY, M. *Sir William Gowers.* London, 1949.
—— MCMENEMEY, W. H., WALSHE, F. M. R., and GREENFIELD, J. G. (eds.). *James Parkinson. Papers dealing with Parkinson's disease.* London, 1955.
CROOKSHANK, F. G. The history of epidemic encephalomyelitis. *P.R.S.M.*, 1918–19, xii, 1–21.
DANDY, W. E. *Selected writings.* Ed. Troland and Otenasek. Springfield, 1957.
FULTON, J. F. *Harvey Cushing. A biography.* Springfield and Oxford, 1946.
—— The contribution of physiology to neurology. *S.M. & H.*, ii, 537–44.
GUILLAIN, G. *Charcot, his life—his work.* Trans. Bailey. London, 1959.
HUGHLINGS JACKSON, J. *Selected writings* (see p. 781).
JEFFERSON, Sir G. *Selected papers.* London, 1960.
MCINTYRE, N. Robert Bentley Todd. *King's Coll. Hosp. Gaz.*, 1956, xxxv, 79–91, 184–98.
NAUNYN, B. Jean Martin Charcot. *Arch. f. Exp. Path.*, 1893, xxxiii, i–x.
NEUBURGER, M. 'Joh. Peter Frank und die Neuropathologie'. *Wien. Klin. Wchnsch.*, 1913, xxvi, 627–31.
PENFIELD, W., and RASMUSSEN, T. *The cerebral cortex of man.* New York, 1950.
RIESE, W. History and principles of classification of nervous diseases. *B.H.M.*, 1945, xviii, 465–512.
ROWNTREE, L. G. James Parkinson. *Bull. Johns Hopkins Hosp.*, 1912, xxiii, 33–45.

TEMKIN, O. *The Falling Sickness, a history of epilepsy.* Baltimore, 1945.
—— Research on epilepsy before Hughlings Jackson, in *Epilepsy (Publications Assoc. Res. Nervous and Ment. Dis.,* xxvi), Baltimore, 1947, 3–7.
UNDERWOOD, E. A. The neurological complications of varicella. *Brit. J. Child. Dis.,* 1935, xxxii, 83–107, 177–96, 241–63.
—— Incidence and control of cerebrospinal fever. *B.M.J.,* 1940, i, 757–63.
WALKER, A. EARL (ed.). *A history of neurological surgery.* London, 1951.

Schools of clinical medicine and clinical teachers (pp. 280–6):

ACKERKNECHT, E. H. Broussais, or a forgotten medical revolution. *B.H.M.,* 1953, xxvi, 320–43.
—— The therapy of the Paris School, 1795–1840. *Gesnerus,* 1958, xv, 151–63.
BELLOT, H. HALE. *University College, London, 1826–1926.* London, 1929.
BROCK, R. C. *The life and work of Astley Cooper.* Edinb. and London, 1952.
BROCKBANK, E. M. *The honorary medical staff of the Manchester Infirmary, 1752–1830.* Manchester, 1904.
BROWNE, O'D. T. D. *The Rotunda Hospital [Dublin], 1745–1945.* Edinb., 1947.
CAMERON, H. C. *Mr. Guy's Hospital, 1726–1948.* London, 1954.
CAWADIAS, A. P. Corvisart. *S.M. & H.,* ii, 256–62.
CHANCE, B. Richard Bright. *A.M.H.,* 1927, ix, 332–6.
CHRISTIAN, H. A. Bright's description of nephritis in the light of modern knowledge. *A.M.H.,* 1927, ix, 337–46.
COPE, Sir Z. *The history of St. Mary's Hospital Medical School.* London, 1954.
DELAUNAY, P. 'Les doctrines médicales au début du XIXᵉ siècle'. *S.M. & H.,* ii, 321–30.
—— *Le monde médicale parisien au XVIIIᵉ siècle.* 2nd ed. Paris, 1906.
—— *La vie médicale aux XVIᵉ, XVIIᵉ, et XVIIIᵉ siècles.* Paris, 1935.
DOWNIE, J. WALKER. *The early physicians and surgeons of the Western Infirmary, Glasgow.* Glasgow, 1923.
FABER, K. *Nosography in modern internal medicine.* New York, 1923.
FRANKLIN, K. J. The Oxford Medical School. *Ann. Sci.,* 1936, i, 431–46.
GIBSON, G. A. *Life of Sir William Tennant Gairdner* [Glasgow School]. Glasgow, 1912.
GIESE, E., and HAGEN, B. VON. *Geschichte der medizinischen Fakultät der Friedrich–Schiller-Universität Jena.* Jena, 1958.
GOLDSCHMID, E. Nosologia naturalis. *S.M. & H.,* ii, 103–22.
GUTHRIE, D. *The Medical School of Edinburgh.* Edinb., 1959.
HALE-WHITE, Sir W. Thomas Addison. *Guy's Hosp. Repts.,* 1926, lxxvi, 253–79.
—— Richard Bright and Bright's disease. *Guy's Hosp. Repts.,* 1921, lxxi, 1–20.
—— Other observations of Richard Bright. *Guy's Hosp. Repts.,* 1921, lxxi, 143–57.
HAY, J. Centenary of the Liverpool School of Medicine. *Liverpool Med.-Chir. J.,* 1934, lxxix, 57–68.
HOLMES, Sir. G. *The National Hospital, Queen Square.* Edin. and London, 1954.
HUNTER, W. *Historical account of Charing Cross Hospital and Medical School.* London, 1914.
KIRKPATRICK, T. P. C. *The book of the Rotunda Hospital.* Dublin, 1913.
—— *History of the medical teaching in Trinity College, Dublin.* Dublin, 1912.
—— *The history of Doctor Steevens' Hospital, Dublin, 1720–1920.* Dublin, 1924.
—— The Schools of Medicine in Dublin in the 19th century. *B.M.J.,* 1933, ii, 109–12.
LANGDON-BROWN, Sir W. *Some chapters in Cambridge medical history.* Cambridge, 1946.
LANGDON-DAVIES, J. *The Westminster Hospital . . . 1719–1948.* London, 1952.
LYLE, H. WILLOUGHBY. *King's and some King's men.* London, 1935.
—— *An addendum to King's and some King's men.* London, 1950.

McDONALD, A. L.   The Aphorisms of Corvisart. *A.M.H.*, 1939, 3rd ser. i, 374–87, 471–6, 546–63; 1940, 3rd ser. ii, 64–69.
MAGNUS-LEVY, A.   The heroic age of German medicine. *B.H.M.*, 1944, xvi, 331–42.
MOORE, Sir N.   *History of St. Bartholomew's Hospital.* 2 vols. London, 1918.
MORRIS, E. W.   *A history of the London Hospital.* London, 1910.
NEUBURGER, M.   *Die Entwicklung der Medizin in Österreich.* Vienna, 1918.
—— *Das alte medizinische Wien in zeitgenössischen Schilderungen.* Vienna, 1921.
—— *British medicine and the Vienna School.* London, 1943.
ORMEROD, H. A.   *The early history of the Liverpool Medical School.* Liverpool, 1955.
OSMAN, A. A. (ed.).   *Original papers of Richard Bright on renal disease.* London, 1937.
PARSONS, F. G.   *History of St. Thomas's Hospital.* 3 vols. London, 1932–6.
PATRICK, J.   *A short history of Glasgow Royal Infirmary.* Glasgow, 1940.
POWER, Sir D'ARCY.   *A short history of St. Bartholomew's Hospital, 1123–1923.* London, 1923.
ROLLESTON, Sir H.   *Internal medicine.* (Clio Medica.) New York, 1930.
—— *The Cambridge Medical School. A biographical history.* Cambridge, 1932.
ROLLESTON, J. D.   F. J. V. Broussais. *P.R.S.M.*, 1938–9, xxxii, 27–35.
SAUNDERS, H. St. G.   *The Middlesex Hospital, 1745–1948.* London, 1949.
SCHÖNBAUER, L.   *Das medizinische Wien. Geschichte, Werden, Würdigung.* Vienna, 1947.
SMITH, G. MUNRO.   *A history of the Bristol Royal Infirmary.* Bristol, 1917.
STERNBERG, M.   *Josef Skoda.* Vienna, 1924.
STOKES, Sir W.   *William Stokes.* London, 1898.
THAYER, W. S.   Richard Bright. *Guy's Hosp. Repts.*, 1927, lxxvii, 253–301.
THÉODORIDÈS, J. (ed.).   The journal of J. V. Audouin, medical student at Paris (1817–18). *Hist. de la méd.*, 1958, viii, Nov., 4–63; Dec., 5–56; 1959, ix, Jan., 5–48.
THOMPSON, H. CAMPBELL.   *The story of the Middlesex Hospital Medical School.* London, 1935.
TURNER, A. LOGAN.   *Story of a great hospital, the Royal Infirmary of Edinburgh.* Edinb., 1937.
TURNER, G. GREY, and ARNISON, W. D.   *Newcastle upon Tyne School of Medicine, 1834–1934.* Newcastle upon Tyne, 1934.
WILKS, Sir S., and BETTANY, G. T.   *A biographical history of Guy's Hospital.* London, 1892.

Joh. Müller; physiology of nerve and muscle (pp. 287–94):
ADRIAN, E. D.   *The basis of sensation.* London, 1928.
—— *The mechanism of nervous action.* London and Phila., 1932.
—— *The physical background of perception.* Oxford, 1947.
HILL, A. V.   The mechanism of muscular contraction. *Physiol. Rev.*, 1922, ii, 310–41.
—— *Muscular activity.* (Herter Lectures.) Baltimore, 1926.
—— *Muscular movement in man.* New York and London, 1927.
—— *Chemical wave transmission in nerve.* Cambridge, 1932.
Keith Lucas. [A memoir by eight of his friends.] Cambridge, 1934.
KOENIGSBERGER, L.   *Hermann von Helmholtz.* Trans. Welby. Oxford, 1906.
LUCAS, KEITH.   *The conduction of the nervous impulse.* Revised by E. D. Adrian. London, 1917.
M'KENDRICK, J. G.   *Hermann von Helmholtz.* London, 1899.
MÜLLER, J.   *Elements of physiology.* Trans. W. Baly. 2 vols. London, 1837–8.
STEUDEL, J.   'Wissenschaftslehre und Forschungsmethodik Johannes Müllers'. *Deut. Med. Wchnsch.*, 1952, lxxvii, 115–18.

Cl. Bernard; Karl Ludwig; gastric digestion (pp. 294–303):
FOSTER, Sir M.   *Claude Bernard.* London, 1899.
IZQUIERDO, J. J.   *Bernard, creador de la medicina científica.* Mexico, 1942.

LOMBARD, W. P. The life and work of Carl Ludwig. *Science*, 1916, 2nd ser. xliv, 363–75.
OLMSTED, J. M. D. *Claude Bernard.* London, 1939.
PAVLOV, I. P. *The work of the digestive glands.* Trans. W. H. Thompson. London, 1902.
YOUNG, F. G. Bernard and the theory of the glycogenic function of the liver. *Ann. Sci.*, 1937, ii, 47–83.
—— Bernard and scientific adventure. *Brit. Med. Bull.*, 1946, iv, 289–90.
—— Bernard and the discovery of glycogen. *B.M.J.*, 1957, i, 1431–7.

Respiration (pp. 303–11):
ACKERKNECHT, E. H. Paul Bert's triumph. *B.H.M.*, 1944, Supp. 3, 16–31.
BARCROFT, J. *The respiratory function of the blood.* 2 pts. Cambridge, 1925–8.
FRANKLIN, K. J. *Joseph Barcroft, 1872–1947.* Oxford, 1953.
HALDANE, J. S. *Respiration.* New Haven, 1922.
—— and PRIESTLEY, J. G. *Respiration.* New ed. Oxford, 1935.
MARCET, W. *A contribution to the history of the respiration of man.* London, 1897.

Circulation; the blood (pp. 311–19):
BAYLISS, Sir W. M. *The vaso-motor system.* London, 1923.
DREYFUS, C. *Some milestones in the history of hematology.* New York, 1957.
EHRLICH, P. 'Beiträge zur Kenntniss der Anilinfärbungen und ihrer Verwendung in der mikroskopischen Technik'. *Arch. f. mikros. Anat.*, 1877, xiii, 263–77.
HILL, Sir L., and BARNARD, H. L. A simple form of sphygmomanometer. *B.M.J.*, 1897, ii, 904.
LONG, E. R. Addison and his discovery of idicpathic anaemia. *A.M.H.*, 1935, 2nd ser. vii, 130–2.
MAJOR, R. H. The history of taking the blood pressure. *A M.H.*, 1930, 2nd ser. ii, 47–55.
—— Karl Vierordt. *A.M.H.*, 1938, 2nd ser. x, 463–73.
RICHARDSON, Sir B. W. William Hewson, in his *Disciples of Aesculapius*, 1900, ii, 532–53.
ROBB-SMITH, A. H. T. The advantages of false assumptions [history of pernicious anaemia]. *Oxf. Med. School Gaz.*, 1949, i, 73–85, 188–202; 1950, ii, 53–75.
—— The Rubicon: changing views on thrombosis and blood coagulation. *Brit. Med. Bull.*, 1955, xi, 70–77.
ROLLESTON, Sir H. D. *Cardio-vascular diseases since Harvey's discovery.* Cambridge, 1928.
—— The history of haematology. *P.R.S.M.*, 1933–4, xxvii, 31–48.
SABINE, J. C. A history of the classification of human blood corpuscles. *B.H.M.*, 1940, viii, 696–720, 785–805.

Biochemistry (pp. 319–20):
DAKIN, H. D. *Oxidations and reductions in the animal body.* 2nd ed. London, 1922.
DRABKIN, D. L. *Thudichum, chemist of the brain.* Phila., 1958.
McILWAIN, H. Thudichum and the medical chemistry of the 1860's to 1880's. *P.R.S.M.*, 1958, li, 5–10.

The Cell Theory (pp. 320–6):
BAKER, J. R. The Cell Theory: a restatement, history, and critique. *Quart. J. Micros. Sci.*, 1948, lxxxix, 103–25; 1949, xc, 87–108, 331; 1952, xciii, 157–90.
CAUSEY, G. *The cell of Schwann.* Edinb., 1960.
GOODSIR, J. *Anatomical memoirs.* 2 vols. Edinb., 1868.
HUGHES, A. *A history of cytology.* London and New York, 1959.
KISCH, B. G. G. Valentin, in *Victor Robinson Memorial Volume*, New York, 1948, pp. 193–212.

KLEIN, M. *Histoire des origines de la théorie cellulaire.* Paris, 1936.
ROBINSON, V. *The life of Jacob Henle.* New York, 1921.
SCHWANN and SCHLEIDEN. Trans. of selected papers. (Sydenham Soc.) London, 1847.
WATERMANN, R. *Theodor Schwann: Leben und Werk.* Düsseldorf, 1960.

Germ Origin of Disease (pp. 326–41); *bacteriology, &c.* (pp. 379–452):

BOYD, J. S. K. Bacteriophage-typing and epidemiological problems. *B.M.J.*, 1952, ii, 679–85.
BRAY, G. W. *Recent advances in allergy.* London, 1931.
BULLOCH, W. *The history of bacteriology.* London, 1938.
BURNET, Sir F. M. *Viruses and man.* 2nd ed. Harmondsworth, 1955.
CHALIAN, W. The history of lockjaw. *B.H.M.*, 1940, viii, 171–201.
CHEYNE, W. WATSON (ed.). *Bacteria in relation to disease.* (New Sydenham Soc.) London, 1886. (Translations of classic papers on bacteriology.)
DALRYMPLE-CHAMPNEYS, Sir W. *Brucella infection and undulant fever in man.* London, 1960.
DUBOS, R. J. *Free Lance of Science* [Pasteur]. London, 1951.
FORD, W. W. *Bacteriology.* (Clio Medica.) New York, 1939.
—— Life and work of R. Koch. *Bull. Johns Hopkins Hosp.*, 1911, xxii, 415–25.
HENLE, J. On miasmata and contagion. Trans. Rosen. *B.H.M.*, 1938, vi, 907–83.
HEYMANN, B. *Robert Koch.* Leipzig, 1932.
MAJOR, R. H. Agostino Bassi and the parasitic theory. *B.H.M.*, 1944, xvi, 97–107.
—— The history of asthma. *S.M. & H.*, ii, 518–29.
MUIR, R., and RITCHIE, J. *Manual of bacteriology.* London, 1897 (and later eds.)
PASTEUR, L. *Œuvres.* Ed. Vallery-Radot. 7 vols. Paris, 1922–39.
RIVERS, T. M. (ed.). *Viral and rickettsial infections of man.* 2nd ed. Phila., 1952.
ROLLESTON, J. D. *Acute infectious diseases.* London, 1925, and 3rd ed. by Rolleston and G. W. Ronaldson, 1940.
SINGER, C. Benjamin Marten, a neglected precursor of Pasteur. *Janus* (Leyden), 1911, xvi, 81–98.
System of bacteriology in relation to medicine. (Various authors.) 9 vols. (Medical Research Council.) London, 1929–31.
TOPLEY, W. W. C., and WILSON, G. S. *Principles of bacteriology and immunity.* London, 1929, especially 3rd ed. (1946) and 4th ed. (1955) by Wilson and A. A. Miles.
TYNDALL, J. *Essays on the floating-matter of the air in relation to putrefaction and infection.* London, 1881.
VALLERY-RADOT, R. *Life of Pasteur.* Trans. Devonshire. 2 vols. London, 1902.
Virus and rickettsial diseases, with especial consideration of their public health significance. Cambridge, Mass., 1940.
WEZEL, K. *Robert Koch.* Berlin, 1912.
WILLIAMSON, R. The Germ Theory of Disease. *Ann. Sci.*, 1955, xi, 44–57.
WOLSTENHOLME, G. E. W., and MILLAR, ELAINE C. P. (eds.). *The nature of viruses.* London, 1957.
ZEISS, H., and BIELING, R. *Behring, Gestalt und Werk.* Berlin and Grünewald, 1940.

Anaesthesia (pp. 341–51):

CARTWRIGHT, F. F. *The English pioneers of anæsthesia* (Beddoes, Davy, and Hickman). Bristol and London, 1952.
COLEMAN, F. The history of nitrous oxide anaesthesia. *Med. Illus.*, 1954, viii, 419–28.
DUNCUM, B. M. *The development of inhalation anaesthesia.* London, 1947.
FULTON, J. F., and STANTON, M. M. *The centennial of surgical anesthesia.* New York, 1946.
GORDON, H. LAING. *Sir James Young Simpson.* London, 1897.

Hickman Centenary Exhibition (Wellcome Museum). London, 1930.
KEYS, T. E. *The history of surgical anesthesia.* New York, 1945.
RAPER, H. R. *Man against pain.* New York, 1945.
ROBINSON, V. *Victory over pain.* New York, 1946.
SNOW, J. *On chloroform and other anaesthetics.* London, 1858.
UNDERWOOD, E. A. Before and after Morton. *B.M.J.*, 1946, ii, 525–31.

Revolution in surgery; modern advances; puerperal fever (pp. 351–75):

ADAMI, J. G. *Charles White and the arrest of puerperal fever.* Liverpool and London, 1922.
BISHOP, W. J. *The early history of surgery.* London, 1960.
BOWMAN, A. K. *The life and teaching of Sir William Macewen.* Glasgow, London, and Edinb., 1942.
CAMERON, H. C. *Joseph Lister, the friend of man.* London, 1948.
COPE, Sir Z. *Pioneers in acute abdominal surgery.* London, 1939.
—— Seventy years of abdominal surgery. *S.M. & H.*, ii, 341–50.
—— *The Royal College of Surgeons of England. A history.* London, 1959.
CROWE, S. J. *Halsted of Johns Hopkins.* Springfield, 1957.
DUKES, C. *Lord Lister.* London and Boston, Mass., 1924.
GODLEE, Sir R. J. *Lord Lister.* 3rd ed. Oxford, 1924.
GRAHAM, H. *Surgeons all.* 2nd ed. London, 1956.
GUTHRIE, D. *Lord Lister, his life and doctrine.* Edinb., 1949.
HELFREICH, F. 'Geschichte der Chirurgie', in Puschmann's *Handbuch*, iii, 1–306.
HOCHBERG, L. A. *Thoracic surgery before the 20th century.* New York, 1960.
LEONARDO, R. A. *History of surgery.* New York, 1943.
LISTER, JOSEPH. *Collected papers.* 2 vols. Oxford, 1909.
Lister Centenary Exhibition (Wellcome Museum). London, 1927.
MEADE, R. H. *A history of thoracic surgery.* Springfield, 1961.
PORTER, I. A. *Alexander Gordon, M.D. of Aberdeen.* Edinb. and London, 1958.
SINCLAIR, Sir W. J. *Semmelweiss, his life and doctrine.* Manchester, 1909.
SOUTH, J. FLINT. *Memorials of the craft of surgery in England.* London, 1886.
WIDDESS, J. D. H. *An account of the Schools of Surgery, Royal College of Surgeons, Dublin, 1789–1948.* Edinb., 1949.
YOUNG, S. *The annals of the Barber-Surgeons of London.* London, 1890.

Radiology and radium therapy (pp. 374–9):

CURIE, EVE. *Madame Curie.* Trans. V. Sheean. London, 1938.
GLASSER, O. *Wilhelm Conrad Röntgen and the early history of the Roentgen rays.* London, 1933.
RÖNTGEN, W. C. 'Ueber eine neue Art von Strahlen'. *S.B. Phys. Med. Ges. Würzburg*, 1895, N.S. xxix, 132–41. Facsimile in *Isis*, 1936, xxvi, 349–69. Eng. trans. in *Nature*, 1896, liii, 274, 377.
UNDERWOOD, E. A. W. C. Röntgen and the early development of radiology. *P.R.S.M.*, 1944–5, xxxviii, 27–36.

Tropical diseases (except plague); parasitology (pp. 452–88; 492–4):

ARTELT, W. 'Deutsche und Niederländer als Pioniere der Tropenmedizin im 17. Jahrhundert'. *Klin. Wchnschr.*, 1938, xvii, 24–27.
BOYD, J. S. K. Fifty years of tropical medicine. *B.M.J.*, 1950, i, 37–43.
BRUMPT, E. *Précis de parasitologie.* Paris, 1910, and later eds.
CARTER, H. R. *Yellow fever: an epidemiological and historical study of its place of origin.* Baltimore, 1931.
COLE, F. J. *The history of protozoology.* London, 1926.

DOBELL, C. The discovery of the intestinal protozoa of man. *P.R.S.M.*, 1919–20, xiii, 1–15.
—— *The amoebae living in man.* London, 1919.
ECKSTEIN, G. *Noguchi.* New York and London, 1931.
FRANCHINI, J. Alphonse Laveran. *A.M.H.*, 1931, 2nd ser. iii, 280–8.
GALTES, F. H., ABASCAL Y VERA, H., and RODRÍGUEZ EXPÓSITO, C. *Finlay en la historia de la medicina.* Havana, 1954.
GORGAS, M. D., and HENDRICK, B. J. *William Crawford Gorgas.* Phila., 1924.
HOARE, C. A. Émile Brumpt. *Trans. Roy. Soc. Trop. Med. & Hyg.*, 1951, xlv, 397–8.
HOEPPLI, R. *Parasites and parasitic infections in early medicine and science.* Singapore, 1959.
JARAMILLO-ARANGO, J. *The British contribution to medicine.* Edinb. and London, 1953.
JONES, W. H. S. *Malaria and Greek history.* Manchester, 1909.
KELLY, H. A. *Walter Reed and yellow fever.* New York, 1906.
LEIPER, R. T. Landmarks in medical helminthology. *J. Helminth.*, 1929, vii, 101–18.
LEUCKART, R. *Die menschlichen Parasiten.* 2 vols. Leipzig and Heidelberg, 1863–76. Trans. Hoyle as *The parasites of man*, Edinb., 1886.
MANSON-BAHR, Sir P. H., and ALCOCK, A. *Life and work of Sir Patrick Manson.* London, 1927.
MÉGROS, R. L. *Ronald Ross.* London, 1931.
RODRÍGUEZ EXPÓSITO, C. *Finlay.* Havana, 1951. (The best book on Finlay.)
Royal Society. *Reports of the Sleeping Sickness Commission.* Especially the first five Reports, London, 1903–5.
RUSSELL, P. L. *Man's mastery of malaria.* London, 1955.
SCOTT, Sir H. H. *History of tropical medicine.* 2nd ed. 2 vols. London, 1942.
TRUBY, A. E. *Memoir of Walter Reed.* New York and London, 1943.
[WATESON, G.] *The cures of the diseased in forraine attempts of the English nation.* London, 1598. Ed. with introduct. and notes by C. Singer. Oxford, 1915.
WENYON, C. M. *Protozoology.* 2 vols. London, 1926.

Plague (pp. 488–92):

BELL, W. G. *The Great Plague in London in 1665.* London and New York, 1924.
CAMPBELL, ANNA M. *The Black Death and men of learning.* New York, 1931.
CRAWFURD, Sir R. *Plague and pestilence in literature and art.* Oxford, 1914.
CREIGHTON, C. *Epidemics* (see p. 794).
GASQUET, F. A. *The Great Pestilence (A.D. 1348–9), now commonly known as the Black Death.* London, 1893.
HIRSCH, A. *Historical and geographical pathology* (see p. 795).
HIRST, L. F. *The conquest of plague.* Oxford, 1953.
MACARTHUR, Sir W. The Plague of Athens. *B.H.M.*, 1958, xxxii, 242–6.
NOHL, J. *The Black Death, a chronicle of the plague.* Trans. Clarke. London, 1926.
SINGER, D. W. Some plague tractates. *P.R.S.M.*, 1915–16, ix, 159–212.
STICKER, G. *Abhandlungen aus der Seuchengeschichte und Seuchenlehre. I. Die Pest.* 2 pts. Giessen, 1908–10.

Insanity and psychology (pp. 494–515):

ACKERKNECHT, E. H. 'Josef Breuer über seinen Anteil an der Psychoanalyse'. *Gesnerus*, 1957, xiv, 169–71.
—— *A short history of psychiatry.* Trans. Wolff. New York and London, 1959.
BELLONI, L. 'Dall'elleboro alla reserpina'. *Arch. psicol. neurol. e psichiat.*, 1956, xvii, 115–48.
GALDSTON, I. The psychiatry of Paracelsus. *S.M. & H.*, i, 408–17.
KRAEPELIN, E. 'Hundert Jahre Psychiatrie'. *Ztsch. f. ges. Neurol. u. Psych.*, 1918, xxxviii, 161–275.

LEWIS, N. D. C. *A short history of psychiatric achievement.* New York, 1942.
NEUBURGER, M. *Johann Christian Reil.* Stuttgart, 1913.
SIGERIST, H. E. *Civilization and disease.* Ithaca, N.Y., 1943 (for tarantism).
UNDERWOOD, E. A. Apollo and Terpsichore. *B.H.M.*, 1947, xxi, 639–73 (for tarantism).
WHITWELL, J. R. *Historical notes on psychiatry.* London, 1936.
ZILBOORG, G., and HENRY, G. W. *A history of medical psychology.* New York, 1941.

Ductless glands (pp. 515–55):
BENJAMIN, H. Eugen Steinach. *Sci. Monthly,* 1945, lxi, 427–42.
BIEDL, A. *The internal secretory organs.* Trans. Forster. London, 1912.
BUCHANAN, J. A. Lugol, his work and his solution. *A.M.H.,* 1928, x, 202–8.
CANNON, W. B. *Bodily changes in pain, hunger, fear and rage.* 2nd ed. New York and London, 1929.
CAWADIAS, A. P. The history of endocrinology. *P.R.S.M.,* 1940–1, xxxiv, 25–30.
—— Théophile de Bordeu. *P.R.S.M.,* 1949–50, xliii, 1–6.
DALE, Sir H. H. Evidence concerning the endocrine function of the neurohypophysis and its nervous control. *Colston Papers,* 1956, viii, 1–9.
DODDS, Sir C. *Biochemical contributions to endocrinology.* Stanford and London, 1957.
LANGERHANS, P. Contributions to the microscopic anatomy of the pancreas (trans. H. Morrison). *B.H.M.,* 1937, v, 259–97.
McCARRISON, Sir R. *The etiology of endemic goitre* (Milroy Lectures). London, 1913.
—— *The thyroid gland in health and disease.* London, 1917.
—— *The simple goitres.* London, 1928.
MacNALTY, Sir A. S. Sir Victor Horsley. *B.M.J.,* 1957, i, 910–16.
MEANS, J. H. *The thyroid and its diseases.* 2nd ed. Phila. and London, 1948.
PAGET, S. *Sir Victor Horsley.* London, 1919.
PAPASPYROS, N. S. *The history of diabetes mellitus.* London, 1952.
RIEPPEL, F. 'John Hunter und die experimentelle Begründung der Endokrinologie'. *Schweiz. Med. Wchnsch.,* 1952, lxxxii, 338–9.
ROLLESTON, Sir H. Caleb Hillier Parry. *A.M.H.,* 1925, vii, 205–15.
—— *The endocrine organs in health and disease.* London, 1936.
SINCLAIR, H. M. (ed.). *The work of Sir Robert McCarrison.* London, 1953.
STENO, N. *Opera philosophica.* Ed. V. Maar. 2 vols. Copenhagen, 1910.
STEVENSON, L. *Sir Frederick Banting.* 2nd ed. London, 1947.

Histamine (pp. 555–64):
DALE, Sir H. H. *Adventures in physiology.* London, 1953.
—— Historical survey of histamine and its functions. *Internat. Assoc. of Allergology Congress, Rio de Janeiro, 6 Nov. 1955.*
—— Autobiographical sketch. *Perspectives in Biol. and Med.,* 1958, i, 125–37.
GADDUM, J. H. Histamine. *B.M.J.,* 1948, i, 867–73.

Chemical transmission of nerve impulse (pp. 564–77):
BROWN, Sir G. L. Transmission at nerve endings by acetylcholine. *Physiol. Rev.,* 1937, xvii, 485–513.
CANNON, W. B. Development of ideas of chemical mediation of nerve impulses. *Amer. J. Med. Sci.,* 1934, clxxxviii, 145–59.
DALE, Sir H. H. *Adventures in physiology.* London, 1953.
FELDBERG, W. Role of acetylcholine in the central nervous system. *Brit. Med. Bull.,* 1949–50, vi, 312–21.
—— Neuromuscular transmission and neuromuscular block. *B.M.J.,* 1951, i, 967–76.
LOEWI, O. Chemical transmission of nerve impulses. *Amer. Scientist,* 1945, xxxiii, 159–74. (Also in *Science in Progress,* ser. iv, New Haven, 1945.)

LOEWI, O. Transmission of nerve impulses. *J. Mt. Sinai Hosp.*, 1945, xii, 803–16, 851–65.

NACHMANSOHN, D. Physiological significance of cholinesterase. *Yale J. Biol. and Med.*, 1939–40, xii, 565–89.

—— (ed.). *Molecular biology. Elementary processes of nerve conduction and muscle contraction.* New York and London, 1960.

Nutrition and metabolism (pp. 578–610):

BOYD ORR, J. *Food health and income.* London, 1936.

CATHCART, E. P. *The physiology of protein metabolism.* 2nd ed. London, 1921.

DRUMMOND, Sir J. C., and WILBRAHAM, ANNE. *The Englishman's food.* London, 1939.

LEATHES, J. B., and RAPER, H. S. *The fats.* 2nd ed. London, 1925.

LIEBIG, J. *Animal chemistry, or organic chemistry in its applications to physiology and pathology.* London, 1842.

LUSK, G. *The elements of the science of nutrition.* Phila. and London, 1906; 4th ed., 1928.

—— Carl von Voit. *A.M.H.*, 1931, 2nd ser. iii, 583–94.

—— *Nutrition.* (Clio Medica.) New York, 1933.

McCOLLUM, E. V. *A history of nutrition.* Boston, Mass., 1957.

MURLIN, J. R. Graham Lusk. *J. Nutrition*, 1932, v, 527–38.

NEEDHAM, J., and BALDWIN, E. (eds.). *Hopkins & biochemistry, 1861–1947.* Cambridge, 1949.

SINCLAIR, H. M. (ed.). *The work of Sir Robert McCarrison.* London, 1953.

Vitamins and Deficiency Diseases (pp. 610–22):

BICKNELL, F., and PRESCOTT, F. *The vitamins in medicine.* 3rd ed. London, 1953.

DALE, Sir H. *Some epochs in medical research.* (Harveian Oration.) London, 1935.

JARAMILLO-ARANGO, J. *The British contribution to medicine (v.a.):* section on vitamins.

McCOLLUM, E. V. *The newer knowledge of nutrition.* New York, 1918. 5th ed., 1939.

MOORE, T. *Vitamin A.* Amst., London, and New York, 1957.

NEEDHAM and BALDWIN. *Hopkins & biochemistry (v.a.).*

Vitamins: A survey of present knowledge. (Medical Research Council.) London, 1932.

Function and diseases of the heart; thermometry (pp. 622–7):

ALLBUTT, Sir T. C. Medical thermometry. *Brit. and For. Med.-Chir. Rev.*, 1870, xlv, 429–41; xlvi, 144–56.

—— *Diseases of the arteries, including angina pectoris.* 2 vols. London, 1915.

DOCK, G. Corrigan and the water-hammer pulse. *A.M.H.*, 1934, 2nd ser. vi, 381–95.

EAST, T. *The story of heart disease.* London, 1958.

FLAXMAN, N. History of aortic insufficiency. *B.H.M.*, 1939, vii, 192–209.

FRANKLIN, K. J. Richard Lower and his 'De corde'. *A.M.H.*, 1931, 2nd ser. iii, 599–602.

—— *A monograph on veins.* Springfield and London, 1937.

—— History of research on the renal circulation. *P.R.S.M.*, 1949, xlii, 27–36.

—— The history of research on the circulation. *Trans. and Studies Coll. Phys. Phila.*, 1952–3, 4th ser. xx, 23–33.

HERRICK, J. B. *A short history of cardiology.* Springfield, 1942.

LEAMAN, W. G., Jr. The history of electrocardiography. *A.M.H.*, 1936, 2nd ser. viii, 113–17.

McMICHAEL, J. (ed.). *Circulation. Proceedings of the Harvey Tercentenary Congress, London, 1957.* London, 1958.

MAJOR, R. H. Raymond Vieussens on the heart. *A.M.H.*, 1932, 2nd ser. iv, 147–54.

MOON, R. O. *Growth of our knowledge of heart disease.* London, 1927.

ROLLESTON, Sir H. D. *Cardio-vascular diseases since Harvey's discovery.* Cambridge, 1928.

ROLLESTON, Sir H. D. *Sir Thomas Clifford Allbutt: a memoir.* London, 1929.
—— History of aortic regurgitation. *A.M.H.*, 1940, 3rd ser. ii, 271–9.
ROY, P. S. History of the circulation and its disorders. *A.M.H.*, 1917, i, 141–54.
WHITE, P. D. *Heart disease.* 4th ed. New York, 1951. (Contains a historical introduction.)
WIGGERS, C. J. *Reminiscences and adventures in circulation research.* New York and London, 1958.
WILLIAMSON, R. T. Sir Dominic Corrigan. *A.M.H.*, 1925, vii, 354–61.
WILLIUS, F. A., and DRY, T. J. *A history of the heart and circulation.* Phila. and London, 1948.
—— and KEYS, T. E. *Cardiac classics.* St. Louis, 1941.
WOODHEAD, Sir G. S., and VARIER-JONES, Sir P. C. On clinical thermometry. *Lancet*, 1916, i, 173–80, 281–8, 338–40, 450–3, 495–502.
WUNDERLICH, C. A. *On the temperature in diseases: a manual of medical thermometry.* (New Sydenham Soc.) London, 1871.

Modern pathology (pp. 627–40):

ACKERKNECHT, E. H. *Rudolf Virchow, doctor, statesman, anthropologist.* Madison, Wis., 1953.
BENIVIENI, A. *De abditis nonnullis . . . morborum causis.* Trans. and ed. Singer and Long. Springfield, 1954.
CAMERON, Sir ROY. *Pathology of the cell.* Edinb. and London, 1952.
COHNHEIM, J. *Lectures on general pathology.* Trans. McKee. 3 vols. (New Sydenham Soc.) London, 1889–90.
DIEPGEN, P. Rudolf Virchow. *Deut. Gesundheitswesen*, 1946, i, 800–9.
FLAXMAN, N. James Hope. *B.H.M.*, 1938, vi, 1–21.
FLEXNER, S. and J. T. *W. H. Welch and the heroic age of American medicine.* New York, 1941.
FRANKLIN, K. J. The earlier history of phlebitis. *Ann. Sci.*, 1939–40, iv, 47–60.
GOLDSCHMID, E. Hermann Lebert. *Gesnerus*, 1949, vi, 17–33.
IRONS, E. E. Théophile Bonet. *B.H.M.*, 1942, xii, 623–65.
LANCISI, G. M. *De aneurysmatibus (1745).* Trans. W. C. Wright. New York, 1952.
MENNE, F. R. Rokitansky. *A.M.H.*, 1925, vii, 379–86.
MORRISON, H. Carl Weigert. *A.M.H.*, 1924. vi, 163–77.
OSLER, Sir W. Virchow. *Boston Med. Surg. J.*, 1891, cxxv, 425–7.
PAGEL, W. *Virchow und die Grundlage der Medizin des 19. Jahrh.* Jena, 1931.
—— Jahn, Virchow and the philosophy of pathology. *B.H.M.*, 1945, xviii, 1–43.
POSNER, C. *Rudolf Virchow.* Vienna, 1921.
RATH, G. Neural pathology, a pathogenetic concept of the 18th and 19th centuries. *B.H.M.*, 1959, xxxiii, 526–41.
RICHARDSON, Sir B. W. Matthew Baillie, in his *Disciples of Aesculapius*, ii, 554–72.
ROBB-SMITH, A. H. T. Clinical pathology, past and future. *Lancet*, 1946, i, 485–8.
ROLLESTON, Sir H. The early history of the teaching of human anatomy and pathological anatomy in Great Britain. *A.M.H.*, 1939, 3rd ser. i, 203–38.
ROLLESTON, J. D. J. B. Bouillaud. *P.R.S.M.*, 1930–1, xxiv, 37–46.
SIGERIST, H. E. The historical development of the pathology and therapy of cancer. *Bull. New York Acad. Med.*, 1932, viii, 642–53.
VIRCHOW, R. *Hundert Jahre allgemeiner Pathologie.* Berlin, 1895.
WELCH, W. H. On the history of pathology. *B.H.M.*, 1935, iii, 1–18.
WELLS, H. GIDEON. *Chemical pathology.* Phila. and London, 1907.
WILKS, Sir S. *Biographical reminiscences of Sir Samuel Wilks.* London, 1911. (This title on spine and in running-heads; title-page has a much expanded title.)
See also works in previous general section on *Pathology* (p. 765).

The eye and its disorders (pp. 640–50):

BOCK, E. *Die Brille und ihre Geschichte.* Vienna, 1903.
CHANCE, B. *Ophthalmology.* (Clio Medica.) New York, 1939.
—— Sir William Bowman, anatomist, physiologist, and ophthalmologist. *A.M.H.*, 1924, vi, 143–58.
DUKE-ELDER, Sir S. *A century of international ophthalmology (1857–1957).* London, 1958.
HIRSCHBERG, J. *Geschichte der Augenheilkunde.* 9 pts. Leipzig, 1899–1918.
JAMES, R. R. *Studies in the history of ophthalmology in England prior to the year 1800.* Cambridge, 1933.
OLDHAM, F. *Thomas Young, philosopher and physician.* London, 1933.
PANSIER, P. *Histoire des lunettes.* Paris, 1901.
SORSBY, A. *A short history of ophthalmology.* 2nd ed. London, 1948.
—— Richard Banister and the beginnings of English ophthalmology. *S.M. & H.*, ii, 42–55.
TURNER, D. M. Thomas Young on the eye and vision. *S.M. & H.*, ii, 243–55.
WOOD, A., and OLDHAM, F. *Thomas Young, natural philosopher.* Cambridge, 1954.
WOOD, C. A. The first scientific work on spectacles. *A.M.H.*, 1921, iii, 150–5.

Paediatrics and orthopaedics (pp. 650–9):

ASTRUC, P. 'Le Traité des maladies des enfants de Billard'. *Progrès méd.* (Paris), 1948, lxxvi, 548–9.
—— 'Le Traité des maladies des enfants de Barthez et Rilliet'. *Progrès méd.* (Paris), 1948, lxxvi, 614–17.
BICK, E. M. *Source book of orthopaedics.* 2nd ed. Baltimore, 1948.
BOKAY, J. VON. *Die Geschichte der Kinderheilkunde.* Berlin, 1922.
GARRISON, F. H. History of pediatrics, in I. A. Abt, *Pediatrics*, Phila. and London, 1923, i, 1–170.
HOLMES, T. *Sir Benjamin Collins Brodie.* London, 1898.
KEITH, Sir A. *Menders of the maimed.* London, 1919.
LE VAY, D. *The life of Hugh Owen Thomas.* Edinb. and London, 1956.
LEVINSON, A. *Pioneers of pediatrics.* 2nd ed. New York, 1943.
MALONEY, W. J. *George and John Armstrong of Castleton.* Edinb. and London, 1954.
PHAIRE, T. *The boke of chyldren.* London, 1553. Reprinted, Edinb., 1955.
RUHRÄH, J. Walter Harris. *A.M.H.*, 1919, ii, 228–40.
—— Thomas Phaer. *A.M.H.*, 1919, ii, 334–47.
—— William Cadogan. *A.M.H.*, 1925, vii, 64–92.
—— *Pediatrics of the past.* New York, 1925.
STILL, Sir G. F. *The history of paediatrics . . . to the end of the XVIIIth century.* London, 1931.

Dental conditions and dentistry (pp. 659–71):

BOISSIER, R. *L'évolution de l'art dentaire.* Paris, 1927.
BREMNER, M. D. K. *The story of dentistry.* 2nd ed. Brooklyn, N.Y., 1946.
CAMPBELL, J. MENZIES. *From a trade to a profession: Byways in dental history.* (Privately printed), 1958.
COHEN, R. A. Methods and materials used for artificial teeth. *P.R.S.M.*, 1959, lii, 775–86 (whole vol. pp.)
COLYER, Sir F. *Old instruments used for extracting teeth.* London, 1952.
FAUCHARD, P. *The surgeon dentist, or treatise on the teeth.* 2nd ed., 1746, trans. Lilian Lindsay. London, 1946.
GUERINI, V. *A history of dentistry.* Phila. and New York, 1909.

LINDSAY, LILIAN. *A short history of dentistry.* London, 1933.
LUFKIN, A. W. *A history of dentistry.* 2nd ed. London, 1948.
STRÖMGREN, H. L. *Index of dental and adjacent topics in medical and surgical works before 1800.* Copenhagen, 1955.
SUDHOFF, K. *Geschichte der Zahnheilkunde.* Leipzig, 1921.
WEINBERGER, B. W. *An introduction to the history of dentistry.* 2 vols. St. Louis, 1948.

Drugs and pharmacology (pp. 671–97):

BENEDICENTI, A. *Malati, medici e farmacisti.* 2nd ed. 2 vols. Milan, 1947–51.
BROCKBANK, W. *Ancient therapeutic arts.* London, 1954.
BROWN, H. M. The beginnings of intravenous medication. *A.M.H.*, 1917, i, 177–97.
CUSHNY, A. R. William Withering. *P.R.S.M.*, 1914–15, viii, 85–94.
DALE, Sir H. H. *Chemistry and medicinal treatment.* (Third Dalton Lecture at the Roy. Inst. of Chemistry.) London, 1948.
—— Advances in medicinal therapeutics. *B.M.J.*, 1950, i, 1–7.
—— Changes and prospects in medicinal treatment. (Harben Lectures.) *J. Roy. Inst. Pub. Health and Hyg.*, 1954, xvii, 39–57, 70–84, 98–109.
—— Paul Ehrlich. *B.M.J.*, 1954, i, 659–63.
—— *Humanity's rising debt to medical research.* (Paget Memorial Lecture.) London, 1955.
EHRLICH, P. *Experimental researches on specific therapeutics.* (Harben Lectures.) London, 1908.
—— *Collected papers.* Ed. F. Himmelweit, asstd. by Martha Marquardt, under the direction of Sir H. Dale. (To be completed in 4 vols.) London and New York, 1956–.
—— and HATA, S. *The experimental chemotherapy of spirilloses.* London, 1911.
FLEMING, Sir A. (ed.). *Penicillin, its practical application.* 2nd ed. London, 1950.
FLOREY, Sir H. W., *et al. Antibiotics.* 2 vols. London, 1949.
—— and ABRAHAM, E. P. The work on penicillin at Oxford. *J.H.M.*, 1951, vi, 302–17.
GADDUM, J. H. Administration of drugs. *Edinb. Med. J.*, 1944, li, 305–19.
GALDSTON, I. *Behind the sulfa drugs.* New York and London, 1943.
GOTFREDSEN, E. On the first intravenous, intramuscular, and subcutaneous injections. *Münch. Med. Wchnsch.*, 1939, lxxxvi, 504–5.
GUNTHER, R. T. *Early British botanists and their gardens.* Oxford, 1922.
HAGGIS, A. W. Fundamental errors in the early history of cinchona. *B.H.M.*, 1941, x, 417–59, 568–92.
HOWARD-JONES, N. The origins and early development of hypodermic medication. *J.H.M.*, 1949, ii, 201–49.
JARAMILLO-ARANGO, J. Critical review of the early history of cinchona. *J. Linn. Soc.* (*Bot.*), 1946–52, liii, 272–311.
—— *The British contribution to medicine* (see p. 788): section on antibiotics.
LANGDON-BROWN, Sir W. *From witchcraft to chemotherapy.* (Linacre Lectures.) Cambridge, 1941.
MARQUARDT, M. *Paul Ehrlich.* London, 1949.
MOGEY, G. A. Centenary of hypodermic injection. *B.M.J.*, 1953, ii, 1180–5.
Pharmacopoeia Londinensis of 1618. Facsimile ed. by G. Urdang. Madison, Wis., 1944.
POWER, Sir D'ARCY. The Oxford Physic Garden. *A.M.H.*, 1919, ii, 109–25.
SCHMIEDEBERG, O. Rudolf Buchheim. *Arch. f. Exper. Path.*, 1912, lxvii, 1–54.
SIGERIST, H. E. Materia medica in the Middle Ages. *B.H.M.*, 1939, vii, 417–23.
THOMAS, Sir H. The Society of Chymical Physitians. *S.M. & H.*, ii, 56–71.
UNDERWOOD, E. A. Introduction to cat. of exhibition illustrating *The history of pharmacy* (Wellcome Museum). London, 1951.

URDANG, G. The mystery about the First London Pharmacopoeia. *B.H.M.*, 1942, xii, 304–13.
—— Biographies as material and as subject of the history of pharmacy. *Amer. J. Pharm. Educ.*, 1943, vii, 326–37.
—— Pharmacopoeias as witnesses of world history. *J.H.M.*, 1946, i, 46–70.
—— The development of pharmacopoeias. *Bull. Wld. Health Org.*, 1951, iv, 577–603.
WAKSMAN, S. A. (ed.). *Streptomycin, nature and practical applications.* London, 1949. (Historical introduction.)
—— (ed.). *Neomycin, its nature and practical application.* London, 1958.
WITHERING, W. *An account of the foxglove.* Birmingham, 1785. Facsimile ed., London, [1948].
See also earlier general section on *Materia Medica, Pharmacy, Pharmacology* (p. 765).

Blood transfusion (pp. 698–701):
JONES, H. W., and MACKMULL, G. Influence of James Blundell on development of blood transfusion. *A.M.H.*, 1928, x, 242–8.
KEYNES, Sir G. L. The history of blood transfusion. *Brit. J. Surg.*, 1943, xxxi, 38–50.
—— (ed.). *Blood transfusion.* Bristol and London, 1949.
MALUF, N. S. R. The history of blood transfusion. *J.H.M.*, 1954, ix, 59–107.

Nursing (pp. 701–10):
ABEL-SMITH, B. *A history of the nursing profession.* London, 1960.
BETT, W. R. *A short history of nursing.* London, 1960.
COOK, Sir E. *Life of Florence Nightingale.* 2 vols. London, 1913.
COPE, Sir Z. *Florence Nightingale and the doctors.* London, 1958.
DOCK, LAVINIA L., and STEWART, ISABEL M. *Short history of nursing.* 4th ed. New York and London, 1938.
JACOBS, H. B. Elizabeth Fry, Pastor Fliedner and Florence Nightingale. *A.M.H.*, 1921, iii, 17–25.
NUTTING, MARY A., and DOCK, LAVINIA L. *History of nursing.* Vols. i and ii, New York and London, 1907; vols. iii and iv by L. L. Dock, 1912.
PAVEY, AGNES E. *The story of the growth of nursing.* 5th ed. London, 1959.
SEYMER, LUCY R. *A general history of nursing.* 3rd ed. London, 1954.
—— *Florence Nightingale's nurses.* London, 1960.
WOODHAM-SMITH, C. *Florence Nightingale.* London, 1950.

Vital statistics; biometry; epidemiology (pp. 710–41):
BROWNLEE, J. *An investigation into the epidemiology of phthisis pulmonalis in Great Britain and Ireland.* Pts. i and ii, 1918; Pt. iii, 1920. Med. Res. Council, London.
—— Periodicity of measles epidemics in London, 1890–1912. *Phil. Trans. Roy. Soc.*, 1919, ccix, 181–90.
CARR-SAUNDERS, Sir A. M. *The population problem.* London, 1922.
COX, P. R. *Demography.* 3rd ed. Cambridge, 1959.
CREIGHTON, C. *A history of epidemics in Britain.* 2 vols. Cambridge, 1891–4.
CROOKSHANK, F. G. *Epidemiological essays.* London, 1930.
—— (ed.). *Influenza, essays by several authors.* London, 1922.
DELAUNAY, P. 'Les doctrines médicales au début du XIXe siècle; Louis et la méthode numérique'. *S.M. & H.*, ii, 321–30.
FARR, W. *Vital statistics.* (Selected writings, ed. N. A. Humphreys.) London, 1885.
FROST, W. H. *Papers of Wade Hampton Frost; a contribution to epidemiological method.* Ed. K. F. Maxey. New York and London, 1941.
GOODALL, E. W. Infectious diseases and epidemiology in the Hippocratic Collection. *P.R.S.M.*, 1933–4, xxvii, 11–20.
—— *William Budd.* London, 1936.

GREENWOOD, M. Galen as an epidemiologist. *P.R.S.M.*, 1920-1, xiv, 3-16.
—— *Epidemiology, historical and experimental.* Baltimore and London, 1932.
—— *Epidemics and crowd-diseases.* London, 1935.
—— *The medical dictator.* London, 1936.
—— Sydenham as an epidemiologist. *P.R.S.M.*, 1918-19, xii (Sect. Epidemiol.), 55-76.
—— *Medical statistics from Graunt to Farr.* Cambridge, 1948.
—— *Some British pioneers of social medicine.* London, 1948.
HALL, A. J. *Epidemic encephalitis.* Bristol, 1924.
HAMER, Sir W. *Epidemiology, old and new.* London, 1928.
—— History of epidemiology during the last 100 years. *Lancet*, 1928, i, 1313-15; ii, 1-4.
HILL, A. BRADFORD. Observation and experiment. (Cutter Lecture.) *New Eng. J. of Med.*, 1953, ccxlviii, 995-1001.
HIRSCH, A. *Handbook of geographical and historical pathology.* Trans. C. Creighton. 3 vols. London, 1883-6.
Ministry of Health. *Report on the pandemic of influenza.* London, 1920.
MACNALTY, Sir A. S. *Epidemic diseases of the central nervous system.* London, 1927.
NEWSHOLME, Sir A. *Elements of vital statistics.* London, 1889. 3rd ed. 1923. Rewritten by B. Benjamin, 1959.
PEARL, R. *The natural history of population.* London, 1939.
PEARSON, E. S. *Karl Pearson. An appreciation of some aspects of his life and work.* Cambridge, 1938.
PEARSON, K. *The life, letters and labours of Francis Galton.* 3 vols. (in 4). Cambridge, 1914-30.
PRINZING, F. *Epidemics resulting from wars.* Oxford, 1916.
RUCKER, W. C. William Budd. *Bull. Johns Hopkins Hosp.*, 1916, xxvii, 208-15.
SCOTT, Sir H. H. *Some notable epidemics.* London, 1934.
SOPER, H. E. The interpretation of periodicity in disease prevalence. *J. Roy. Statist. Soc.*, 1929, N.S. xcii, 34-73.
STALLYBRASS, C. O. *The principles of epidemiology.* London, 1931.
STICKER, G. *Abhandlungen aus der Seuchengeschichte und Seuchenlehre. II. Die Cholera.* Giessen, 1912.
TEMKIN, O. 'Die Krankheitsauffassung von Hippokrates und Sydenham in ihren "Epidemien"', *Arch. Gesch. Med.*, 1928, xx, 327-52.
THOMPSON, T. *Influenza or epidemic catarrhal fever. An historical survey of past epidemics in Great Britain from 1510 to 1890.* New ed. by E. S. Thompson. London, 1890.
UNDERWOOD, E. A. The history of the 1832 cholera epidemic in Yorkshire. *P.R.S.M.*, 1934-5, xxviii, 5-18.
—— Charles Creighton, scholar, historian and epidemiologist. *P.R.S.M.*, 1948, xli, 7-14.
—— The history of cholera in Great Britain. *P.R.S.M.*, 1948, xli (Sect. Epidemiol.), 1-9.
—— History of the quantitative approach in medicine. *Brit. Med. Bull.*, 1951, vii, 265-74.
WINSLOW, C.-E. A. *The conquest of epidemic disease.* Princeton, 1944.
ZINSSER, H. *Rats, lice and history.* [History of typhus.] Boston, Mass., 1935.

INDEX OF PERSONS

In this index, so far as forenames are concerned, index and text are complementary. Full forenames—including in certain cases forenames which the bearers never used—are generally given in the text. In the index only those forenames are given by which the bearers are best known, or with which they signed their writings. In certain cases where the forenames are very numerous, some were either omitted, or indicated by initials, in the text; in such cases the full forenames are given in the index.

Dates of birth and death will usually be found to correspond in text and index. At least two authorities, and in many cases several, were consulted before entering these dates. Justifiable variations in dates are. however, found in different authorities. In the case of discrepancy between dates in the text and in the index respectively, those in the index are on the whole to be preferred.

Where a name is followed by more than one entry, the entry which gives biographical particulars is printed in italics.

Abderhalden, Emil (1877–1950), 32c, *596*, 619.

Abel, J. J. (1857–1938), 440, 538, 555, 560, 597, *685*.

Abulcasis [Abul Qasim] (d. *c.* 1013), *76*, 77, 523, 660, 662.

Ackermann, Otto Heinrich Rudolf Dankwart (1878–), *557*, 558.

Addison, Thomas (1793–1860), *284–5*, 318, 365, 517, 540, 621, 632.

Adler, Alfred (1870–1937), 514.

Adrian, E. D., 1st baron Adrian of Cambridge (1889–), *290–2*.

Aesculapius, 6, 20, 21, 22, 24, 25, 26, 57.

Agamemnon, 1.

Agramonte y Simoni, Aristides (1868–1931), 469.

Airy, Sir George Biddell (1801–92), 643.

Aitken, Sir William (1825–92), 626.

Albinus, B. S. (1697–1770), 150.

Albrecht, Heinrich (1866–1922), 409.

Albucasis, *see* Abulcasis.

Alcmaeon of Croton (*c.* 500 B.C.), 244.

Alderotti, *see* Thaddeus.

Aldrich, T. B. (1861–?), 538.

Alexander III, the Great, king of Macedon, 41.

Alexander of Tralles (525–605), 68, 71, 240.

Alexandra, consort of Edward VII, 378.

Alibert, J. L. (1766–1837), 281.

Allbutt, Sir Clifford (1836–1925), *625*, 626. 627.

Allen, Edgar (1892–1943), 551.

Allen, Willard Myron (1904–), 551.

Almquist, H. J. (1903–), 621.

Anderson, Sir Hugh Kerr (1865–1928), 262.

Anderson, John F. (1873–1958), 421.

Anderson, Rudolph John (1879–1961), *591*, 594.

Andral, Gabriel (1797–1876), *282*, 286.

André, Nicolas (1658–1742), 657.

Andrewes, Sir C. H. (1896–), 449.

fra Angelico, painter, 67.

Angle, E. H. (1855–1930), 671.

Antoninus Pius, emperor of Rome, 56.

Antony, Saint, of Padua, 495.

Antrim, 12th earl of, *see* M'Donnell, R. M. K.

Apollo, 26, 106.

Aran, François Amilcar (1817–61), 274.

Archibald, E. W. (1872–1945), 373.

Arculanus, Joannes (?–1484), 668.

Aretaeus of Cappadocia (A.D. 81–138?), *239*, 428, 552, 650.

Argyll Robertson, Douglas [Moray Cooper Lamb] (1837–1909), 275.

Aristophanes, 43.

Aristotle (384–322 B.C.), 16, 28, *41–47*, 48, 77, 91, 118, 122, 135, 143, 146.

Arkwright, Sir Joseph A. (1864–1944), *402*, 405, 409.

Armstrong, George (1720–89), *652*, 656.

Arnold of Villanova (1235–1311), 522.

Arnott, Neil (1788–1874), 209, *210*, 213, 214.

Arrhenius, Svante (1859–1927), 413.

Artemis, 26.

Arthus, Maurice (1862–1945), 421.

Aschheim, Selmar (1878–?), *547*, 551.
Aschner, Bernard (1883–1960), 547.
Aschoff, Ludwig (1866–1942), 318, 601, 638.
Asclepiades of Bithynia (*c*. 124–*c*. 40 B.C.), *51*, 53.
Aselli, Gaspare (1581–1626), 123.
Ash, Claudius (fl. 1838), 665.
Ashley, Lord, *see* Cooper, Antony Ashley.
Ashurbanipal, king of Assyria, 10.
Askanazy, Max (1865–1940), 537.
Asklepios, *see* Aesculapius.
Astor, Waldorf, 2nd viscount Astor of Hever Castle (1879–1952), 229.
Astwood, E. B. (1909–), *530*, 534.
Atkins, John (1685–1757), 482.
Atwater, Wilbur Olin (1844–1907), 583, *588*–9, 593, 605, 607.
Auenbrugger, Leopold (1722–1809), *172*, 280, 281, 286, 653.
Auer, John (1875–1948), *430*, 561.
Auerbach, Leopold (1828–97), 260.
Augustus, emperor of Rome, 52.
Aveling, James H. (1828–92), 699.
Avery, Oswald Theodore (1877–1955), 401.
Avicenna (980–1037), *76*, 77, 79, 80, 88, 100, 116.

Babbage, Charles (1792–1871), 289.
Babinski, Joseph (1857–1932), *277*, 544.
Bacharach, A. L. (1891–), 622.
Bacon, Roger (1214?–94), 641.
Bacot, A. W. (1866–1922), 490.
Bacq, Z. M. (1903–), 571.
Baelz, Erwin von (1849–1913), 611.
Baer, Karl Ernst von (1792–1876), *237*, 321.
Baeyer, Adolf von (1835–1917), 567.
Bagellardo, P. (?–1492), 650.
Baglivi, Giorgio (1668–1707), *503*–4.
Baillie, Matthew (1761–1823), *169*–71, 629.
Baillou, Guillaume de (1538–1616), *106*, 110.
Baker, Sir George (1722–1809), 204.
Balfour, Francis Maitland (1851–82), 237.
Ballonius, *see* Baillou.
Bancroft, Joseph (1836–94), 492.
Bang, Bernhard (1848–1932), 385.
Banister, Richard (1570?–1626), 647.
Banting, Sir Frederick (1891–1941), *554*–5, 754.

Barcroft, Sir Joseph (1872–1947), *304*–6, 308–11.
Bardeleben, Adolf von (1819–95), 519.
Barger, George (1878–1939), *527*, 557, 558, 570, 682.
Barlow, Sir Thomas (1845–1945), 655.
Barnard, J. E. (1869–1949), 446.
Barrington, F. J. F. (1884–1956), 263.
Barthez, Ernest (1811–91), 654.
Bartholin, Caspar (1585–1629), 538, *627*.
Bartholin, Thomas (1616–80), 123, *627*.
Bartholow, Roberts (1831–1904), 257.
Bartisch, Georg (1535–1605), 644, *646*.
Bary, Anton de (1831–88), 325.
Basch, Samuel von (1837–1905), *311*–12.
Basedow, Carl Adolph von (1799–1854), *530*, 532, 534.
Bassi, Agostino (1773–1856), 327.
Bastian, Henry Charlton (1837–1915), *257*, 277.
Bastianelli, G. (1862–1959), *459*, 462, 463.
Bateman, Thomas (1778–1821), *204*, 281.
Batten, Frederick Eustace (1865–1918), 276.
Bauer, Ferdinand Lucas (1760–1826), 321.
Baumann, Eugen (1846–96), 526.
Bayle, A. L. J. (1799–1858), 507.
Bayle, G. L. (1774–1816), *282*, 630.
Bayliss, Sir William M. (1860–1924), 302, *518*–19, 555, 558.
Bayon, H. P. (1876–1952), 637.
Beaumont, William (1785–1853), *157*, 159, 302, 578.
Beauté, professional faster, 590, 600.
Becher, J. J. (1635–82), 143.
Becquerel, Henri (1852–1908), 377.
Behring, Emil von (1854–1917), *411*–12, 436, 442.
Beijerinck, M. W. (1851–1931), 445.
Bell, Benjamin (1749–1806), *341*–2.
Bell, Sir Charles (1774–1842), *154*, 250, 251, 270, 272, 273, 288.
Benda, Carl (1857–1933), 543.
Benedict, Francis Gano (1870–1957), *588*–9, 590, 591, 593, 600.
Benivieni, Antonio (1443–1502), 627.
Bennett, Alexander Hughes (1848–1901), *349*, 368.
Bennett, John Hughes, (1812–75), 634.
Bentham, Jeremy (1748–1832), 194, *208*, 209, 211.
Berengario da Carpi, *see* Carpi.
Berger, Hans (1873–1941), 292.

Bergmann, Ernst von (1836–1907), *365*, 367, 370, 392.

Bernard de Gourdon (d. *c.* 1320), 83.

Bernard, Claude (1813–78), 261, 262, 285, 287, *294*-9, 304, 320, 335, 351, 517, 546, 553, 602, 637, 676, 680.

Bernheim, Hippolyte (1840–1919), *510*, 513.

Bert, Paul (1833–86), *304*, 307, 308.

Bertheim, Alfred, 689.

Berthelot, Marcellin (1827–1907), 602.

Berthold, A. A. (1803–61), *516*, 549.

Bertillon, Jacques (1821–83), 715.

Bertrand, Alexandre (1795–1831), 509.

Besredka, Alexandre (1870–1940), 561.

Best, C. H. (1899–), *554*-5, 560, 754.

Bezold, Albert von (1836–68), 313.

Bichat, Xavier (1771–1802), 281, *320*, 6;0.

Bidder, Friedrich (1810–94), 261, 301, 314, *582*-3, 584, 589.

Biedl, Artur (1869–1933), *539*, 549, 557.

Bier, August (1861–1949), 350.

Bigelow, Henry Jacob (1818–90), 659.

Biggs, Herman M. (1859–1923), 236.

Bignami, Amico (1862–1929), *459*, 462, 463.

Billard, Charles Michel (1800–32), 653.

Billroth, Theodor (1829–94), *364*, 523, 535.

Bini, Lucio (1908–), 511.

Binz, Carl (1832–1913), 684.

Bischoff, Theodore Ludwig Wilhelm von (1807–82), *583*, 584, 598, 602.

Bishop, Katharine Scott (1889–), 618.

Bismarck, Prussian statesman, 635.

Bizzozero, Giulio (1846–1901), 318.

Black, Greene Vardiman (1836–1915), 668.

Black, Joseph (1728–99), *163*-4.

Blackley, C. H. (1820–1900), *428*-9.

Blacklock, J. W. S., 399.

Blane, Sir Gilbert (1749–1834), *187*, 188.

Blankaart, Steven (1650–1702), 628.

Bleuler, (Paul) Eugen (1857–1939), 511.

Blix, Magnus Gustav (1849–1904), 269.

Bloor, Walter Ray (1877–), 602.

Blundell, James (1790–1877), 699.

Bock, Hieronymus (1498–1554), 103.

Bodington, George (1799–1882), 228.

Boë, Franz De le, *see* Sylvius, Franciscus.

Boerhaave, Hermann (1668–1738), 134, 148, *149*-50, 151, 163, 169, 184, 280.

Bohr, Christian (1855–1911), 308.

Boissier de Sauvages, François (1706–67), 280.

Bollinger, Otto von (1843–1909), *390*, 391.

Bonet [Bonetus], Théophile (1620–89), *168*, 542, 627.

Bontius [De Bondt], Jacobus (1598–1631), 610.

Boot, Arnold (1600?–1653?), 613.

Boothby, Walter M. (1880–1953), 532.

Bordet, Jules (1870–1961), 391, 403, 413, *414*-17, 418.

Bordeu, Théophile de (1722–76), *516*, 549.

Borelli, G. A. (1608–79), 50, *140*-1, 144.

Boring, E. G. (1886–), 271.

Borovsky, P. F. (1863–1932), 487.

Borries, Bodo Julius Heinrich Hermann Adalbert von (1905–56), 446.

Borsook, H. (1897–), 601.

Bostock, John (1773–1846), 428.

Botallo, Leonardo (1530–?), 427.

Bouchard, [Henri] Abel (1833–99), 274.

Bouchut, J. Eugène (1818–91), 654.

Bouillaud, Jean Baptiste (1796–1881), 632.

Bourdillon, R. B. (1889–), 615.

Boussingault, Jean Baptiste [Joseph Dieudonné] (1801–87), 579.

Bowditch, Henry P. (1840–1911), 314.

Bowman, Sir William (1816–92), 301–2, *641*.

Boycott, A. E. (1877–1938), 639.

Boyd, Sir John (1891–), *443*, 444.

Boyd Orr, *see* Orr, J. B.

Boyle, Robert (1627–91), 47, 111, 132, *136*, 137, 144, 161, 254.

Braconnot, Henri (1780–1855), 595.

Brahe, Tycho (1546–1601), *112*, 145.

Braid, James (1795–1860), 509.

Bramwell, Sir Byrom (1847–1931), *278*, 524.

Bramwell, John Byrom (1822–82), 524.

Brandes, Rudolph (1795–1842), 681.

Braunschweig, H., *see* Brunschwig.

Brehmer, Hermann (1826–89), 228.

Bretonneau, Pierre Fidèle (1778–1862), *204*, 282, 381, 531, 655.

Breuer, Josef (1842–1925), 513.

Bright, Richard (1789–1858), *284*, 365, 553, 632.

Brissaud, Édouard (1852–1909), 543.

Brisseau, Michel (1670?–1743), 645.

Broca, Paul (1824–80), *256*, 276, 277, 542.

Brodie, Sir Benjamin Collins (1783–1862), 658.

Brodmann, Korbinian (1868–1918), 248.

Broom, J. C. (1902–60), 477.
Broster, L. R. (1889–), 541.
Broussais, F. J. V. (1772–1838), 281–2, 283.
Brown, John (1735–88), 148, 280.
Brown, Sir Lindor (1903–), 573, 574, 576, 577.
Brown, Robert (1773–1858), 321.
Brown, Thomas Graham, see Graham Brown.
Browne, Sir Thomas (1605–82), 7.
Browning, C. H. (1881–), 417.
Brownlee, John (1868–1927), 733, 736, 737.
Brown-Séquard, Charles Édouard (1817–94), 261, 316, 518, 538, 539, 542, 549.
Bruce, Sir David (1855–1931), 384–5, 443, 482–3, 484, 485.
Brumpt, Émile (1877–1951), 487.
Brunfels, Otto (1490?–1534), 103, 104.
Brunner, Johann Conrad (1653–1727), 552.
Bruno, Giordano (1548–1600), 111–12, 115.
Bruns, Victor von (1812–83), 356.
Brunschwig, H. (1450–1533), 181–2, 675.
Brunt, E. H. (?–1922), 451.
Brunton, see Lauder Brunton.
Bruschettini, A. (1868–1932), 440.
Buchanan, Sir George (1831–95), 223, 232.
Buchheim, Rudolf (1820–79), 684.
Buchner, Hans (1850–1902), 396, 599.
Budd, William (1811–80), 493, 731.
Budin, Pierre (1846–1907), 227.
Bulloch, William (1868–1941), 396, 441, 541.
Bunge, Gustav von (1844–1920), 319.
Bunsen, Robert [Wilhelm Eberhard] von (1811–99), 319.
Burdach, Karl Friedrich (1776–1847), 248.
Burdon-Sanderson, see Sanderson.
Burnet, Sir (Frank) Macfarlane (1899–), 449.
Burr, George O. (1896–), 618.
Butenandt, Adolf (1903–), 550, 551.

Cadogan, William (1711–97), 651.
Caelius Aurelianus (fl. 5th cent. A.D.), 240.
Caesar, Gaius Julius (102–44 B.C.), 55.
Cagniard-Latour, Charles, baron (1777–1859), 330.
Caius, John (1510–73), 740, 741.
Cajal, see Ramón y Cajal.
Calmeil, L. F. (1798–1895), 507.

Calmette, Albert (1863–1933), 426–7.
Calvin, Protestant Reformer, 119.
Cameron, Sir Roy (1899–), 639.
Campbell, A. W. (1868–1937), 248.
Campbell Swinton, see Swinton.
Camus, Jean (1872–1924), 546.
Cannon, Walter Bradford (1871–1945), 303, 375, 539, 570–1.
Cardan, Jerome (1501–76), 428.
Carmichael Low, see Low.
Carpenter, Mary (1807–77), 709.
Carpi, Jacopo Berengario da (?–1550), 241.
Carr, Francis Howard (1874–), 682.
Carrel, Alexis (1873–1944), 320, 448.
Carroll, James (1854–1907), 469–70.
Carson, James (1772–1843), 372.
Carswell, Sir Robert (1793–1857), 275, 633.
Carter, Henry R. (1852–1925), 470.
Castellani, Aldo (1877–), 484–5.
Castle, William Bosworth (1897–), 621.
Cathcart, E. P. (1877–1954), 583, 590, 593, 596, 599–601, 605, 607–8.
Cavendish, Henry (1731–1810), 164.
Caventou, J. B. (1795–1877), 681.
Cawley, Thomas (fl. 1778), 553.
Celli, Angelo (1857–1914), 459.
Celsus, A. C. (fl. A.D. 10–37), 53–55, 643, 650, 668.
Cerletti, Ugo (1877–), 511.
Cesalpino, Andrea (1524–1603), 119.
Cetti, professional faster, 590, 591.
Chadwick, Sir Edwin (1800–90), 194, 209–19.
Chagas, Carlos (1879–1934), 487.
Chain, E. B. (1906–), 695–6.
Chamberlen, Peter (?–1631), 176.
Chantemesse, André (1851–1919), 399, 443.
Charcot, Jean Martin (1825–93), 258, 272, 274–5, 276, 277, 278, 510, 513.
Charles V (1500–58), emperor, 92.
Charles I (1221–85), king of Naples, 75.
Charlesworth, E. P. (1783–1853), 500.
Charlton, Willy (1889–), 437, 438.
Chaucer, Geoffrey, poet, 676.
Chémant, see Dubois de Chémant.
Cheselden, William (1688–1752), 151, 648.
Chesney, Alan Mason (1888–), 529–30.
Chevreul, Michel Eugène (1786–1889), 319, 552.
Cheyne, George (1671–1743), 505.
Cheyne, John (1777–1836), 535, 653.

Chiarurgi, Vincenzo (1739–1820), 505.
Chick, Dame Harriette (1875–), 615.
Chittenden, R. H. (1856–1943), 605–6.
Christian, Walter, 620.
Christy, Cuthbert (1863–1932), 484.
Chvostek, Franz (1835–84), 535.
Clark, Alfred Joseph (1885–1941), 685.
Clarke, J. A. Lockhart, see Lockhart Clarke.
Clarke, John (1761–1815), 535.
Clarke, William E., of Rochester, U.S.A., 343.
Claudius, emperor of Rome, 57.
Clay, Rev. John (1796–1858), 216.
Cleopatra, queen of Egypt, 48, 51.
Clerk Maxwell, see Maxwell.
Clift, William (1775–1849), 171.
Clover, J. T. (1825–82), 347–8, 349.
Clowes, William (1544–1604), 182–3.
Coats, Joseph (1846–99), 636–7.
Cockburn, W. (1669–1739), 186.
Cohn, Ferdinand [Julius] (1828–98), 324, 336.
Cohnheim, Julius (1839–84), 353, 392, 595, 636, 637.
Cohnheim [Kestner], Otto (1873–1953), 595.
Coindet, J. F. (1774–1834), 523.
Cole, Sydney William (1876–1951), 596.
Coleridge, S. T., poet, 466.
Colles, Abraham (1773–1843), 284.
Collier, James S. (1870–1935), 276.
Collip, J. B. (1892–), 536–7, 548, 555.
Colombo, Realdo (1516?–59), 119, 244.
Comte, Louis (1870–), 547.
Conolly, John (1794–1866), 499–501.
Conradi, Heinrich (1876–), 408.
Constantine the African (1010?–87), 71–72.
Cook, James (1728–79), explorer, 187.
Cook, James Wilfred (1900–), 638.
Cooper, Antony Ashley, 7th earl of Shaftesbury (1801–85), 218, 502.
Cooper, Sir Astley Paston (1768–1841), 284, 520.
Cooper, William White (1816–86), 531, 533.
Cope, Edward Drinker (1840–97), 237.
Copernicus, Nicholas (1473–1543), 92, 112.
Coram, Thomas (1668?–1751), captain, 656.
Corbet, Ruth E. (1910–), 617.
Cori, Carl (1896–), 294, 296.

Cori, Gerty (1896–1957), 294, 296.
Corner, G. W. (1889–), 548, 551.
Corning, J. Leonard (1855–1923), 350.
Corrigan, Sir Dominic (1802–80), 245, 283, 625, 628.
Corti, Alfonso (1822–88), 250.
Corvisart [-Desmarets], J. N., baron (1755–1821), 172, 281, 286, 535, 630.
Corvisart, Lucien (1824–82), 535, 552.
Cosmas, Saint, 67–68.
Cotugno, Domenico (1736–1822), 249.
Courtois, Bernard (1777–1838), 522.
Coward, Katharine Hope (1885–), 617.
Cowell, S. J. (1891–), 563, 616.
Coxeter, instrument manufacturer, 686.
Cramer, William (1878–1945), 441.
Crawford, Albert Cornelius (1869–1921), 538.
Creighton, Charles (1847–1927), 741.
Cremer, Max (1865–1935), 604.
Crichton-Browne, Sir James (1840–1938), 606.
Croce, Andrea della (fl. 1573), 358.
Crookes, Sir William (1832–1919), 374.
Cruveilhier, Jean (1791–1874), 273, 275, 282, 631–2.
Cullen, William (1710–90), 148, 151, 251, 280.
Curie, Marie (1867–1934), 377.
Curie, Pierre (1859–1906), 377.
Curling, T. Blizard (1811–88), 521.
Cushing, Harvey [Williams] (1869–1939), 350, 367, 371, 543, 545, 546, 549.
Cushny, Arthur R. (1866–1926), 302, 685.
Cuvier, Georges, baron (1769–1832), 236, 726.
Cyon, Elie von (1842–1912), 314.
Czermak, Johann Nepomuk (1828–73), 249.

Dakin, Henry Drysdale (1880–1952), 320, 570, 603.
Dale, Sir Henry (1875–), 545, 546, 555–60, 562–70, 572, 575–7, 682.
Dalrymple, John (1803–52), 533.
Dalton, John (1766–1844), 649.
Dam, Henrik (1895–), 621, 622.
Damian, Saint, 67–68.
Dandy, Walter Edward (1886–1946), 279, 371.
Darwin, Charles (1809–82), 237, 333, 513.
Davaine, Casimir (1812–82), 328, 336.
Daviel, Jacques (1696–1762), 645.
Davies, H. Morriston (1879–), 373.

3 F

Davis, John Bunnell (1780–1824), 656.
Davis, Marguerite, 612.
Davy, Sir Humphry (1778–1829), 342, 343, 377.
De Bondt, J., see Bontius.
de Graaf, Regnier (1641–73), 297, 298, 516, 551.
De Haen, Anton (1704–76), 280.
Dejerine, Joseph J. (1849–1917), 279.
Dejerine-Klumpke, Augusta (1859–1927), 279.
Delafield, Francis (1841–1915), 456.
Delpech, Jacques Matthieu (1777–1832), 658.
Demarquay, Jean Nicolas (1811–75), 492.
Democritus (c. 400 B.C.), 49, 51.
Denis, Willey Glover (1879–1929), 597.
Denys, Jean Baptiste (1625 ?–1704), 698–9.
Denys, Joseph (?–1932), 418.
Derosne, Charles (1780–1846), 680.
Desault, Pierre Joseph (1744–95), 523.
Descartes, R. (1596–1650), 50, 112, 113, 138–40, 143, 250, 251, 264, 748.
Deventer, see Van Deventer.
Dick, George (1881–), 438.
Dick, Gladys (1881–), 438.
Diderot, D. (1713–84), 142.
Dieffenbach, J. F. (1792–1847), 648.
Diocletian, emperor of Rome, 67.
Dioscorides (fl. middle of 1st cent. A.D.), 53, 60, 671, 673.
Dittmar, Carl (1844–1920), 316.
Dix, Dorothea Lynde (1802–87), 502.
Dixon, Walter Ernest (1870–1931), 566, 569.
Dobell, Clifford (1886–1949), 493.
Dobson, Matthew (1745 ?–84), 552.
Dochez, Alphonse (1882–), 401.
Dodds, Sir Charles (1899–), 551.
Doering, Michael (?–1644), 203.
Doisy, E. A. (1893–), 551, 621, 622.
Domagk, Gerhard (1895–), 693.
Donath, W. F. (1889–), 619.
Donders, Frans Cornelis (1818–89), 643.
Donné, Alfred (1801–78), 317.
Donovan, Charles (1863–1951), 487.
Dopter, Charles (1873–1950), 402.
Douglas, C. G. (1882–), 306, 307, 309, 590.
Douglas, S. R. (1871–1936), 419.
Dragstedt, C. A. (1895–), 563.
Dran, H. F. Le, see Le Dran.
Drigalski, Karl Wilhelm von (1871–1950), 408.

Drummond, Sir Jack (1891–1952), 612, 616.
Dryander, Johannes (1500–60), 241.
Dubini, Angelo (1813–1902), 493.
Du Bois, Delafield (1880–), 590.
Du Bois, Eugene Floyd (1882–1959), 590.
Dubois de Chémant, N. (1753–1824), 665, 667.
Du Bois Reymond, Emil (1818–96), 161, 289, 564–5.
Dubos, René J. (1901–), 696.
Duchâteau (fl. 1774–88), 665.
Duchenne, G. B. A., de Boulogne (1806–75), 273, 658.
Ducrey, Augusto (1860–1940), 391, 393.
Dudgeon, Robert Ellis (1820–1904), 313, 622.
Dudley, Harold Ward (1887–1935), 546, 560, 570, 683.
Dürer, Albrecht, painter, 88.
Duhamel du Monceau, H. L. (1700–82), 657.
Dujardin, Félix (1801–60), 321, 324, 327.
Dumas, Jean Baptiste (André) (1800–84), 681.
Dumortier, Barthélemy Charles (1797–c. 1840), 326.
Dunant, Henri (1828–1910), 185.
Dunbar, W. P. (1863–1922), 429.
Duncan, William Henry (1805–63), 219.
Dunhill, Sir Thomas (1876–1957), 534.
Dunkin, George W. (1886–1942), 449.
Dunluce, viscount, see M'Donnell, R. M. K.
Dupuytren, Guillaume, baron (1777–1835), 184–5, 658.
Durham, Herbert Edward (1866–1945), 400, 418.
Dusch, Theodor von (1824–90), 329.
Dusser de Barenne, J. G. (1885–1940), 266.
Dutrochet, Henri (1776–1847), 321.
Dutton, Joseph Everett (1874–1905), 483–4, 485.

Eberth, Carl Joseph (1835–1926), 387, 391, 399.
Eccles, Sir John C. (1903–), 573.
Edinger, Ludwig (1855–1918), 249.
Edward VI, king of England, 702.
Edward VII, king of Great Britain and Ireland, 378.
Edwards, A. Tudor (1890–1946), 373.

Egas Moniz, Antonio C. de (1874–1955), 512.
Ehrenberg, C. G. (1795–1876), 327.
Ehrlich, Paul (1854–1915), 318, 394, 412, 413, 415–16, *687*–90, 691, 692.
Eijkman, Christiaan (1858–1930), *611*, 612.
Einthoven, Willem (1860–1927), *625*, 754.
Eliot, George, novelist, 683.
Elliot Smith, *see* Smith, Sir Grafton Elliot.
Elliotson, John (1791–1868), 342, 428, *509*, 523.
Elliott, T. R. (1877–1961), *565*, 566, 570.
Elvehjem, C. A. (1901–), 620.
Embden, Gustav (1874–1933), 294.
Engle, Earl Theron (1896–1957), 547.
Epicurus (342–270 B.C.), 49.
Erasistratus of Chios (*c.* 300–250 B.C.), 48, *49*, 50, 51, 239.
Erb, Wilhelm (1840–1921), *252*, 274.
Erdheim, Jakob (1874–1937), 537.
Erlanger, Joseph (1874–), *290*–1.
Ermengem, Émile P. van (1851–1932), 391, *394*.
Escherich, Theodor (1857–1911), 391, *392*, 399.
Esdaile, James (1808–59), 342.
Esmarch, Friedrich von (1823–1908), 185.
d'Espine, Jacob Marc (1806–60), 715.
Esquirol, J. E. D. (1772–1840), *501*, 505.
Estienne, Charles (1504–64), *242*, 276.
Euler, Ulf von (1905–), 572.
Eustachi [Eustachius], Bartolommeo (1520–74), *243*–4, 260, 538.
Evans, Sir Charles Lovatt, *see* Lovatt Evans.
Evans, Conway (1830–92), *715*–16.
Evans, Griffith (1835–1935), 481.
Evans, Herbert M. (1882–), *547*, 618.
Evelyn, John (1620–1706), 188.
Ewing, James (1866–1943), 639.
Ewins, A. J. (1882–1957), *566*, 568.

Fabbroni, Adamo (fl. 1787), 329.
Faber, Knud [Helge] (1862–1956), 439.
Fabricius, Hieronymus, ab Aquapendente (*c.* 1533–1619), *97*–98, 118–19, 120, 125, 640, 645, 668.
Fabricius Hildanus, *see* Fabry, W.
Fabrizio, Girolamo, *see* Fabricius, H.
Fabroni, *see* Fabbroni.
Fabry, Wilhelm, of Hilden (1560–1634), 183.
Fagge, C. Hilton (1838–83), *522*, 524.

Faier, *see* Phaer.
Fairley, Sir Neil Hamilton (1891–), *464*, 466.
Fallopio, Gabriele (1523–62), 244.
Falstaff, 40.
Fantham, Harold B. (1875–1937), 486.
Faraj ben Salīm (fl. 1280), 74, 75, *76*.
Farr, William (1807–83), 213, 714, 715, 717, 732–3.
Farrar, John Nutting (1839–1913), 671.
Fauchard, Pierre (1678–1761), 662, *663*, 665, 668, 669.
Fehleisen, Friedrich (1854–1924), 391, *392*.
Feldberg, Wilhelm S. (1900–), *563*, 569, 572, 573, 574, 575, *576*, 577.
Feldman, William Hugh (1892–), 697.
Felix, Arthur (1887–1956), 404, *405*, 443, 444.
Fergusson, Sir William (1808–77), 352.
Fernel, Jean (1497–1558), *98*, 100.
Ferri, Alfonso (1515–95), 182.
Ferriar, John (1761–1815), 189.
Ferrier, Sir David (1843–1928), *257*–8, 606.
Ferrus, Guillaume (1784–1861), 501.
Fick, Adolf (1829–1901), 592.
Fieser, Louis Frederick (1899–), 621.
Fildes, Sir Paul (1882–), *396*, 441.
Findlay, George Marshall (1893–1952), *477*–8.
Findlay, Leonard (1878–1947), *614*, 655.
Finlay, Carlos ['Carlos Juan'] (1833–1915), *468*–9, 471, 472, 476, 478.
Finsen, Niels R. (1860–1904), *377*–8.
Fischer, Emil (1852–1919), 320, *595*.
Fisher, Sir Ronald A. (1890–), 727.
Fitz, Reginald Heber (1843–1913), 365.
Flack, Martin W. (1882–1931), 623.
Flagg, Josiah Foster (1789–1853), 668.
Flechsig, Paul E. (1847–1929), 249.
Fleming, Sir Alexander (1881–1955), *694*–5, 696, 754.
Fletcher, Thomas, British dentist (fl. 1880), 668.
Fletcher, Sir Walter Morley (1873–1933), *292*, 293.
Fletcher, William (1874–1938), 611.
Flexner, Simon (1863–1946), 449.
Fliedner, Friederike (1800–42), 703.
Fliedner, Theodor (1800–64), 703.
Florey, Sir Howard (1898–), 638, *695*–6.
Flourens, Pierre (1794–1867), 252, *255*–6, 260.

Floyer, Sir John (1649–1734), *171*, 428.
Foix, Charles (1882–1927), 272.
Folin, Otto (1867–1934), *320*, 596, 597, 599, 600.
Fontana, Felice (1720–1805), 320.
Fonzi, Giuseppangelo (1768–1840), *665*, 667.
Forde, Robert Michael (1861–1948), 483.
Forestier, Jacques (1890–), 375.
Forlanini, Carlo (1847–1918), *372*, 373.
Foster, Goodwin LeBaron (1891–), 547.
Foster, Sir Michael (1836–1907), *262*, 305, 314, 555, 564.
Fothergill, John (1712–80), *190*, 203.
Fox, Edward Lawrence (1859–1938), 526.
Fracastoro, Girolamo (1478–1553), *105*–8, 729, 731.
Fraenkel, Albert (1848–1916), 391, *393*.
Fraenkel, Carl (1861–1915), 411.
Frampton, John (fl. 1577–96), 103.
Francia [Raibolini], Francesco (1450–1517), painter, 78.
Francis, Thomas (1900–), 449.
Frank, Johann Peter (1745–1821), *197*–8, 273, 280, 545.
Frankland, Sir Edward (1825–99), 586.
Franklin, Benjamin (1706–90), *190*, 643.
Fraser, Henry (1873–1930), 611.
Frazer, Sir James George (1854–1941), 27.
Frederick the Great, of Prussia, 666.
Frederick William, elector of Brandenburg (1620–88), 183.
Freeman, John (1877–1962), 430.
Frerichs, Friedrich Theodor von (1819–85), *275*–6, 553.
Freud, Sigmund (1856–1939), *513*–15.
Frey, Max von (1852–1932), 269.
Friedberger, Ernst (1875–1932), 562.
Friedemann, Ulrich (1877–1949), 562.
Friedländer, Carl (1847–87), 391, *392*.
Fritsch, Gustav Theodor (1838–97), 257.
Fröhlich, Alfred (1871–1953), 544.
Frölich, Theodor C. B. (1870–1947), 618.
Frosch, Paul (1860–1928), *408*, 445.
Fry, Elizabeth (1780–1845), *190*, 703, 704.
Fuchs, Leonhart (1501–66), *103*–4, 105.
Fulton, John F. (1899–1960), 260.
Funk, Casimir (1884–), *612*, 613, 618.
Funke, Otto (1828–79), 303.

Gaddum, J. H. (1900–), *569*, 570, 572, 573.
Gaertner, August (1848–1934,) 391, *393*.
Gaffky, Georg (1850–1918), *387*, 392, 399.

Gaine, Charles, dentist, of Bath (fl. 1858), 670.
Gale, Thomas (1507–87), 182.
Galé [Galle], Philipp (1537–1612), 109.
Galen (129–99), 16, 50, *59*–66, 68, 71, 74, 77, 84, 88, 89, 90, 91, 93, 94, 98, 100, 104, 111, 116, 118, 122, 146, 242–3, 519, 542, 629, 640, 644, 671, 673, 728.
Galilei, Galileo (1564–1642), 112, *113*–15, 116, 124, 135, 138, 140, 144, 145, 147, 171.
Gall, F. J. (1758–1828), *254*–5, 256.
Gallegos, F. (1461?–1550), Spanish painter, 67.
Galton, Sir Francis (1822–1911), *725*, 726.
Galvani, Luigi (1737–98), 158, *159*, 289.
Gamgee, Arthur (1841–1909), 685.
Garcia, Manuel [Patricio Rodriguez] (1805–1906), 249.
Gariopontus (d. *c.* 1050), 71.
Garnham, P. C. C. (1901–), 464.
Gaskell, Walter Holbrook (1847–1914), *262*, 314–15, 316, 555, 565.
Gasser, Herbert Spencer (1888–), *290*–1, 575, 576.
Gaubius, Hieronymus David (1705–80), 134.
Gaucher, Ernest (1854–1918), 319.
Gauss, K. F. (1777–1855), 725.
Gauvain, Sir Henry (1878–1945), 378.
Gay, Frederick Parker (1874–1939), 561.
Gay-Lussac, Joseph (1778–1850), 237, *680*.
Gegenbaur, Karl (1826–1903), 237.
Geiger, Ernest (1896–), 574.
Geiger, Philipp Lorenz (1785–1836), 681.
Generali, Francesco (fl. 1896), 536.
Gengou, Octave (1875–1957), 391, *416*.
George II, king of Great Britain and Ireland, 648.
Georget, Étienne Jean (1795–1828), 505.
Gerard of Cremona (1114–87), 76.
Gerhard, William Wood (1809–72), 387.
Gerhardt, Carl Adolph Christian Jacob (1833–1902), 654.
Gersdorff, Hans von (fl. 1490–1520), 182.
Ghon, Anton (1866–1936), 409, *426*.
Gilbert, Sir Joseph H. (1817–1901), 603.
Gilbert, William (1544–1603), 112, *185*–6.
Gilford, Hastings (1861–1941), *366*, 544.
Glenny, A. T. (1882–), *436*, 442.
Gley, Eugène (1857–1930), 536.
Glisson, Francis (1597–1677), *123*, 153, 613–14, 655.

Glover, J. Alison (1876–), 409.
Gmelin, Leopold (1788–1853), 297.
Godlee, Sir Rickman J. (1849–1925), 356, 368.
Goldberger, Joseph (1874–1929), 620.
Goldblatt, Harry (1891–), 617.
Goldscheider, Johannes Karl [August Eugen Alfred] (1858–1935), 269.
Golgi, Camillo (1843–1926), 247–8, 249, 270, 459.
Goll, Friedrich (1829–1903), 249.
Goltz, Friedrich (1834–1902), 258.
Goodpasture, Ernest W. (1886–1960), 448.
Goodsir, John (1814–67), 325.
Goodyear, Charles (1800–60), 667.
Gordon, Alexander (1752–99), 361, 362.
Gordon, Mervyn H. (1872–1953), 402, 403.
Gorgas, William Crawford (1854–1920), 471–4.
Gosset, William Sealy ['Student'] (1876–1937), 727.
Gotch, Francis (1853–1913), 289–90.
Gowers, Sir William (1845–1915), 249, 278–9, 318.
Gowland Hopkins, see Hopkins.
Graaf, R. de, see de Graaf.
Graefe, Albrecht von (1828–70), 533, 647, 648.
Graham, George (1801–88), 717.
Graham, John Henry Porteus (1869?–1957), 451.
Graham, Thomas (1805–69), 319.
Graham Brown, Thomas (1882–), 259.
Graham-Smith, G. S. (1875–1950), 409.
Grassi, Battista (1854–1925), 462, 463, 493.
Graunt, John (1620–74), 179–80, 712.
Graves, R. J. (1796–1853), 283, 530, 531, 532.
Green, Harry Norman (1902–), 617.
Greenfield, W. S. (1846–1919), 532, 637.
Greenwood, Major (1880–1949), 444, 607, 736, 738–9.
Greig, Edward David Wilson (1874–1950), 485.
Grew, Nehemiah (1641–1712), 320.
Griesinger, Wilhelm (1817–68), 506.
Griffith, Arthur Stanley (1875–1941), 399.
Griffith, Fred (1879?–1941), 399, 402.
Grijns, Gerrit (1865–1944), 611.
Gruber, Max (1853–1927), 418.
Gruby, David (1810–98), 481.

Grünbaum [Leyton], A. S. (1869–1921), 259, 418.
Guérin, Camille (1872–1961), 426–7.
Guillemeau, Jacques (1550–1613), 646, 663, 668.
Guiscard, Robert, duke of Apulia, 71.
Gull, Sir William Withey (1816–90), 273, 276, 285, 524.
Gulliver, George (1804–82), 538.
Gullstrand, Allvar (1862–1930), 648.
Guthrie, G. J. (1785–1856), 184.
Guthrie, Samuel (1782–1848), 344.
Guttmann, Paul (1834–93), 689, 691.
Guy de Chauliac (1298?–1368), 83–84, 669.
Gwathmey, James T. (1863–1944), 350.

Haagen, Eugen, 479.
Haen, A. De, see De Haen.
Händel, Ludwig (1869–1939), 401.
Haeser, Heinrich (1811–84), 741.
Haffkine, Waldemar M. (1860–1930), 439, 484, 491.
Halban, Josef von (1870–1937), 550.
Haldane, John Scott (1860–1936), 304–7, 309–11, 590.
Hales, Stephen (1677–1761), 154, 155, 156, 189, 194, 251, 311.
Hall, Marshall (1790–1857), 252.
Haller, Albrecht von (1708–77), 123, 148, 151–4, 163, 288, 314.
Halley, Edmund (1656–1742), 180.
Halliburton, W. D. (1860–1931), 524, 557.
Halsted, W. S. (1852–1922), 349, 370, 529, 534, 536.
Hamer, Sir William (1862–1936), 729, 740.
Hamilton, John, abp. of St. Andrews, 428.
Hammurabi, king of Assyria, 10–12.
Hancock, Henry (1809–80), 365.
Hansemann, David von (1858–1920), 614.
Hansen, Gerhard (1841–1912), 390, 391.
Hare, Edward Selleck (1812–38), 261.
Harington, Sir Charles R. (1897–), 527, 532.
Harless, Emil (1820–62), 583.
Harnack, Erich (1852–1915), 566.
Harris, Walter (1647–1732), 651.
Hartley, Sir Percival Horton-Smith- (1867–1952), 407.
Harvey, William (1578–1657), 45, 112, 119, 120–3, 124, 125, 138, 144, 145, 628, 698.
Haslam, John (1764–1844), 507.

Hasselbalch, K. A. (1874–), *307*, 308.
Hata, Sahachiro (1873–1938), 690.
Haworth, Sir Norman (1883–1949), 619.
Hayem, Georges (1841–1933), 317.
Head, Sir Henry (1861–1940), 262, 269, *270*–1, 277, 291.
Heberden, William, the Elder (1710–1801), *36*, 625, 629, 653.
Heberden, William, the Younger (1767–1845), 653.
Hebra, Ferdinand von (1816–80), 286.
Hecker, J. F. K. (1795–1850), 741.
Heidelberger, Michael (1888–), 401.
Heidenhain, Rudolph (1834–97), *302*, 595.
Heilbron, Sir Ian Morris (1886–1959), 617.
Heine, Jacob von (1799–1879), *272*, 655.
Helmholtz, Hermann von (1821–94), 161, *288*–9, 319, 325, 643, 649.
Helmont, J. B. van (1577–1644), 142.
Hench, Philip Showalter (1896–), 540.
Henderson, Yandell (1873–1944), *309*, 310.
Hendrick, E. G., 619.
Henle, Jakob (1809–85), 247, *321*, 322, 326, 328, 336, 729–30.
Henoch, Eduard (1820–1910), 654.
Henri de Mondeville (1260?–1325), 80.
Henry, prince of Portugal (1394–1460), 'the Navigator', 185.
Henry, T. A. (1873–1958), 682.
Herbert, Sidney, 1st baron Herbert of Lea (1810–61), 706, 708.
d'Herelle, Félix (1873–1949), 391, *395*, 406, 407, 696.
Hering, Heinrich Ewald (1866–1948), 314.
Hering, [Karl] Ewald [Constantin] (1834–1918), 287.
Hermann, Ludimar (1838–1914), 601.
Hermes, 5.
Herodotus, Greek historian, 4.
Herophilus of Alexandria (fl. *c.* 300 B.C.), *48*, 239.
Herring, P. T. (1872–), *539*, 546.
Herschel, Sir John, astronomer, 649.
Heusner, Ludwig (1846–1916), 366.
Hewitt, Sir Frederic W. (1857–1916), 349.
Hewson, William (1739–74), *316*–17.
Hickman, Henry Hill (1800–30), 342.
Hildanus, Fabricius, *see* Fabry, W.
Hildebrandt, Fritz (1887–), 551.
Hill, Sir A. Bradford (1897–), 738.
Hill, A. V. (1886–), *292*–3, 308.
Hill, R. Gardiner (1811–78), 500.

Hilton, John (1804–78), 658.
Himsworth, Sir Harold P. (1905–), 534.
Hindhede, Mikkel (1862–1945), 606.
Hindle, Edward (1886–), *477*, 478.
Hippocrates (*c.* 470–*c.* 400), 16, 22, 27, *28*, 29, 30, 31, 36, 77, 104, 280, 440, 728, 746.
Hippolytus, 26.
Hirsch, August (1817–94), 741.
His, Wilhelm, Senior (1831–1904), *247*, 451.
His, Wilhelm, Junior (1863–1934), 451, *623*.
Hitch, Samuel (1801–81), 502.
Hitzig, Eduard (1838–1907), 257.
Hodgkin, Thomas (1798–1866), *285*, 632.
Hoelzel, professional faster, 591.
Hoffmann, Friedrich (1660–1742), 148.
Hoffmann, (Paul) Erich (1868–1959), 391, *395*, 689.
Hofmeister, Franz (1850–1922), 595.
Hohenheim, Philip Bombast von, *see* Paracelsus.
Holmes, Sir Gordon (1876–), *279*, 541.
Holmes, Harry Nicholls (1879–), 617.
Holmes, Oliver Wendell (1809–94), *351*, 361.
Holmes, Timothy (1825–1907), 523.
Holmgren, Frithjof (1831–97), 649.
Holst, Axel (1861–1931), 618.
Holt, Luther Emmett (1855–1924), 655.
Home, Sir Everard (1756–1832), 629.
Homer, Greek poet, 7, 18, 341, 494.
Hooke, Robert (1635–1703), *132*, 320.
Hope, James (1801–41), *632*–3.
Hopkins, Sir Frederick Gowland (1861–1947), 292, 293, 319, 596, 598, 606, *611*–12.
Hoppe-Seyler, Felix (1825–95), *303*–4, 319.
Horace [Quintus Horatius Flaccus], 55.
Horner, Johann Friedrich (1831–86), 261.
Horsley, Sir Victor (1857–1916), 257, 279, 368, *525*, 535, 536, 545.
Horton-Smith-Hartley, *see* Hartley.
Horus, 5.
Houssay, Bernardo A. (1887–), *548*–9.
Houston, Sir A. C. (1865–1933), *232*, 400.
Howard, John (1726?–90), *189*, 190, 194, 198, 199.
Howe, Percy Rogers (1864–1950), 617.
Howell, William Henry (1860–1945), *545*, 596.
Hughes Bennett, *see* Bennett.

Hughlings Jackson, John (1835–1911), *256*–7, 258, 276, 277, 556.
Huldschinsky, Kurt (1883–?), 615.
Hume, E. Margaret, 617.
Hunt, George Herbert (1884–1926), 451.
Hunt, Reid (1870–1948), 567.
Hunter, Charles (1835–78), 687.
Hunter, John (1728–93), 171, 174, 176, *177*–9, 183, 200, 316, 543, 629, 637, 657, 670, 737.
Hunter, William (1718–83), 176.
Hunter, William (1861–1937), 665.
Hurst [Hertz], Sir Arthur (1879–1944), 639.
Hutchinson, Sir Jonathan (1828–1913), 544.
Hutchinson, Woods (1862–1930), 543.
Hutchison, Sir Robert (1871–1960), 655.
Huxham, John (1692–1768), 204.
Huxley, Thomas Henry (1825–95), 325.
Hyrtl, Josef (1810–94), 286.

Ibn an-Nafis (1210–88), 119.
Ido, Yutaka (1881–), 475.
Imhotep, 5, 6, 20.
Inada, Ryūkichi (1874–1950), 475.
Ingrassia, Giovanni Filippo (1510–8c), *202*–3, 244.
Innocent VIII, Pope, 698.
Isaac Judaeus (*c.* 832–932), *76*, 77.
Isidore of Seville [Isidorus Hispalensis] (570?–636), 69.
Isis, 5.
Israel, James (1848–1926), *390*, 391.
Ivanowski, Dmitri Alexievitch, 445.

Jackson, John Hughlings, *see* Hughlings Jackson.
Jacobi, Abraham (1830–1919), 655.
Jameson, Sir Wilson (1885–), *223*, 224.
Jansen, Barend Coenraad Petrus (1884–), 619.
Jenner, Edward (1749–1823), 188, *200*–2, 433, 448, 530, 632, 655, 737.
Jenner, Sir William (1815–98), 387.
Jerome, Saint, 58.
Joffroy, Alexis (1844–1908), 272, *275*, 533.
Johne, Heinrich Albert (1839–1910), 391, *392*.
Johnson, James McIntosh (1883–1953), 538.
Johnson, Samuel, lexicographer, *170*–*1*, 629.
Joll, Cecil Augustus (1885–1945), 534.
Jones, Sir Robert (1857–1933), 659.

Jung, Carl G. (1875–1961), 514.
Junker [von Langegg], Ferdinand Adalbert (*c.* 1830–1900), 363.
Jupille, Jean Baptiste, 339.
Justinian I, emperor of Constantinople, 56.
Juvenal, Latin poet, 55, 520.

Karrer, Paul (1889–), 617.
Kaufmann, Eduard (1860–1931), 638.
Kay-Shuttleworth, Sir James Phillips (1804–77), *210*–11, 213.
Keen, William W. (1837–1932), 277.
Keith, Sir Arthur (1866–1955), 543, *623*.
Kellaway, C. H. (1889–1952), 563.
Kellie, George, of Leith (1770?–1830), 535.
Kendall, Edward Calvin (1886–), *526*, 540.
Kennaway, Sir Ernest L. (1881–1958), 638.
Kennedy, Thomas Henry, 530.
Kent, A. F. Stanley (1863–1958), 623.
Kepler, J. (1571–1630), *112*, 113, 135, 145, 641.
Kerckring, Theodor (1640–93), 628.
Kestner, *see* Cohnheim.
Kimball, O. P. (1889–), 529.
King, Charles Glen (1896–), 619.
King, T. Wilkinson (1809–47), 520.
Kinghorn, Allan (?–*c.* 1955), 486.
Kingsley, Norman W. (1829–1913), 670.
Kinnier Wilson, S. A. (1878–1937), 276.
Kinyoun, Joseph J. (1860–1919), 234.
Kirkbride, Thomas Story (1809–83), 501.
Kitasato, S. (1852–1931), 381, 387, 391, 392, *393*, 394, 411–12, 439, 440, 442, 489.
Kjeldahl, Johann (1849–1900), 320.
Klebs, Edwin (1834–1913), 339, *381*, 391, 636.
Klein, Emanuel (1844–1925), 398.
Kleine, Friedrich Karl (1869–1951), 486.
Kleitman, Nathaniel (1895–), 591.
Knapp, Paul (1874–1954), 616.
Knauer, Emil (1867–1935), 550.
Knoop, Franz (1875–1946), 603.
Koch, Robert (1843–1910), 234, 235, *336*–41, 379, 380, 381, 387, 390, 391, 392, 393, 394, 396, 397, 398, 408, 411, 412, 422–4, 426, 427, 486, 586, 688, 746.
Kocher, Theodor (1841–1917), *374*, 523–4, 525, 534, 535.
Kölliker, Albert von (1817–1905), *247*, 270, 326, 595.
Kohn, Alfred (1867–1959), 536.

Koller, Carl (1857–1944), 349.
Koppe, Richard, 565.
Kossel, Albrecht [Karl Ludwig Martin Leonhard] (1853–1927), 595.
Kraemer, Heinrich, Dominican monk, 495.
Kraepelin, Emil (1856–1926), 511.
Kraft-Ebing, Richard von (1840–1902), 507.
Kraus, Rudolf (1868–1932), *418*, 557.
Krause, Wilhelm (1833–1910), 269.
Krönlein, Rudolph Ulrich (1847–1910), 366.
Krogh, August (1874–1949), *307*, 308, 309, 594.
Kromayer, Ernst [Franz] (1862–1933), 378.
Kubota, Bennosuke (1885–), 560.
Kühne, Willy (1837–1900), *270*, 552, 565, 595.
Kützing, Friedrich T. (1807–93), 330.
Kuhn, Richard (1900–), *620–1*.
Kupffer, Karl von (1829–1902), 318.
Kutscher, Friedrich (1866–1942), 557.

Laennec, R. T. H. (1781–1826), *172–4*, 281, 282, 283, 286, 428, 625, 630, 631, 653.
Laguesse, G. E. (1861–1927), 553.
Laidlaw, Sir Patrick Playfair (1881–1940), *449*, 557, 559.
Lancefield, Rebecca C. (1895–), 402.
Lancisi, Giovanni Maria (1654–1720), *196–7*, 456, 628.
Landsteiner, Karl (1868–1943), 437, 449, *700–1*.
Lane, Sir (William) Arbuthnot (1856–1943), *370*, 371.
Langdon-Brown, Sir W. (1870–1946), 549.
Langerhans, Paul (1847–88), 553.
Langley, J. N. (1852–1925), *262*, 539, 555, 565.
Laplace, Pierre Simon (1749–1827), *166*, 168, 725.
Laquer, Fritz (1888–1954), 550.
Larrey, Dominique Jean, *baron* (1766–1842), *184*, 185.
Lauder Brunton, Sir Thomas (1844–1916), *684–5*.
Laveran, Alphonse (1845–1922), *456–7*, 459, 460.
Lavoisier, Antoine Laurent (1743–94), *166–8*, 237, 578, 579, 581.
Lavosier, Marie A. P., Mme (1758–1836), 167, 168.

Lawes, Sir John Bennet (1814–1900), 603.
Lazear, Jesse W. (1866–1900), *469–70*.
Leathes, J. B. (1864–1956), 596.
Leclef, Joseph (fl. 1895), 418.
Ledingham, Sir John C. G. (1875–1944), 409.
Le Dran, Henri François (1685–1770), 183.
Leeuwenhoek, Antoni van (1632–1723), 50, 124, *126*–31, 320, 327, 395.
Legallois, César (1770–1814), 252.
Le Gras, [Louise de Marillac] Mme (1591–1662), 702.
Lehmann, Curt (fl. 1893), 591.
Leishman, Sir William B. (1865–1926), *419*, 487.
Lenard, Philipp (1862–1947), 374.
Leo X, Pope, 641.
Leonardo da Vinci, *see* Vinci.
Lesseps, Ferdinand, *vicomte de* (1805–94), 473.
Lester Smith, E. (1904–), 621.
Lettsom, John Coakley (1744–1815), 190.
Levaditi, Constatin (1874–1953), *417*, 437.
Levi, Ettore, of Florence (fl. 1908), 544.
Lewis, Paul A. (1879–1929), *430*, 450, 561.
Lewis, Sir Thomas (1881–1945), 560, *624*, 625.
Lewis, Timothy R. (1841–86), 481, *492*, 493.
Leydig, Franz von (1821–1908), 325.
Leyton, A. S., *see* Grünbaum.
Liddell, E. G. T. (1895–), 266.
Liébeault, Ambroise Auguste (1823–1904), *510*, 513.
Liebig, Justus von (1803–73), *237–8*, 319, 331, 344, 579–81, 582, 583, 592, 595, 598, 681.
Linacre, Thomas (1460?–1524), 103.
Lind, James (1716–94), *186–7*, 188, 189, 194, 196.
Lindhard, Johannes (1870–1947), 594.
Linnaeus, *see* Linné.
Linné, Carl (1707–78), 280.
Lisfranc, Jacques (1790–1847), 364.
Lister, Sir F. Spencer (1876–1939), 401.
Lister, Joseph, baron Lister of Lyme Regis (1827–1912), 317, 335, *352–60*, 365, 366, 367, 370, 374, 520, 637, 647.
Lister, Joseph Jackson (1786–1869), 352.
Lister, Thomas Henry (1800–42), 717.
Liston, Robert (1794–1847), *344*, 351.
Little, William John (1810–94), *658–9*.
Livingstone, David (1813–73), 482.

Lloyd, Wray Devere Marr (1902–36), 480.
Lobstein, Jean Georges Chrétien Frédéric Martin (1777–1835), 631.
Lockhart Clarke, J. A. (1817–80), *249*, 276.
Loeb, Jacques (1859–1924), 540.
Loeffler, Friedrich (1852–1915), 381, 391, *392*, 411, 445.
Lösch, Friedrich (fl. 1875), 493.
Loewi, Otto (1873–1961), *568*, 569, 570, 574, 577.
Loewy, Adolf (1862–1937), 593.
Long, Crawford Williamson (1815–78), 343.
Long, Esmond R. (1890–), 638.
Long, Joseph Abraham (1879–?), 547.
Longet, François Achille (1811–71), 428.
Looss, Arthur (1861–1923), 493.
Lorain, Paul (1827–75), 543.
Lorrain Smith, J. (1862–1931), 305.
Louis, P. C. A. (1787–1872), 282, 286, 631, 633, *721*, 722.
Lovatt Evans, Sir Charles A., *316*, 519.
Low, G. Carmichael (1872–1952), 484.
Lowe, Peter (1560–1610), 183.
Lower, Richard (1631–91), 698.
Lucas, Keith (1879–1916), 289–90.
Lucas-Championnière, Just (1843–1913), 371.
Luciani, Luigi (1842–1919), *260*, 590.
Lucretius, Latin poet, 51, 104–5.
Ludwig, Karl (1816–95), 287, *299–302*, 311, 314, 316, 320, 592, 637.
Lugol, J. G. A. (1786–1851), 523.
Luke, Saint, 70.
Lundsgaard, Christen (1883–1930), 307.
Lunin, Nicolai Ivanovitch (1853–1937), 610.
Lusk, Graham (1866–1932), 583, 590, 591, *594*, 604, 605, 607.

McBurney, Charles (1845–1913), 366.
MacCallum, W. G. (1874–1944), 461, 536, 553, *639*.
McCance, R. A. (1898–), 606.
McCarrison, Sir Robert (1878–1960), *527*–8, 530, 608.
McCay, David (1873–1948), 606.
McCleary, G. F. (1867–1962), 227.
McCollum, E. V. (1879–), 598, *612*, 616.
MacConkey, Alfred T. (1861–1931), 400.
M'Donnell, Randal Mark Kerr, viscount Dunluce and later 12th earl of Antrim (1878–1932), 607.

McDowell, Ephraim (1771–1830), 362.
Macewen, Sir William (1848–1924), 350, *366–70*, 371, 614, 659.
McFarlane, William Douglas (1900–), 621.
M'Gonigle, G. C. M. (1888–1939), *609*–10.
Machado, A. L. (fl. 1943), 577.
McIntosh, James (1883–1948), 396.
Mackenzie, Sir Hector [William Gavin] (1856–1929), 526.
Mackenzie, Ivy (1877–1959), 417.
Mackenzie, Sir James (1853–1925), 313, *623*, 624, 625, 684.
McLeod, James Walter (1887–), 403.
Macleod, J. J. R. (1876–1935), *554*–5.
MacNalty, Sir Arthur S. (1880–), *223*, 224.
McNee, Sir John W. (1887–), *451*, 452.
Madhava, Krishna Bindu (1895–), 528.
Madsen, Thorvald (1870–1957), 413.
Magendie, François (1783–1855), *154*, 250, 251, 256, 297, 353, 578, 637, 680, 681.
Magnus, Heinrich Gustav (1802–70), 579.
Magnus, Rudolf (1873–1927), 266.
Magnus-Levy, Adolf (1865–1955), *589*–90.
Mair, William, *427*, 438.
Maître-Jan, Antoine (1650?–1730), 645.
Malacarne, Vincenzo (1744–1816), 521.
Malassez, Louis Charles (1842–1909), 318.
Malcolmson, John Grant (?–1844), 611.
Malpighi, Marcello (1628–94), 121, *124*–6, 140, 515.
Malthus, T. R. (1766–1834), 712.
Mandl, Felix (1892–1957), 537.
Mansfield, E. R. (fl. 1904), 604.
Manson, Sir Patrick (1844–1922), *460*–3, 469, 492–3.
Mantoux, Charles (1877–1947), *425*, 426.
Marchand, Felix (1846–1928), 318.
Marchi, Vittorio (1851–1908), 248.
Marchiafava, Ettore (1847–1935), 457.
Marey, Étienne Jules (1830–1904), *313*, 622.
Maria Theresa, empress of Austria, 280.
Marie, Auguste Charles (1864–1935), 440.
Marie, Pierre (1853–1940), 274, *277*, 542, 543.
Marine, David (1880–), *529*–30.
Marinesco, Georges (1864–1938), 277.
Marmorek, Alexander (1865–1923), 401.
Marrian, G. F. (1904–), 551.

Marryat, Frederick, captain, R.N., and novelist, 466.
Marsh, Sir Henry (1790–1860), *530*, 532.
Martin, Sir Charles (1866–1955), 490.
Martin, H. Newell, *see* Newell Martin.
Mather, Cotton (1663–1728), 200.
Mather, Increase (1639–1723), 200.
Mattioli, Pietro Andrea (1501–77), 671.
Mauriceau, François (1637–1709), 177.
Maxwell, James Clerk (1831–79), 649.
Mayerne, Sir Theodore Turquet de (1573–1655), 672.
Mayo, Charles Horace (1865–1939), *370*, 532.
Mayo, Herbert (1796–1852), 251.
Mayo, William James (1861–1939), 370.
Mayo Robson, *see* Robson, Sir A. W. Mayo.
Mayow, John (1641–79), *136*–7, 161–3, 237, 614.
Mazzoni, Vittorio (fl. 1891), 269.
Mead, Richard (1673–1754), *200*, 656, 657.
Means, J. H. (1885–), *532*, 534.
Medin, Oscar (1847–1927), *272*, 655.
Meduna, Ladislas Joseph (1896–), 511.
Meeh, K. (fl. 1879), 587, 590.
Meige, Henri (1866–1940), 543.
Meigs, Arthur Vincent (1850–1912), 655.
Meigs, Charles Delucena (1792–1869), 654.
Meigs, John Forsyth (1818–82), 655.
Meissl, Emmerich (1855–1905), 603.
Meissner, Georg (1829–1903), 269, 271.
Meister, Joseph, 339.
Mellanby, Sir Edward (1884–1955), 559, *614*–15, 617.
Mellanby, Lady May, 670.
Meltzer, Samuel J. (1851–1920), 430.
Mendel, Lafayette Benedict (1872–1935), 598, *612*.
Mennell, J. B. (1880–1957), 371.
Mercurialis, Hieronymus (1530–1606), 651.
Mering, Joseph von (1849–1908), 553.
Merkel, Friedrich (1845–1919), 269.
Merlatti, professional faster, 591.
Merry, Charles (fl. 1850), 669.
Mesmer, Franz Anton (1734–1815), 507–9.
Mesuë, the Elder (777?–857), 549.
Metchnikoff, Élie [Ilya Ilyich] (1845–1916), 406, *410*–11, 417, 418.
Metzger, Johann Georg (1838–1909), 371.
Meyer, Gustav Morris (1875–), 597.

Meyer, Lothar (1830–95), 303.
Meyerhof, Otto (1884–1951), 293.
Michaelangelo, Italian painter, 88.
Michael Scot, *see* Scot.
Middleton, T. (1570?–1627), dramatist, 84.
Mill, John Stuart (1806–73), 208.
Milton, John, poet, 676.
Minkowski, Oscar (1858–1931), *542*, 553.
Minot, G. R. (1885–1950), *621*, 622.
Mintz, Beatrice (1909–), 619.
Mitchell, Silas Weir (1829–1914), *185*, 277, 643.
Möbius, Paul Julius (1854–1907), *532*, 533.
Mohl, Hugo von (1805–72), *324*, 326.
Mohr, Bernhard (fl. 1840), 544.
Moir, J. Chassar (1900–), 683.
Moivre, Abraham de (1667–1754), *180*, 725.
Molière, French dramatist, 552.
Monakow, Constantin von (1853–1930), 249.
Monardes, Nicolas (1493–1588), 103.
Monceau, *see* Duhamel du Monceau.
Mondino de' Luzzi [Mundinus] (1275?–1326), *80*–83, 241.
Moniz, Egas, *see* Egas Moniz.
Monro, Alexander, *primus* (1697–1767), *150*–1, 280, 642.
Monro, Alexander, *secundus* (1733–1817), *151*, 245.
Monro, Alexander, *tertius* (1773–1859), *151*, 325.
Montagu, Lady Mary Wortley (1689–1762), 200.
Moore, Joseph Waldron (1879–), 507.
Moore, Samson (1866–1940), 227.
Moore, Thomas, of Cambridge, 618.
Morax, Victor (1866–1935), 440.
Morel, Benedict (1809–73), *506*, 511.
Morgagni, Giovanni Battista (1682–1771), *169*, 628, 629.
Morgan, John (1797–1847), 285.
Morgenroth, Julius (1871–1924), 415.
Morley Fletcher, *see* Fletcher.
Moro, Ernst (1874–1951), 425.
Morse, Thomas H. (1855–1921), 366.
Morton, Richard (1637–98), 203.
Morton, Thomas George (1835–1903), 366.
Morton, W. T. G. (1819–68), *344*, 345, 346, 351.
Mott, Sir Frederick W. (1853–1926), *260*, 557.

Mouton, Claude (?–1786), 665.
Moynihan, Berkeley, 1st baron Moynihan of Leeds (1865–1936), 370.
Mudrow [-Reichenow], Lili (1908–), 464.
Müller, Heinrich (1820–64), 533.
Müller, Johannes (1801–58), 42, 269, 287–8, 289, 299, 320, 321, 322, 582, 595, 634, 637.
Müller, Otto Friedrich (1730–84), 327.
Muir, Sir Robert (1864–1959), 637, 638–9.
Mundinus, see Mondino de' Luzzi.
Munk, Immanuel (1852–1903), 590, 602.
Murchison, Charles (1830–79), 731.
Murlin, John Raymond (1874–), 605.
Murphy, J. B. (1857–1916), 370.
Murphy, Joseph, London dentist (fl. 1837), 668.
Murphy, William Parry (1892–), 621, 622.
Murray, Mrs. A. M. T., 607.
Murray, E. G. D. (1890–), 403.
Murray, George Redmayne (1865–1939), 526.

Nabarro, David (1874–1958), 484–5.
Nachmansohn, David (1899–), 577.
Nägeli, Karl Wilhelm von (1817–91), 324.
Nagelschmidt, Karl [Franz] (1875–1952), 378.
Nageotte, Jean (1866–1948), 248.
Napoleon I, emperor of France, 73, 172.
Nasmyth, James (1808–90), 669.
Needham, John Turberville (1713–81), 328.
Neisser, Albert (1855–1916), 390, 391, 417.
Nelmes, Sarah, 201.
Nero, emperor of Rome, 675.
Neufeld, Fred (1861–1945), 401.
Neuschlosz, Simon M. (1893–), 575.
Newell Martin, Henry (1848–96), 375, 545.
Newman, Sir George (1870–1948), 223, 224.
Newsholme, Sir Arthur (1857–1943), 223.
Newton, Sir Isaac (1642–1727), 113, 145–7, 205, 641, 642, 748.
Nicolaier, Arthur (1862–?), 386, 391, 392.
Nicolle, Charles (1866–1936), 451.
Nightingale, Florence (1820–1910), 226, 503, 704–9.
Nocard, Edmond (1850–1903), 397.
Noguchi, Hideyo (1876–1928), 406, 428, 475–6, 478, 507.
Noon, Leonard (1878–1913), 430.

North, Elisha (1771–1843), 272.
Nothnagel, Günther (fl. 1894), 567.
Nott, Josiah Clark (1804–73), 468.
Nuttall, George H. F. (1862–1937), 410, 418.
Nye, Robert Nason (1892–1947), 448.

Obermeier, Otto (1843–73), 390, 391.
O'Brien, Irish giant, 543.
O'Dwyer, Joseph P. (1841–98), 655.
Ogston, Sir Alexander (1844–1929), 391, 392, 448.
Oliver, George (1841–1915), 538, 545, 556.
Opie, Eugene L. (1873–), 553, 639.
Ord, William Miller (1834–1902), 524.
Oré, Pierre Cyprien (1828–89), 350.
Oribasius (325–403), 68, 240.
Orr, John Boyd, 1st baron Boyd Orr of Brechin Mearns (1880–), 605, 609.
Osborne, Thomas Burr (1859–1929), 598, 612.
Osler, Sir William (1849–1919), 317, 367, 524.
Otto, Richard Ernst Wilhelm (1872–1952), 421.
Overton, Charles Ernest (1865–1933), 325.
Owen, Sir Richard (1804–92), 237, 535.
Owen Thomas, see Thomas, H. O.

Pacini, Filippo (1812–83), 270.
Paget, Sir James (1814–99), 636.
Palm, Theobald Adrian (1848?–1928), 614.
Panizza, Bartolomeo (1785–1867), 256.
Papanicolaou, George Nicholas (1883–1962), 550.
Paracelsus (1493–1541), 100–1, 108, 142, 504, 521, 672.
Paré, Ambroise (1510–90), 95–97, 175, 182, 240, 371, 646, 648, 649, 662.
Park, William H. (1863–1939), 436.
Parker, Frederic (1890–), 448.
Parkinson, James (1755–1824), 272.
Parmly, Levi Spear, American dentist working in London c. 1820, 670.
Parona, Corrado (1848–1922), 493.
Parona, Ernesto (1849–1902), 493.
Parry, Caleb Hillier (1755–1822), 273, 530, 532.
Pasteur, Louis (1822–95), 156, 235, 330–6, 337–41, 354, 379, 381, 395, 403, 410, 432, 433, 439, 647, 694.
Paterson, Marcus (1870–1932), 228.

Paul of Aegina (fl. 7th cent.), *68*, 71, 240–1.

Pavlov, Ivan Petrovitch (1849–1936), *266*–9, 302, 303, 600.

Pavy, Frederick William (1829–1911), *232*, 285, 296, 319.

Pearson, Karl (1857–1936), *726*, 733, 736.

Pecquet, Jean (1622–74), 123.

Pelletier, Pierre Joseph (1788–1842), *680*, 681.

Penfield, Wilder G. (1891–), 260.

Percival, Thomas (1740–1804), *189*, 194.

Perroncito, Edoardo (1847–1936), 493.

Peters, Sir Rudolph Albert, 308, 619.

Petit, F. Pourfour du, *see* Pourfour du Petit.

Petri, Richard Julius (1852–1921), 340.

Petroncellus (d. *c*. 1050), 71.

Pettenkofer, Max [Josef] von (1818–1901), *231*, 396, 583, 584–6, 588, 592, 604.

Petty, Sir William (1623–87), *179*–80.

Peyer, Johann Conrad (1653–1712), *204*, 631.

Pézard, Albert (?–1927), 550.

Pfaff, Philipp (1716–80), 666.

Pfeiffer, Richard F. J. (1858–1945), 391, *393*, 414, 459.

Pfiffner, Joseph John (1903–), 539.

Pflüger, Eduard (1829–1910), *237*, 309, 581, 589, 592, 598–9, 604.

Pfolspeundt, Heinrich von (fl. 1460), 181.

Phaer [Phayre], Thomas (1510?–1560), 651.

Philip II, king of Macedon, 41.

Philip, Sir Robert W. (1857–1939), 229.

Philiscus, 39.

Phipps, James, 200.

Phryesen, Laurentius (?–*c*. 1532), 241.

Physick, Philip Syng (1768–1837), *351*, 659.

Pilleau, Pezé (fl. 1715–55), 666.

Pinel, Philippe (1745–1826), 281, 282, *497*, 499, 501, 505, 630.

Piorry, Pierre Adolphe (1794–1879), 283.

Pirogoff, Nikolai Ivanovich (1810–81), 350.

Pirquet, Clemens von (1874–1929), *424*–5, 429.

Pitcairn, David (1749–1809), 632.

Pitcairne, Archibald (1652–1713), 280.

Pitres, Albert (1848–1927), 275.

Pitt, R. Margaret, 405.

Place, Francis (1771–1854), 712.

Plater, Felix (1536–1614), 497.

Plato, Greek philosopher, 28, 41, 43.

Plimmer, R. H. A. (1877–1955), 597.

Pliny the Elder (A.D. 23–79), 520, 522.

Plummer, Henry Stanley (1874–1937), *532*, 534.

Poiseuille, Jean Léonard Marie (1799–1869), 311.

Pollender, Franz Aloys Antoine (1800–79), 328, *336*, 391.

Polykleitos, 24.

Popielski, Leon, of Lemberg, 557, 558.

Popper, Erwin, 449.

Portal, Antoine, *baron* (1742–1832), 276.

Porterfield, William (fl. 1717–59), *641*–2.

Pott, Percivall (1714–88), 179.

Pouchet, Félix Archimède (1800–72), 329.

Poulton, E. P. (1883–1939), *306*, 307.

Pourfour du Petit, François (1664–1741), *260*–1.

Power, Frederick B. (1853–1927), 678.

Power, Sir William H. (1842–1916), 223.

Prásěk, Emil (1884–1934), 437.

Prausnitz, Wilhelm (1861–1933), 591.

Pravaz, C. G. (1791–1853), 686.

Price-Jones, Cecil (1863–1943), 318.

Prichard, J. C. (1786–1848), 506.

Priestley, J. G. (1880–1941), *306*–7.

Priestley, Joseph (1733–1804), *164*–6, 208.

Pringle, Sir John (1707–82), *184*, 185, 189, 194.

Prochaska, Georgius (1749–1820), 251.

Propertius, Latin poet, 55.

Proskauer, Bernhard (1851–1915), 400.

Prout, William (1785–1850), *157*, 297, 522.

Prowazek, Stanislaus von (1875–1915), *450*, 451.

Ptolemy I, Soter, king of Egypt, 48.

Ptolemy VI, Philometor, king of Egypt, 8.

Purkinje, Johannes Evangelista von (1787–1869), *246*, 321, 323, 324, 326, 552, 637.

Purmann, Matthäus Gottfried (1648–1721), 183.

Purves, Herbert Dudley, 530.

Pylarini, Giacomo (1659–1718), 200.

Pythagoras, Greek mathematician (*c*. 530 B.C.), 31.

Quetelet, Adolphe (1796–1874), *181*, 725.

Quincke, Heinrich (1842–1922), 249.

Raistrick, Harold (1890–), 695.

Ramazzini, Bernardino (1633–1714), 197.

Ramon, Gaston (1886–), *436*, 442.

Ramón y Cajal, Santiago (1852–1934), *248*, 250.

Ranke, Karl Ernst (1870–1926), 426.
Rankin, Allan Coats (1877–1959), 451.
Ranvier, Louis Antoine (1835–1922), 318.
Raphael, Italian painter, 88, 641.
Rayleigh [John William Strutt], 3rd baron (1842–1919), 649.
Reagh, A. L. (1871–1949), 404.
Réaumur, René A. F. de (1683–1757), 155–6, 157.
Recklinghausen, Friedrich von (1833–1910), 553, 636.
Redfern, Peter (1821–1912), 659.
Redi, Francesco (1626–97), 328.
Reed, Walter (1851–1902), 469–70, 476.
Regnault, Victor (1810–78), 581, 582, 587.
Rehn, Ludwig (1849–1930), 531, 534.
Reichstein, Tadeus (1897–), 540.
Reil, Johann Christian (1759–1813), 501.
Reiset, Jules (1811–?), 581, 582, 587.
Remak, Robert (1815–65), 246, 301, 314.
Rembrandt Harmensz van Rhyn, Dutch painter, 610.
Renshaw, Arnold, 451.
Retzius, Gustaf (1842–1919), 246.
Reverdin, Auguste (1848–1908), 525.
Reverdin, Jacques Louis (1842–1929), 373, 524, 525, 535.
Rhazes (d. c. 923), 74, 75, 77.
Richard of Accerra, 72.
Richard, Eugène (1844–1926), 457.
Richards, Alfred Newton (1876–), 302, 559.
Richardson, Sir Benjamin Ward (1828–96), 355.
Richet, Charles (1850–1935), 420–1.
Rickes, Edward Lawrence (1912–), 621.
Ricketts, Howard Taylor (1871–1910), 450–1.
Riddoch, George (1889–1947), 262.
Riesser, Otto L. M. (1882–1949), 575.
Rilliet, Frédéric (1814–61), 654.
Rindfleisch, Eduard (1836–1908), 636, 637.
Ringer, Sydney (1835–1910), 315, 626.
Riolan, Jean (1580–1657), 538.
Risien Russell, James Samuel (1863–1939), 276.
Ritchie, James (1864–1923), 639.
Riva-Rocci, Scipione (1863–1936), 312.
Rivers, Thomas Milton (1888–), 448.
Rivers, W. H. R. (1864–1922), 270.
Roberts, J. E. H. (1881–1948), 373.
Robertson, D. M. C. L. Argyll, see Argyll Robertson.
Robiquet, Pierre Jean (1780–1840), 681.

Robson, Sir Arthur W. Mayo (1853–1933), 370.
Rocha-Lima, Henrique da (1879–1956), 451.
Roe, John (1795–1874), 215.
Röntgen, Wilhelm Conrad (1845–1923), 374, 375, 376, 754.
Roger of Palermo (fl. c. 1170–1200), 522.
Rogers, Sir Leonard (1868–), 488, 494.
Rogoff, Julius Moses (1884–), 539.
Rokitansky, Karl von (1804–78), 171, 285–6, 633–4, 635, 636.
Rolando, Luigi (1773–1831), 255.
Rolleston, Sir Humphry Davy (1862–1944), 626.
Rollett, Joseph Pierre Martin (1824–94), 270.
Rollier, Auguste (1874–1954), 378, 379.
Romberg, Moritz Heinrich (1795–1873), 273, 274, 278.
Rosa, E. B. (1861–1921), 588.
Rosen von Rosenstein, Nils (1706–73), 652.
Rosenau, Milton J. (1869–1946), 234, 421.
Rosenblueth, Arturo Stearns (1900–), 571.
Rosenheim, Otto (1871–1955), 616.
Rosenthal, Isidor (1836–1915), 304.
Ross, Sir Ronald (1857–1932), 460–3, 470, 737.
Rouget, Jules (1864–1936), 441.
Roussy, Gustave (1874–1948), 262, 546.
Roux, Émile (1853–1933), 394, 397, 406, 411–12.
Rubner, Max (1854–1932), 583, 586–8, 599, 604, 605.
Rudbeck, Olof (1630–1702), 123, 628.
Rueff, Jacob (1500–58), 175.
Ruffini, Angelo (1864–1929), 270.
Runge, Friedlieb Ferdinand (1795–1867), 681.
Rush, Benjamin (1745–1813), 184, 190–1, 468, 501.
Ruska, Ernst August (1906–), 446.
Russell, J. S. Risien, see Risien Russell.
Ruysch, Frederik (1638–1731), 516, 628.
Ruzicka, Leopold (1887–), 550.

Sacco, Luigi (1769–1836), 202.
Saint-Yves, Charles de (1667–1736), 645.
Sakel, Manfred Joshua (1900–57), 511.
ben Salim, see Faraj ben Salim.
Salter, Hyde (1823–71), 428.
Sanctorius [Santorio Santorio] (1561–1636), 115–18, 138, 171, 313, 578.

Sanderson, Sir John S. Burdon (1828–1905), 232.

Sandifort, Eduard (1742–1814), 629.

Sandström, Ivar (1852–89), *535*, 536.

Santorio, Santorio, *see* Sanctorius.

Sargent, Sir Percy [William George] (1873–1933), 541.

Sargon, king of Assyria, 10.

Saucerotte, Nicolas (1741–1814), 542.

Sauerbruch, Ferdinand (1875–1951), 373.

Sauvages, François Boissier de la Croix de, *see* Boissier de Sauvages.

Savage, Sir William G. (1872–1961), 230.

Sawyer, Wilbur Augustus (1879–1951), *478–9*, 480.

Scarpa, Antonio (1747?–1832), *245–6*.

Schäfer, Edward Albert, *see* Sharpey-Schafer.

Schaudinn, Fritz (1871–1906), 391, *394*, 463, 689.

Scheele, Carl Wilhelm (1742–86), *165–6*.

Schick, Bela (1877–), 429, *434*.

Schiff, Moritz (1823–96), *520*, 525, 535.

Schleiden, Matthias Jacob (1804–81), *322*, 323, 324, 326.

Schmidt, Carl (1822–94), *582–3*, 584, 589.

Schmidt-Mülheim, Adolf (fl. 1880), 556.

Schmiedeberg, Oswald (1838–1921), 314, 565, *684*, 685.

Schneider, Conrad Viktor (1614–80), 542.

Schoenheimer, Rudolf (1898–1941), *320*, 601, 603.

Schönlein, Lucas (1793–1864), 328.

Schottmüller, [Adolf Alfred Louis George] Hugo (1867–1936), 391, *394*, 401, 402.

Schröder, Heinrich (1810–85), 329.

Schultz, Werner (1878–1944), *437*, 438.

Schultz, William Henry (1873–1955), 562.

Schultze, Max (1825–74), 325.

Schulze, Franz (1815–73), 329.

Schwann, Theodor (1810–82), 246, 288, *322–4*, 326, 329, 330, 333, 578, 635.

Schwarzbach, Saul (1902–), 548.

Schwenk, Erwin (1887–), 551.

Scot, Michael (1175?–1234?), 77.

Scot, Reginald (1538?–1599), 496.

Scott, Sir Harold (1874–1956), 620.

Scribonius Largus (*c.* A.D. 1–50), 669.

Seaton, Edward Cator (1815–80), 223.

Sebastian, Saint, 68.

Seebeck, Ludwig Friedrich W. A. (1805–49), 649.

Sellards, Andrew Watson (1884–1942), 477.

Semmelweis, Ignaz Philipp (1818–65), *360–1*.

Semon, Sir Felix (1849–1921), 525.

Sennert, Daniel (1572–1637), 203.

Sequeira, J. H. (1865–1948), *396*, 541.

Sertürner, Friedrich (1783–1841), 680.

Serveto [Servetus], Miguel (1511–53), *119*, 244.

Severino, Marco Aurelio (1580–1656), 628.

Shaftesbury, 7th earl of, *see* Cooper, Antony Ashley.

Shakespeare, William, dramatist, 40.

Shanks, Margaret, 607.

Sharpey, William (1802–80), 258, *352*.

Sharpey-Schafer, Sir Edward Albert (1850–1935), *258*, 260, 538, 539, 545, 546, 556.

Shattuck, Lemuel (1793–1859), 235.

Sherren, James (1872–1945), 270.

Sherrington, Sir Charles Scott (1857–1952), 253, 259, 260, *263–6*, 270, 442, 556.

Shiga, Kiyoshi (1870–1957), 391, *394*.

Shipway, Sir Francis (1875–), 348.

Shorb, Mary Shaw (1907–), 621.

Shortt, H. E. (1887–), 464.

Shovell, Sir Clowdisley (1650–1707), 186.

Sicard, J. A. (1872–1929), 375.

Sick, Paul (1836–1900), 523.

Simmonds, Morris (1855–1925), 544.

Simmonds, Nina (1893–), 616.

Simon, Gustav (1824–76), 365.

Simon, Sir John (1816–1904), *219–20*, 223, 231, 520, 717.

Simonart, André (1903–), 576.

Simond, Paul Louis (1858–1947), 490.

Simpson, Sir James Young (1811–70), *344*, 659.

Sims, James Marion (1813–83), 362.

Skoda, Josef (1805–81), 285, *286*, 633.

Slyke, D. D. Van, *see* Van Slyke.

Smellie, William (1697–1763), 176.

Smith, Ernest Lester, *see* Lester Smith.

Smith, Sir Grafton Elliot (1871–1937), 246.

Smith, James Lorrain, *see* Lorrain Smith.

Smith, Morris Isidore (1887–1951), 619.

Smith, Philip Edward (1884–), *547*, 548.

Smith, Theobald (1859–1934), 398, 404, *420–1*, 561.

Smith, T. Southwood (1788–1861), 194, *210*, 213, 214, 215, 217, 218, 219.

Smith, Wilson (1897–), 449.

Snellen, Herman (1834–1908), 643.
Snow, John (1813–58), 219, 345–7, 350, 729, 730–1.
Soames, Katharine Marjorie, 617.
Soboleff, L. V. (1876–1919), 554.
Soemmerring, Samuel Thomas von (1755–1830), 245.
Sommerkamp, Hermann (fl. 1928), 575.
Soper, H. E. (1865–1930), 737.
Soranus of Ephesus (fl. A.D. 98–138), 239–40, 241, 494, 650.
Soubeiran, Eugène (1793–1858), 344.
Southard, Elmer Ernest (1876–1920), 561.
Southwood Smith, see Smith, T. Southwood.
Spallanzani, Lazaro (1729–99), 156–7, 328, 395, 578.
Spencer Wells, see Wells, Sir T. Spencer.
Spiro, Karl (1867–1932), 682.
Sprenger, Jakob, Dominican monk, 495.
Spurzheim, Johann [Christoph] Caspar (1776–1832), 254–5, 256.
Stahl, G. E. (1660–1734), 143–4, 148, 163, 504.
Stanley, W. M. (1904–), 447.
Stannius, Hermann (1808–83), 314.
Stannus, H. S. (1877–1957), 620.
Stanton, Sir (Ambrose) Thomas (1875–1938), 611.
Starling, E. H. (1866–1927), 302, 315, 316, 518–19. 555, 556, 558.
Steinach, Eugen (1861–1944), 549–50.
Stellwag von Carion, Carl (1823–1904), 533.
Stensen [Steno], Niels (1638–86), 516.
Stephens, J. W. W. (1865–1946), 459, 486.
Stepp, Wilhelm Otto (1882–), 616.
Stewart, G. N. (1860–1930), 539.
Stewart, Matthew J. (1885–1956), 639.
Still, Sir George Frederick (1868–1941), 655.
Stockard, Charles R. (1879–1939), 550.
Stohmann, Friedrich (1832–97), 587.
Stokes, Adrian (1887–1927), 476–7.
Stokes, Sir George Gabriel (1819–1903), 319.
Stokes, William (1804–78), 283, 531, 532, 533, 534, 653.
Stoll, Arthur (1887–), 682.
Stoll, Maximilian (1742–87), 280.
Stolz, Friedrich (1860–1936), 539.
Stradanus, see Van der Straet.
Strohmer, Friedrich (fl. 1883), 603.
Stromeyer, Louis (1804–76), 185, 658.

Strutt, J. W., see Rayleigh, 3rd baron.
'Student', see Gosset, W. S.
Succi, professional faster, 590.
Süssmilch, Johann Peter (1707–67), 180–1.
Swammerdam, Jan (1637–80), 50, 129, 133–5, 149, 153.
Swieten, G. L. B. van, see van Swieten.
Swingle, Wilbur Willis (1891–), 539.
Swinton, A. A. Campbell (1863–1930), 375.
Sydenham, Thomas (1624–89), 106, 110–11, 203, 272, 280, 455, 505, 655, 728–9, 735.
Sylvius, Franciscus [F. De le Boë] (1614–72), 142–3, 144, 149, 297, 651.
Syme, James (1799–1870), 344, 351–2, 659.
Symonds, Sir Charles (Putnam) (1890–), 279.
Szent-Györgyi, Albert (1893–), 619, 622.

Tagliacozzi, Gaspare (1545–99), 98, 99, 373.
Tait, Lawson (1845–99), 362.
Takaki, K., baron (1849–1915), 611.
Takamine, J. (1854–1922), 538.
Talbert, G. A. (1865–1947), 258.
Taveau, René de M., 567.
Taylor, John, 'Chevalier' (1703–72), 648.
Thackeray, W. M. novelist, 467.
Thackrah, Charles Turner (1795–1833), 197.
Thaddeus of Florence [Taddeo Alderotti] (1223–1303), 79, 80.
Theiler, Max (1899–), 477–8, 479, 480.
Theodoric, bp. of Cervia (1205–98), 79.
Theophrastus (372–287 B.C.), 47.
Theseus, 26.
Thiersch, Karl (1822–95), 373.
Thoma, Richard (1847–1923), 636.
Thomas, Hugh Owen (1834–91), 659.
Thomson, John (1856–1926), 655.
Thorn, George Widmer (1906–), 540.
Thorne-Thorne, Sir Richard (1841–99), 223.
Thorpe, William Veale (1902–), 560.
Thoth, 5.
Thucydides, Greek historian, 488.
Thudichum, Ludwig (1829–1901), 319.
Tiberius, emperor of Rome, 52.
Tiedemann, Friedrich (1781–1861), 297.
Timoni, Emanuel (fl. 1713–21), 200.
Tissandier, Gaston (1843–99), 304.
Todd, Edgar William (1889–1950), 402.

Todd, John Lancelot (1876–1949), *483*–4.
Todd, Robert Bentley (1809–60), 273.
Töpfer, Hans Willi (1876–?), 452.
Töpler, —, 305.
Tomes, Sir Charles Sissmore (1846–1928), 668.
Tomes, Sir John (1815–95), *663*, 668.
Tooth, Howard H. (1856–1925), 275.
Topley, W. W. C. (1886–1944), *738*–9.
Torre, Marcantonio della (1473–1506), 89.
Tragus, H., *see* Bock, H.
Traube, Ludwig (1818–76), 637.
Trembley, Abraham (1710–84), 321.
Trendelenburg, Friedrich (1844–1924), 350.
Treves, Sir Frederick (1853–1923), 366.
Trotter, Thomas (1761–1832), *187*–8, 505.
Trotter, Wilfred (1872–1939), 270.
Trousseau, Armand (1801–67), 274, *282*, 517, 531, 535, 614, 654.
Truman, Edwin (1809–1905), 667.
Türck, Ludwig (1810–68), *248*–9, 273.
Tuke, Henry (1755–1814), 500.
Tuke, William (1732–1822), *497*, 499, 500.
Tulloch, W. J. (1887–), 441.
Tulp, Nicolaas (1593–1674), 610.
Twort, F. W. (1877–1950), 391, *395*, 406, 407, 696.
Tyndall, John (1820–93), 335.

Uhlenhuth, Eduard (1885–), 548.
Underwood, Michael (1736–1820), *226*, 272, 652, 653.
Urey, H. C. (1893–), 601.

Vaillard, Louis (1850–1935), 441.
Valentin, G. G. (1810–83), 324, 326, *481*.
Valsalva, Antonio Maria (1666–1723), 246, *628*–9.
Van der Straet [Stradanus], Jan (1523 [or 1536] –1605), 108, 109.
Van Deventer, H. (1651–1724), 177.
Van Slyke, D. D. (1883–), 310–11, *597*.
van Swieten, Gerard L. B. (1700–72), 183, *280*.
Vaquez, Henri (1860–1936), 317.
Varolio, Costanzo (1543–75), 244.
Varrier-Jones, Sir Pendrill (1883–1941), *230*.
Vartiainen, Armas (1901–), 573.
Vassale, Giulio (1862–1912), 536.
Vaughan, V. C. (1851–1929), 561.
Vedder, E. B. (1878–1952), 494.
Velpeau, A. A. L. M. (1795–1867), 341.

Vesalius, Andreas (1514–64), 81, *90*–95, 97, 98, 101, 145, 150, 242–3, 244, 497, 640.
Vesling, Johann (1598–1649), 516.
Vespasian, emperor of Rome, 53.
Vianna, Gaspar de (1885–1914), 487.
Vierordt, Karl (1818–84), *313*, 318, 622.
Vieussens, Raymond (1641–1715), *245*, 628.
Vieusseux, Gaspard (1746–1814), 272.
Vigo, Giovanni da [John of Vigo] (1460–1520), 182.
Villemin, Jean Antoine (1827–92), *396*–8.
Vincent de Paul, Saint (1576–1660), 702.
Vinci, Leonardo da (1452–1519), *89*–90, 241.
Vines, H. W. C. (1893–), 541.
Virchow, Rudolf [Ludwig Karl] (1821–1902), 247, 288, 303, 325, 326, 353, 381, 387, 535, *634*–5, 636, 637, 640, 749, 750.
Vives, Juan Luis (1492–1540), 496.
Voegtlin, Carl (1879–1960), 536.
Voges, O. (fl. 1898), 400.
Vogt, Marthe (1903–), 575.
Vogt, W. (fl. 1907), 557.
Voit, Carl von (1831–1908), *583*–6, 588, 590, 591, 592, 594, 598, 599, 600, 602, 603, 604, 605.
Voit, Erwin (1852–1932), 583, *591*, 604.
Volkmann, Alfred Wilhelm (1800–77), *261*, 313, 428.
Volkmann, Richard von (1830–89), 365.
Volta, Alessandro (1745–1827), *159*–61, 289.
Voronoff, Serge (1866–1951), 550.

Wagner, Richard (1813–83), 466.
Wagner, Rudolph (1805–64), 321.
Wagner-Jauregg, Julius von (1857–1940), 511.
Waksman, S. A. (1888–), 697.
Waldeyer-Hartz, Wilhelm (1836–1921), 247.
Waller, Augustus Volney (1816–70), *249*, 353.
Walshe, Sir Francis (1885–), 279.
Walther, Otto (1853–1919), 228.
Warburg, Otto (1883–), *620*, 622.
Wardrop, James (1782–1869), 646.
Wassermann, August von (1866–1925), *390*, 417.
Waterhouse, Benjamin (1754–1846), 202.
Watson, Sir Patrick Heron (1832–1907), 534.

Waugh, W. A., 619.
Wawra, Cecil Z., 622.
Webb, J. Leyden (1914–), 622.
Weber, Eduard Friedrich (1806–71), *313*, 568.
Weber, Ernst Heinrich (1795–1878), *313*, 568.
Webster, L. T. (1894–1943), 740.
Wecker, Louis de (1832–1906), 648.
Weddell, Graham, 271.
Weichselbaum, Anton (1845–1920), 391, *393*.
Weigert, Carl (1845–1904), 636.
Weil, Adolf (1848–1916), 475.
Weil, Edmund (1880–1922), 404.
Weil, Richard (1876–1917), 563.
Welch, William Henry (1850–1934), 391, *394*, 637.
Wellcome, Sir Henry S. (1853–1936), 555.
Wells, Harry Gideon (1875–1943), 562, *638*.
Wells, Horace (1815–48), *343*, 349.
Wells, Sir T. Spencer (1818–97), *362*, 363, 364.
Wells, William Charles (1757–1817), 632.
Welsh, D. A. (1865–1948), 536.
Wenyon, C. M. (1878–1948), *488*, *493.*
Wepfer, J. J. (1620–95), *271*–2, 542, 628.
Werner, Heinrich (1874–?), 451.
Wernicke, Carl (1848–1905), 277.
West, Charles (1816–98), *653*, 657.
Westphal, Carl (1833–90), *252*, 275.
Wharton, Thomas (1614–73), *516*, 519.
Whipple, George Hoyt (1878–), *621*, 622.
Whistler, Daniel (1619–84), 613.
White, Charles (1728–1813), 361.
Whytt, Robert (1714–66), *251*, 655.
Widal, Fernand (1862–1929), 399, *418*.
Wiggers, Carl John (1883–), 627.
Wilder, Russell Morse (1885–1959), 538.
Wilkins, John (1614–72), 698.
Wilks, Sir Samuel (1824–1911), *285*, 517, 637.
Willan, Robert (1757–1812), *204*, 281.
William of Saliceto (c. 1210– c. 1280), 79.
Williams, Robert R. (1886–), 619.
Willis, Thomas (1621–75), 242, *245*, 254, 260, 272, 428, 507, 545, 552.

Wilson, Sir G. S. (1895–), 738.
Wilson, S. A. Kinnier, *see* Kinnier Wilson.
Windaus, Adolf (1876–1959), *557*, 619.
Winslow, J. B. (1669–1760), *245*, 260.
Winterbottom, T. M. (1765?–1859), 482.
Wirsung, Georg (1600–43), 516.
Wiseman, Richard (1622?–76), 183.
Withering, William (1741–99), 683.
Wöhler, Friedrich (1800–82), *238*, 319, 336, 681.
Wolbach, Simeon Burt (1880–1954), *451*, 617.
Wollaston, William Hyde (1766–1828), 595.
Wood, Alexander (1817–84), 686, *687*.
Woodall, John (1556?–1643), 186.
Woodruff, Alice Miles, 448.
Woodruff, H. B., 697.
Woods, Charles Dayton (1856–1925), 604.
Woodworth, John M. (1837–79), *233*–4.
Woollard, H. H. (1889–1939), 271.
Wren, Sir Christopher (1632–1723), 698.
Wright, Sir Almroth (1861–1947), *419*, 444.
Wright, James Homer (1870–1928), 487.
Wunderlich, Carl A. (1815–77), 626.
Wyer [Weyer], Johann (1515–88), 496.

Yamagiwa, K. (1863–1930), 637.
Yersin, Alexandre (1863–1943), 381, 391, *394*, 411–12, 489, 491.
Yorke, Warrington (1883–1943), 486.
Young, F. G. (1908–), 549.
Young, Thomas (1773–1829), 300, *642*, 648–9.
Yule, G. Udny (1871–1951), 444.

Ziegler, Ernst (1849–1905), *636*, 638.
Zilva, S. S., 617, 618, 622.
Zingher, Abraham (1885–1927), *434*, 436.
Zoeller, Christian (1888–1934), 442.
Zondek, Bernhard (1891–), *547*, 551.
Zoser, king of Egypt, 6.
Zuelzer, Georg L. (1870–1949), 554.
Zuntz, Nathan (1847–1920), *309*, 589, 590, 591, 593.

3 G

INDEX OF SUBJECTS AND PLACES

abator, 25.
Abdominal surgery, 362–6.
Abdominal tumours, 284, 317.
Aberdeen, 210, 257, 361, 392, 659.
Abscess of lung, *see* Lung.
Acacia, 673.
Académie de Médecine, Paris, 335, 397.
Académie des Sciences, Paris, 329, 334, 509, 645.
Acapnia, 309.
Accessory food factors, 612. *See also* Vitamins.
Acclimatization at high altitudes, 308–10.
Acetylcholine, 566–77; leech test for, 573.
Achaeans, 18.
Achilles, tendon of, 185, 658.
Achondroplasia, 36.
Achorion Schönleinii, 328.
Acids, 142, 143, 157, 165; in therapeutics, 676.
Acromegaly, 542–3, 548.
A.C.T.H., *see* Adrenocorticotropic hormone.
Actinomyces bovis, 391.
Actinomycin, 697.
Actinomycosis, 390, 391, 392.
Action current, in nerves, 290.
Active principles, of drugs, 676, 679–84.
Acute yellow atrophy of liver, *see* Liver.
Addison's anaemia, *see* Pernicious anaemia.
Addison's disease, 517.
Adenosine diphosphate, 294.
Adenosine triphosphate, 294.
Adipose tissue, 324.
Adrenal glands, 285, 396, 517–18, 538–41, 545, 548, 566.
Adrenaline, 316, 538, 545, 565, 566, 568, 570, 571, 572.
'Adrenergic' fibres, 572.
Adrenocorticotropic hormone (A.C.T.H.), 548.
Adreno-genital syndrome, 540–1.
Aëdes aegypti, 469, 471, 472, 473–4.
Aëdes mosquitoes, 461, 469–74, 476–8.
Aegina, 68.
Aerotonometer, Pflüger's, 309.
Agar-agar, 340.

Agglutination, 405, 417; in blood transfusion, 700–1.
Agglutinins, 417–18, 420.
Agriculture, 191, 196.
Ague, *see* Malaria.
Air, composition of, 161–8; effects of vitiated, 305; weight of, 136.
Air-pump, of Boyle, 136–7, 161.
Akron, Ohio, U.S.A., 529.
Alabama, U.S.A., 468, 471.
Alanine, 597.
Alchemy, 135, 522.
Alcohol, as anaesthetic, 341.
Alexandria, 59, 68; School of, 48–51.
Alkali, 143.
Alkaloids, 679–83.
Allergic diseases, 427–30, 563.
Allergy, 427, 429.
'All-or-none' law, 289, 314.
All Saints Sisterhood, 704.
Almond oil, 673.
Aloes, 673.
Alton, Hants, 378.
Alum, 673.
Alum precipitated toxoid (A.P.T.), 436.
Alveolar air, 306.
Amboceptor, *see* Immune body.
Ambulance, of Larrey, 184.
American Civil War, 185, 277, 709.
American Physiological Society, 554.
Amiens, France, 98.
Amino-acids, 275, 320, 595, 596, 597, 598, 601; conversion of, into glucose, 604.
Ammonia, 165.
Ammoniacum, 673, 674.
Amoebiasis, 493–4.
Amputation, 96, 182, 183, 184, 352, 356–7.
Amsterdam, Holland, 516, 610, 628.
Amyl nitrite, 685.
Amyotrophic lateral sclerosis, 274.
Anabolism, 578.
Anaemia, 282; experimental, 639; pernicious, *see* Pernicious anaemia.
Anaerobic organisms, 387, 395–6.
Anaesthesia, 341–51, 352; origin of the word, 351.
Anaesthetics, in the *Pharmacopoeia*, 678.
Analytical Psychology, School of, 514.

Anaphylatoxin, 562, 563.
Anaphylaxis, 420–2, 430, 561–4; cellular theory of, 562; humoral theory of, 562.
Anatomical injection, 242, 516.
Anatomy, 4, 12, 48–50, 150–1, 236–7, 241–50, 286, 322, 325, 351, 497; comparative, 41, 178, 236–7, 287, 325; of Galen, 59, 61–62; medieval, 78–83; of nervous system, 241–50; renaissance of, 88–95, 97–98.
Anatomy Act (1832), 210.
Ancoats and Ardwick Dispensary, Manchester, see Hospitals.
Androsterone, 550.
Aneurine, see Vitamin B₁.
Aneurysm, 178, 184, 197, 284, 285, 352, 630.
Angina pectoris, 278, 530, 625–6, 629, 684–5, 721.
Angiography, 752.
Aniline dyes, 318, 688, 689, 692.
Animalcules, 327, 328.
Animal electricity, 158, 159.
Animal magnetism, 509.
Animal remedies, 14–15.
Animism, 17, 29; of Stahl, 504.
Aniseed, 673.
Ankylostomiasis, see Hookworm disease.
Ann Arbor, see Michigan, University of.
Annuities, 180.
Annular bodies, see Malaria parasite.
Anopheles mosquitoes, 461, 462.
Anoxaemia, 307, 308.
Anthrax, 335–9, 379, 380, 390, 391.
Anthrax bacillus, 336–8, 391, 403, 417, 432, 696.
Antibiotics, 491, 688, 693–7.
Antibody, 420.
Antigen, 420.
Antihistaminic drugs, 564.
Antimeningococcal serum, 403.
Antimony, 8, 677.
Antiphlogistic treatment, 282.
Antiscorbutics, see Lemon juice, Lime juice, Vegetables.
Antiseptic surgery, 335, 352, 357–8. See also Surgery, Listerian revolution in.
Antiseptics, 184.
Antitoxins, 411–14, 420, 679. See also Diphtheria antitoxin.
Antityphoid vaccine, 419.
Aorta, 283, 373.
Aortic disease, 245, 283, 628.

Aosta, Italy, 521.
Aphasia, 276–7, 632.
Aphorisms, of Hippocrates, 36–38, 386.
Apnoea, 304, 306.
Apoplexy, 38, 76, 239, 240, 272, 273, 278, 754.
Appendicitis, 365–6, 638.
Apulia, Italy, 71, 503.
Aquapendente, Italy, 97.
Aqueduct, of Fallopius, 244.
Aqueducts of Rome, 56.
Arabian medicine, see Medicine.
Arachis oil, 674.
Archaeus, of Paracelsus, 100–1.
Archaei, of van Helmont, 142.
Archangel, U.S.S.R., 493.
Areolar tissue, 324.
Arezzo, Italy, 328.
Argyll Robertson pupil, 275.
Arles, France, 53.
Armies, disease in, see Medicine, military.
Arnott's smokeless grate, 210.
Arnott's valve, 210.
Arrow-poison, of Java, 680.
Arsenic, 673, 689.
Art, renaissance of, 88.
Arterenol, see nor-adrenaline.
Arteries, 48, 49.
Arteriocapillary fibrosis, 285.
Arthritis, 275. See also Rheumatoid arthritis.
Arthus phenomenon, 421.
Artificial eyes, 649.
Artificial limbs, 96–97.
Artificial pneumothorax, 230, 372–3.
Artificial teeth, 661–2, 663–7, 670.
Arytenoid cartilages, 241.
Asafetida, 674.
Ascorbic acid, see Vitamin C.
Aseptic surgery, 354–60, 366–7.
Asklepieia, 24–25, 57–58.
Aspirin, 683.
Assyria, 10, 15, 20. See also Mesopotamia.
Asthma, bronchial, 428, 430, 753; cardiac, 632.
Astigmatic lenses, 643.
Astigmatism, 642, 643.
Astor Committee, 229.
Astrology, 61.
Astronomy, 20, 60–61, 92, 112, 113–14, 145–6.
Asylums, for insane, 496, 502, 503.
Atebrine, see Mepacrine.

Athens, Greece, 26, 28, 41, 45.
Atmospheric pressure, effect of, on body functions, 304.
Atomic theory, of Democritus, 49, 51.
Atoxyl, 689.
Atrio-ventricular groove, 315.
Atrio-ventricular node, 301.
Atropine, 567, 571, 573, 680, 681.
Attenuation, of virulence, 432.
Augsburg, Germany, 516.
Augustinian sisters, 702.
Aura, in epilepsy, 239.
Aureomycin, 697.
Auricular fibrillation, 624.
Auriculo-ventricular, see Atrio-ventricular.
Auscultation, of chest, 172–4, 283, 286.
Australian Q fever, 451.
Autogenous vaccines, 419.
Autonomic ganglia, 260, 262, 566.
Autonomic nervous system, 260–2, 565, 566, 573. See also Sympathetic nervous system.
Avignon, France, 83.
Axon, of nerve-fibre, 246, 247.

Babylonia, 15, 20. See also Mesopotamia.
Bacilli, 331, 333; of cholera, diphtheria, dysentery, gas-gangrene, influenza, leprosy, paratyphoid, plague, tetanus, typhoid, whooping-cough, see under the individual diseases.
Bacillus, of contagious abortion, see Brucella abortus; of tuberculosis, see Tubercle bacillus.
Bacillus abortus, see Brucella abortus; B. aerogenes, 399; B. anthracis, see Anthrax bacillus; B. coli, 387, 391, 393, 399–400; B. icteroides, 474; B. mallei, 391; B. proteus X19, 404.
Bacteria, 131, 327, 328, 331, 333; types and varieties of, 396.
Bacterial endocarditis, 285, 317.
Bacterial mutation and variation, 403–6.
Bacteriology, 231, 326–41, 379–409.
Bacteriolysins, 420.
Bacteriolysis, 393, 401–2, 406–7, 414–16.
Bacteriophage, 391, 395, 406–7, 696.
Baghdad, 74.
Balloon ascents, 304.
Baltimore, Maryland, U.S.A., 317, 367, 424, 532; association of, parathyroid hypertrophy with renal rickets and dwarfism, first shown at, 536; —, diabetes with degeneration of islets, shown at, 553; desoxycorticosterone implantation developed at, 540; ex-flagellation in malaria parasite first seen at, 461; goitrogenic action of cabbage first shown at, 529–30; Institute for the History of Medicine established at, 394; isolated mammalian heart first studied at (1880), 315; nerve block as anaesthetic method first used at, 349; pharmacology chair established at, 685; pneumoencephalography and ventriculography introduced at, 279; pressor effect of posterior pituitary extract shown at, 545; yellow fever at, 467. See also Hospitals, Johns Hopkins University.
Bandaging, 34–35.
Baquet, of Mesmer, 508, 509.
Barber-Surgeons, of London, 186; of York, 101–2.
Barbiturates, 350.
Barcelona, Spain, 67.
Barium meal, 375.
Barmen, Germany, 366.
Base, chemical, 142, 143.
Basedow's disease, 532. See also Hyperthyroidism.
Basle (Basel), Switzerland, 247, 638; anatomical and botanical classics published at, 91, 103; anatomical theatre and botanical garden established at, 497; apoplexy, shown due to cerebral haemorrhage at, 271–2; lectures in vernacular at, 100; natural diets shown (1881) to contain unknown substances at, 610.
Batavia, Dutch East Indies, 610, 611.
Bath, Somerset, 273, 530, 625, 670.
Bathurst, Gambia, 483.
Battersea, London, 227.
'Bayer 205', see Suramin.
B.C.G. vaccine, 230, 426–7.
Beer, 7, 330–2, 335.
Belladonna, 674.
Belle Isle, expedition to, 183.
Bell's palsy, see Facial paralysis.
'Bends', in muscles, 311.
Benzoic acid, 603.
Benzyl penicillin, 696.
Bergen, Norway, 390.

Beri-beri, 527, 610–11, 612, 613, 618, 619.
Berkeley, California, U.S.A., 547.
Berkeley, Glos., 200.
Berlin, 246, 378, 437, 620, 741; bacteriologists at, 387, 392, 393, 394, 395, 400; chemists at, 329, 550, 595–6; diphtheria antitoxin first used at, 434; first virus pictures made at, 446; histologists at, 543, 553; ophthalmologists at, 647; pathologists at, 303, 599, 614, 634; physicians at, 273, 275, 328, 393, 451, 554, 615, 654; physiologists at, 287, 289, 309, 321, 322, 563, 579, 586, 589, 593, 602, 634; surgeons at, 365, 373, 390, 392. See also Hospitals.
Bermuda, 467.
Bern, Switzerland, 374, 481, 520, 523.
Bethesda, Maryland, 235.
Bethlehem Hospital ('Bedlam'), 496, 499, 507.
Bethnal Green, London, 213.
Betz cells, 259.
Beveridge Report, 743.
Bible, The, 494.
Bibliotheca Osleriana, 317.
Bidder's ganglion, 314.
Bile, 46, 138, 552, 583.
Bile pigments, 319.
Bills of Mortality, 180, 189.
Biochemistry, 231, 237–8, 287, 288, 319–20; textbooks of, 319, 581.
Biometry, 721–7.
Bird malaria, see Malaria.
Birmingham, 193, 619, 683.
Birth control, 712.
Birth palsy (Erb-Duchenne), 274.
Birth-rate, 718, 720.
Births, notification of, 226–7; registration of, 714.
Births and Deaths Registration Act (1874), 714.
Bithynia, province of Roman Empire, 51, 53.
Black Death, see Plagues.
Bladder, nervous control of, 262–3; stone in, see Vesical calculus.
Blindness, 225, 650.
Blood, 46, 49, 50, 138, 316–19, 596, 597, 639; circulation of, 65, 118, 119–23, 129, 142, 155, 244, 311–16, 698; coagulation of, 317, 318, 699–700; red corpuscles of, see Erythrocytes.
Blood count, 318.

Blood gas pump, mercurial, 301, 590; of Töpler, 305.
Blood groups, 700–1.
Blood-letting, 282. See also Venesection, Leeching.
Blood platelets, 317–18.
Blood pressure, 155, 311–13.
Blood sugar, 548–9, 552.
Blood transfusion, 698–701.
Blood velocity, 155, 310, 311, 313.
Board of Admiralty, 187, 188.
Board of Control, 503.
Board of Education, 224–5.
Board of Sick and Wounded Seamen, 187.
Boards of Guardians, 213.
Body constituents, dynamic state of, 320, 601.
Body posture, control of, 266.
Boer War, 444.
Bologna, Italy, 83, 169, 651; 'animal electricity' discovered at, 159; early anatomy at, 78–80; medical faculty at, since 1156, 78; microscopical research at, 124; Montpellier derived traditions from, 80; pharmacopoeia published at (1574), 672; research on ear at, 628–9; surgical school established at (c. 1270), 79.
Bolton, Lancs., 229, 716.
Bombay, 484.
Bone grafting, 366, 659.
Bone, growth of, 152, 368, 657, 659; —, pathology of, 636.
Bone marrow, 542, 639.
Bones, see Osteology.
Bonn, Germany, 321, 638, 655; animal cell, nature of first clearly defined at, 325; lymph gland infection in syphilis shown at, 395; pathological anatomy at, 636; pharmacological institute founded at (1869), 684; respiration, essential role of tissues in, shown at, 237.
Bony labyrinth, 239. See also Labyrinth.
Bordeaux, France, 53.
Boston, Mass., U.S.A., 371, 597, 600, 621, 659; early use of general anaesthetics at, 343, 344, 351; health department at, 235; Marine Hospital at, 233; yellow fever at, 467. See also Hospitals.
Botanical gardens, see Physic gardens.
Botany, 47, 69, 103, 104.
Botrytis bassiana, 328.
Botulism, 391.

Boulogne, France, 273, 274.
Boyle's law, 136.
Bradford, Yorks., 224.
Brain, 62, 93, 239, 319; 'erysipelas' of the, 240; views on, of Aristotle, 43; —, of Herophilus and Erasistratus, 48, 50, 239; —, of Leonardo da Vinci, 90. *See also* Cerebral convolutions, Cerebral cortex, Cerebral hemispheres, Cerebral localization, Cerebral peduncles, Neurology.
Brain abscess, 240, 367, 368, 628.
Brain tumour, 368, 371, 507.
Brandenburg, Germany, 394.
Breast feeding, 652.
Breslau, Silesia, 240, 336, 390, 393, 424, 637.
Bridgwater, Somerset, 455.
Bright's disease, *see* Nephritis.
Bristol, Glos., 284, 731.
British Pharmaceutical Codex (B.P.C.), 674-5.
Broad Street pump, 730.
Bronchiectasis, 631.
Bronchiole constriction, 557, 561
Bronchitis, 721, 753.
Bronze Age, 1.
Brown Institution, London, 395, 525.
Brucella abortus, 385.
Brucellosis, 384-6, 453.
Brucine, 681.
Brunner's glands, 552.
Brunonian theory, 148.
Brussels, Belgium, 90, 142, 414, 715.
Buboes, 492.
Bucharest, Romania, 277.
Buchner tube, 396
Buckinghamshire, England, 226.
Budapest, Hungary, 511.
Buenos Aires, Argentine, 548.
Bugs, as transmitters of Chagas's disease, 487, 488.
Bundle of His, 452, 623.
Burial grounds, 55, 217.
Burnley, Lancs., 623.
Butter, 330, 578, 602, 608, 612, 613.
Byzantium, 68, 73. *See also* Constantinople.

Cabbage, as goitrogen, 530.
Cachexia strumipriva, 525.
Caesarean section, 55.
Caffa, Crimea, 488.

Caffeine, 681.
Cairo, Egypt, 119, 493.
Caisson disease, 304, 305.
Caius College *see* Gonville and Caius.
Cajuput, 674.
Calciferol, 615.
Calcination, 166.
Calcium, 536-7.
Calcium cyanide, 490.
Calculating machine, of Babbage, 289.
Calculi, 628.
Calcutta, 461.
Caledonia, H.M.S., 221.
California Institute of Technology, 601.
California, University of, 602, 618.
Calomel, 677.
Calorimeter, Atwater-Rosa, 588-9, 591, 593, 594; bomb, 586; ice, 166; physiological, 581, 585-7; Thomson, 585.
Cambridge, England, 120, 275, 315, 409, 618; foundation of Gonville and Caius College at, 740; physiology at, 555, 564; regius professors of physic at, 123, 626; research on the autonomic system at, 262; —, foodstuffs at, 606; —, muscle at, 292; —, the nerve impulse at, 289, 290; —, respiration at, 304, 305 ff.; —, vitamins at, 619.
Canada, 232, 236.
Cancer, 754; death-rates from, 1896-1955, 720; in chimney sweeps, 179; in X-ray workers, 377; of liver, mentioned in the *Aphorisms*, 37; recent increase in, 721; surgery of, 363-5.
Cancer research, 637-8, 751-2.
Cannabis indica, 673, 674. *See also* Indian hemp.
Cannes, France, 425.
Cannstadt, Germany, 272.
Cantharides, 674.
Capillaries, 261, 262; action of H-substance (of Lewis) on, 560; demonstrated by Malpighi, 121, 124-5; effect of histamine on, 557, 559; illustrated by Leeuwenhoek, 130; Krogh's work on, 307; shown to possess power of constricting and dilating, 155.
Capillary electrometer, 289, 290.
Capsicum, 674.
Caraway, 674.
Carbohydrate metabolism, 296.
Carbohydrates, 578, 579, 581, 583, 585, 587, 591, 593, 601; as source of

Carbohydrates (*cont.*)
muscular energy, 594; conversion of, into fat, 603; conversion of protein into, 604; requirement of, in normal diet, 604, 608, 609.
Carbolic acid, 354–5.
Carbolic acid spray, of Lister, 355–6, 363, 367.
Carbon, 238, 584.
Carbon dioxide, 142, 163–4, 168, 238, 304–9, 581, 582, 584; used as 'anaesthetic' by Hickman, 342.
Carbon monoxide, 165, 298, 305.
Carboxyhaemoglobin, 308.
Cardamoms, 673.
Cardiac catheterization, 752.
Cardiac dilatation, 197.
Cardiac murmurs, *see* Heart murmurs.
Cardiac muscle, 134, 316.
Cardiazol, 511.
Cardiff, Wales, 607, 608.
Carnegie Institution, Boston, Mass., 600.
Carotene, 616.
Carotenoid pigments, 319.
Carotid sinus, 314.
Carpo-pedal spasm, 535.
Carrel-Dakin solution, 320.
Carriers, 407–9.
Carthage, 71.
Cartilage, 323.
Cascara sagrada, 674.
Casein, 598.
Cassia, 673, 674.
Castor-oil, 673.
Castration, 516, 517, 550.
Cataract, 83, 640, 643–5, 646, 647.
Catechu, 674.
Catgut, 359.
Cathode-ray tube, as amplifier, 290.
Cattle plague, 732.
Caudate nucleus, 243.
Cauterization, 8, 76, 79, 96–97, 182, 668.
Cell division, 323, 326.
Cell membrane, 321, 326.
Cell theory, 320–6, 635.
Cells, of plants and animals, 132, 320–5.
Cells of Purkinje, 246.
'Cellular Pathology', of Virchow, 325, 326, 635, 749.
Census, 181, 712–13, 718.
Census Day, 713.
Central Midwives Board, 227.
Centrifuge, high-speed, 446.

Cephalins, 319.
Cerebellar ataxy, 279.
Cerebellar syndrome, 279.
Cerebellum, 50, 243, 246, 255; ablation of, 256, 260.
Cerebral abscess, *see* Brain abscess.
Cerebral convolutions, 50, 241, 256.
Cerebral cortex, 246, 248, 256, 291–2; ablation of, 257–8; motor area of, 254, 257, 259, 260; sensory area of, 291–2; stimulation of, 154, 257–8.
Cerebral degeneration, 506.
Cerebral hemispheres, 246, 255, 256; ablation of, 255, 264.
Cerebral localization, 254–60, 275, 279.
Cerebral peduncles, 243.
Cerebral sulci, 243.
Cerebral tumour, *see* Brain tumour.
Cerebral ventricles, 50, 90, 241, 242, 243, 245, 279.
Cerebrospinal fever, 272, 391, 402–3, 409, 693, 728.
Cerebrospinal fluid, 249, 484–5.
Cerebrum, 50; ablation of, 258. *See also* Cerebral convolutions, Cerebral cortex, Cerebral hemispheres, Cerebral localization, Cerebral peduncles, Neurology.
Cerro de Pasco, Andes, 310.
Cervia, Italy, 79.
Cervical sympathetic, 260–2.
Cesspools, 193, 215, 220.
Chagas's disease, *see* Trypanosomiasis, American.
Chalcedon, Asia Minor, 48.
Chalk, 163.
Chamomile, 673, 674.
Charcot's joints, 274.
Chatham, Kent, 188.
Chauliac, France, 83.
Chemical affinity, 142.
Chemical physiology, *see* Biochemistry.
Chemical remedies, 672.
Chemistry, 136–7, 149, 161–8; organic, 238, 579–81.
Chemotherapy, 678, 687–97, 749.
Chest, diseases of, 7, 283; —, physical signs in, 172, 173, 281; —, surgery in, 230, 368–9, 372–3. *See also* Bronchitis, Emphysema, Phthisis, Pneumonia, &c.
Chest, military medical, 183.
Chester, Cheshire, 199.
Cheyne-Stokes respiration, 39, 283, 653.
Chicago, Illinois, U.S.A., 438, 451, 638.

Chick embryo tissue culture, 448–9.
Chicken cholera, 339, 432.
Chicken-pox, *see* Varicella.
Child hygiene, 198, 224–8, 650–7 *passim*.
Child welfare centres, 226, 227.
Children's diseases, *see* Paediatrics.
Children's hospitals, 655–7.
Chimney-sweep's cancer, 179.
Chios, Greece, 48, 49.
Chi-square test, of Pearson, 726.
Chloral hydrate, 350.
Chloramphenicol, 697.
Chloroform, 344–8.
Chloroguanide, 692.
Chloroquin, 692.
Cholecystotomy, 362.
Cholera, causative organism, discovery of, 340, 391. *See also* Cholera vibrio; epidemic outbreaks, in Great Britain, 730–1, 734; —, effect of, on public health reform, 87, 209, 211; —, in Exeter (1832), 215; —, in Munich, 231; etiology of, miasmatic theory, 231; —, effect of height of ground water in, 231; —, hypothesis of infected water-supply, 219; treatment of, in marine hospitals in U.S.A., 233.
Cholera vibrio, 231, 391, 414, 418.
Cholesterol, 616.
Cholinacetylase, 577.
Choline, 565, 567, 570.
'Cholinergic' fibres, 572, 573.
Cholinesterase, 577.
Chorda tympani nerve, 243, 244, 571.
Chorea, 257, 272, 273, 278.
Choroid, of the eye, 642.
Choroid plexus, 241, 242, 243.
Christianity, effect of, on science, 69.
Chronic diseases, 240, 753. *See also* Geriatrics.
Chvostek's sign, 535.
Chyle, 62, 123.
Chyluria, 492.
Cider, 204.
Ciliary muscle, 642.
Cinchona, 103, 454–5, 674, 681, 687.
Cinchonine, 681.
Cinnamon, 668, 673, 678.
Circulation of the blood, *see* Blood, Heart.
Circulus arteriosus, of Willis, 242.
Circumcision, 8.
Cirrhosis of liver, 37, 276, 628, 633.
Civil War, in America, *see* American Civil

War; in England, *see* Great Rebellion; in Spain, *see* Spanish Civil War.
Classification, Linnaean system of, 280.
Clavicle, 61.
Cleft palate, 352.
Cleveland, Ohio, U.S.A., 539, 627, 685.
'Climbing boys', 218.
Clinical medicine, founded by Sydenham, 111; Schools of, 280–6; anatomico-pathological school of, 282; English School, 284–5; French School, 280–3, 286; Irish School, 283–4; teaching of, 147–51; Vienna School, 280, 285–6. *See also* Dublin, Edinburgh, Glasgow, Leyden, Medicine, Paris, Vienna.
Clinical Society of London, 525.
Cloaca Maxima, Rome, 55.
Clostridium botulismum, 391.
Clostridium tetani, *see* Tetanus bacillus.
Clostridium welchii, *see* Gas gangrene bacillus.
Clover's inhaler, 347–8.
Cloves, 673, 674.
Club-foot, 185, 658.
Cnidos, Greece, 18, 19, 22.
Cocaine, 349, 680.
Cocci, 331, 333.
Coccidia, 459.
Cochlea, 244, 250.
Code of Hammurabi, 10–12.
Codex Theodosianus, 494.
Cod-liver oil, 612, 614, 615, 617.
Coffee, 681.
Colchester, Essex, 185.
Colchicine, 682.
Coli-typhoid organisms, 399–400.
Collective medical data, 710–41.
Collège de France, Paris, 550.
Colles's law, 284.
Colmar, Alsace, 241.
Colocynth, 673, 674, 677.
Colour blindness, 649.
Colour vision, 288, 289, 648–9.
Columbia University, New York, 601.
Combustion, 137, 143, 161–3, 165, 166, 238; of foodstuffs, 586.
Commissioners in Lunacy, 502.
Common cold, 446, 753.
Communal diseases, 196–8.
Complement, 414–16; fixation of, 416–17.
Conditioned reflexes, 266–9.
Congenital pyloric stenosis, 652.

Conjunctivitis, 650; granular, *see* Trachoma.
Conservation of energy, *see* Energy.
Conservative surgery, 352.
Constantinople, 67, 200, 488.
Consultation de nourrissons, 227.
Contagionists, 489, 729–30.
Contagious abortion of cattle, 385.
Contagium vivum, of Fracastor, 105–6, 729.
Contracted pelvis, 176.
Contracture, of Dupuytren, 185, 658.
Convulsions, 239.
Convulsive therapy, in mental diseases, 511.
Coonoor, India, 527.
Copaiba, 674.
Copenhagen, 307, 308, 377, 378, 413, 516, 621.
Copper, 8, 673, 677.
Cordova, Spain, 76.
Coriander, 673.
Cori ester, 294.
Cork, structure of, 132.
Cornea, 642.
Cornell University Medical College, New York, 550, 589, 590, 594, 639.
Coronary disease, 625, 721.
Coronary vessels, 245.
Corpora quadrigemina, 243.
Corporin, *see* Progesterol.
Corpus callosum, 243.
Corpus luteum, 550–1.
Correlation, 725–6.
Corrosive sublimate, 108.
Cortin, 540.
Cortisone, 540, 548.
Corynebacterium diphtheriae, *see* Diphtheria bacillus.
Cos, Greece, 18, 19, 22, 24, 28.
Coventry treatment of goitre, 522.
Cow-pox, 200–2, 446.
Cranial nerves, 242, 243, 244, 245, 251, 272.
'Crases', Rokitansky's theory of, 634.
Creatine, 319, 600, 601.
Creatinine, 540, 599, 600.
Cremona, Italy, 76, 123.
Creosote, 674.
Crescent forms, *see* Malaria parasite.
Crete, 18, 19.
Cretinism, 101, 521–2, 525, 526, 527.
Crimean War, 384, 704–8.

Cripples, 225.
Crippling conditions, 228.
Crocus, 673.
Crookes tube, 374.
Croton, Italy, 244.
Croton oil, 674, 677.
Croup, 631. *See also* Diphtheria.
Crown and bridge work (dental), 663, 665.
Crusades, 491.
Cubebs, 674.
Culex mosquitoes, 461, 462.
Curare, 298–9, 351, 573, 575, 577.
Cushing's syndrome, 545.
Cutaneous plantar reflex (Babinski's sign), 277.
Cutaneous sensation, 246–7, 269–71, 279.
Cyanocobalamine, *see* Vitamin B_{12}.
Cyanosis, 309, 310, 317.
Cyprus, 488.
Cystine, 595.
Cytology, 639.

Dakar, Senegal, 477.
Damascus, 119.
'Damps', in mines, 311.
Dancing mania, *see* Tarantism.
Dandelion, 674.
Dark Ages, 65–66.
Datura, 673.
Davos, Switzerland, 593.
DDT, 465, 491.
Deaf-mutism, 225.
Death certificates, 714–15.
Death-rates, 194, 221, 714–15, 720.
Decerebrate rigidity, 264, 279.
Defibrination, of blood, 700.
Deficiency diseases, 610–22.
Delhi boil, 487.
Delirium, 37, 38, 39.
Dementia praecox, *see* Schizophrenia.
Demography, 710–14; definition of, 712.
Demonic possession, 3, 6, 7, 14–15, 494.
Dengue, 453.
Dental caries, 225, 668–70.
Dental clinics, school, 225.
Dental crowns, 663, 665.
Dental drill, 669.
Dental elevator, 662.
Dental engine, 669.
Dental fillings, 668–9.
Dental impressions, 663, 666, 667.
Dentistry, 55, 659–71.
'Dephlogisticated air', 165, 166.

Depressor nerve, 301, 314.
Depressor substances, 557, 560.
Derbyshire neck, 521.
Dermacentroxenus rickettsi, see Rickettsia rickettsi.
Dermatology, 204. *See also* Skin diseases.
Design of experiments, 727.
Desoxycorticosterone, 540.
Desquamation, 203.
Deuterium (H²), 601.
Devonshire colic, 204.
Diabetes insipidus, 544–5, 552.
Diabetes mellitus, 232, 245, 285, 296, 548–9, 552–5, 639.
Diabetogenic hormone, 549.
Dialysis, 319.
Diarrhoea, 37, 38, 240.
Dick test, 438–9.
Dienoestrol, 551.
Diet, 50, 68; of Broussais, 282; in Hippocratic practice, 41; in fever, 187; normal, 604–10; relation of, to nutrition, 608; Voit's Standard, 604.
Dietetics, *see* Diet.
Digestion, 581; gastric, 141, 142, 152, 155–7, 159.
Digestive tract, movements of, 303.
Digitalis, 674, 683–4, 685.
Digitoxin, 683.
Digoxin, 684.
Dill, 674.
Diphtheria, 38, 203, 231; first description of, 204, 631; first tracheotomy in, 204; immunity to, 433; intubation for, 655; laryngeal, 435; specific prophylaxis of, 434–6.
Diphtheria antitoxin, 412–13, 420, 421, 427, 434, 687.
Diphtheria bacillus, 382, 411, 696; carriers of, 409; discovery of, 381, 391, 392; variant strains of, 403, 404.
Disease, etiology of, 6, 46–47, 50, 98, 100.
Disease, occupational, *see* Occupational diseases.
Disinfectants, 678.
Disinfection, 189.
Dislocations, 55, 179, 284.
Dispensary for the Infant Poor, London, 652, 656.
Dispensatory, the Florentine, 672.
Dissection, *see* Anatomy, Post-mortem examinations.
Disseminated sclerosis, 275, 632, 754.

District Registrar, 713, 714.
Divination, 12–13, 20.
Diviners, 10.
Dog distemper, 449.
Dog-fish, 42–43.
Domesday Book, 712.
Dorians, 18, 19.
Dorpat (Tartu), 475, 582, 684.
Douglas bag, 307, 590.
Drainage, 84, 193, 214, 215, 235; of land, 191.
Drain-tests, 231.
Dreadnought, H.M.S., 221–2.
Dresden, Saxony, 392, 646.
Drill, surgical, 79–81.
Dropsy, 284.
Drug resistance, 693, 697, 750.
Drugs, 7, 8, 14, 20, 35, 53, 59–60, 103, 671–87; administration of, 685–6.
Dublin, 476, 530, 535, 653, 731; fatal scarlet fever at (1801–4), 204; high death-rate in Foundling Hospital at (1775–96), 225; Irish School of, 283–4; Park Street School of Medicine at, 283. *See also* Hospitals, Pharmacopoeia.
Ducrey's bacillus, 391, 393.
Ductless glands, 515–55. *See also* Adrenal glands, Gonads, Pancreas, Parathyroid glands, Pituitary body, Thyroid gland.
Düsseldorf, Germany, 58.
Dum-dum fever, *see* Kala-azar.
Dumfries, 503.
Duodenal ulcer, 639, 749.
Dupuytren's contracture, *see* Contracture.
Dupuytren's fracture, *see* Fracture.
Durham, 526.
Durham tube, 400.
Dwarfism, 536, 544.
Dynamic state, of body constituents, 320, 601.
Dysentery, amoebic, *see* Amoebiasis; bacillary, 185, 452, 472, 473.
Dysentery bacillus, 407, 409; of Shiga, 391.
Dystrophia adiposo-genitalis, *see* Fröhlich's syndrome.

Ear, 245, 246, 629.
Ear, nose, and throat, diseases of, 225.
Earl's Court, London, 177, 178.
East India Company, 186, 342.
Ebers Papyrus, 4–5.

Edinburgh, 210, 257, 284, 349, 351, 394, 632, 637, 655, 659, 685, 731; amyl nitrite first used for angina pectoris at, 684; anatomists at, 150–1, 325; chloroform first used as anaesthetic at, 344; early lectures on histology at, 634; histology of thyroid studied at, 532; hypodermic syringe first used at, 687; Medical School, 150–1; —, foundation of, 280; physicians at, 148, 278, 642; physiologists at, 251, 258; surgeons at, 344, 351–3, 534; tuberculosis dispensary system founded at, 229. *See also* Hospitals, Pharmacopoeia.
Edmonton, Alberta, 536.
Education, 211, 213.
Education Act (1902), 224.
Education (Administrative Provisions) Act (1907), 224.
Edwin Smith Surgical Papyrus, 4.
Eel, circulation in, 128, 129.
Effort syndrome, 625.
Egg albumen, 447, 595, 597.
Egg yolk, 612.
Ego, of Freud, 513–14.
Egypt, 3–9, 10.
Einsiedeln, Switzerland, 100.
Electricity, 160–1; animal, 158, 159.
Electrocardiograph, 624–5, 754.
Electron microscope, 446.
Electrotherapy, 246, 274.
Element, chemical, 136.
Elements, the four, 46, 102, 135.
Elephantiasis, 460.
Embalming, 3–4.
Embolism, 636, 654.
Embryology, 133, 152, 237, 246, 287, 326, 583; of chick, 44, 97, 125–6; discovery of mammalian ovum, 321; first textbook of comparative embryology, 247; of human foetus, 90.
Emetics, 7, 680.
Emetine, 494, 680, 681, 687, 691.
Emphysema, 170, 311, 631.
Encephalitis lethargica, 453, 729.
Encephalogram, 292, 752.
Endocarditis, 629.
Endocrine glands, *see* Ductless glands.
Endotoxin, 439.
Endotracheal anaesthesia, 350.
End-plates, in muscle, 574, 576.
Enemata, 7.
Energy, conservation of, 289, 588.

Energy requirements of human subjects, 604, 605, 607, 608.
'English Hippocrates', 111.
English key, 660, 662.
English Sweat, *see* Sweating sickness.
Enophthalmos, 260.
Entamoeba coli, 493.
Entamoeba histolytica, 493.
Enteric fever, *see* Typhoid fever.
Enterokinase, 298.
Enzymes, 294, 296, 311, 518.
Ephesus, 239.
Epicritic, *see* Protopathic.
Epidaurus, Greece, 24–26.
'Epidemic constitution', of Hippocrates, 106, 280, 728–9.
Epidemics, control of, 198–204; history of, 740–1; periodicity of, 737; spread of, 84, 85, 87, 732–7.
Epidemic wave, 733–6.
Epidemiology, 727–41; experimental, 737–40; historical, 740–1.
Epilepsy, 50, 76, 239, 240, 273, 278; Jacksonian, 3, 256–7, 258. *See also* Sacred Disease.
Epinephrine, *see* Adrenaline.
Epithelium, 322.
Epsom salts, *see* Magnesium sulphate.
Erepsin, 595.
Ergometrine, 683.
Ergosterol, 615.
Ergot, 546, 555–8, 566–8, 682–3.
Ergotamine, 682.
Ergotine, 682.
Ergotinine, 682.
Ergotism, 278, 682.
Ergotoxine, 571, 682.
Erlangen, Germany, 237, 373.
Errors of refraction, 641–3.
Erysipelas, 86, 354, 391, 682, 693.
Erythrocytes, 129, 133, 311, 317, 353, 700; in malaria, 456; measurements of, 318.
Eschatin, 539.
Eserine (physostigmine), 569, 572, 573, 575–7.
Essences, *see* Elements.
Essential (volatile) oils, 678.
Ether, anaesthetic, 343, 344, 346, 350.
Ether frolics, 343.
Ethmoid bone, 241.
Etruria, 13.
Eustachian tube, 244.
Evipan, 350.

Exeter, Devon, 215.
Exflagellation, 461, 462.
Exophthalmic goitre, *see* Goitre.
Exophthalmos, 530, 531; causes of, 533–4; tests for, 533.
Exorcism, 14.
Exorcists, 10.
Exotoxins, 411.
Experimental medicine, 120, 294.
Extrasystoles, cardiac, 623.
Eye, 640–50; anatomy of, 97, 239, 640–2, 648; pathology of, 646–7; physiology of, 139, 641, 642, 648–9.
Eye diseases, in ancient Egypt, 7; in Mesopotamia, 15; school clinics for, 225.
Eye-ball, enucleation of, 646.

Facial hemiatrophy, 273.
Facial nerve, 251, 272.
Facial paralysis, 272.
Factories, health of children in, 210, 217.
Factory Acts, 217.
Faeces, 579, 583, 584, 602.
Fallopian tubes, 244.
Falx cerebri, 243.
Fasters, professional: Beauté (1907), 590, 600; Cetti (1893), 590, 591; Hoelzel (1926), 591; Merlatti, 591; Succi (1890), 590.
Fat, 294, 319, 578, 581, 601; amount of, destroyed during starvation, 585, 591; calorie value of, 586–7; digestion of, by pancreatic juice, 298; metabolism of, 579, 602–3; —, influence of muscular work on, 593; production of, from carbohydrate, 603–4; requirement of, in normal diet, 604, 607, 608; as source of muscular energy, 594.
Fatty acids, 298, 319, 602, 603.
Fatty degeneration, 635.
Fatty infiltration, 635.
Faulhorn, Switzerland, ascent of, 592.
Favus, 328.
Feathers, 323.
Fécamp, France, 227.
Federal health service (of U.S.A.), 232.
Fennel, 674.
Fermentation, 143, 156–7, 238, 329–30, 331–2, 354, 395.
Fermentation tests, for organisms, 400, 402.

Ferments, 143, 331, 337; of van Helmont, 142.
Ferricyanide method (blood gases), 305, 310.
Fertility, 718.
Fever, 38, 39, 288.
Fever hospitals, *see* Hospitals, isolation.
Fevers, 76, 111, 185, 283, 522; 'essential', of Pinel, 282; notification of, *see* Infectious diseases; stationary and intercurrent, of Sydenham, 728. *See also* Infection, London.
Fibrinogen, 317.
Fibroid phthisis, 101, 284.
Filaria bancrofti, 460, 492.
Filaria sanguinis hominis, 492.
Filariasis, 460, 469, 492–3.
Filterable viruses, *see* Viruses.
Filters, bacteriological, 445. *See also* Water, filtration of.
Final common path, of efferent nerve impulses, 264, 265.
Finsen Light, 378.
'Fire air', 165.
Firearms, 181, 182. *See also* Gun-shot wounds.
First Dutch War, 613.
First field dressing, for war wounds, 185.
First intention, healing by, 79.
First World War, 285, 667, 709, 728–9; D.A.H. and V.D.H. studied during, 625; decrease in rate of growth of population after, 713; effect of, on quinine supplies, 691; results obtained during, with tetanus antitoxin, 443; —, with typhoid vaccine, 444; slum clearance after, 609; storage of blood during, 701; studies made during, of amoebiasis, 493; —, of rickets, 613, 614–15; —, of surgical shock, 558; surgical advances during, 371, 373; tetanus incidence during, 441, 443; trench fever first described during, 451–2.
Fissure of Rolando, 257, 258.
Five-day fever, *see* Trench fever.
'Fixed air', 163, 165, 166. *See also* Carbon dioxide.
Flagella, of malaria parasite, 456–7, 458, 460, 461, 462.
Flagellar antigens, 404–5.
Florence, Italy, 29, 79, 260, 505, 520, 544, 627, 672.
Fluxes, 185. *See also* Dysentery.

'Flying Ambulance', see Ambulance.
Flying Dutchman, 466.
Foetal rickets, 638.
Food, in metabolism, 581, 582, 578–622 passim.
Food poisoning, 391.
Foodstuffs, calorie values of, 585, 586, 587; chemical composition of, 606; quantities of, used in normal diets, 607–10.
Food supply, control of, 56, 223.
Foot-and-mouth disease, 392, 445.
Foramen, interventricular, 245; of Winslow, 245.
Forceps, dental, 662–3; obstetric, 176; surgical, 8, 9, 362–3.
Formol toxoid, 436.
Fornix, 242, 243.
Foundling hospitals, 198, 225, 651–2, 655–6.
Fourth ventricle, of brain, 546.
Fowl cholera, see Chicken cholera.
Foxglove, see Digitalis.
Fracture, of Colles, 284; of Dupuytren, 185, 658; of Pott, 179.
Fractures, 2, 55, 179, 185, 241, 254, 284, 355, 369, 371.
Franco-Prussian War, 335, 336, 358, 392, 699.
Frankfort-on-Main, 249, 294, 531, 687.
Frankfort-on-the-Oder, 392, 393.
Free association, of Freud, 513–14.
Freiburg-im-Breisgau, Germany, 325, 601, 636, 638.
Frequency curves, 733–4.
Fröhlich's syndrome, 544, 546.
Fruits, as drugs, 8, 14.

Gall, 7.
Gall bladder, 362, 370.
Gall stones, 638.
Galvanism, 159.
Gaol fever, see Typhus fever.
'Gas', of van Helmont, 142.
Gas analysis, 319.
Gases, estimation of, in blood, 305, 306; R. Boyle on, 136. See also names of individual gases.
Gas gangrene, 391.
Gas gangrene bacillus, 391, 395.
Gastric juice, 143, 155–7, 159, 266–7, 302.
Gastric ulcer, 366, 639, 749.
Gastroenteritis, of Broussais, 282.

Gastroenterostomy, 370.
Gaucher's disease, 319.
Gelatine, 340, 578, 598.
General Board of Health (1848), 210, 218, 219, 220, 715.
General Medical Council, 672, 673.
General Nursing Council, 710.
General paralysis of the insane (G.P.I.), 507, 511.
General practitioner, 746.
General Register Office, 713, 714.
Generalized osteitis fibrosa cystica, 537.
Generation, Aristotle on, 44–45; Harvey on, 45.
Geneva, Switzerland, 520, 715; cachexia strumipriva first described at, 525; cerebrospinal fever first described at (1805), 272; generalized osteitis associated with parathyroid tumour at, 537; iodine in treatment of goitre at (1820), 523; Red Cross founded at, 185.
Geneva Convention, 185.
Geriatrics, 275, 752.
Germ origin of disease, 326–41.
Germinal epithelium, 247.
Germinal vesicle, 246, 321.
Gerontology, see Geriatrics.
Ghent, Belgium, 394.
Ghon's focus, 426.
Gibraltar fever, see Brucellosis.
Giessen, Germany, 583, 631; laboratory for practical chemistry established at, 237, 580; oestradiol discovered at, 551; research in, and teaching of, pharmacology at, 684.
Gigantism, 543, 547.
Ginger, 678.
Glanders, 391, 396.
Glands, secretory, stimulation of, 267.
Glasgow, 148, 417, 599, 633, 697; antiseptic system of surgery, founded at, 352–3; —, scientific basis of, worked out at, 353–4, 358–9; aseptic surgery, early establishment at, 366–7; excision of lung at (1895), 368–9; Hunterian Museum and Library at, 176; Medical School founded at (1751), 151; metabolic and nutritional research at, 600–1, 607–8; neurological surgery founded at, 367–8; pathological chair at, founded, 637; —, held by Muir for thirty-seven years, 639; pioneer work at, on rachitic deformities, 369, 614; —, on transplantation

of bone, 659; researches at, on growth
of bone, 368; —, on rickets, 614; Royal
Faculty of Physicians and Surgeons
founded at (1599), 183; surgery at,
during Listerian revolution, 354–9. See
also Hospitals.
'Glass-chamber' experiment, of Barcroft,
310.
Glaucoma, 646–7.
Globus pallidus, 243.
Glossina morsitans, 482, 486.
Glossina palpalis, 483, 485.
Gloucester, Glos., 502.
Glucose, 295, 316, 552, 587, 594, 683.
Glucose-1-phosphate, 296.
Glucose-6-phosphate, 296.
Glycerol, 298, 319, 602.
Glycine, 595, 597, 603.
Glycogen, 293, 294–6, 316, 591, 593.
Glycosides, 679, 680, 683–4.
Glycosuria, 245, 552, 553.
Goats' milk, 384–5.
Gobelin tapestry works, 552.
Goerbersdorf, Silesia, 228.
Göttingen, Germany, 321, 336, 392, 516,
549, 638.
Goitre, 54; endemic, 101, *and see* simple;
exophthalmic, 283, 530–4, *see also*
Hyperthyroidism; simple, 520–30; —,
artificial production of, 528; —, pro-
phylaxis of, 529–30; —, surgical treat-
ment of, 523–4.
Goitrogens, 528, 529–30.
Golgi apparatus, 247.
Golgi-Mazzoni corpuscles, 269.
Gonadotrophic hormone, of anterior
pituitary, 547.
Gonads, 549–51.
Gonococcus, 390, 391, 696.
Gonorrhoea, 391, 693.
Gonville and Caius College, Cambridge,
740.
Goschen, Connecticut, U.S.A., 272.
Gout, 110, 275, 652.
Graafian follicles, 297, 547.
Gradacol membranes, 446.
Graduated exercise, in treatment of
tuberculosis, 228.
Grampus, H.M.S., 221.
Graves's disease, 531–2. See also Hyper-
thyroidism.
Gravitation, 145–7.
Graz, Austria, 550, 568, 591.

Great Rebellion, 110, 183.
Great Windmill Street School, 176.
Greece, 1, 18–47 *passim*.
Greeks, 1, 6, 8, 9, 16–45. *See also* Medi-
cine.
Greenwich, London, 188, 221, 222.
Greenwich Palace, 188.
Greifswald, Germany, 350, 392.
Ground itch, 493.
Ground-water, 231.
Guaiac, 108–10, 674.
Guillotine, tonsillar, 351.
Gull's disease, *see* Myxoedema.
Gun-shot wounds, 96, 97, 181–5, 371; of
nerves, 185.
Gymnastics, ancient, 651.
Gynaecology, 239.
Gyri, cerebral, 246.

Haematology, 316–19.
Haemochromatosis, 636.
Haemochromogen, 319.
Haemocytometer, 318.
Haemoglobin, 303, 310, 319.
Haemoglobinometer, 278, 306.
Haemoglobinuria, 285.
Haemolysis, 415–17, 700.
Haemolytic disease, of new born, 701.
Haemophilia, 396.
Haemophilus ducreyi, *see* Ducrey's bacillus.
Haemophilus influenzae, *see* Influenza
bacillus.
Haemophilus pertussis, *see* Whooping cough
bacillus.
Haemoptysis, 50.
Haemorrhage, control of, 96, 183.
Haffkine's plague vaccine, 439, 491.
Hague, The, Holland, 280.
Halifax, Yorks., 224.
Halle, Germany, 365, 391, 596.
Hallucinations, 505; in epilepsy, 239.
Hamburg, Germany, 451, 544, 595.
Hamburg-Eppendorf, Germany, 394.
Hare lip, 352.
Hartford, Connecticut, U.S.A., 343.
Harvard University, 361, 420, 477, 540,
602; early investigation (1896) by X-
rays of movements of gastro-intestinal
tract at, 303; first professor of medicine
at, 202; introduction of micro-methods
in biochemistry at, 596; successful
investigation of cause of pernicious
anaemia at, 621.

Haslar Hospital, see Hospitals.
Havana, Cuba, 468, 471-4, 492.
Hay fever, 427-9.
Hayling Island, Hants, 378.
Health of Towns Association, 210, 217.
Health of Towns Commission, 214, 217.
Health visitors, 226, 656.
Health Visitors Certificate, 226, 710.
Hearing, 288.
Heart, 119, 155, 245; change in volume of, on contraction, 134; development of, 44; dilatation of, 197; diseases of, see Heart disease; functions of, 43, 48, 120-1, 622, 625. See also Blood, circulation of, Bundle of His; innervation of, 245, 262, 314; interventricular septum of, 64, 65, 89, 93, 119, 301, 314; irregularity of, 623-5; isolated mammalian, 315; Law of the, 315-16; metabolism of, 316; surgery of, 373; valves of, 64-65, 89, 120-1, 197, 241; views on, of Aristotle, 43, 44; —, of Leonardo, 89-90.
Heart-beat, 623, 624, 625, 627; theories of, 314-15.
Heart disease, 197, 283, 622-7, 630, 632; congenital, 373, 653; statistics of, 720-1. See also under individual diseases.
Heart–lung preparation, of Starling, 315.
Heart murmurs, 625, 627.
Heat production, in body, 168, 587. See also Metabolism.
Heat stroke, 240.
Heat value, of foodstuffs, see Foodstuffs, calorie values of.
Heidelberg, Germany, 321, 475, 583, 595, 596, 620.
Heliotherapy, 377-9. See also Sunlight.
Hemicrania, 240.
Hemispheres, cerebral, see Cerebral hemispheres.
Henry Phipps Institute, Philadelphia, 553, 639.
Hepatoscopy, 12-13.
Herbal, 103-4; of Dioscorides, 53.
Hereditary cerebellar ataxia, 277.
Hernia, 83, 179, 246, 284, 368, 629.
Herpes simplex, 448.
Herpes zoster, 446.
Hexoestrol, 551.
Hexuronic acid, 619.
Hilden, Germany, 183.
Hippocratic anatomy, 239.

Hippocratic Collection, 22, 23, 27-41, 53, 59, 60, 386, 454, 494.
Hippocratic Constitutions, 728-9.
Hippocratic facies, 40.
Hippocratic Oath, 31-32.
Hippocratic practice, 32-41.
Hippocratic succussion, 40.
Hippuric acid, 603.
Histamine, 430, 555-64, 569, 570.
Histidine, 558, 596.
Histology, 125, 247, 269-71, 288, 318-19, 320, 321, 323-6, 352, 398.
Hodgkin's disease, 285.
Hog cholera, 404.
Holmgren's wools, 649.
Homeostasis, 303.
Honey, 7.
Hong Kong, 381.
Hookworm disease, 493.
Hormones, 518-19, 679.
Horner's syndrome, 261.
Horse serum, 421-2, 429.
Hospital fever, see Typhus fever.
Hospital gangrene, 354.
Hospitals, foundations of the London, 194; foundling, see Foundling hospitals; isolation, for infectious diseases, 189, 190, 194, 223; medieval, 84, 85; military, 183, 184, 706; naval, 188; nursing in, see Nursing; Roman, 56-59; the Royal, of England, 702.
Hospitals, and institutions, named: Allgemeines Krankenhaus, Vienna, 197, 280, 286, 360, 633; Ancoats and Ardwick Dispensary, Manchester, 210; Bellevue, New York, 589, 590; Bethlehem Hospital, London, 496, 499, 507; Bicêtre, Paris, 497, 499, 501; Charing Cross, London, 365, 541, 665; Charité, Berlin, 390, 634, 654; Charité, Paris, 227; Crichton Royal Institution, Dumfries, 503; Edinburgh Royal Infirmary, 344, 352; the Foundling Hospital, Dublin, 225; the Foundling Hospital, London, 651-2, 656; Glasgow Royal Infirmary, 353, 366, 367, 637; Gloucester Asylum, 502; Guy's, London, 232, 284-5, 418, 476, 522, 632, 658, 699, 704; Haslar, 186, 188; Hospital for Sick Children, Great Ormond Street, London, 656-7; Hospital for Tropical Diseases, London, 223; Hôtel-Dieu, Paris, 85, 95, 283,

702; Johns Hopkins, Baltimore, *see* Johns Hopkins University, Baltimore; King's College, London, 257, 273, 352, 353, 524, 704; Leeds General Infirmary, 626; the London Hospital, London, 194, 256, 378, 395, 541, 544, 500, 655, 736; London Fever, 731; Manchester Royal Infirmary, 189; Massachusetts General, Boston, U.S.A., 343–4, 534, 597; Maudsley, London, 260; Mayo Clinic, Rochester, U.S.A., 370, 532; Meath, Dublin, 283; Middlesex, London,'251, 551, 653, 663; Middlesex Asylum, Hanwell, 499, 500; National Hospital for Nervous Diseases, Queen Square, London, 279, 541; Orthopaedic, London, 658; Radcliffe Infirmary, Oxford, 702; Retreat, York, 498–9; Royal Cancer Hospital, London, 638; Royal Waterloo, for Children and Women, London, 656; St. Bartholomew's, London, 179, 182, 186, 194–5, 402, 535, 632, 685; St. Boniface, Florence, 505; St. George's, London, 632, 642; St. Mary's, Paddington, London, 419, 430, 531, 694; St. Thomas's, London, 151, 187, 284, 395, 456, 524, 525, 632, 648, 708; Salpêtrière, Paris, 274, 275, 497, 510; Stonehouse, Plymouth, 188; 'The United', London, 284; University College Hospital, London, 344, 352, 509, 534, 624, 640, 704; Val-de-Grâce, France, 281, 396, 441, 456; West Riding Asylum, Wakefield, 257, 606; Western Infirmary, Glasgow, 637; York County Asylum, 497, 499.

'Houses of recovery', 189.

Housing, 189, 214, 216, 235.

'Houssay dogs', 549.

H-substance, of Lewis, 560.

Huddersfield, Yorks., 227.

Huddersfield Corporation Act (1906), 227.

Humoral theory, 98, 101, 138, 286. *See also* Humours.

Humours, the four, 40, 46–47, 101, 102.

Hunterian Museum, Glasgow, 176.

Hunterian Museum, London, 171, 178–9, 543.

Huskisson, barque, 466.

Hydrocephalus, 279, 653.

Hydrochloric acid, 157, 165, 677.

Hydrocyanic acid, 490.

Hydrogen, 165.

Hydrogen-ion concentration, 307, 310, 316.

Hydrophobia, *see* Rabies.

Hydrothorax, 39–40.

Hygiene, Alexandrian, 50; communal, 197–8; military, 183, 184, 190; Mycenaean, 19; naval, 185, 186–8; personal, 73; prison, 189, 190; Roman, 55–56; urban, 193–4.

Hygienic Laboratory, United States Public Health Service, 234, 562.

Hyoscyamus, 341, 669, 674.

Hyperglycaemia, 552, 553.

Hypersensitiveness, 420–2, 429.

Hypertension, 754.

Hyperthyroidism, 530–4; histology of thyroid in, 532; treatment of, 534.

Hypnotic state, 509, 513.

Hypnotics, 678.

Hypnotism, 509–10, 513.

Hypochondria, 505.

Hypoglycaemia, 554.

Hypophysis cerebri, *see* Pituitary body.

Hypothalamus, 546.

Hypothyroidism, 520–30.

Hysterectomy, 239.

Hysteria, 275, 495, 505, 510, 513.

iatreia, 57.

Iatrochemistry, 142–3, 144.

Iatrophysics, 138–42, 144, 250, 503, 504.

Id, of Freud, 514.

ignis sacer, 682.

β–iminazolylethylamine, 557. *See also* Histamine.

Immune body, 414–16.

Immune sera, 411–18, 419.

Immunity, 409–45, 563, 731–2; active, 431–3; antitoxic, 393, 411–16; artificial, 202, 432, 739–40; cellular theory of, 411; herd, 735–6, 738–40; humoral theory of, 410, 411; natural, 431; passive, 431–2, 433; practical applications of, 433–45; types of, 430–3.

Improvement Acts, for towns, 193.

Indestructibility of energy, *see* Energy.

Indian hemp, 341. See also *Cannabis indica*.

Indian Medical Service, 460, 462, 463, 485, 527.

Individual Psychology, School of, 514.

Industrial dwellings, 210.

Industrial Revolution, 189, 191–6, 683.

Infant mortality, 180, 223, 226, 227, 228, 656, 711, 712.

3 H

Infant mortality rate, 228, 715, 720.
Infantalism, 543-4.
Infarcts, 631, 636.
Infection, theories of, 84, 85, 86-87, 104-6, 111, 197, 739; pythogenic (miasmatic) theory of, 197, 214-15, 231, 328, 489, 729-30; sublethal and latent, 739.
Infectious diseases, 220, 231, 283, 716, 727-41, 742; of central nervous system, 224; notification of, 189, 715-16; and water-supplies, 231-2. See also Fevers.
Infectious Diseases (Notification) Acts, 716.
Infectivity, 733-5, 736.
Inferiority complex, 514.
'Inflammable air', see Hydrogen.
Inflammation, 183, 352, 629, 635, 636, 639; cardinal signs of, 54; Cohnheim on, 637; chronic, of Broussais, 281-2; Lister's researches on, 353-4.
Influenza, 391, 446, 449, 729, 741, 753-4; pandemic of (1918-19), 735-6; virus of, 447, 448, 449.
Influenza bacillus, 391, 393, 449.
Infundibulum, see Pituitary body.
Inhalations, of drugs, 7, 686.
Injection, anatomical, see Anatomical injection; hypodermic, 686-7.
Inkermann, battle of, 706.
Innate heat, 43, 238.
Inoculation, smallpox, see Smallpox.
Insanity, see Mental diseases.
Insects, 155; minute anatomy of, 125, 133.
Insensible perspiration, 117.
Institute for Hygiene, Berlin, 393, 586.
Institute for Infectious Diseases, Berlin, 387, 392.
Institute of Nursing Sisters, 704.
Instruments, surgical, see Surgical instruments.
Insulin, 548, 554-5, 754; in treatment of schizophrenia, 511.
Intention tremor, 275.
'Intercostal nerve', of Willis, 260-1.
Internal environment, 299, 320.
Internal secretion, 515-55; demonstration of, 516; origin of the term, 295, 517.
International List of Causes of Death, 715.
International Medical Congress, London (1881), 258, 340, 356.
International Red Cross Committee, 709.
International Sanitary Commission, Washington (1881), 468.

Interventricular foramen, see Foramen.
Interventricular septum, 64, 65, 89, 93, 119, 301, 314.
Intestinal mucosa, isolation of histamine from, 558.
Intestines, 364-5; movements of, 301, 303.
Intracranial tumour, 278. See also Brain tumour.
Intravenous anaesthesia, 350.
Intubation of larynx, 655.
Inunction of drugs, 685.
Involuntary nervous system, of Gaskell, 262.
Iodides, 677.
Iodine, 522-3, 526, 527-9, 534, 681; Lugol's solution of, see Lugol's solution.
Iodized salt, 527.
Ionians, 18, 19.
Ipecacuanha, 103, 674, 680, 687.
Iridectomy, 647.
Iris, 645.
Iron, 639, 677.
Irritability, see Muscles, Tissues.
Islam, 61, 74, 76.
Islets of Langerhans, 549, 552, 553.
Isodynamic law, of proximate principles, 586.
Isoniazid, 697.
Itch, 86. See also Scabies.

Jail fever, see Typhus fever.
Jalap, 674, 677.
Jamaica, 467, 620.
Jaundice, 37, 638, 639; infectious, 475-6; malignant familial, 652.
Jefferson, Georgia, U.S.A., 343.
Jena, Germany, 292, 322, 393, 654.
Jesuit's bark, see Cinchona.
Johne's bacillus, 391.
Johne's disease, 391, 392.
Johns Hopkins University, Baltimore, 367, 424; first professor, of medicine at, 317; —, of pathology at, 394; —, of pharmacology at, 685; —, of surgery at, 349; isolated mammalian heart first studied at, 315; malaria parasite, sexual cycle of, first demonstrated at, 461; pressor effects of pituitrin shown due to posterior pituitary at, 545; research on, desoxycorticosterone acetate at, 540; —, diabetes at, 553; —, tetany at, 536, 639; —, thyroid gland at, 529, 532. See also Hospitals.

Joints, 61; excision of, 351–2; tuberculosis of, 183, 378.
Juniper, 673, 674.
Junker inhaler, 363.

Kairouan, Tunis, 71, 76.
Kaiserswerth, Germany, 703, 704.
Kaiserswerth Deaconesses, 703–4.
Kala-azar, 419, 453, 462, 487, 488.
Katabolism, 578.
Kell antigen, 701.
Keratitis, 646.
Kidney, 284, 301–2, 365, 638, 639, 641.
Kiel, Germany, 293, 318.
King's College, London, 352–3, 524.
Kino, 674.
Knee-jerk, 252, 275.
Koch's phenomenon, 422–3, 429.
Koch's postulates, 379–80.
Königsberg, Germany, 318, 393, 601; association of acromegaly with enlarged pituitary noted at, 542; calorie value of diets at, 605; fasciculus cuneatus described at, 248.
Krause's end-bulbs, 269.
Kromayer lamp, 378.
Kuala Lumpur, Malaya, 611.
Kupffer cells, 318.
Kymograph, 300, 311.

Laboratories, 142, 149, 235, 314, 580, 684–5.
Labouring Population, Sanitary Conditions of, Report by Chadwick, 214, 215, 217.
Labyrinth, of ear, 244, 246.
Lactacidogen, 294.
Lacteals, 123.
Lactic acid, 292–4, 296.
Lactose-fermenters, 400.
Ladder of Nature, of Aristotle, 41–42.
Ladies' Sanitary Reform Association of Manchester and Salford, 226.
Ladysmith, siege of, 444.
Lagos, 477.
Lanarkshire, 177.
Larissa, Greece, 28.
Laryngoscope, 249.
Larynx, 94.
Latrines, 56, 184.
Laudable pus, 522.
Laudanum, 101.
Laughing gas, see Nitrous oxide.
Lausanne, Switzerland, 394.

Lavender oil, 674.
Law of the Heart, 315–16.
Laws, natural, 145–6.
Lazarettos, 198–9.
Lead, 101, 677.
Lead colic, 204.
Lead poisoning, 223.
Leeching, 282.
Leeds, Yorks., 370, 626, 639; foundation of Medical School at, 197; variant strains of Corynebacterium diphtheriae investigated at, 403. See also Hospitals.
Leipzig, Germany, 247, 249, 318, 373, 532; early studies of body temperature at, 626; physiological research at, 299, 313; studies of pathology of inflammation at, 637.
Leishman-Donovan bodies, see Leishmania.
Leishmania donovani, 419, 487; L. tropica, 487.
Leishmaniasis, 454, 487–8.
Leishman's stain, 419.
Leith, Midlothian, 535.
Lemberg, Poland, 557.
Lemon juice, 187, 188.
Lenard tube, 374.
Lens, of eye, 244, 640, 642, 643–5.
Lenses, for visual defects, 641, 643.
Lenticular nucleus, 243.
Leprosy, 86, 106, 174, 390, 391, 452.
Leprosy bacillus, 391.
Leptospira icterohaemorrhagiae, 475; L. icteroides, 475.
Lesser circulation, 119.
Lethargy, 240.
Leucin, 275, 595.
Leucocytes, 317, 318, 353, 354, 410–11.
Leucotomy, prefrontal, 512.
Leukaemia, 634, 635, 754.
Leyden, Holland, 134, 297, 395, 651; anatomical research at, 150; clinical medicine first taught at, 148–9; electrocardiograph invented at, 625; first chemical laboratory at, 142; Leeuwenhoek microscopes preserved at, 128; museum of morbid anatomy at, 629; physicians at, 148–9, 280; rickets first described in thesis at, 613; School of, as model for Old Vienna School, 280; teaching at, of anatomy, 150; —, of chemistry, 142–3; —, of medicine, 148–9; —, of physiology, 149.

Leysin, Switzerland, 378.
Libido, 514.
Lice, as transmitters of disease, 451, 452.
Liège, Belgium, 322, 571.
Ligation of arteries, 98, 183.
Ligatures, 351, 358–9.
Light, theories of, 642.
Lille, France, 330, 395, 553.
Lime juice, 188.
Lincoln, Lincs., 500.
Linseed, 674.
Lipase, 602.
Lipiodol, 376.
Liquorice, 674.
Lisbon, Portugal, 512.
Lister Institute, London, 396, 400, 599, 612, 617.
Lithotomy, 54, 151, 183, 352.
Liver, 12–13, 62, 65, 123, 125, 556, 596, 618, 634; acute yellow atrophy of, 275, 284, 633; glycogenic function of, 294–6; in treatment of pernicious anaemia, 621; models of, 12–13.
Liver abscess, 493.
Liverpool, 263, 659; artificial pneumo-thorax first suggested at, 372; diabetic urine, nature of, shown at, 552; first local authority in Great Britain to appoint a medical officer of health, 219, 232.
Liverpool School of Tropical Medicine, 483, 486, 689.
Local Education Authorities, 224.
Local Government Board, 220, 223, 232.
Locomotor ataxia, see Tabes dorsalis.
Lodging houses, 189, 217.
London, 45, 189, 200, 227, 249, 345, 374, 375, 394, 485, 533, 598, 599, 613, 740; ague in, 456; anatomical teaching in, 120, 124, 151, 176, 177, 273, 740; bac-teriologists at, 231–2, 395, 396, 398; Bills of Mortality for (1603–1661), 180; black rat in, incidence of, 492; chest hospitals established at, 229; children's dispensaries established at, 652, 656; cholera in, 730–1; circulation of blood discovered at, 120–3; City of, first medical officer of health, appointment of, 219; —, —, work and *Reports* of, 220; —, Improvement Act (1766), 193; 'con-tinued fevers' studied in, 731; County of, appoints medical officer to examine school children (1890), 224; —, first

medical officers of health in area of, 232; —, first to enforce standard of training for health visitors (1908), 226; dentistry in, 668, 670; dermatology in, 204, 396; diseases prevalent in (1804–16), 204; fevers in, causes of (1838), 213–14; —, types of, prevalent in 17th cent., 728; garden at Upton near, 190; general anaesthesia, first introduced in England at, 344; Great Plague of, 489; Great Windmill Street School at, 176; influenza virus investigated at (1932–3), 449; malaria research at, 463; Medical Society of, 190; medical statistics de-veloped at, 722; nursing in, in 18th cent., 702; obstetrics in, 176; ortho-paedic hospital founded at, 658; paediatric works published at, 651–3, 655; parathyroids first discovered at, 535; pathologists at, 629, 632, 633, 636, 638, 639–40; plague in, 489; physicians at, 110, 120, 123, 170, 187, 190, 210, 256, 257, 272, 273, 279, 284–5, 499; physiologists at, 120–4, 154, 251, 258, 302, 518–19, 538; pure culture, method of, demonstrated at, 340; Royal College of Physicians of, founded 1518, 103; scarlet fever in, 203; sur-geons at, 151, 154, 177, 179, 182, 344, 353, 362, 365, 687; sweating sickness in, 740; tubercle bacilli, difference between human and bovine announced at, 398; University of, 210, 344, 499; urology at, 263; water bacteriology and purification, research at, 231; yellow fever research at, 477. *See also* Hospitals, Hunterian Museum, Inter-national Medical Congress, King's College, Pharmacopoeia, Royal College of Physicians, Royal College of Sur-geons, Royal Society, University College.
London County Council, 226, 232.
London School Board, 224.
London School of Hygiene and Tropical Medicine, 695, 736, 738.
Long thoracic nerve, of Bell, 272.
Louvain, Belgium, 90, 322, 394, 418.
Lugol's solution, 523.
Lumbar puncture, 249.
Lund, Sweden, 325.
Lung, 89, 119, 124, 460; abscess of, 368; excision of, 230, 368–9.
Lupus ,377, 378.

Lyme Regis, Dorset, 352.
Lymphadenoma, *see* Hodgkin's disease.
Lymph, 123.
Lymph vessels, 123, 516, 520, 628.
Lymphatic glands, 242, 317.
Lyons, France, 53, 633.
Lysis, *see* Bacteriolysis.

Macaca, 62, 476.
Macedon, Greece, 41.
Madras, 611.
Madrid, 467.
Magic, 77, 494. *See also* Medicine, magico-religious.
Magnesia, 522.
Magnesium sulphate, 677.
Magnet, 112, 185-6, 507.
Malaria, 54, 380, 452, 453, 711, 736; accurately described in 1st cent. A.D., 54; bird, 462, 463-4; control of, 464-6; decrease of, during Industrial Revolution, 191; described in Hippocratic Collection, 728; history of, 454-6; methylene blue in treatment of, 689; miasma as cause, 197, 730; mosquito suggested as transmitter (1717), 197; mosquito net used in Roman times, 55; prevalence in Havana, 471-2; quinine used to treat (1630), 688; used for shock therapy, 511. *See also* Malaria parasite, *Plasmodium*.
Malaria parasite, 456-64, 639, 687, 691; exoerythrocytic and pre-erythrocytic forms, 463-4. *See also Plasmodium*.
Male fern (*Felix mas*), 674.
Malformations, congenital, 629, 633-4.
Malignant disease, *see* Cancer.
Malleus maleficarum, 496.
Malnutrition, 609-10, 615.
Malocclusion, dental, 670.
Malta, 384-5.
Malta fever, *see* Brucellosis.
Maltose, 298.
Mammary gland, 548.
Manchester, 210, 403, 509, 526, 738; condition of cotton operatives at, 211; fever wards opened at (1794), 189; Improvement Act (1776), 193; medical ethics first described at, 189; puerperal fever studied at (1773), 361; typhus fever at, 189; voluntary health visitors first introduced at, 226.
'M. & B. 693', 693.

Mandragora (Mandrake), 341.
Mania, 497, 504.
Man midwife, 176.
Manometer, 155, 311.
Mantoux test, 425.
Mantua, Italy, 672.
Marburg, Germany, 299, 592; acetylcholine synthesized at (1894), 567; anatomy of head studied at, 241; research, on biochemistry and the cell nucleus at, 596; —, on nutrition at, 586.
Margarine, 608.
Marine cycle, 520.
Marine Hospital Service, 232-4; Surgeon General of, 233-4.
Marriages, 714.
Marseilles, France, 53, 198, 489.
Marsh's disease, 532. *See also* Hyperthyroidism.
Marshes, diseases associated with, 184, 197.
Massachusetts, Sanitary Commission of State of, 235.
Massage, 26, 371-2.
Materia medica, 53, 151. *See also* Drugs.
Maternal mortality rate, 720.
Maternity and child welfare, 225-8.
May-fly, 133.
Mayo Clinic, Rochester, Minn., U.S.A., 370, 532.
Measles, 203, 445, 446, 626, 728; differentiated from smallpox, 74; epidemics of, periodicity of, 737; —, hypothetical cause of, 740.
Meat, dried, 586.
Meat extract (Liebig), 238.
Mediastinum, 244.
Medical Acts, 672, 673.
Medical bibliographies, 744.
Medical education, 51-53, 56, 78, 79, 81, 91, 147-51, 177, 280-6. *See also* Clinical medicine.
Medical ethics, 10, 20, 31-32, 189.
Medical journals, 744-5.
Medical officers of health, 217, 218, 219-20, 224, 227; in London area, 232.
Medical police, 198.
Medical Research Council, 221, 292.
Medical Society of London, 190.
Medical statistics, 721-7.
Medicine, Alexandrian, 8, 48-51, 239, 643; Arabian, 73-76, 523, 549; Assyrian and Babylonian, 9-15, 20; Byzantine,

Medicine (*cont.*)
67–68, 240–1; of Dark Ages, 68–73; Egyptian, 3–9, 20; Greek, 8, 9, 16–45, 239–41, 494, 626, 650, 671; Hippocratic, 27–41; internal, 53, 84, 101–3, 110; medieval, 76–87, 488, 494–6, 626, 650; military, 181–5; naval, 182, 185–8; prehistoric, 1–3; preventive, *see* Hygiene, Preventive medicine, Public health; prison, 189–90; Renaissance, 88–110, 241–4, 626, 627, 651; Roman, 51–66, 643; temple, in Greece, 22–26.
Medicine, magico-religious, 4, 5, 10–15, 17, 22, 51.
Medicine, Schools of, *see* Clinical medicine, Dublin, Edinburgh, Glasgow, Leyden, Paris, Vienna.
Medico-Psychological Association, 502.
Mediterranean fever, *see* Brucellosis.
Medulla oblongata, 243, 252, 316.
Megrim, *see* Migraine.
Meissner's corpuscles, 269, 271.
Melanin, *see* Pigment.
Melun, France, 339.
'Membranes', of Bichat, 320.
Meninges, 50.
Meningioma, 368, 371.
Meningococcus, 391, 393, 402–3, 409, 696.
Mental deficiency, 225, 503.
Mental diseases, 191, 239, 240, 494–512; certification of, 501, 502, 512; classification of, 497, 506.
Mental faculties, cerebral localization of, 254–5, 256.
Mepacrine, 466, 691.
Mercuric chloride, 677.
Mercuric oxide, 165.
Mercury, 108, 174, 522, 668, 673, 687, 688, 691; of Paracelsus, 101.
Mercury manometer, 311.
Merkel's disks, 269.
Merozoites, *see* Malaria parasite.
Merseburg, Germany, 530.
Mesentery, 242.
Mesmerism, 504, 507–9; as anaesthetic, 342.
Mesopotamia, 9–15, 20.
Messina, Italy, 410.
Metabolism, 117, 168, 578–622; basal, 531, 582, 590, 593; calcium, 536; carbohydrate, 285, 316, 548–9; chemical regulation of, 303; endogenous and exogenous, 599; fat, 579, 593, 602–4;

see also Fat; influence on, of anterior pituitary, 547–8; —, of muscular work, *see* Work; intermediate, 582; Lavoisier's experiments on, 168; origin of word, 578; pre-fasting level of, 591; protein, 586, 587, 594–602.
Methaemoglobin, 319.
Methyl methacrylate, 667.
Methylene blue, 689, 691.
Metrazol, *see* Cardiazol.
Metropolitan Management Act (1855), 232.
Metropolitan Water Board, 231.
Miasmatic theory, *see* Infection.
Michigan, University of, (Ann Arbor), 685.
Micrococcus catarrhalis, 393.
Micrococcus melitensis, 384–5.
Micro-organisms, 143, 326–41, 354–5.
Microscope, 113, 124–35, 171, 320; in pathology, 288, 634.
Microtome, 635–6.
Microtonometer, of Krogh, 309.
Micturition, 263.
Midwifery, *see* Obstetrics.
Midwives, 176, 227.
Midwives Act (1902), 227.
Migraine, 190, 240.
Migration of races, 246.
Milan, 87, 202, 655.
Military surgeons, 53, 56, 57, 58, 95–97, 181–5.
Milk, 7, 385, 610, 612, 618, 653, 654; effect of, on growth, 609; secretion of, 548; souring of, 331; tuberculous, 230–1.
Milk centres, 227.
Milk supply, control of, 223; pasteurization of, 231.
Ministry of Health, 220, 223, 225, 716.
Minoans, 19–20, 23.
Mites, as transmitters of disease, 451.
Mitral disease, of heart, 245, 624, 628, 632.
MNS antigen, 701.
Modena, Italy, 197, 536.
Mollusca, Aristotle on, 42.
Monasteries, medicine in, 69.
Montecassino, Italy, 71.
Monte Rosa, Switzerland, 309.
Montpellier, France, 83, 516, 631; burnt sponge and seaweed early used for goitre at, 522; heart diseases studied at, 245; nervous diseases studied at, 245;

orthopaedic hospital established near, 658; tenotomy for club foot first successful at, 658; traditions of, derived from Bologna, 80.

Montreal, Canada, 317, 395, 536.

Moral insanity, 506.

Morbid anatomy, 168–71, 282–3, 284, 285–6, 627–34; chairs of, 631. *See also* Pathology.

Moro's test, 425.

Morphine, 680, 681.

Mosquito, 197, 460–5, 468–78.

Mosquito-malaria theory, 460, 463.

Mosquito net, 55.

Motion, laws of, 145–6; planetary, 145–6.

Motor area, of cerebral cortex, *see* Cerebral cortex.

Motor impulses, 139, 154, 263–5.

Mountain sickness, 308–9, 310.

Multiple neurofibromatosis, 636.

Mummification, *see* Embalming.

Mummy, as drug, 7.

Mummies, Egyptian, 246.

Mumps, 445, 446, 728.

Munich, Germany, 390, 392, 396, 425, 591, 599, 605; outbreaks of cholera and typhoid at, 231; physiological institute at, 583, 605.

Muscardine, 327–8.

Muscarine, 565, 566, 567, 573.

Muscle sense, 263, 265, 270.

Muscle spindles, 270.

Muscle tone, 266.

Muscles, 61, 62; anatomical illustrations of, 90, 94, 150; cardiac, *see* Cardiac muscle; chemical transmission of nerve impulse in voluntary, 574–7; distension by animal spirits as causes of contraction of, 50; electrical stimulation of, 274; 'inherent muscular force' as cause of contraction of, 153; innervation of voluntary, 263; 'irritability' as cause of contraction of, 123; mechanistic theory of action of, 90, 98, 140–1, 142; microscopic structure of voluntary, 131; proof that no increase in volume of, on contraction, 133–4; theory of increase in volume of, on contraction, 50.

Muscular contraction, theories of, 133–4, 153; heat generated in, 289, 292; mechanism of, 292–4.

Mustard, 674.

Mutation, in bacteria, 403–6.

Myasthenia gravis, 245.

Mycenaeans, 17–20, 23.

Mycobacterium leprae, see Leprosy bacillus.

Mycobacterium tuberculosis, see Tubercle bacillus.

Myelins, 319.

Myelin sheath, 246, 248.

Myenteric plexus, 260.

Myogenic theory, of heart-beat, *see* Heart-beat.

Myosin, 294.

Myrrh, 673, 674.

Myxoedema, 285, 524–7.

Nagana, 482, 483.

Nancy, France, 510, 513.

Naphthaleine, 691.

Naples, Italy, 72, 75, 628.

Napoleonic War, 184, 467.

Narceine, 681.

Narcotics, 84.

National Board of Health (U.S.A.), 234.

National Health Insurance Act (1911), 223, 229, 670, 743, 747.

National Health Service Act (1946), 670, 743, 747.

National Institute of Health, Bethesda, Maryland, U.S.A., 234–5.

National Institute for Medical Research, Hampstead, 555.

Nautical Almanac, 642.

Navy, Royal, *see* Royal Navy; United States, 233.

Near East, 1, 198. *See also* Assyria, Babylonia, Mesopotamia.

Neisseria gonorrhoeae, see Gonococcus.

Neisseria meningitidis, see Meningococcus.

Neoarsphenamine, 690.

Neoplasms, *see* Cancer, Tumours.

Neosalvarsan, *see* Neoarsphenamine.

Nepenthe, of Homer, 341.

Nephritis, 275, 278, 284.

Nerve cells, 246, 247.

Nerve compression, as anaesthetic, 341, 342.

Nerve fibre, structure of, 246, 247, 248.

'Nerve force', of Haller, 153.

Nerve impulse, 154; chemical transmission of, 555, 556, 564–77; electrical theory of, 564, 565; speed of, 288–9.

Nerve-muscle preparation, 133–4, 159.

Nerve regeneration, 248.

Nerve roots, 154, 248, 251, 253, 288.

Nerve tracts, in spinal cord, 248, 249, 255, 279.

Nerves, gun-shot wounds of, 277.

Nerves, 48, 49; accelerator, 314; of heart, 245; inhibitory action of, 313; peripheral, function of, 48; —, nature of, 50; resting current in, 289, 290.

Nervous co-ordination, 256. See also Nervous integration.

'Nervous energy', 148.

'Nervous ether', 148.

Nervous fluid, 139–40, 152–3.

Nervous integration, 253–4, 263–6.

Nervous system, microscopic anatomy of, 246, 260.

Nervous system, anatomy of, 62, 241–50, 279; central, diseases of, 224; —, role of acetylcholine in, 577; pathology of, 271 ff; physiology of, 48–50, 65, 138–40, 152, 241–50, 250–71, 564–77. See also Autonomic nervous system, Sympathetic nervous system.

Nestorians, 74.

Netley, Hants, 419.

Neuralgia, trigeminal, 371.

Neurogenic theory, of heart-beat, see Heart-beat.

Neuroglia, 247.

Neurolemma, 246.

Neurology, 239–80; textbooks of, 273, 278–9.

Neuron theory, 247, 248.

Neuropathology, see Nervous system.

Neurophysiology, see Nervous system.

Neurosis, 505, 506, 507, 510, 514.

New-born infant, salting of, 240.

New Haven, Connecticut, U.S.A., 612.

New Lanark, 225.

New Stone Age (Neolithic), 1–3.

New Testament, 494.

New York, 236, 366, 456, 471, 563, 655; diphtheria immunization early introduced at, 436; first children's hospital in U.S.A. established at (1854), 657; first diagnostic laboratory under a local authority established at (1892), 235; influenza virus B isolated at (1940), 449; national Hygienic Laboratory established at (1887), 234; physiological calorimeters constructed at, 589; public health department established at, 235; Schick test data for city of, 434–5; spinal anaesthesia studied at, 350; toxin-

antitoxin mixture widely used in prophylaxis of diphtheria at, 436; tuberculosis notification introduced at (1893), 229; vesico-vaginal fistula, first satisfactory operation for, performed at (1852), 362; yellow fever at, 467. See also Cornell University, Columbia University, Rockefeller Institute.

New York Medical College, 655.

New Zealand, 530, 709.

Nicotine, physiological action of, 262, 565–7, 574.

Nicotinamide, 620.

Nicotinic acid (niacin), 620.

Night-blindness, 618, 629.

Nîmes, France, 53.

Nineveh, 10.

Nitre, 165.

Nitric acid, 677.

Nitric oxide, 165.

Nitro-aerial particles, 163.

Nitrogen, 305, 310; amount of, excreted in starvation, 584; continuous exchange of, between different tissues, 601–2; derived by plants from ammonia in atmosphere, 238; excretion of, after muscular exercise, 592; —, after protein ingestion, 599; in formation of urea, 582; Kjeldahl method for determination of, 320; micromethod for determination of, 596; production of, from tissue disintegration, 601; in urine, as measure of protein destruction, 581–2, 592; —, in relation to nitrogen in diet, 599.

Nitrogen cycle, 238.

Nitrogen equilibrium, 584, 605.

Nitrous oxide, 165, 343, 348–9.

Nobel Prizes: Banting (1923), 555; Bordet (1919), 414; Butenandt (1939), 550; Cajal (1906), 248; Cori, C. F. and G. T. (1947), 294; Dale (1936), 577; Dam (1943), 622; Doisy (1943), 622; Eijkman (1929), 612; Finsen (1903), 378; Fischer (1902), 595; Golgi (1906), 248; Gowland Hopkins (1929), 612; Haworth (1937), 619; Hench (1950), 540; Hill, A. V. (1922), 293; Houssay (1947), 549; Karrer (1937), 619; Kendall (1950), 540; Kocher (1909), 374; Kossel (1910), 596; Krogh (1920), 307; Laveran (1907), 459; Loewi (1936), 577; Macleod (1923), 555; Metchnikoff (1908), 410; Meyerhoff (1922), 293; Minot (1934), 622;

Murphy (1934), 622; Nicolle (1928), 451; Ross (1902), 463; Reichstein (1950), 540; Ruzicka (1939), 550; Stanley (1946), 447; Szent-Györgyi (1937), 622; Theiler (1951), 477; Warburg (1931), 622; Whipple (1934), 622. *See also* Appendix.
Nociceptive reactions, 263.
nor-adrenaline, 571.
Nordrach-in-Baden, Germany, 228.
Normal curve, 722–5, 732, 733.
North Shields, Northumb., 524.
North-western University, Illinois, U.S.A., 563.
Norwich, Norfolk, 366, 651, 740.
Nosology, systems of, 280–1.
Notification, *see* Births, Infectious diseases, Tuberculosis.
Notification of Births Acts (1907, 1915), 227.
Notochord, 321, 323.
Novocaine, 350.
Nucleolus, 322.
Nucleus, cell, 247, 320–5, 596.
Nucleus dorsalis, 249.
Nuisances, abatement of, 213, 231; Inspectors of, 219.
Nuisances Removal Act (1848), 218.
Numerical Method, of Louis, 721–2.
Nurses, State Registration of, 709.
Nursing, 194, 701–10; of infants, 651, 652.
Nursing Orders, 702.
Nutmeg, 674.
Nutrition, 225, 228, 604–10.
Nux vomica, 681.
Nyctalopia, *see* Night blindness.
Nystagmus, 275.

Oatmeal, 608.
Obstetrics, 96, 174–7, 239–40, 344, 345, 360–2.
Occupational diseases, 101, 179, 197.
Occupational therapy, 501.
Odessa, U.S.S.R., 410.
Odontological Society, 663.
Oesophagus, 364.
Oestradiol, 551.
Oestriol, 551.
Oestrogens, 551.
Oestrone, 551.
Oestrous cycle, 547, 550–1.
Offensive trades, 220.

Ointments, 7, 14, 79, 101.
Oldham, Lancs., 229.
Old Stone Age (Palaeolithic), 1.
Old Testament, 494.
Olfactory nerves, 542.
Olive oil, 578.
Ontario, Canada, 236.
Oocyst, 458, 461, 462.
Open-air schools, 225.
Ophthalmia neonatorum, 650.
Ophthalmoscope, 289, 643, 647, 654.
Opium, 341, 680.
Opsonins, 419, 420.
Optic chiasma, 241, 242.
Optic nerve, 244, 288.
Optic thalamus, 243, 291.
Optics, 641–3.
Oral deformities, 670.
Organ of Golgi, 270.
Organs of special sense, 244, 245.
Orthodontics, 670–1.
Orthopaedics, 185, 657–9.
Osler-Vaquez disease, 317.
Osmic acid stain, 248.
Osmosis, 319, 321, 325.
Osteology, 59, 61, 93–94, 150, 151.
Osteomalacia, 537, 636.
Osteotomy, 366, 369–70.
Ostia, Italy, 29.
Oswaldo Cruz Institute, Brazil, 487.
Ovarian tumour, 362, 628.
Ovary, 550–1.
Ovum, 321.
Oxford, 110, 179, 266, 613, 651; physicians at, 232, 317; physiology at, 132, 232, 263, 266, 289, 304; research on, nerve currents at, 289–90; —, nervous integration at, 263–6; —, the sensory cortex at, 266; —, penicillin at, 695–6; —, respiration and blood gases at, 304–11; —, the tricarboxylic acid cycle and aneurine at, 619. *See also* Hospitals.
Oxford, County of, 229.
Oxidation, 320, 578, 603.
Oxygen, 303–10; alveolar, 306; in blood, estimation of, 305; discovery of, 165–6; in metabolism, 579, 581, 585, 586; secretion, theory of, 309–10.
Oxygen-debt, 293.
Oxygen-dissociation curve, 308–10.
Oxyhaemoglobin, 304, 308, 319.
Oxytocin, 546.

3 I

'Pace-maker' of heart, *see* Sino-auricular node.
Pacinian corpuscles, 270.
Paddington, London, 232.
Padua, Italy, 105, 120, 148, 149, 516, 740; anatomical teaching at, 90–92, 97–98; anatomists at, 89, 90, 97–98, 118, 169, 244; connexion of lymphatics with thoracic duct discovered by student at, 123; first printed work on paediatrics published at, 650; morbid anatomy at, 169; physicians at, 115; valves in veins described at, 118.
Paediatrics, 68, 226, 240, 650–9.
Pain stimuli, 252, 291.
Palermo, Italy, 203.
Palmaris brevis muscle, 62, 63.
Paludrine, 692.
Panama, malaria in, 464–5; yellow fever in, 473–4.
Pancreas, 143, 548, 551–5, 628, 639.
Pancreatic duct, 297, 515–16.
Pancreatic juice, 296–8, 551–2, 602.
P antigen, 701.
Papworth Colony, Cambs., 230.
Papyrus, 3.
Papyri, Egyptian, 4, 5, 6, 7, 671, 673.
Paracentesis thoracis, 98.
Paragonimus westermanii, 460.
Paralysis, 169, 239, 240, 278; Little's spastic, 658–9. *See also* Apoplexy, General paralysis of the insane.
Paralysis agitans, 272.
Paraplasma flavigenum, 474–5.
Paraplegia, 65, 239, 285.
Parasympathetic nerve fibres, 566, 568, 570–2.
Parathormone, 537, 538.
Parathyroid glands, 534–8; discovery of, 535.
Parathyroidectomy, 537.
Paratyphoid bacillus, 391, 409, 444.
Paratyphoid fever, 391, 394.
Parenchyme, 324.
Paris, 83, 90, 237, 394, 613, 633, 659, 731; anaphylaxis, first described at, 420; —, mechanism of, studied at, 561; anatomy at, 90, 242, 255, 272, 279; bacteriology founded at, 330–9; electrotherapy founded at, 274; endocrinology founded by Bordeu at, 516; eye diseases, early treatise on, published at, 646; eye sign, in exophthalmic goitre, introduced at, 533; heart diseases studied at, 281, 283; immunity studied at, 401, 410, 414, 417, 442; Institut Pasteur at, 395, 397–8, 401, 410, 411, 414, 417, 426, 440, 442, 561; Lugol's solution introduced at, 523; lunatics freed from chains by Pinel at Bicêtre at, 497; mesmerism practised widely at, 509; metabolism research carried out at, 581; morbid anatomy at, 282, 631–2; —, chair of, founded (1836) at, 631; neurology at, 254, 274–5, 279, 513; nosology at, 281; obstetrics at, 177; parathyroids studied early at, 536; percussion developed at, 283; phrenology at, 254; physicians at, 98, 173, 274–5, 279, 281–3, 513, 533, 632, 657, 721–2; physiology at, 154, 248, 255, 262, 294–9, 536; porcelain teeth first made at, 665; rejuvenation by testicular transplants performed at, 550; School of, 280–3, 286; society for study of Numerical Method founded at, 721; stethoscope invented at, 172–3; surgery at, 95; tetanus, active immunization against, at, 442; tissue pathology founded at, 320. *See also* Hospitals.
Parotid duct (of Stensen), 516.
Parotid gland, 242.
Parry's disease, 532. *See also* Hyperthyroidism.
PAS (para-aminosalicylic acid), 697.
Pasteurella pestis, see Plague bacillus.
Pasteurization of milk, 231, 386.
Pathology, 46, 53, 84, 100, 197, 287, 321, 325, 627–40; cellular, 326. *See also* 'Cellular Pathology'; comparative, 380; experimental, 629, 637–8, 751–2; humoral, 138, 281. *See also* Morbid anatomy.
Pavia, Italy, 159, 197, 372, 428.
Pavlov's pouch, 302–3.
Pébrine, 335.
Pelican (dental instrument), 660.
Pellagra, 619–20.
Pelvis, 176, 177.
Pendulum-myograph, 288.
Penicillin, 694–6, 754.
Penicillium notatum, 694, 695.
Peppermint, 678.
Peptides, 595.
Peptones, 595.
Perception, *see* Sensory impressions.
Percussion, 172, 281, 283, 286.

Pergamon, Asia Minor, 59, 68.
Pericardium, 628.
Periosteum, 657, 659.
Periostitis, 636.
Peritoneum, 244.
Peritonitis, 365.
Perityphlitis, 365.
Pernicious anaemia, 276, 284–5, 621, 751.
Peru, 349.
Petri dish, 340.
Petrograd (St. Petersburg), U.S.S.R., 600.
Peyer's patches, 204.
Pfeiffer's reaction, 414.
Pfeifferella mallei, see B. mallei.
Phagocytosis, 411, 418–19.
Pharmaceutical Society of Great Britain, 674.
Pharmacology, 679, 684–5.
Pharmacopoeia, 53, 671–9; British, 672–5, 677–9; contents of a modern, 676–9. *See also British Pharmaceutical Codex,* Dispensatory.
Pharmacopoeia Commission, 672, 673.
Pharmacopoeia Edinburgensis, 672.
Pharmacopoeia Londinensis, 672.
Phenaceturic acid, 603.
Phenolphthalein, 677.
Phenylacetic acid, 603.
Phenylbutyric acid, 603.
Phenylpropionic acid, 603.
Phenylvaleric acid, 603.
Philadelphia, Pennsylvania, U.S.A., 190, 317, 553; appendicitis, early operations for, performed at, 365, 366; health department established before 1800 at, 235; orthopaedic surgery, early development at, 659; surgery chair divorced from anatomy chair at, 351; typhoid and typhus first distinguished at, 337; University of Pennsylvania at, 351, 659; yellow fever outbreaks at, 191, 467, 468.
Phlebitis, 632, 635.
Phlebograph, 623.
Phlebotomus, 488.
Phlegm, 46, 138.
Phlogiston, 143, 163, 165, 166.
Phosphates, 294, 540.
Phosphoric acid, 294.
Phosphorus, 166.
Phosphorylase, 296.
Phrenitis, 240.
Phrenology, 254–5, 256.
Phthisis, 37, 54, 86, 179, 203, 306, 373,

381, 721; fibroid (miners'), 101, 284, 306; notification of, 229; pathology of, 282, 631, 633. *See also* Tuberculosis.
Physic gardens, 497.
'Physician's Pulse Watch', 171.
'Physiological medicine', of Broussais, 282.
Physiology, 50, 98, 101, 115–17, 119–23, 138–43, 149, 287–320, 515–55 *passim,* 555–77, 578–622; of circulation, 119–23, *see also* Blood; of digestion, 155–9; Galenic, 62, 64–65, 118–19; medieval, 81, 84, 88; of metabolism, 578–610; of muscle, 123, 152–4, 292–4; of nervous system, 241–71, 287–92; Renaissance, 94, 98; of respiration, 303–11; of vascular system, 118–23, 124, 155, 311–16, 622–7 *passim. See also* under individual organs, systems, and tissues.
Physiotherapy, 371–2.
Physostigmine, *see* Eserine.
Pigment, in malaria, 456, 457.
Pigment cells, 323.
Pike's Peak, Colorado, 309.
Pineal body, 138–9, 241, 242, 243.
Pirquet test, 424–5, 429.
Pisa, Italy, 113, 244, 393, 651.
Pituita, 43, 239, 241, 243, 542.
Pituitary body, 43, 241, 242, 243, 277, 371; anterior lobe of, 541, 542–4, 545, 546–9; posterior lobe of, 545–6.
Pituitary extract, 546.
Pituitrin, 546.
Placenta praevia, 176.
Plague, 83, 104, 202, 452, 454, 736; bubonic, 492; campestral, 492; discovery of bacillus of, 381, 391; history of, 488–90; immunological reactions in, 418; pneumonic, 492; prevalence of, in London (1590–1665), 489; —, in Russia (1709), 198;—, in Toulon (1720), 198; quarantine for, 198; restrictive measures against, in Middle Ages, 86; saints associated with, 68; transmission of, 384, 489–90; treatment of, 491–2; —, by sera, 491; vaccines against, 439, 491.
Plague bacillus, 383, 393, 489–90; discovery of, 381, 391; immunological test using, 416–17; involution forms, 404.
Plagues, historic: of Athens (430 B.C.), 488; Black Death (1347–8), 86–87, 488, 741; in Egypt (1834), 489; Great Plague of London (1665), 489; of

Plagues, historic (*cont.*)
Justinian (A.D. 542), 488; of Marseilles (1720), 198, 489; in Rome, (293 B.C.), 25; —, (A.D. 683), 68.
Plain muscle, action of histamine on, 557, 562–3.
Plasmochin, 691.
Plasmodium falciparum, 459, 462; *P. malariae,* 459, 462; *P. ovale,* 459; *P. vivax,* 459, 463. *See also* Malaria parasite.
Plaster of Paris, for bandages, 371; for dental impressions, 666.
Plasters, 101.
Playing fields, 217.
Plethora, 50.
Pleura, 244.
Pleuritic rub, 40.
Plymouth, Devon, 188.
pneuma, 49–50, 62, 64.
'Pneumatic chemistry', 162, 164–5.
Pneumatism, 49.
Pneumobacillus, 391.
Pneumococcus, 391, 401, 696.
Pneumoencephalography, 279.
Pneumonectomy, *see* Lung, excision of.
Pneumonia, 50, 169, 391, 474, 633, 693, 697, 721.
Pneumothorax, artificial, *see* Artificial pneumothorax; spontaneous, 631.
Podophyllum, 674, 677.
Poisons, 285.
Poland, 115, 203.
Poliomyelitis, 272, 275, 445–7, 652, 729; virus of, 449–50.
Political arithmetic, 179.
Pollen sensitivity, 429, 430.
Polygastrica, 327.
Polygraph, 622; Mackenzie's ink, 623–4.
Polyneuritis, 279.
Polypeptides, 595.
Polypharmacy, 286, 676.
Polyps of heart, 628.
Polypus, nasal, 54.
Polyuria, 546, 552.
Pomegranate, 674.
Pompeii, Italy, 54, 55, 58.
Pons Varolii, 242, 243, 244.
Poor Law, 209–14.
Poor Law Commission 210 212, 213, 214, 218.
Poppy, 673.
Population, 181, 191–2, 711–13, 718–20.
Population Act (1800), 712.

Portal vein, 62, 295.
Portsmouth, Hants, 188.
Posen, Germany, 393.
Postganglionic neurons, 262.
Post-mortem examinations, 78–79, 149, 168–9, 170, 171, 280, 286. *See also* Pathology.
Post-partum haemorrhage, 239.
Potassium iodide, 522–3.
Pott's disease, 179.
Pott's fracture, 179.
Poultices, 14.
Poverty, effect of, on food consumption, 609–10.
Prague, Czechoslovakia, 392, 539, 595; nerve cells first described at, 246; parathyroids recognized as distinct from thyroid at, 536; primary tuberculous lung focus described at, 426.
Precipitins, 417–18, 420, 563.
Pregnancy, 551; Zondek-Aschheim test for, 547.
Pregnanediol, 551.
Preventive medicine, 181; in Great Britain, 208–32; in United States and Canada, 232–6. *See also* Hygiene, Public health.
Preventive Police, 211.
Priest of Artemis, 26–27.
Primary complex, tuberculous, 426.
Primary tuberculous focus, 426.
Primordial utricle, *see* Utriculus primordialis.
Printing of medical texts, 88.
Prisons, 155. *See also* Medicine.
Privy Council, 211, 220, 232, 319.
Probability, 722–7.
Progeria, 544.
Progesterol (progestin), 551.
Prognosis, 69; Hippocratic, 40.
Progressive bulbar paralysis, 274.
Progressive lenticular degeneration, 276.
Progressive muscular atrophy, 274, 618.
Prolactin, 548.
Prolans, 547.
Prontosil red, 693.
Proprioceptive nerve fibres, 263.
Proprioceptive receptors, 270.
Prostate, 551, 638, 753.
Protein, 294, 583, 603; amount of, destroyed during starvation, 585, 591; breakdown products of, 238, 595; calorie value of, 586–7; certain types of,

necessary for life, 578; circulating, 590, 598; consumption of, relative to muscular work, 592–3; conversion of, to carbohydrate and fat, 604; destruction of, measured by nitrogen in urine, 581–2; ingestion of, relation to nitrogen equilibrium, 584; metabolism of, 594–602; —, influence of muscular work on, 579; organized ('tissue'), 590, 598, 601; requirement of, in normal diet, 604–10; specific dynamic action of, 587–8, 599. *See also* Amino-acids.
Proteosoma, 462.
Protopathic and epicritic nerve fibres, 270–1.
Protoplasm, 247, 321, 324, 325.
Protozoology, 327, 487, 488. *See also* under names of diseases and parasites.
Proximate principles, 578–9, 585–6; calorie value of, 587; interconversion of, 603–4.
Prussic acid, 681.
Pseudohypertrophic paralysis, 272.
Pseudomuscarine, 566, 567.
Pseudotuberculosis, of cattle, *see* Johne's disease; of guinea-pigs, 391.
Psittacosis, 447.
psyche, of Aristotle, 44, 45, 46, 143.
Psychoanalysis, 504, 512, 514–15.
Psychology, 287, 512–15.
Psychoneurosis, 504.
Psychoses, 504, 506, 507, 510–11.
Psychosomatic diseases, 749.
Ptosis, 239, 260.
Public health, 55–56, 208–36.
Public Health Acts: of 1848, 218; of 1875, 220, 223, 236; of Ontario, 236.
Public Health and Marine Hospital Service, of U.S.A., 234.
Public medical service, in Rome, 53, 56.
Puerperal fever, 177, 245, 360–2, 693.
Pulmonary artery, 64, 119.
Pulmonary vein, 62, 64, 89, 119.
Pulse, 49, 115–16; 'water-hammer', 245, 283, 628.
Pulse measurers, 171. *See also* Pulsilogium.
Pulse wave, 313.
Pulsilogium, 115–16, 171.
Pulvinar, 243.
Pupil, light reflex of, 250.
Pure cultures, 338–40.
Purgatives, 7, 677.
Purified protein derivative (P.P.D.), 425.

Purpura, of Henoch, 654.
Putamen, 243.
Putrefaction, 156, 157, 184, 238, 328–9, 331, 354.
Pyaemia, 354, 635.
Pyonephrosis, 638.
Pyrethrum, 465.
Pythogenic theory, of fevers, *see* Infection.

Qualities, the four, 46.
Quarantine, 87, 190, 198–9, 210, 215, 220, 223, 236, 490.
Quarantine Acts, of U.S.A., 233–4.
Quassia, 674.
Quebec, Canada, 236.
Quicklime, 163.
Quinine, 454, 680, 681, 687, 688, 691.
Quinsy, 38.

Rabies, 240, 339, 445, 446.
Racemic acid, 330.
Radicles, chemical, 238, 681.
Radioisotopes, 752, 753.
Radiology, 370, 374–7.
Radium therapy, 377.
Ragusa, Yugoslavia, 87.
Rape seed, as goitrogen, 530.
Rat, as plague transmitter, 490, 491, 492.
Rat-flea, as plague transmitter, 490, 491.
Ray, Persia, 74.
Reading, Berks., 366, 607, 608.
Rebreathing, in anaesthesia, 349.
Reciprocal innervation, 263–4.
Recreation grounds, 217.
Rectal anaesthesia, 350.
Rectum, nervous control of, 262.
Red Cross, 185.
Reductions, chemical, 320.
Reflex, conditioned, 266–9; extensor, 264; flexion, 263, 264; knee-jerk, 252; refractory phase of, 265; scratch, 264; stretch, 266; unconditioned, 267.
Reflex action, 250–4, 263–6.
Reflex arcs, 252, 264–5.
Reflex inhibition, 263–4.
Refraction, errors of, 643.
Refuse removal, 215.
Regeneration of tissue, 248, 636, 639.
Regimen sanitatis, of Salerno, 73, 522.
Registrar General, 212–13, 220, 713–18.
Registration Act (1836), 212.
Regression, 726.
Rehabilitation therapy, 55.

Rejuvenation, 549–50.
Relapsing fever, 391; African, 484.
Remittent fever, 731.
Renal rickets, 536.
Rennet, 143, 157.
Reserpine, 682.
Resins, synthetic, 667.
Respiration, 94, 152, 155, 250; air necessary for, 136, 137, 161; effect of altitude on, 309; essential changes in tissues during, 168, 237; experiments with small animals on, 162, 165; foetal, 311; haemoglobin, role of, in, 303–4; in metabolism, 582; oxygen consumption in, variations of, 168; regulation of, 306–7; is slow combustion, 166; vital substance in air necessary for, 163, 165, 166. *See also* Oxygen, Oxygen-dissociation curve, Oxyhaemoglobin, Respiratory quotient.
Respiration apparatus, 585–7; portable, 589.
Respiratory centre, 252, 304, 306.
Respiratory diseases, 720, 721.
Respiratory quotient (R.Q.), 581–2, 585–6, 593.
Restraint, physical, in mental diseases, 497, 499, 500–2, 505.
rete mirabile, 65, 241, 242–3.
Reticulo-endothelial system, 318–19, 638.
Retina, 139, 250, 278, 289, 641, 642, 643, 648.
Rheims, France, 642.
Rhesus monkey, 62.
Rheumatism, 110, 753; acute (rheumatic fever), 540, 629, 632; chronic articular, in children, 655.
Rheumatoid arthritis, 540, 548.
Rh-factor, 701.
Rhubarb, 674.
Riboflavin, 620.
Ribs, 61.
Rice, 611, 612, 613.
Ricettario Fiorentino, 672.
Rickets, 196, 225, 636; bony deformities in, 369, 613; —, operations for, 369–70; calciferol in, 615–16; cod-liver oil in, 614, 615; considered a chronic infectious disease, 614; a deficiency disease (food and sunlight), 611, 612, 615; early history of, 613; first descriptions of, 123, 240, 613–14, 650; in Glasgow, 369; sunlight in, 614, 615; vitamins D_2

and D_3 in, 615–16; in Vienna (1919), 615.
Rickettsia burneti, 451; *R. prowazeki*, 451; *R. quintana*, 452; *R. rickettsi*, 451.
Rickettsiae, 450–2.
Rickettsial diseases, 450–2.
Ringer's solution, 315, 568.
Ring forms, *see* Malaria parasite.
Ringworm, 225.
Rochester, Minn., U.S.A., 343, 370, 548, 602, 621, 697.
Rockefeller Commission on Yellow Fever, 475, 476.
Rockefeller Foundation, 476–80, 561.
Rockefeller Institute for Medical Research, 310, 401, 420, 447, 449, 475, 597, 696.
Rocky Mountain spotted fever, 451.
Romberg's sign, 273.
Rome, 112, 124, 182, 197, 243, 244, 260, 393, 512; infected mosquitoes sent from, to London, 463; malaria research at, 457; pharmacopoeia published at (1580), 672.
Rome, Ancient, 59; aqueducts at, 56; *asclepieion* on Insula Tiberina at, 25, 57; hospitals (*valetudinaria*) at, 58; medical teaching at, 51–53; plague at, (293 B.C.), 25; —, (A.D. 683), 68; public health at, 55–56; public medical service at, 53, 56.
Rosemary, 674.
Rothamsted Experimental Research Station, 603.
Rough and smooth variants, 405.
Round ligaments, *see* Uterus.
Royal College of Physicians of Edinburgh, 280, 642.
Royal College of Physicians of London, 110, 123, 519, 532, 613; foundation of (1518), 103; *Pharmacopoeia Londinensis* of (1618), 672; committee of, responsible for classification of diseases, 715.
Royal College of Surgeons of England, 178–9, 543.
Royal Commissions: on a Constabulary Force, 217; on Health of the Army, 708; on Health of Towns, 217–18; on Lunatic Asylums in Scotland, 502; on Poor Laws, 211–12; on Population, 718; on State of Children in Factories, 217; on Tuberculosis, 398–9.
Royal Faculty of Physicians and Surgeons of Glasgow, 183.
Royal Institution, London, 335.
Royal Naval College, 188.

Royal Navy, 186.

Royal Society of London, 113, 123, 180, 232, 272, 555; *Catalogue of Scientific Papers* of, 743–4; Copley Medal of, awarded for research on animal cell, 322; discovery of oxygen communicated to (1775), 166; early experiments on blood transfusion at, 698; first Curator of Experiments to, 132; incorporated by Charles II (1662), 136; Malta Fever Commission of, 384; mechanism of eye communicated to, 642; papers on smallpox inoculation read to, 200; published works by foreign scientists, 124; Sleeping Sickness Commissions of, 484–5.

Rubber gloves, in surgery, 370.

Russia, plague in, 198.

Saarbrücken, Sarre, 408.

Sacred Disease, 494. *See also* Epilepsy.

Sacrum, 61.

Sailors, diseases of, *see* Medicine, naval.

St. Andrews, Fife, 428, 441, 607, 608.

St. Bartholomew, Island of (Insula Tiberina), Rome, 57.

St. Francis, Third Order of, 701.

St. Gall, Switzerland, 58.

St. Gothard tunnel, 493.

St. Helens, Lancs., 227.

St. John's House Nurses, 704, 706.

St. Louis, U.S.A., 551, 553, 639, 669.

Saints, healing, 67–68.

Salerno, Italy, 71–73; School of, 73, 522.

Salford, Lancs., 224, 226.

Saliceto, Italy, 79.

Salicin, 683.

Salicylic acid, 683.

Saliva, 143, 267–9.

Salivary glands, 267; of mosquito, 462. *See also* Parotid gland, Submaxillary gland.

Salmonella enteritidis, 391, 393.

Salmonella paratyphi, *see* Paratyphoid bacillus.

Salmonella typhi, *see* Typhoid bacillus.

'Salt', of Paracelsus, 101.

'Salting' of new-born infant, 240, 650.

Salts, composition of, 142.

Salvarsan, 688, 690, 691.

Salzburg, Austria, 100, 521.

Sanatoria, for tuberculous, 228–9.

Sandfly-fever, *see* Leishmaniasis.

San Domingo, W. Indies, 108.

Sanitary Idea, of Chadwick, 211.

Sanitary inspectors, 219, 220, 226.

Sanitation, domestic, 55, 214; military, 183, 184.

Sapienzia, Rome, 197.

Saragossa, Spain, 53.

Sarcode, 321, 324.

Sardinia, 255.

Sauerkraut, 188.

Sausages, 608.

Scabies, 730, 737. *See also* Itch.

Scammony, 674, 677.

Scarlatina (scarlet fever), 190, 202–4, 284, 436–9, 735.

Scarlet-fever antitoxin, 439.

Schaffhausen, Switzerland, 204.

Schick test, 434–5.

Schizogony, 459.

Schizophrenia, 511.

Schneider's membrane, 542.

Scholasticism, 77.

School Boards, 224.

School children, medical inspection of, 224–5.

School clinics, 225.

School dental clinics, 225, 670.

School meals, 224.

School medical officers, 224.

School medical service, 223, 224–5.

School nurses, 225.

Schultz-Charlton test, 437–8.

Sclerema, 652.

Scotoma, 240.

Scrub typhus, 475.

Scurvy, 185, 186, 187, 188, 196, 611, 612, 618; infantile, 655.

Scutari, 706–7.

Seamen's Hospital Society, 221.

Seaweed, burnt, in treatment of goitre, 522.

Sebastopol, 705.

Second intention, healing by, 522.

Second World War, 436, 563–4, 609, 617, 649; DDT introduced during, 491; growth of gerontology since, 752; increase of pulmonary tuberculosis during, 381; institution of blood banks during, 701; malaria research during, 464, 465–6; Medical History of the, 224; need for synthetic antimalarials during, 692; tetanus incidence in troops during, 443; various researches since, 753.

Secretin, 302, 518, 558.
Secretion, 301.
Sedatives, 148.
'Seiriasis', 650.
Semen, 549.
Semicircular canals, of ear, 256, 266.
Senegal, 466.
Senile dementia, 507.
Senna, 674.
Sensation, 153.
'Sensitive soul', of Stahl, 143.
Sensorium commune, 251.
Sensory area, see Cerebral cortex.
Sensory impressions, 139, 154, 269–71, 289–92.
Septicaemia, 38, 354.
Septum lucidum, 243.
Serpent, as medical symbol, 19, 24, 25, 57.
Serpentaria, 674.
Serpentarius, 113.
Serum globulin, 447, 595.
Serum sickness, 421–2, 429
Sesame, 674.
Seton, 182.
Seville, Spain, 69, 103.
Sewage, 193; disposal of, 193, 216, 231.
Sewerage, 55, 193, 218, 220.
Sewers, Commissioners of, 215; design of, 215.
Sex, 514.
Sex characters, 547.
Sex glands, 549–51.
Sex organs, 396.
Shaking palsy, see Paralysis agitans.
Sheffield, Yorks., 229, 596, 614.
Shigella shigae, see Dysentery bacillus (Shiga).
Shipway's inhaler, 348.
Shock therapy, 511.
Sicily, 75, 77, 488.
Sick children, hospitals for, 225, 655–7.
Sick poor, 212, 214.
Side-chain theory, 413, 687, 692.
Siena, Italy, 260, 671.
Sierra Leone, 463, 466, 467, 482.
Silk-worms, 328, 337.
Silver chromate, 247, 248.
Simmonds's disease, 544.
Sino-auricular node, 623.
Sinus venosus, 314.
Sinuses, cerebral, 243.
Sister tutor diploma, 710.

Sisters of Charity, 702.
Skin, histology of, 125, 269, 271.
Skin diseases, 7, 204, 225, 286, 377; nosology of, 281, 286.
Skin grafting, 373.
Skodaic resonance, 286.
Slaked lime, 163.
Sleeping sickness, see Trypanosomiasis.
Sleeping Sickness Commissions, 484–6.
Sleepy sickness, see Encephalitis lethargica.
Slit-lamp, 648.
Smallpox, 233, 711, 728; Chester outbreak (1774), effects of, 199; differentiated, from chicken-pox, 629; —, from measles, 74; inoculation of, 199–200; vaccination against, 200–2; a virus disease, 446. See also Vaccination, Vaccine, Vaccinia.
Smell, sense of, 292.
Smyrna, Asia Minor, 59.
Snake-venom, 420, 475, 563.
Snakes, in healing temples, 25.
Snellen's types, 643.
Snow's chloroform inhaler, 346, 347.
Social medicine, 743.
Societies, scientific, 113.
Society of Medical Officers of Health, 715.
Sodium bicarbonate, 673.
Sodium carbonate, 163, 673.
Sodium citrate, 700.
Sodium phosphate, 700.
Soft chancre, 391, 393.
Soldiers, diseases of, see Medicine, military.
Solferino, battle of, 185.
Somatic antigens, 404–5.
Soporific sponge, 341.
Soul, Aristotle's three types of, 45–46; seat of, 138, 152.
Spain, 76–77.
Spanish–American War, 471.
Spanish Armada, 182, 186.
Spanish Civil War, 701.
Spastic paraplegia, 279.
Spearmint, 674.
Specialism in medicine, 746.
Special schools, 225.
Specific dynamic action, 587–8, 599.
Specific nerve energies, law of, 287–8, 291.
Spectacles, 641–3; provision of, for school children, 225, 650.
Spectrum analysis, 319.
Speech centre, 256, 276.

Spermatozoa, 129.

Sphygmograph, 313, 622, 623.

Sphygmomanometer, 311–13.

Spinal accessory nerve, 245.

Spinal anaesthesia, 350.

Spinal cord, 252, 273; diseases of, 278; nerve tracts in, see Nerve tracts; transection of, 65, 94, 239, 249, 252, 263. See also Reflex action.

Spinal shock, 263.

Spine, curvature of, 98, 179.

Spirit, animal, 50, 64, 138; natural, 62, 64, 138; vital, 49, 64, 138.

Spirits of disease, 14.

Spirochaeta duttoni, 484.

Spirochaete, 333, 406, 475.

Spirochaetosis icterohaemorrhagica, see Weil's disease.

Spleen, 94, 125, 311, 317, 362, 542, 634.

Sponge, burnt, in treatment of goitre, 522.

Spontaneous generation, 327, 328–9, 332, 333–6, 635.

Spores, bacillary, 336, 337, 403–4, 441.

Sporozoites, see Malaria parasite.

Squill, 674.

Squint, see Strabismus.

Staining, for microscopical examination, 247, 248, 636.

Standard deviation, 723–4.

Stannius ligature, 314.

Stapes, 244.

Staphylococcus, 391, 392, 406–7.

Starch, 586.

Starvation, physiology of, 584–6, 590–2, 600, 601.

Staten Island, New York, 234.

Stavesacre, 674.

Steam carbolic spray, of Lister, see Carbolic acid spray.

Stegomyia fasciata, see *Aëdes aegypti*.

Stepney, London, 213.

Sterility, 618.

Sterilization, of instruments, &c., 358, 365, 367, 370.

Sternum, 61.

Steroids of adrenal cortex, 540.

Stethoscope, 172–4, 283, 625, 752. See also Auscultation.

Stigmata diaboli, 494.

Stilboestrol, 551.

Stimulants, 148.

Stockholm, Sweden, 272, 652.

Stockton-on-Tees, Durham, 609.

'Stoffwechsel', see Metabolism, origin of word.

Stoic philosophy, 60–61.

Stokes' disease, 532. See also Hyperthyroidism.

Stokes–Adams disease, 283.

Stomach, 42, 143, 157, 159, 302–3, 364, 375. See also Digestion, gastric.

Stonehouse, Plymouth, naval hospital at, 188.

Stovaine, 350.

Strabismus, 647–8.

Strasbourg, Alsace, 182, 304, 595; diabetes shown due to lesion of pancreas at, 553; first chair of pathological anatomy founded at (1819), 631; pathology at, 636; pharmacology at, 684; typhoid carrier at, 408.

Streptococcus, 391, 392, 401–2, 437; *S. erysipelatis*, 391, 392; *S. pneumoniae*, see Pneumococcus.

Streptomyces griseus, 697.

Streptomycin, 491, 621, 697.

Stretch reflex, see Reflex.

'Stromuhr', of Ludwig, 313.

Strychnine, 680, 681.

Student's *t*, 727.

Subacute combined degeneration, 276.

Subarachnoid haemorrhage, 279.

Subconscious mind, 513, 514.

Subdural haematoma, 367.

Submaxillary gland, 261, 301, 306; duct of (of Wharton), 516.

Sucrose, 587.

Sudan, 467.

Sudden deaths, 197.

Suez Canal, 473, 474.

Sugar, 294, 295, 320, 578, 586.

Suggestion, 504.

Sulci, cerebral, 243.

Sulphadiazine, 491, 693.

Sulphanilamide, 693.

Sulphapyridil, 491.

Sulphathiazole, 491, 693.

Sulphonamides, 491, 688, 693.

Sulphur, 14, 599, 601, 673; of Paracelsus, 101.

Sulphur dioxide, 165.

Sulphuric acid, 677.

Sulphuric ether, see Ether, anaesthetic.

Sulphurous acid, 677.

Sumerians, 10.

Sunlight, 378–9; in rickets, 614–16.

Suppositories, 7.

Suppuration, 79, 182, 354, 391.

Suprarenal glands, *see* Adrenal glands.

Suramin, 691.

Surface area, law of, 581, 587; formula for, 587, 590.

Surgeon General, of American Armed Forces, 233; of Marine Hospital Service, 233-4.

Surgeon-General's Library, Index Catalogue of the, 744-5.

Surgery, 51, 53, 68, 80, 174; abdominal, 362, 364-6, 370; antiseptic, 335, 352-9; Arabian, 76, 644; aseptic, 356, 366-7; Assyrian and Babylonian, 15; of bones and joints, 352, 356-7, 369-70; cardiac, 373, 753; conservative, 352; development of modern, 362-74; Egyptian, 4, 8; eighteenth century, 177-9; gastric, 366; Graeco-Roman, 54-55; Hippocratic, 32-34; Listerian revolution in, 351-60; medieval, 79, 83-84; military, *see* Medicine, military, Military surgeons; naval, 182, 186; neurological, 367-8, 370-1; orthopaedic, 370; plastic, 54, 98-99, 352, 373; Renaissance, 95-98; Roman, *see* Graeco-Roman; sixteenth century, 360; thoracic, 230, 368-9, 372-3; of thyroid, *see* Thyroidectomy. *See also* Amputation, Appendicitis, Cancer, Dislocations, Fractures, Guillotine, Gun-shot wounds, Ligatures, Steam carbolic spray, Trephination, Wounds.

Surgical instruments, Arabian, 76; Babylonian, 14, 15; Egyptian, 8-9, 20; Graeco-Roman, 33-34, 54-55.

Surgical shock, 558-9, 563.

Surra, 482.

Suspended animation, 342.

Sutton Coldfield, Warwicks., 228.

Sweat glands, of cat, 572.

Sweating sickness, 740-1.

Sympathetic nerve fibres, 246.

Sympathetic nervous system, 243, 245, 262, 539, 565, 572.

'Sympathin', of Cannon, 571.

'Sympathomimetic' action, 570.

Synapse, 264; liberation of acetylcholine at, 573, 576.

Synthetic organic drugs, 678-9.

Syphilis, 380, 390, 529, 630, 730; aortic aneurysm due to, 285; of brain, first description of (1770), 169; country of origin of, 108; general paralysis of insane due to, 507; guaiac in treatment of, 108-10; history of, 106-8; mercury in treatment of, 108, 174, 687, 688; salvarsan in treatment of, 689, 690, 692; spirochaete of, 391, 395, 689; —, first transmission of, to anthropoid apes, 406; —, pure culture of, 406; tabes dorsalis due to, 274; Wassermann reaction as evidence of infection with, 417. *See also* Aneurysm, General paralysis of the insane, Tabes dorsalis, *Treponema pallidum*, Wassermann reaction.

Syringe, hypodermic, 686-7.

Syringomyelia, 242, 276.

T.A.B. vaccine, 444.

Tabes dorsalis, 273, 274, 278.

Tarantism (Dancing Mania), 503-4, 741.

Tartaric acid, 330.

Tartu, *see* Dorpat.

Teddington, Middlesex, 155.

Teeth, 61, 659-71.

Teleology, of Galen, 60.

Telescope, 113, 124.

Temperaments, the four, 47, 101, 102.

Temperature, in disease, 116, 626.

Temple medicine, *see* Medicine.

Tendon division, 658.

Tendon transplantation, 659.

Teneriffe, 309.

Tensor tympani muscle, 243.

Tentorium cerebelli, 243.

'Terra pinguis', *see* Phlogiston.

'Testaceous Medicines', 651.

Testes, extracts of, 549; transplantation of, 517, 549, 550.

Testosterone, 550.

Tetania thyreopriva, 535.

Tetanus, 278; in the classical writers, 37, 386, 440, 650; discovery of bacillus of, 386-7, 391; immunology of, 439-43; specific prophylaxis in, 442-3.

Tetanus antitoxin, 412, 440, 442.

Tetanus bacillus, 387, 388, 391, 392, 393, 696.

Tetanus neonatorum, 468.

Tetanus toxin, 412.

Tetanus toxoid, 442.

Tetany, 535, 537, 639.

Texas, State of, 235.

Thasos, Greece, 28, 38, 728.

Thebaine, 681.
Therapeutic nihilism, 286.
Therapeutics, 53, 100.
Theriac, 675-6.
Thermometer, 116, 155, 171; clinical, 116, 171, 280, 626-7.
Thiamine, see Vitamin B₁.
Thiouracil, 530, 534.
Thiourea, 530, 534.
Third ventricle, of brain, 546.
tholos, 24.
Thong drill, 79-80, 81.
Thoracic duct, 123, 520, 628.
Thoracoplasty, 230, 369, 373.
Thorshavn, The Faeroes, 377.
Thrombosis, 635, 638.
Thymus gland, 241, 242, 317.
Thyroid blocking agents, 530, 534.
Thyroid gland, 516, 519-34, 542, 548, 638, 753; excision of, see Thyroidectomy; life-line of the, 528.
Thyroidectomy, 54, 374, 520, 523-4, 525, 531, 534, 535; subtotal, 531, 534.
Thyrotoxicosis, 532. See also Hyperthyroidism.
Thyrotropic hormone, of anterior pituitary, 529, 534, 548.
Thyrotropin, 548.
Thyroxine, 527, 532.
Tic douloureux, 190.
Tinctures, 522.
Tissues, 49, 123, 153, 320, 630.
Tobacco, 103, 566.
Tobacco mosaic, 445, 447.
Tocopherol, 618.
Tokyo, Japan, 393, 394, 611.
'Tonics', of Hoffmann, 148.
Tonsillectomy, 54.
Tonsillitis, 50.
'Tonus', of Hoffmann, 148.
Tooth extraction, 659-63.
Toronto, Canada, 554.
Torticollis (wry neck), 98, 278, 658.
Toulon, France, 198.
Toulouse, France, 658.
Tours, France, 204, 381, 631.
Toxic adenoma, of thyroid, 532. See also Hyperthyroidism.
Toxicology, first English book on, 285.
Toxin, 409, 411-14; of diphtheria, 411-12; of tetanus, 412.
Toxoid, 413, 436.
Tracheotomy, 204, 350, 655.

Trachoma (granular conjunctivitis), 86, 475, 650.
Tragacanth, 674.
Tralles, Asia Minor, 68.
Translation and translators, 71, 74, 76-77, 78, 80, 88, 103.
Traumatic shock, see Surgical shock.
Tremor-rigidity syndrome, 279.
Trench fever, 451-2.
Trephination, 1-3, 8, 32-34, 40, 79, 80, 358, 360, 367.
Treponema, see Spirochaete.
Treponema pallidum, 260, 391, 395, 406, 417, 475, 507, 689, 690, 696. See also Syphilis.
Treponema recurrentis, 391.
Tri-acid stain, of Ehrlich, 318.
Trichinosis, 392.
Trier, Germany, 408.
Trigeminal nerve, 251.
Trinity College, Dublin, 476.
Triple response, of Lewis, 560.
Tropical diseases, 452-94.
Tropical ulcer, see Delhi boil.
Trousseau's sign, 535.
Troy, 18.
Trypanosome fever, 483, 485.
Trypanosomes, 481-2, 488, 689; *T. brucei*, 483, 486; *T. cruzi*, 487; *T. evansi*, 482; *T. gambiense*, 483, 484, 485, 486; *T. lewisi*, 481; *T. rhodesiense*, 486.
Trypanosomiasis, African, 340, 453, 454, 481-7, 689, 690, 692; American, 487.
Trypsin, 298, 552, 553.
Trypsinogen, 298.
Tryptophane, 596, 598.
Tsetse-fly, 482, 483, 485, 486.
Tubal pregnancy, 177.
Tubercle bacillus, 379; avian, bovine, and human strains differentiated, 397-9; discovery of, 340, 391, 396; incidence of, in raw milk, 230; injection of, produces Koch's phenomenon, 422-3; streptomycin, action of, on, 697.
Tuberculin, 423-7, 429, 511.
Tuberculin tests, 230, 423-5. See also Mantoux, Moro, Pirquet.
Tuberculosis, 223, 224, 390, 393, 523, 626, 628; of bones, 378; British Congress of (1901), 398-9; cause of, 340, 396; cutaneous, 378; death-rates from, 720; Finsen Light and sunlight in, 378; in Great Britain, control, treatment, and

Tuberculosis (cont.)
prevention, 228–31; human and bovine, distinction between, 398–9; immunity to, 426–7; of joints, 183, 378; of kidney, first described (1760), 169; of larynx, 284; miliary, 636; notification of, 229; pathology of, 203, 282, 426, 631, 636, 638, 639; transmissibility of proved, 396–7, 398; treatment of, 228–30; —, with streptomycin, PAS, and isoniazid, 697; of vertebrae, 179. See also Artificial pneumothorax, B.C.G., Phthisis, Sanatoria, Surgery, thoracic, Thoracoplasty, Tuberculin.

Tuberculosis contacts, 230.

Tuberculosis dispensaries, 228, 229.

Tuberculosis officer, 229.

Tübingen, Germany, 304, 313, 636; research on plant and animal cells at, 324, 325; sphygmograph invented at, 622; word 'protoplasm' popularized at, 324.

Tulane University, 597.

Tumours, 284, 288, 639; of adrenal, 279, 541; of bone, 636; of brain, 169, 368, 371; of spinal cord, 368.

Tunis, N. Africa, 75, 451.

Turin, Italy, 493, 521.

Turpentine, 673.

Twort-d'Herelle phenomenon, see Bacteriophage.

Typhlitis, 365.

Typhoid bacillus, 231, 389; carriers of, 407–9; complement-fixation test for, 417; discovery of, 387, 391, 399; Rough and Smooth variants, 405; Vi reaction in, 405–6.

Typhoid (enteric) fever, 215, 433, 452, 469; agglutination test for (Widal), 418; antitoxic sera in treatment of, 443; carriers, 407–9; chloramphenicol in treatment of, 697; death-rates from, 453; discovery of causative organism of, 387, 391, 399; in Havana (1898), 471–2; immunization against (T.A.B.), 444–5; infected water and spread of, 731; miasmatic theory of, held in Munich, 231; treatises on, 204, 631, 721, 731; and typhus first distinguished, 387.

Typhoid state, 38–39.

Typhus (jail) fever, 187, 192, 204, 215, 446, 452, 731; chloramphenicol in treatment of, 697; discovery of causative organism of (Rickettsia prowazeki), 450–1; first scientific description of, 108; high incidence in England (1838), 213; identified with hospital fever, 184; Manchester outbreaks of, 189; in prisons, 155, 190; transmitted by lice, 451.

Tyrocidine, 696.

Tyrosine, 275, 595, 598.

Ultra-violet rays, 377–8, 617. See also Sunlight.

Unconditioned reflexes, see Reflex.

Undulant fever, see Brucellosis.

United States Public Health Service, 234.

Universities, medical schools at, 148, 280–6; medieval, 78–79.

University College, London, 499; adrenaline discovered at, 538; chair of, physiology at, 258, 352, 519; —, pathological anatomy at, 633; —, pharmacology established at (1905), 685; research on, biometry and statistics at, 726; —, histology at, 352–3; —, pathology of the cell at, 639–40; secretin discovered at, 518–19. See also Hospitals.

University College Hospital, London, see Hospitals.

Uppsala, Sweden, 535, 648, 652.

Upton, Essex, 190, 352.

Ur, Mesopotamia, 10.

Urbanization, 191–4.

Urea, 238, 302, 582, 587, 596, 597, 691.

Uric acid, 599.

Urinary pigments, 319.

Urine, 245, 338, 545, 579, 581–2, 584, 592, 599, 600, 685; diabetic, 245, 552; theories of secretion of, 301–2.

Uterine version, 96, 240.

Uterus, 42–43, 90, 177, 239, 362; round ligaments of, 244.

Utilitarianism, 207–8, 210.

Utrecht, Holland, 266.

Utriculus primordialis, 324.

Vaccination, 190, 200–2, 213; Act enforcing (1853), 223; introduced to Royal Navy, 188.

Vaccine, 419, 433, 444–5, 679.

Vaccinia, 202, 445; virus of, 445, 446, 448.

Vaginal smear test, 550.

Vagus apnoea, 304, 306.

Vagus centre, 313.

Vagus nerve, 261, 304, 313, 428, 566, 568, 569, 572, 637.

'Vagus substance', of Loewi, 568–9.

Valerian, 674.

valetudinaria, 58.

Valves, *see* Heart, Veins.

Valvulae conniventes, 628.

Vapour baths, 50.

Variation, in bacteria, 403–6.

Varicella, 203, 446, 629.

Vascular system, 89, 118–23, 245; ancient views on, 42, 48–49, 62.

'Vasodilatin', 557, 558.

Vasodilator fibres, 316.

Vasomotor centre, 316.

Vasomotor nerves, 261–2, 298, 518.

Vegetable bitters, 678.

Vegetables, as drugs, 8, 14; as antiscorbutics, 187, 196.

Veins, 48, 49, 118; valves in, 118, 120–1.

Vena cava, 64.

Venereal disease, 174, 198. *See also* under names of individual diseases.

Venesection, 35, 50. *See also* Bloodletting.

Venice, Italy, 87, 488, 672.

Venous pulse, 313.

Ventilation, 155, 156, 185, 189; in hospitals, 194; in prisons, 155, 189; in ships, 155.

Ventricles, of brain, *see* Cerebral ventricles; of heart, 64–65, 89–90, 93, 119, 120–1, 245, 623.

Ventriculography, 279.

Veratrine, 681.

Vermiform appendix, 241, 242. *See also* Appendicitis.

Verona, Italy, 105.

Vertebrae, 61.

Vesical calculus, 54, 151, 183, 352.

Vesico-vaginal fistula, 362.

Vibrio cholerae, see Cholera vibrio.

Vienna, 251, 299, 364, 374, 392, 393, 394, 401; 'Animal magnetism' used in treatment at, 507–9; bacterial agglutination discovered at, 418; cocaine first used as local anaesthetic at, 349; ductless glands first comprehensively discussed at, 539; encephalitis lethargica first appeared at, 729; Fröhlich's syndrome discovered at, 544; New Vienna School at, 285–6, 633; neuro-logical researches at, 248; Old Vienna School at, 280; ovarian hormone first demonstrated at, 550; pathological anatomy at, 171, 633; percussion invented at, 172; phrenology devised at, 254; psychoanalysis at, 513; puerperal fever overcome at, 360–1; rickets investigated in (1919–22), 615; scarlet fever transmitted to monkeys at, 437; Schick test discovered at, 434; serum sickness first studied at, 429; sign found in tetany described at, 535; thyroidectomy developed at, 523; tuberculin sensitivity first widely studied at, 424–5. *See also* Hospitals.

Village settlements, for the tuberculous, 230.

Vinegar, 188, 330.

Virilism, 541.

Virulence, 733–5.

Vi[rulence] antigen, 405–6, 444.

Virus diseases, 445–50.

Viruses, 407, 445–50, 748, 750.

'vis medicatrix naturae', 51, 101, 111.

Vision, mechanism of, 139, 255, 256, 279, 640–3.

Vitalism, 45, 143–4, 148.

Vital registration, 714–21.

Vital statistics, 179–81, 710–11, 714–21.

Vitamins, 609, 610–22, 670, 679.

Vitamins (named): A, 612, 615, 616, 617; B, 613; B_1, 619; B_2, 619, 620; B_{12}, 621, 751; C, 613, 618, 619; D, 615, 616, 617; D_1, 615; D_2 (Calciferol), 615; D_3, 616; E (Tocopherol), 618; K, 621; K_2, 622; P, 622.

Vividiffusion, 597.

Vivisection, 65, 92, 94, 120.

Voges-Proskauer reaction, 400.

Voice, 288.

Volhynian fever, *see* Trench fever.

Voltaic pile, 159–61.

Vomiting, 680.

Vorticella, 129.

Votive offerings, 25.

Wallerian degeneration, 249.

Wapping, London, 213.

War gases, 311.

Warsaw, Poland, 203.

Washington, D.C., U.S.A., 294, 562, 567.

Washington Point, Virginia, U.S.A., 233.

Wassermann reaction, 390, 417.

Water, 578; bacteriological examination of, 400; filtration of, 730.

Water-closets, 193.

Water-hammer pulse, 245, 283, 628.

Water-supplies, 55, 56, 84, 193, 215–16, 218, 220, 231–2, 235; filtration of, 231–2, 730.

Wax, for dental impressions, 666.

Wax injection, of anatomical specimens, 628.

Weil's disease, 475, 476.

Wellcome Historical Medical Museum, 68, 378.

Wellcome Physiological Research Laboratories, 555.

West Indies, 467.

Western Reserve University, Cleveland, Ohio, 627.

Westminster, 193, 666.

West Riding Asylum, Wakefield, Yorks., see Hospitals.

Wheat, 56.

Wheat embryo, 613, 618.

Whitechapel, London, 213.

White matter, of brain, 255; of cord, 248.

White swelling, see Tuberculosis, of joints.

Whooping cough, 110, 391.

Whooping cough bacillus, 391.

Wiggers-Dean recorder, 627.

Wine, 7, 329–30, 331.

Wintergreen, oil of, 683.

Witches, 494, 495, 496.

Wittenberg, Germany, 203, 542, 687.

Witte's peptone, 556, 558, 561.

Wollstein, Posen, Germany, 336.

Work, muscular, influence on metabolism, 592–4, 600; metabolism during, 585–6.

World War, see First World War, Second World War.

Wounds, 8, 32, 79, 96, 97, 101, 181;

effects of, experimentally produced, 261. See also Gun-shot wounds.

Writer's cramp, 278.

Wry-neck, see Torticollis.

Würzburg, Germany, 391, 392, 583, 595; exophthalmos studied experimentally at, 533; embryology and histology, first treatises on, written at, 247; Fröhlich's syndrome, earliest case of, described at, 544; morbid histology at, 636; large treatise on paediatrics edited at, 654; pathological anatomy, first chair of, in Germany founded at, 634; research on biophysics at, 592; X-rays discovered at, 374.

Wynne's Act (1808), 501.

Xerophthalmia, 616, 617.

X-rays, 374–7, 749, 752, 754.

Yale University, 260, 266, 394, 395, 605.

Yeast, 143, 330, 331, 613, 620.

Yellow fever, 210, 233, 446, 453, 454, 464; causative organism of, 474–8; history of, 191, 466–8; jungle type of, 480–1; mouse protection tests in, 479–80; vaccines against, 478–9, 480–1.

Yellow Fever Commission, 469–73, 474.

'Yellow jack', see Yellow fever.

York, Yorks., 101, 102, 497–9, 500.

Zein, 598.

z test, of Fisher, 727.

Zürich, Switzerland, 299, 391, 592, 601, 636; cell membrane first suggested at, 325; diphtheria bacillus discovered at, 381; early work on general anatomy written at, 321; male sex hormones first synthesized at, 550; surgery developed at, 364.

Zygote, of malaria parasite, 458, 462.